I0060971

# Genomics III
## Methods, Techniques and Applications

Genomics III – Methods, Techniques and Applications

Publisher: iConcept Press Ltd.
Cover design: Pineapple Design Ltd.
Interior design: iConcept Press Ltd.
Typesetting and copy editing: iConcept Press Ltd. and Pineapple Design Ltd.

ISBN:

This work is subjected to copyright. All rights are reserved, whether the whole or part of the materials is concerned, specifically the rights of translation, reprinting, re-use of illustrations, recitation, broadcasting, reproduction on microfilms or in other ways, and storage in data banks. Duplication of this publication or parts thereof is only permitted under the provisions of the authors, editors and/or iConcept Press Ltd.

Printed in the United States of America

Copyright © iConcept Press 2014

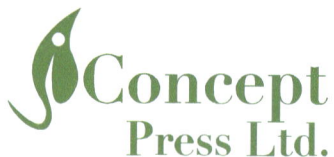

Concept
Press Ltd.

www.iconceptpress.com

# Contents

**Preface** . . . . . . . . . . . . . . . . . . . . . . . . . . . . . . . . . . . . . . . . . . . . . . . . vii

**1   Exome Sequencing and Biomedical Implications** . . . . . . . . . . . . . . . . . . . . 1
Esra Asilmaz (*University College London Hospital, United Kingdom*), Terry Gaasterland (*University of California, San Diego, USA*) and Bahar Taneri (*Eastern Mediterranean University, Famagusta, North Cyprus / Maastricht University, Maastricht, The Netherlands*)

**2   Whole Genome Amplification: Technologies and Applications** . . . . . . . . . . . . . . 21
Daniel W.H. Ho (*The Hong Kong Polytechnic University, Hong Kong SAR, China*) and Shea Ping Yip (*The Hong Kong Polytechnic University, Hong Kong SAR, China*)

**3   Whole Genome Microarray Gene Expression Profiling of Atherosclerosis Genes after Treatment with Captopril** . . . . . . . . . . . . . . . . . . . . . . . . . . . . . . 39
Joshua Abd Alla (*ETH Zürich, Switzerland*) and Ursula Quitterer (*ETH Zürich, Switzerland*)

**4   Utilization of Large-insert Libraries to Genome Analysis of Genetically Uncharacterized Organisms** . . . . . . . . . . . . . . . . . . . . . . . . . . . . . . . . . . . . . . . . . 63
Yuji Yasukochi (*National Institute of Agrobiological Sciences, Japan*)

**5   Application of a Real-Time qPCR Methodology to Identify Microorganisms as Indicators of Biogas Production During Anaerobic Digestion** . . . . . . . . . . . . . . . . 79
Deborah Traversi (*University of the Study of Turin, Italy*), Valeria Romanazzi (*University of the Study of Turin, Italy*) and Giorgio Gilli (*University of the Study of Turin, Italy*)

**6   Quantitative Analysis of DNA Transposon-mediated Gene Delivery: the *Sleeping Beauty* System as an Example** . . . . . . . . . . . . . . . . . . . . . . . . . . . . . . . 97

Orsolya Kolacsek (*Hungarian Academy of Sciences, Hungary*), Zsuzsanna Izsvák (*Max-Delbrück Center for Molecular Medicine, Germany*), Zoltán Ivics (*Paul Ehrlich Institute, Germany*), Balázs Sarkadi (*Semmelweis University and National Blood Center, Hungary*) and Tamás Orbán (*Hungarian Academy of Sciences, Hungary*)

**7    Prediction of Protein Function based on Machine Learning Methods: An Overview** . . . .    125

Kiran Kadam (*University of Pune, Pune, India*), Sangeeta Sawant (*University of Pune, Pune, India*), Urmila Kulkarni-Kale (*University of Pune, Pune, India*) and Jayaraman K. Valadi (*University of Pune Campus, Pune, India / Shiv Nadar University, Chithera (Gautam Budh Nagar), India*)

**8    Analysis and Characterization of Alu Insertion Sites: A Statistical Method and a Data Mining Solution** . . . . . . . . . . . . . . . . . . . . . . . . . . . . . . . . . . .    163

Kun Zhang (*Xavier University of Louisiana, USA*), Wei Fan (*Huawei Noah Ark's Lab, China*), Andrea Edwards (*Xavier University of Louisiana, USA*), Augustine Orgah (*Xavier University of Louisiana, USA*) and Prescott Deininger (*Tulane University, USA*)

**9    Identification of Coevolving Amino Acids Using Mutual Information** . . . . . . . . . . . . .    185

Elin Teppa (*Fundación Instituto Leloir, Buenos Aires, Argentina*), Diego Javier Zea (*Universidad Nacional de Quilmes, Buenos Aires, Argentina*) and Cristina Marino Buslje (*Fundación Instituto Leloir, Buenos Aires, Argentina*)

**10    Evaluation of Multiple-locus Variable-number Tandem-repeat Analysis for Typing Polyclonal Hospital- and Community-acquired Methicillin-resistant Staphylococcus Aureus Populations** . . . . . . . . . . . . . . . . . . . . . . . . . . . . . . . . . . .    209

Belinda Rivero-Pérez (*Hospital Universitario Ntra. Sra. de Candelaria, Santa Cruz de Tenerife, Spain*), Julia Alcoba-Florez (*Hospital Universitario Ntra. Sra. de Candelaria, Santa Cruz de Tenerife, Spain*) and Sebastian Méndez-Álvarez (*Hospital U. Ntra. Sra. de Candelaria, Spain / Universidad de La Laguna, Spain*)

**11    Sorting Genomes by Rearrangements and Its Application to Phylogeny Reconstruction** . .    229

Chin Lung Lu (*National Tsing Hua University, Taiwan*) and Chuan Yi Tang (*Providence University, Taiwan / National Tsing Hua University, Taiwan*)

**12    Optimization of Sequence Alignment for Microsatellite Regions** . . . . . . . . . . . . . . .    245

Abdulqader Jighly (*International Center for Agricultural Research in the Dry Areas (ICARDA), Syria*), Khaled El-Shamaa (*International Center for Agricultural Research in the Dry Areas (ICARDA), Syria*), Reem Joukhadar (*International Center for Agricultural Research in the Dry Areas (ICARDA), Syria*), Al-addin Hamwieh (*University of Aleppo, Syria*) and Francis Ogbonnaya (*Grains Research and Development Corporation (GRDC), Australia*)

**13  Regulation of Endosomal Membrane Trafficking with RUN Domain Proteins** . . . . . . . .  263

Yasuko Kitagishi (*Nara Women's University, Japan*), Satoru Matsuda (*Nara Women's University, Japan*) and Mayumi Kobayashi (*Nara Women's University, Japan*)

**14  Decoding the Cis-Regulatory Grammar Behind Enhancer Architecture** . . . . . . . . . . .  277

Jacqueline Dresch (*Harvey Mudd College, USA*) and Robert Drewell (*Harvey Mudd College, USA*)

**15  Strategies for Genetic Screening of Multiple Samples Using PCR-Based Targeted Sequence Enrichment** . . . . . . . . . . . . . . . . . . . . . . . . . . . . . . . . . . . .  305

Paola Benaglio (*University of Lausanne, Switzerland*) and Carlo Rivolta (*University of Lausanne, Switzerland*)

**16  Finding and Characterizing Small Group I Introns in rRNA Genes** . . . . . . . . . . . . .  327

Lorena B. Harris (*Bowling Green State University, USA*) and Scott O. Rogers (*Bowling Green State University, USA*)

**17  Variant Antigen Expression Control in *Plasmodium* Parasites** . . . . . . . . . . . . . . . .  343

Fernanda Janku Cabral (*University of São Paulo, Brazil*), Wesley Luzetti Fotoran (*University of São Paulo, Brazil*) and Gerhard Wunderlich (*University of São Paulo, Brazil*)

# Preface

Genomics is the study of the genomes of organisms. The field includes intensive efforts to determine the entire DNA sequence of organisms and fine-scale genetic mapping efforts. It is a discipline in genetics that applies recombinant DNA, DNA sequencing methods, and bioinformatics to sequence, assemble, and analyse the function and structure of genomes. Genomics III - Methods, Techniques and Applications is the last volume of our Genomics series.

There are totally 17 chapters in this book. Chapter 1 presents an overview of exome sequencing technology and details its use in identification of molecular bases of rare diseases in human. Chapter 2 describes and compares different methods of whole genome amplification (WGA) for replenishing DNA samples for genetic studies. It also discussed the applications of WGA products in different DNA-based assays, sample sources of DNA for WGA, and other related aspects of WGA. Chapter 3 ilustrates the method of whole genome microarray gene expression profiling and its application to study the treatment effect of a widely used cardiovascular drug. The approach proved suitable to elucidate pathomechanisms of atherosclerosis and identify a potential new target involved in atherosclerotic plaque development. Chapter 4 describes a brief history of large-insert libraries and their utility in exploring organisms with poor genetic and genome information. Lepidoptera, butterflies and moths, is a good example of less analyzed organisms due to their great diversity, and large-insert libraries play a critical role.

Chapter 5 proposes a bio-molecular approach for the evaluation of the anaerobic digestion performance. Significant microorganism groups such as methanogens and sulphate reducing bacteria are proposed as bio-indicators of optimized processes, during the digestion they can be quickly detected by qRT-PCR methods. In Chapter 6, quantitative issues of the transposon-based gene delivery methods are addressed. Using the *Sleeping Beauty* transposon system as a prominent example, special detailed focus is given to copy number determination and to transposon excision efficiency quantification by real-time PCR based methodologies. Chapter 7 provides an overview of extraction of a compendium of sequence and structural features, as well as the methodology for function prediction based on the techniques from Artificial Intelligence and Machine learning. Chapter 8 presents a statistical method and a data mining solution for the problem of insertion site analysis and characterization of Alu elements, which is an important problem in primate-specific bioinformatics research.

Chapter 9 investigates how Mutual Information (MI) can be used to improve methods of predicting functional residues and enhance structural data to describe the topological properties of amino acid coevolution networks within a protein and their interactions. Chapter 10 attempts to validate MLVA to see if it could predict MRSA clones that were previously characterized by PFGE, MLST, and staphylococcal cassette chromosome mec (SCCmec) typing and to establish possible criteria of clustering MLVA patterns, looking for high concordance levels. In addition, this chapter also tries to introduce MLVA as a routine typing method in hospital. Chapter 11 introduces a web server which allows the user to perform genome rearrangement analysis using reversals, block-interchanges (also called generalized transpositions) and translocations (including fusions and fissions). The web server also allows the user to infer phylogenetic trees of genomes being considered based on their pairwise genome rearrangement distances and further evaluate statistical reliability of tree branches. Chapter 12 discussed an algorithm which is used to optimally align simple sequence repeat (microsatellite) regions as they evolve uniquely through a process called polymerase slippage. This process allows higher chance for insertion/deletion mutations over SNP mutations which created a need for a new tool to compare microsatellites.

Chapter 13 possesses a background of the RUN domain research with an emphasis on the interaction between RUN domain protein including RUFY proteins and small GTPases with respect to the cell polarity and membrane trafficking. In Chapter 14, the authors detail recent advances in understanding mechanisms of gene regulation in Drosophila. A combination of molecular genetics and mathematical modelling approaches reveals the emerging evidence for an underlying architecture of transcription factor binding sites in cis-regulatory modules. Chapter 15 provides guidelines for human molecular geneticists to perform genetic screenings using next generation sequencing. Two target enrichment strategies based on tagged or untagged pools of long-range PCRs are described in detail and discussed. Chapter 16 describes the process that was used to locate and characterize small group I introns in the rRNA gene locus of fungi. The establishment and evolution of these small introns is discussed.

Chapter 17 summarizes recent insights in the biology of variant gene transcription in human and murine malaria species and addresses the molecular mechanisms at work which regulate the expression of important virulence factors.

Editing and publishing a book is never an easy task. Each chapter in this book has gone through a peer review, a selection and an editing process so as to guarantee its quality. Without the supports and contributions of the authors and reviewers, this book can never be able to complete. We would like to thank all of the authors in this book and all of the reviewers who participated in the reviewing process: Ana Afonso, Heather A Amthauer, Razvan Anistoroaei, Taeok Bae, Elke S Bergmann-Leitner, Parbati Biswas, Teresia J Buza, Yudong Cai, Enrico Casalone, Tien-Hao Chang, Virander Singh Chauhan, Davide Corá, Patrizia D'Adamo, Aaron Farnsworth, Anna-Sophie Fiston-Lavier, Martin C. Frith, Kseniya A Golovnina, Felix Grewe, Fan Jin, Nicolas Joannin, Sung-Chul Jung, Fabienne Lesueur, Quan Long, Martin A. Lysak, Stefan Moisyadi, Lilia Montoya, Achuthsankar S. Nair, Cécile Neuvéglise, Ferenc Olasz, Christopher Potter, Guy A. Rouleau, Unitsa Sangket, Christoph D. Schmid, Peidong Shen, Takahito Shikano, Aleksander L Sieroń, Shaneen M Singh, Guy Tsafnat, Gert Jan C. Veenstra, Chung-Hsiung Wang, Liya Wang, René Wintjens, Ka-Chun Wong, Stephen S.-T. Yau, Chenggang Zhang, Xing-Ming Zhao and Xiaoyong Zou. We hope that you, the reader, will find this book interesting and useful. Any advices please feel free and are always welcome to tell us.

iConcept Press Ltd
February 2014

# Exome Sequencing and Biomedical Implications

Esra Asilmaz
*University College Lodon Hospital,United Kingdom*

Terry Gaasterland
*Scripps Genome Center, Scripps Institution of Oceanography*
*University of California, San Diego, USA*

Bahar Taneri
*Department of Biological Sciences*
*Eastern Mediterranean University, Famagusta, North Cyprus*
*Institute of Public Health Genomics*
*Maastricht University, Maastricht, The Netherlands*

# 1   Introduction

In the recent years, high-throughput sequencing of whole genomes, targeted exome sequencing and RNA sequencing technologies have accelerated biomedical discovery and applications. Next-generation sequencing technologies enable sequence data output at very high rates. Combined sequencing approaches enable correct identification of mutations and their impact on messenger RNA transcripts (Srirangalingam & Chew, 2012). The era of Personal Genome sequencing brings personalized DNA, RNA diagnostics and thus personalized healthcare and medicine. Personal genome and personal exome sequencing yield rapid sequence data from patients and controls, and thus provide an invaluable source for variant calling and comparative mutation analysis. It is expected that personal genomics will be of common use in medical practice in the future (Gonzaga-Jauregui *et al.*, 2012). Needless to say sequencing goes hand in hand with computational analysis. Effective translation of the accumulating high-throughput sequence data into meaningful biomedical knowledge and application relies in its interpretation. High-throughput sequence analyses are only made possible via intelligent computational systems designed particularly to decipher meaning of the complex world of nucleotides (Zhang *et al.*, 2011). In this chapter, we particularly discuss the advance brought specifically by exome sequencing to rare mutation identification in various diseases (Taneri *et al.*, 2012).

# 2   High-throughput Sequencing Methods and Exome Sequencing

In the last few years, targeted sequencing of coding regions of the genome from particular individuals has yielded significant discoveries of rare mutations in various disease states (Taneri *et al.*, 2012). In this section, we discuss next-generation sequencing in general and targeted exome sequencing in particular. Compared to conventional sequencing, high-throughput next-generation sequencing technologies produce much more data at an unprecedented rate of speed (Pareek *et al.*, 2011). Currently, the three widely used next-generation sequencing platforms are SOLiD, Roche 454 and Illumina. Briefly, Roche 454 Genome Sequencer uses pyrosequencing, Illumina Genome Analyzer applies a sequencing-by-synthesis approach and ABI SOLiD platform employs a sequencing-by-ligation approach (Zhang *et al.*, 2011). Zhang *et al.* provides a detailed overview for these three most popular sequencing platforms as well as others. Pareek *et al.* present an extensive overview on how next-generation sequencing technologies impacted different aspects of biomedical sciences. These include but are not limited to; whole genome genotyping, re-assembly of the human genome, genome-wide variation detection, and advances in cancer genomics (Pareek *et al.*, 2011). Within the scope of this chapter, we focus on personal exome sequencing as part of the advancements brought by next-generation sequencing to biomedical sciences, medicine and healthcare.

With the emergence of the personal genome era, a personalized approach in medicine was set in motion. Personalized medicine begins with DNA sequence analysis and molecular diagnostics. Importance of personal genomics in healthcare and medicine will become more and more evident as the cost of personal sequencing decreases and availability to the public increases as foreseen by the scientific community (Mardis, 2010). In parallel, ongoing development of sophisticated analysis for interpretation of the personal sequence data would eventually enable proper interpretation of genomic variations (Gonzaga-Jauregui *et al.*, 2012). A cost-effective and time-efficient alternative to whole-genome sequencing is targeted sequencing of the coding regions of the genome, i.e. exome sequencing (Biesecker, 2010). The

180,000 exons cover only 1% of the human genome. However, they encompass 85% of disease causing mutations (Choi *et al.*, 2009). Since it was first reported in 2009, exome sequencing has opened a new era in identifying disease causing mutations in over 100 rare Mendelian conditions, in addition to the identification of gene variants, which may be significant in common complex conditions. With the help of powerful bioinformatics analysis, exome sequencing proved to be very useful in identifying mutations in very rare conditions. A recent review, which reported to be up to date as of May 2012, by Rabbani *et al.* summarized 102 Mendelian conditions, where exome sequencing was used to identify disease causing genetic variants (Rabbani *et al.*, 2012). However, several more genes have since been identified and publications in this field accumulate at a very high rate. In addition, several new studies report the use of this technology on its own or in combination with other more classical methods to study complex diseases as well as rare conditions.

## 3   Computational Tools and Analysis of Exome Sequencing

Exome sequencing allows the capture of protein coding regions of the genome, i.e. only 1% of the genome (Teer & Mullikin, 2010). This method enables a targeted approach for mutation profiling within a small, restricted section of the genome and thus provides an advantage as currenlty much of the genome function remains to be elucidated. As with any sequencing data, with exome sequencing challenge remains in the interpretation process. Interpretation of the data is critical in terms of valid knowledge discovery and has certain limitations. Therefore, computational tool development is a critical phase of the exome sequence analysis. Inferring meaningful mutations from the generated datasets becomes only possible with computational analysis.

Mutation profiling of an individual requires statistical and computational analysis. Main computational challenges in the field reside in structured data handling, analysis and knowledge discovery from large datasets. Particularly, challenges arise in quantity of the data to manage as large amount of variants are detected per exome, alignment of short reads to reference sequences, identification of false negatives, i.e. failing to identify true single nucleotide polymorphisms (SNPs), or false positives, read depth, development of specific software and obtaining biologically meaningful results. Main computational efforts in the field reside in SNP calling and deletion/insertion polymorphism (DIP) identification. Efficient SNP calling from high-throughput sequence data, which also apply to exome sequences, is the target for several recent computational analyses (Altmann *et al.*, 2012). As stated by Altmann *et al.* SNP calling from exome data requires "many processing steps and the application of a diverse set of tools." (Altmann *et al.*, 2012).

There are several existing computational pipelines for variant calling in exome sequence data. Here, we provide a general overview for some of the existing computational tools. Challis *et al.* offers an integrative variant analysis pipeline (Challis *et al.*, 2012). Specifically, this pipeline includes logistic regression models particularly trained on whole exome data, which enables identification of true SNPs, as well as short INDELs (insertions-deletions). This tool, termed as Atlas2 Suite, was tested on 92 samples from the 1000 Genomes Exon Pilot Project and was shown to effectively call SNPs and INDELs within tens of base pairs (Challis *et al.*, 2012).

Other available variant calling tools include SAMtools mPileup (Li *et al.*, 2009), VarScan (Koboldt *et al.*, 2009), Dindel (Albers *et al.*, 2010), and GATK (DePristo *et al.*, 2011). Albers *et al.* focused on INDELs and generated a Bayesian method for the purpose of identification of such polymorphisms within short sequences. The authors reported a probabilistic realignment model, named as Dindel, which was implemented on the 1000 Genomes Project data to efficiently call INDEL variations. Dindel can retrieve INDELs that are less than 50 nucleotides in length (Albers *et al.*, 2010). In another study, DePristo *et al.* desgined a computational pipeline for discovery of genotypic variations across mutiple samples at a time. The 3-phase pipeline reported by the authors is presented as part of the Genome Analysis Toolkit (GATK), and has been applied to whole-exome capture data, as well as other sequence datasets including 1000 Genome Trio and HiSeq. GATK has been tested across five sequencing technologies and was shown to be effective in variant calling and genotyping (DePristo *et al.*, 2011).

Li *et al.* (2009) developed the Sequence Alignment/Map (SAM) format, which allows alignment of reads generated by different platforms. SAM format is a common alignment format which enables alignment of various sequence types and separates the alignment step from the analysis. Associated SAMtools enables various types of analysis on the aligned sequence data including variant calling. As well as mapping, aligning and variant calling, the visualization of sequences requires attention. A recent article by Popendorf and Sakakibara indicate that visualization tools such as that of SAMtools, i.e. samtools ivew, are restricted to certain genomic regions and therefore may be limited for high-throughput datasets. The authors propose SAMSCOPE which provides an interface for large-scale complex data browsing and visualization. SAMSCOPE enables flexible visualization and interactive analysis of reads (Popendorf & Sakakibara, 2012). In a different study, Fischer *et al.* generated a computational pipeline named SIMPLEX, which performs alignment, variation detection as well as functional annotation of the variants. SIMPLEX makes use of cloud computing to solve some of the data handling and computational infrastructure problems of experimental laboratories. The authors state that their tool overcomes the installation and configuration steps, which could be difficult for researchers without advanced bioinformatics experience. Fischer *et al.* evaluated SIMPLEX by analyzing raw exome sequencing data from 10 different Kabuki Syndrome patients. The authors report identification of loss-of-function mutations in MLL2 concurring with the analysis by Ng *et al.* from whom the data was obtained (Fischer *et al.*, 2012 & Ng *et al.*, 2010).

VarScan is another tool developed by Koboldt *et al.* VarScan detects SNPs and indels from sequence data generated on different sequencing platforms. Variant calling requires alignment of reads to a reference sequence, which is particularly problematic with short reads. One of the advantages of VarScan relies in its compatibility with different read aligners. Koboldt *et al.* tested their tool on both individual and pooled data. They demonstrated that VarScan calls variants with 97% specificity from individual sequences and with 93% specificity from pooled sequences (Koboldt *et al.* 2009). In a followup software named VarScan2, Koboldt *et al.* took their variant analysis to another level and identified copy number variations as well as single nucleotide mutations utilizing cancer exome sequencing. VarScan2 compared exome sequences from normal and tumor data. From ovarian tumors, single nucleotide variations were identified with 93% sensitivity. In addition, deletion of tumor suppressor genes and oncogene amplifications were deciphered. Copy number variations were found in 582 genes (Koboldt *et al.*, 2012). As VarScan and improved VarScan2 clearly demonstrate computational technologies for genome and exome sequence analysis, assembly, alignment and variant calling tools are certainly rapidly developing and evolving. Therefore, at the time of publication this book chapter might not cover all released tools.

It should be noted that more analysis tools tailored specifically for exome data are needed to be generated in order to tackle this technology, which is soon to be in regular use. In a 2012 article, El-sharawy *et al.* evaluated various SNP analysis tools for next-generation sequence data. Importantly, the authors showed that quality of the SNPs identified is largely affected by the software tools and parameters used. Elsharawy *et al.* recommend a novel integrative approach involving "two-step mapping" in order to efficiently call novel SNPs (Elsharawy *et al.*, 2012). Particularly, tools deployed on platforms easy to be used by scientists with minimal bioinformatics experience, such as Atlas2 Suite Web Interface (Challis *et al.*, 2012), would make the data analysis from exome to mutation identification much more feasible. Finally, it is also forseen that generation of large online databases with the emerging novel mutations would illuminate and fasten future comparative exome studies.

## 4   Exome Sequencing and Rare Diseases

One of the main goals of exome analysis is medical sequencing for identification of disease causing genetic variation (Teer & Mullikin, 2010). Although there are some other applications such as those in population genetics and evolution (Yi *et al.*, 2010), in this chapter we particularly focus on biomedical applications. In the recent years, exome sequencing has yielded identification of various rare novel mutations. In this section, we firstly discuss splicing relevant mutations and also mention other rare mutations identified by exome sequencing.

### 4.1   Splicing and Disease Causing Mutations Identified Through Exome Sequencing

Identification of rare splice-site mutations provides an excellent example for use of exome sequencing in molecular diagnostics. In this section, we choose to highlight splicing relevant mutations since this is a widespread cellular process, which affects the majority of human genes and is therefore crucial in execution of proper gene expression in cells (Taneri *et al.*, 2004, 2005, 2009, 2011). Splicing is an evolutionarily conserved eukaryotic cellular phenomenon, by which non-coding intronic sequences are removed from the premature messenger RNA (pre-mRNA) molecule and coding exonic sequences are ligated to form the mature messenger RNA (mRNA). Splicing is a process, which is coupled with transcription and affects all human genes with multiple exons (Montes *et al.*, 2012). This process is guided by a complex protein-RNA machinery called the spliceosome. Due to its widespread presence across the human genome, splicing is crucial for proper RNA regulation and thus proper gene expression. Furthermore, an additional level of complexity is brought to the eukaryotic gene expression regulation by alternative splicing. Alternative splicing enables differential use of splice-sites on the pre-mRNA and thus leads to generation of different mRNA transcripts from a single gene (Taneri *et al.*, 2004, 2005, 2009, 2011). Splicing related mutations could result in severe diseases (Douglas & Wood, 2011, Taneri *et al.*, 2012). In the recent years, exome sequencing enabled identification of rare splice-site mutations.

Molecular diagnosis of some rare diseases with splicing related mutations was made possible by exome sequencing studies. As we have highlighted in a recent review, Gilissen *et al.* has identified a splice-site mutation in WD repeat domain 35 (WDR35) gene, which is implicated in Sensenbrenner syndrome (Glissen *et al.*, 2010). Sensenbrenner syndrome also known as cranioectodermal dysplasia displays an autosomal recessive inheritance. This is a syndrome where phenotype varies with usual skeletal, facial and ectodermal abnormalities. Glissen *et al.* identified a novel splice-site mutation in exomes of two unrelated Sensenbrenner patients. In particular this mutation was spotted in exon 2 of the WDR35 gene in one of the affected individuals. This splice-site mutation generates an mRNA product with a 58 base-pair insertion, which contains a premature stop codon. In addition to this specific splice-site mutation, exome sequencing yielded in discovery of two other missense mutations in WDR35 gene as well as a single nucleotide deletion, which generates a frameshift mutation leading to premature termination (Glissen *et al.*, 2010).

Another implementation of exome sequencing revealed a splice-site mutation in stromal interaction molecule 1 (STIM1) gene, which leads to Kaposi sarcoma (Byun *et al.*, 2010). Kaposi sarcoma is a human herpes virus 8 associated inflammatory neoplasm. Byun *et al.* were able to identify the single base substitution mutation in STIM1 gene through massively parallel sequencing of the exome from a single patient. Specifically, the novel mutation resides at a consensus splice acceptor site at the intron–exon junction of exon 8 of STIM1. As a result, STIM1 protein was absent in cells of this patient due to lack of transcripts of STIM1 containing consecutive exons 7, 8 and 9. Rather the transcriptome covered several different aberrant splice forms (Byun *et al.*, 2010).

Guergueltcheva *et al.* (2012) used exome sequencing in Roma patients and identified two variants in GRM1 gene, which encodes the metabotropic glutamate receptor mGluR1. The variants cause autosomal recessive congenital cerebellar ataxia, a form of congenital cerebellar ataxia, which are rare heterogenous neurological conditions involving both central and peripheral nervous systems. Patients in this study had global developmental delay in addition to cerebellar signs such as an ataxic gait, dysarthria, dysdiadokinesia, dysmetria and tremors. Brain imaging showed hypoplasia of the inferior vermis of the cerebellum as well as generalized cerebellar atrophy. GRM1 gene variants identified are suggested to affect a critical site for alternative splicing.

In addition, Wadt *et al.* used whole-exome sequencing in a multiple-case Danish family with multiple different cancers including uveal or cutaneous malignant melanoma, mesothelioma and meningioma These authors were able to identify a missense mutation in BRCA1 associated protein 1 (BAP1), and went on using bioinformatics together with splicing assays to show that this mutation generates a truncating frame-shift mutation by causing aberrant splicing (Wadt *et al.*, 2012). Other mutations which do not directly affect splice-sites could as well generate spliceopathies. In a recent study, Liu *et al.* used exome sequencing in a Chinese family with autosomal dominant retinitist pigmentosa and they were able to identify a novel missense mutation in a highly conserved position in SNRNP200 gene, a gene which encodes for a helicase crucial for pre-mRNA splicing (Liu *et al.*, 2012).

X-exome sequencing has been used in five affected individuals of a large Dutch family affected by X-linked learning disability, obesity, gynaecomastia, hypogonadism and unusual face, which the authors state as a distinct but similar disorder to Wilson-Turner Syndrome. In this study, an intronic variant was identified in the histone deacetylase 8 (HDA C8) gene, which is part of a family of genes involved in epigenetic gene silencing during development. Furthermore, they showed that the variant identified affects splicing of exon 2 and causes exon skipping, which results in a premature stop in the protein sequence (Harakalova *et al.*, 2012).

## 4.2    Other Rare Mutations Identified Through Exome Sequencing

This section includes a brief overview of the most recent disease causing mutations identified using exome sequencing. Mainly the very recent studies reported during May – October 2012 are included. Table 1 provides a list of recently identified mutations and their associated diseases. These diseases are further discussed below. It is inevitable that in view of the current rate of publications in this field, at the time of publication this summary will not be exclusive.

Lin *et al.* used whole-exome sequencing in an autosomal recessive condition called pure hair and nail ectodermal dysplasia, which causes nail dystophy and hypotrichosis in affected individuals. The authors were able to identify a homozygous nonsense mutation in HOXC13 gene originally in a consan

| Disease Condition | Gene(s) Implicated | References |
|---|---|---|
| Adult-onset Leukoencephalopathy | CSF1R | Mitsui *et al.* 2012 |
| Alternating Hemiplegia of Childhood | ATP1A3 | Heinzen *et al.* 2012, Rosewich *et al.* 2012 |
| Alpers Encephalopathy | FARS2 | Elo *et al.* 2012 |
| Amyotrophic Lateral Sclerosis | PFN1 | Wu *et al.* 2012 |
| Autosomal Dominant Retinitis Pigmentosa | SNRNP200 | Liu *et al.* 2012 |
| Autosomal Recessive Cerebellar Ataxia | SACS SPG11 APOB | Hammer *et al.* 2012 |
| Brown-Vialetto-Van Laere Syndrome | SLC52A2 | Haack *et al.* 2012 |
| Congenital Non-syndromic Hydrocephalus | CCDC88C | Drielsma *et al.* 2012 |
| Dysosteosclerosis | SLC29A | Campeau *et al.* 2012 |
| Essential Tremor | FUS | Merner *et al.* 2012 |
| Fanconi Anaemia | SLX4/FANCP | Schuster *et al.* 2012 |
| Frontotemporal Dementia-like Syndrome Wthout Bone Involvement | TREM2 | Guerreiro *et al.* 2012 |
| Leber Congenital Amaurosis | NMNAT1 | Chiang *et al.* 2012, Falk *et al.* 2012 Koenekoop *et al.* 2012 |
| Osteogenesis Imperfecta Type V | IFITM5 | Cho *et al.* 2012, Semler *et al.* 2012 |
| Paroxysmal Kinesigenic Dyskinesia Episodic Ataxia Hemiplegic Migraine | PRRT2 | Wang *et al.* 2011, Gardiner *et al.* 2012 |
| Primary Ciliary Dyskinesia | HEATR2 | Horani *et al.* 2012 |
| Pure Hair and Nail Ectodermal Dysplasia | HOXC13 | Lin *et al.* 2012 |
| Putative Stargardt Disease | ABCA4 (RDS, ELOVL, CRB1) | Strom *et al.* 2012 |
| Recessive Retinal Degeneration | CDHR1 | Duncan *et al.* 2012 |
| Spinal Muscular Atropy | DYNC1H1 | Tsurusaki *et al.* 2012 |
| Warsaw Breakage Syndrome | DDX11 | Capo-Chichi et a. 2012 |
| Wiedemann-Steiner Syndrome | MLL | Jones *et al.* 2102 |

**Table 1:** Certain rare mutations identified through exome sequencing.

guineous Chinese family and then identified a further microdeletion in the first exon of HOXC13 gene in an affected Afghan female. They suggest a loss of function as the cause of this condition (Lin *et al.*, 2012). Duncan *et al.* used exome sequencing in eight members of a family with recessive retinal degeneration, where affected members have night blindness, progressive visual acuity and field loss leading to significant central vision loss. The authors were able to identify a novel nonsense mutation in exon 13 of the CDHR1 gene (Duncan *et al.*, 2012).

Guerreirro *et al.* used whole-exome sequencing and whole-genome genotyping in 44 Turkish patients with frontotemporal dementia-like syndrome. These authors were able to identify different homozygous mutations in the triggering receptor expressed on myeloid cells 2 gene (TREM2) in three probands with this condition (Guerreirro *et al.*, 2012). In another recent study, Hammer *et al.* used high-density single-nucleotide polymorphism genotyping together with exome sequencing in an attempt to identify causative gene in a heterogenous group of neurodegenerative disorders called autosomal recessice cerebellar ataxia (ARCA). In this study, the authors were able to identify one new mutation in the SACS gene as well as a previously identified mutation in SPG11 and a homozygous variant in the APOB gene (Hammer *et al.*, 2012).

Using homozygosity mapping together with exome sequencing in two unrelated families with congenital non-syndromic hydrocephalus, a heterogenous condition with no single specific cause, Drielsma *et al.* identified a novel mutation. The authors were able to identify a novel homozygous mutation in the coiled-coil domain containing 88C (CCDC88C) (Drielsma *et al.*, 2012). In a separate study, Horani *et al.* used whole-exome capture and sequencing in two related affected individuals in two separate Amish communities as well as their unaffected parents. These authors were able to identify an autosomal recessive missense mutation in a previously uncharacterized gene called HEATR2. Then they performed a number of functional studies and suggested that this gene may have a role in dynein arm transport or assembly (Horani *et al.*, 2012). Mitsui *et al.* used exome sequencing in four affected individuals in three families with adult onset autosomal dominant leukoencephalopathy. They were able to identify two heterozygous mutations in CSF1R gene in three families as the likely cause for this condition (Mitsui *et al.*, 2012).

Campeau *et al.* used whole exome sequencing in dysosteosclerosis, which is a form of osteopetrosis, to identify mutations in a nucleoside transporter gene called SLC29A, as the cause in this rare condition. They reported a homozygous and a compound heterozygous missense mutation in two individuals with this condition. Further studies are needed to understand the exact mechanism of action of this gene in osteoclast differentiation and function as implicated by the early studies in vivo and in mice (Campeau *et al.*, 2012). In another recent study, Haack *et al.* used exome sequencing in a single affected individual with Brown-Vialetto-Van Laere syndrome (BVVLS) to identify SLC52A2 as the cause of this rare condition. BVVLS is a neurological condition, which causes ponto-bulbar palsy and sensorineural deafness in affected infants. Previously, mutations in SLC5A3 gene, which codes for riboflavin transporter 2, were also correlated with this condition suggesting the importance of riboflavin metabolism in this particular condition (Haack *et al.*, 2012).

In two simultaneous studies, both Semler *et al.* and Cho *et al.* were able to identify a de novo mutation in the 5-UTR of interferon induced transmembrane protein 5 (IFITM5) as the cause for autosomal-dominant osteogenesis imperfecta Type V, using whole-exome sequencing of a single affected individual together with her two unaffected parents. Osteogenesis imperfecta is a heterogenous disease of bones, which makes them fragile hence susceptible to fractures. Mutations in the type 1 collagen genes COL1A1 and COL1A2 were previously shown to cause other types of osteogenesis imperfect (Semler *et al.*, 2012. & Cho *et al.*, 2012).

Merner *et al.* used exome sequencing in a large family affected by essential tremor (ET) and identified a missense mutation in FUS gene as the cause for this common neurodegenerative disororder. They were then able to identify two further missense mutations in this gene by studying 270 additional affected individuals (Merner *et al.*, 2012). Rosewich *et al.* used whole exome sequencing in three proband-parent trios with alternating hemiplegia of childhood (AHC) and were able to identify heterozygous de novo missense mutations in ATP1A3 gene. Further sequencing of 21 individuals revealed additional disease-associated mutations in this gene. This gene is also implicated in patients with rapid-onset dystonia-parkinsonism, which has some overlapping clinical features (Rosewich *et al.*, 2012). In another study by Heinzen *et al.* used exome sequencing in seven patients as well as their unaffected parents and identified mutations in the ATP1A3 gene (Heinzen *et al.*, 2012).

Using whole-exome sequencing in two affected siblings and their mother, Tsurusaki *et al.* identified a heterozygous DYNC1H1 mutation in dominant spinal muscular atrophy with lower extremity dominance (Tsurusaki *et al.*, 2012). Three different studies used exome sequencing in Leber congenital amaurosis, an autosomal recessive retinal dystrophy, which causes severe vision loss and were able to identify mutations in the nicotinamide adenine dinucleotide synthase gene (NMNAT1) (Chiang *et al.*, 2012, Koenekoop *et al.*, 2012 & Falk *et al.*, 2012). Elo *et al.* used whole-exome sequencing in two patients with fatal infantile Alpers encephalopathy to identify mutations in the mitochondrial phenylalanyl-tRNA synthetase gene (FARS2) (Elo *et al.*, 2012). In a different study, Wu *et al.* used exome sequencing in two large families with familial amyotrophic lateral sclerosis (ALS) to identify disease causative mutations in the profilin 1 gene (PFN1) (Wu *et al.*, 2012). Using whole-exome sequencing in a cohort of individuals with Wiedemann-Steiner Syndrome, Jones *et al.* were able to identify de novo mutations in MLL gene, which codes for a histone methyltransferase (Jones *et al.*, 2012).

Researchers are also using genes identified by whole-exome sequencing as leads in identify mutations in related conditions. In one such study, Gardiner *et al.* showed that proline-rich transmembrane protein (PRRT2) gene is associated with episodic neurologic disorders such as episodic ataxia and hemiplegic migraine, in addition to the autosomal dominant paroxysmal kinesigenic dyskenisia (PKD) with or without infantile convulsions, which was originally identified by Wang *et al.* using exome sequencing (Wang *et al.*, 2011, & Gardiner *et al.*, 2012).

In addition, certain mutations have been identified in putative conditions. Strom *et al.* (2012) used whole exome sequencing in nine patients with putative Stargardt Disease in order to identify 3 previously missed mutations in ABCA4 gene, as well as likely disease causing mutations in other genes such as RDS, ELOVL and CRB1. This is a condition, which causes juvenile or early adult onset macular degeneration and previously recessive mutations have been identified in ABCA4 gene in association with this disease. Shamseldin *et al.* (2012) studied the genetic cause of recurrent fetal loss in a couple, who were first cousins and had two previous fetal losses. In this single couple, the authors used exome sequencing together with autozygome analysis and were able to identify a novel mutation in CHRNA1, which was previously associated with fetal akinesia and multiple pterygium. The authors suggest further studies especially in consaginous couples, which will help identify genetic causes of a heterogenous and complex phenotype as fetal loss.

Although, the majority of studies used whole-exome sequencing in an attempt to identify disease-causing variants in rare conditions, there are a number of other studies emerging. These are using chromosome-specific exome sequencing, mainly X-chromosome exome sequencing, as well as exome sequencing in combination with other analyses, such as haplotype analysis and linkage analysis in order to dissect the genetics of both rare and complex conditions. Below are some recent examples of studies, which applied exome sequencing in combination with more conventional analyses.

Puffenberger *et al.* (2012) identified a homozygous missense mutation in HERC2 as the cause of cognitive delay, autistic behaviour and gait instability. The authors initially used genome wide mapping followed by exome sequencing within the mapped interval in two affected children. Then they included another unrelated affected child in order to narrow the mapped interval and were able to identify a missense mutation in HERC2, which is suggested to cause protein aggregation hence reducing protein levels. In another study, Pillay *et al.* studied a rare malignant bone tumor called chordoma, which has a non-Mendelian mode of inheritance. They initially conducted an association study followed by whole-exome and Sanger sequencing of transcription factor T. They were able to identify a strong association with a common nonsynonymous SNP in this transcription factor and chondroma risk (Pillay *et al.*, 2012).

A recent study by Rossi *et al.* (2012) combined whole-exome sequencing with copy-number analysis in order to identify mutations responsible for a type of B cell lymphoma called splenic marginal zone lymphoma (SMZL). In this study, the authors were able to identify mutations in NOTCH2 as well as other most frequently occurring mutations, which could potentially be used as a diagnostic marker in this type of lymphoma. In another study, Andrade *et al.* (2012) used whole genome sequencing in combination with homozygosity mapping in a multiplex family with autosomal recessive teenage-onset progressive myoclonus epilepsy and were able to identify a mutation in CLN6 as the cause for this rare condition.

Thomas *et al.* (2012) used a combination of exome sequencing together with homozygosity mapping to identify truncating mutations in TCTN3 gene, which is proposed to be involved in sonic hedgehog signal transduction, as the causative mutation in orodaciodigital syndromes. Avila-Fernandez *et al.* (2012) used exome sequencing, homozygosity mapping, mutational screening as well as haplotype analysis to identify mutations in RP1 as the cause for early-onset autosomal recessive retinitis in Spanish patients. Ishiura *et al.* (2012) used exome sequencing together with haplotype analysis to show an identical causative mutation in the TRK-fused gene (TFG) in four Japanese families with hereditary motor and sensory neuropathy with proximal dominant involvement.

Using linkage analysis followed by whole-exome sequencing and next-generation sequencing in a family with congenital myopathy, Maljczenko *et al.* (2012) identified a dominant mutation of a splice variant acceptor site in a previously uncharacterized gene called CCDC78. Boileau *et al.* (2012) used genome-wide linkage analysis followed by whole exome sequencing in two large unrelated families with familial thoracic aortic aneurysms and dissections to identify disease causing mutations in TGFB2 gene.

Certain studies used exome sequencing on X-chromosome only in an attempt to identify the causative genes in X-linked conditions. X-exome sequencing was used in a family with X-linked congenital cerebellar ataxia to identify missense mutations in the plasma membrane Ca2+ ATPase isoform 3 as the possible cause for this condition (Zanni *et al.*, 2012). Takano *et al.* used exome capture and deep sequencing of genes on the X-chromosome of patients with intellectual disability, seizures and cardiac problems and were able to identify a mutation in the Chloride intracellular channel 2 (CLC2) gene (Takano *et al.*, 2012).

## 4.3   Exome Sequencing beyond Rare Diseases

Exome sequencing has biomedical and clinical implications beyond rare diseases. Since common complex diseases show both phenotypic and genetic heterogeneity, often they pose more challenges in identification of novel disease causing SNPs. Nonetheless rare alleles have been shown to be significantly associated with such diseases (Prabhu & Pe'er 2009). There is increasing interest in using exome sequencing in order to identify candidate genes in common complex conditions. Recently, exome sequencing is used to identify disease variants for such conditions. One example is a study by Bi *et al.* where mutations in ANK3 were identified, which are implicated in autism spectrum disorders (ASDs). In this study, they initially used whole exome sequencing in a cohort of 20 affected patients, where they were able to identify novel mutations in seven candidate genes. Then the authors went on to sequence another 47 affected individuals and were able to identify three separate missense mutations in four unrelated individuals. The authors suggest the importance of this gene in ASD, as mutations in this gene were also associated with other neurological disorders such as bipolar disease as well as schizophrenia (Bi *et al.* 2012).

In another recent study, Dewan *et al.* used whole-exome sequencing in a family with several members affected with asthma in an attempt to identify any family-specific variants, which may be causing asthma susceptibility. Asthma is a common airways disease. Despite several association studies, which suggested numerous genes associated with asthma, there has not been any causal variants identified up to date. Dewan *et al.* (2012) were able to identify several likely functional variants in asthma candidate genes, however, as they point out, further work is necessary in order to be able to determine which of these variants may be important. In another recent study, Tsurasaki *et al.* (2012) used whole-exome sequencing in five families with Joubert Syndrome related disorders (JSRD). This is a heterogenous syndrome where a total of seventeen causative genes have been identified. The authors were able to identify causative mutations in three separate genes and they suggest the potential use of exome sequencing as a diagnostic tool in identifying these mutations in view of its cost effectiveness and speed compared to Sanger sequencing.

In a recent study, de Ligt *et al.* (2012) used exome sequencing in an attempt to identify new causative mutations in severe intellectual disability. This study involved 100 individuals with an IQ below 50 as well as their unaffected parents. The authors explored the possibility of using exome sequencing as a diagnostic tool in a heterogenous condition. They were able to identify a number of de novo mutations, some in previously predicted candidate genes as well as others in new candidate genes. The authors conclude that exome sequencing may be a useful diagnostic tool in detecting de novo mutations in a heterogenous condition such as severe intellectual disability.

## 5    Biomedical, Clinical and Ethical Implications

Genetic counseling remains crucial for individuals and families, for whom these studies are being considered or performed on, in order for these individuals to be fully informed regarding the implications of the results and their consequences. Guidelines and counseling approaches are needed given that exome and whole genome sequencing are forseen to be used as clinical tests. At present, we may identify a large number of disease causing variants however, further studies are required to decipher distinctly how these variants or genes may be involved in the disease processes, as well as how this information can be used to treat these conditions.

With the development of exome sequencing, it has been relatively easier and quicker to identify disease-causing genes in over 100 rare Mendelian conditions, compared to traditional methods. Up to date, a large number of mutations have been identified for rare conditions, which will pave a new way in our understanding of these genes, their functions as well as their mechanisms of actions in these rare diseases. However, at present, we are not that much closer in our understanding of these conditions and the exact mechanisms of actions of the genes identified. Interestingly, a number of mutations have been identified in the same genes for a number of overlapping as well as non-overlapping conditions. Therefore, it remains crucial that further studies look into the mechanisms of actions, as well as the pathways in which these genes are involved prior to translating all this information for the benefit of the patients with these rare conditions. Understanding of the pathogenesis of these diseases at the molecular level will help with the management of these rare conditions.

In addition to rare Mendelian conditions, exome sequencing is also being used in attempts to identify gene variants that are important in common complex diseases. Even though this is proving to be much harder than identifying disease causing mutations in rare Mendelian conditions, there are studies emerging, which report identification of gene variants considered to significantly contribute to the complex disease phenotypes. However, there are reports in other conditions such as idiopathic generalized epilepsy, where exome sequencing followed by large-scale genotyping failed to identify significant rare variants (Heinzen *et al.* 2012). In a study, Need *et al.* used exome sequencing followed by large-scale genotyping in 166 patients with schizophrenia or schizoaffective disorder, and failed to identify a single variant predisposing to this condition (Need *et al.* 2012). Powerful tools of data analysis and bioinformatics have crucial roles in identifying such significant gene variants in the setting of common complex conditions.

Another important area where exome sequencing is currently being used is the identification of genetic variants in different types of cancers. Exome sequencing has the potential to improve early detection, to offer personalized treatment and to enable molecular classification of various types of common and rare cancers. Studies are being done in cancers such as melanomas, where Krauthammer *et al.* identified RAC1 mutations by utilizing exome sequencing in 147 melanomas. Identification of such genes and understanding their mechanisms of action will help develop ways of preventing and or treating these cancers (Krauthammer *et al.* 2012). Other studies are using whole-exome sequencing in conjunction with a number of other techniques including high-resolution single nucleotide polymorphism arrays in cancers such as primary central nervous system lymphomas in an attempt to identify mutations that would shed light to the pathogenesis of these tumors, hence generating potential therapeutic targets (Gonzalez-Aguilar *et al.* 2012). Studies are also ongoing in other cancers such as medulloblastomas, where exome sequencing has identified mutations in a number of known as well as new genes. These studies are critical in the identification of the genetic drivers of these cancer types in order to be able to diagnose and treat these cancers (Pugh *et al.* 2012). Zhou *et al.* used exome sequencing in conjunction with digital PCR analysis in a patient with metastatic pancreatic ductal adenocarcinoma in an attempt to do genomic profiling in order to understand the mechanism of metastasis in this cancer type (Zhou *et al.* 2012). Another example of a rare cancer is SMZL, where the pathogenesis is not known. Therefore, at present there is no targeted treatment available. However, with the identification of specific pathways involved in the pathogenesis of this and other conditions, treatments targeting these pathways can be used. Furthermore, the mutations identified can be used as diagnostic markers for different types of diseases as in the above case, where Notch2 can be used as a potential marker differentiating this type of lymphoma from others.

Exome sequencing can be used for improving diagnosis and patient management as well as for genetic testing in affected families. In one such study, Hanchard *et al.* used whole exome sequencing in a 3 year old and her parents, where previous traditional diagnostic work-up was inconclusive. In this individual, they were able to identify a mutation in a calcium channel gene CACNA 1S, which was also shown to be associated with hypokalaemic periodic paralysis in another single case. Even though previous clinical, laboratory and standard clinical molecular testing were performed on this individual they were all negative (Hanchard *et al.* 2012). In another example, Futema *et al.* used targeted exome sequencing in 48 patients affected with familial hypercholesterolaemia with no conventionally identified mutations. Using exome sequencing, the authors were able to identify 17 LDLR mutations, two APOB mutations, two novel LDLR variants as well as 5 APOB variants and a heterezygous mutation in LDLRAP1, which was not identified in these individuals previously. As these authors pointed out, this method was useful in identifying mutation in well-covered DNA regions and may be able to replace conventional methods in the future. However, more work still needs to be done in order to provide better coverage of sequences such as promoter areas as well as GC-rich regions and in order to validate the identified variants (Futema *et al.* 2012).

In parallel with advancing sequencing technology and generation of associated computational tools, more and more personal genotype and phenotype data will accumulate. Needless to say, ethical rules and regulations must be in place in terms of several issues that could be associated with this data. These ethical issues include, individual consent, use of sequence data, storage of sequence data and access to any kind of personal sequence data and its associated inference including the molecular diagnoses. There are a number of ethical issues and considerations that are needed to be taken very seriously in view of the amount of emerging individual and family based genetic data. All this new disease related genetic information will have a psychological impact on the individuals as well as their families, and will have implications for health insurance purposes in countries such as the United States of America, where this will become a significant issue if not well thought. Efforts with regards to developing ethical guidelines in personal genomics directly apply to exome sequence data analysis and its implications (Borry, 2009, Gurwitz *et al.*, 2009, Gibson *et al.*, 2010, Cassa *et al.*, 2012, & Oliver *et al.*, 2012).

# References

Srirangalingam, U. & Chew, S.L. (2012). DNA diagnostics and exon skipping. Methods Mol Biol, 867, 3-16.

Gonzaga-Jauregui C, Lupski JR, Gibbs RA. (2012). Human genome sequencing in health and disease. (2012) Annu Rev Med. 63, 35-61.

Zhang, J., Chiodini, R., Badr, A., & Zhang G. (2011). The impact of next-generation sequencing on genomics. Journal of Genetics and Genomics, 38, 95-109.

Taneri, B., Asilmaz, E., & Gaasterland, T. (2012). Biomedical Impact of Splicing Mutations Revealed through Exome Sequencing. Molecular Medicine, 18, 314-319.

Pareek CS., Smoczynski R., & Tretyn, A. (2011). Sequencing technologies and genome sequencing. Journal of Applied Genetics, 52, 413-435.

Mardis ER. (2010). The $1000 genome, the $100,000 analysis? Genome Medicine, 2, 84.

Biesecker LG. (2010). Exome sequencing makes medical genomics a reality. Nature Gen. 42:13–4.

Choi M, Scholl UI, Ji W, Liu T, Tikhonova IR, Zumbo P, et al. (2009). Genetic diagnosis by whole exome capture and massively parallel DNA sequencing. PNAS 106, 19096-19101.

Rabbani B., Mahdieh, N., Hosomichi, K. Nakaoka, H., & Inoue, I. (2012). Next-generation sequencing: impact of exome sequencing in characterizing Mendelian disorders. Journal of Human Genetics, doi: 10.1038/jhg.2012.91. [Epub ahead of print]

Teer JK, & Mullikin JC. (2010). Exome sequencing: the sweet spot before whole genomes. Human Molecular Genetics, 19:R145-R151.

Atlmann A., Weber P., Bader D., Preuss M., Binder EB, Muller-Myhsok, B. (2012). A beginners guide to SNP calling from high-throughput DNA-sequencing data. Human Genetics, 131, 1541-1554.

Challis D., Yu J., Evani US., Jackson AR, Paithanker S., Coarfa C., Milosavlijevic A., Gibbs RA., & Yu F. (2012). An integrative variant analysis suite for whole exome next-generation sequencing data. BMC Bioinformatics, 13, 1-12.

Li H., Handsaker B., Wysoker A., Fenel T., Ruan J., Homer, N., Marth G., Abecasis G., & Durbin, R. (2009). The Sequence Alignment/Map format and SAMtools. Bioinformatics, 2078-2079.

Koboldt DC., Chen K., Wylie T., Larson DE., McLellan MD., Mardis ER., Weinstock GM., Wilson RK, Ding L. (2009). VarScan: Variant detection in massively parallel sequencing of individual and pooled samples. Bioinformatics. 25(17):2283-5.

Albers CA, Lunter G, MacArthur DG, McVean G, Ouwehand WH, Durbin R. (2010). Dindel: accurate indel calls from short-read data. Genome Research, 21(6);961-973.

DePristo MA, Banks E, Poplin R, Garimella KV, Maguire JR, Hartl C, Phillipakis AA, del Angel G, Rivas MA, Hanna M, et al. (2011). A framework for variation discovery and genotyping using next-generation DNA sequencing data. Nature Genetics, 43(5):491-498.

Popendorf K, & Sakakibara Y. (2012). SAMSCOPE: an OpenGL-based real-time interactive scale-free SAM viewer. Bioinformatics, 28:1276-7.

Fischer M, Snajder R, Pabinger S, Dander A, Schossing A, et al. (2012). SIMPLEX: Cloud-enabled pipeline for the comprehensive analysis of exome sequencing data. PLOS One, 7:e41948.

Ng SB, Turner EH, Robertson PD, Flygare SD, Bigham AW et al. (2009). Targeted capture and massively parallel sequencing of 12 human exomes. Nature, 461:272-276.

Koboldt DC, Zhang Q, Larson DR, Shen D, McLellan MD, Lin L, Miller CA, Mardis ER, Ding L, & Wilson RK. (2012). VarScan2: Somatic mutation and copy number alteration discovery in cancer by exome sequencing. Genome Research, 22:568-576.

Elsharawy A, Forster M, Schracke N, Keller A, Thomsen I, et al. (2012). Improving mapping and SNP-calling performance in multiplexed targeted next-generation sequencing. BMC Genomics, 13:417.

Yi X, Liang Y, Huerta-Sanchez E, Jin X, Cuo ZXP et al. (2010). Sequencing of 50 human exomes reveals adaptation to high altitude. Science, 329:75-78.

Taneri B, Snyder B, Novoradovsky A, Gaasterland T. (2004). Alternative splicing of mouse transcription factors affect their DNA-binding domain architecture and is tissue specific. Genome Biology, 5(10): R75.

Taneri B, Novoradovsky A, Snyder B, Gaasterland T. (2005). Databases for comparative analysis of human-mouse orthologous alternative splicing. Lecture Notes in Computer Science, 3388:123-131.

Taneri B, Novoradovsky A, Gaasterland T. (2009). Identification of shadow exons: mining for alternative exons in human, mouse and rat comparative databases. BIOKDD 2009 – Biological Knowledge Discovery from Databases - DEXA 2009 – 20th International Workshop on Database and Expert Systems Application; IEEE Computer Society, 208-212.

Taneri B, Snyder B, & Gaasterland T. (2011). Distribution of Alternatively Spliced Transcript Isoforms within Human and Mouse Transcriptomes. Journal of OMICS Research,1: 1: 1-5.

Montes, M., Becerra, S., Sanchez-Alvarez M, & Sune C. (2012). Functional coupling of transcription and splicing. Gene, 501, 104-117.

Douglas AG, & Wood MJ. (2011). RNA splicing: disease and therapy. Brief Funct Genomics, 10, 151-64.

Gilissen C, et al. (2010). Exome sequencing identifies WDR35 variants involved in Sensenbrenner syndrome. Am. J. Hum. Genet. 87:418–23.

Byun M, et al. (2010). Whole exome sequencingbased discovery of STIM1 deficiency in a child with fatal classic Kaposi sarcoma. J. Exp. Med. 207:2307–12.

Guergueltcheva V, Azmanov DN, Angelicheva D, Smith KR, Chamova T, Florez L, Bynevelt M, Nguyen T, Cherninkova S, Bojinova V,Kaprelyan A, Angelova L, Morar B, Chandler D, Kaneva R, Bahlo M, Tournev I, & Kalaydjieva L. (2012). Autosomal-Recessive Congenital Cerebellar Ataxia Is Caused by Mutations in Metabotropic Glutamate Receptor 1. Am J Hum Genet. [Epub ahead of print]

Wadt K, Choi J, Chung JY, Kiilgaard J, Heegaard S, Drzewiecki KT, Trent JM, Hewitt SM, Hayward NK, Gerdes AM & Brown KM. (2012). A cryptic BAP1 splice mutation in a family with uveal and cutaneous melanoma, and paraganglioma. Pigment Cell Melanoma Res. doi: 10.1111/pcmr.12006. [Epub ahead of print]

Liu T, Jin X, Zhang Z, Yuan H, Cheng J, Lee J, Zhang M, Wu J, Wang L, Tian G, Wang W. (2012). A novel missense SNRNP200 mutation associated with autosomal dominant retinitis pigmentosa in a Chinese family. Plos One. 7(9):e45464. doi: 10.1371/journal.pone.0045464. [Epub ahead of print]

Harakalova M, van den Boogaard MJ, Sinke R, van Lieshout S, van Tuil MC, Duran K, Renkens I, Terhal PA, de Kovel C, Nijman IJ, van Haelst M, Knoers NV, van Haaften G, Kloosterman W, Hennekam RC, Cuppen E, Ploos van Amstel HK. (2012). X-exome sequencing identifies a HDAC8 variant in a large pedigree with X-linked intellectual disability, truncal obesity, gynaecomastia, hypogonadism and unusual face. J Med Genet. 49, 539-43.

Lin Z, Shi L, Lee M, Giehl KA, Tang Z, Wang H, Zhang J, Yin J, Wu L, Xiao R, Liu X, Dai L, Zhu X, Li R, Betz RC, Zhang X, Yang T. (2012). Loss-of-Function Mutations in HOXC13 Cause Pure Hair and Nail Ectodermal Dysplasia. Am J Hum Genet. doi: 10.1016/j.ajhg.2012.08.029 [Epub ahead of print]

Duncan JL, Roorda A, Navani M, Vishweswaraiah S, Syed R, Soudry S, Ratnam K, Gudiseva HV, Lee P, Gaasterland T, Ayyagari R. (2012). Identification of a novel mutation in the CDHR1 gene in a family with recessive retinal degeneration. Arch Ophthalmol. 130(10): 1301-8.

Guerreiro RJ, Lohmann E, Bras JM, Gibbs JR, Rohrer JD, Gurunlian N, Dursun B, Bilgic B, Hanagasi H, Gurvit G, Emre M, Singleton A, Hardy J. (2012). Using Exome Sequencing to Reveal Mutations in TREM2 Presenting as a Frontotemporal Dementia-Like Syndrome Without Bone Involvement. Arch Neurol.doi: 10.1001/archneurol.2013.579. [Epub ahead of print]

Hammer MB, Eleuch-Fayache G, Gibbs JR, Arepalli SK, Chong SB, Sassi C, Bouhlal Y, Hentati F, Amouri R, Singleton AB. (2012). Exome sequencing: an efficient diagnostic tool for complex neurodegenerative disorders. Eur J Neurol. doi: 10.1111/j.1468-1331.2012.03883.x. [Epub ahead of print]

Drielsma A, Jalas C, Simonis N, et al. (2012). Two novel CCDC88C mutations confirm the role of DAPLE in autosomal recessive congenital hydrocephalus. J. Med. Genet., 39:708-12.

Horani A, Druley TE, Zariwala MA, Patel AC, Levinson BT, Van Arendonk LG, Thornton KC, Giacalone JC, Albee AJ, Wilson KS, Turner EH, Nickerson DA, Shendure J, Bayly PV, Leigh MW, Knowles MR, Brody SL, Dutcher SK, Ferkol TW. (2012). Whole-exome capture and sequencing identifies HEATR2 mutation as a cause of primary ciliary dyskinesia. Am J Hum Genet. doi: 10.1016/j.ajhg.2012.08.022. [Epub ahead of print]

Mitsui J, Matsukawa T, Ishiura H et al. (2012). CSF1R mutations identified in three families with autosomal dominantly inherited leukoencephalopathy. Am. J. Med. Genet. B. Neuropscyiatr. Genet., 159B:951-7.

Campeau PM, Lu JT, Sule G, Jiang MM, Bae Y, Madan S, Högler W, Shaw NJ, Mumm S, Gibbs RA, Whyte MP, & Lee BH. (2012). Whole-exome sequencing identifies mutations in the nucleoside transporter gene SLC29A3 in dysosteosclerosis, a form of osteopetrosis. Hum Mol Genet. [Epub ahead of print]

Haack TB, Makowski C, Yao Y, Graf E, Hempel M, Wieland T, Tauer U, Ahting U, Mayr JA, Freisinger P, Yoshimatsu H, Inui K, Strom TM, Meitinger T, Yonezawa A, & Prokisch H. (2012). Impaired riboflavin transport due to missense mutations in SLC52A2 causes Brown-Vialetto-Van Laere syndrome. J Inherit Metab Dis. [Epub ahead of print]

Semler O, Garbes L, Keupp K, Swan D, Zimmermann K, Becker J, Iden S, Wirth B, Eysel P, Koerber F, Schoenau E, Bohlander SK, Wollnik B, & Netzer C. (2012). A Mutation in the 5'-UTR of IFITM5 Creates an In-Frame Start Codon and Causes Autosomal-Dominant Osteogenesis Imperfecta Type V with Hyperplastic Callus. Am J Hum Genet. 91, 349-57.

Cho TJ, Lee KE, Lee SK, Song SJ, Kim KJ, Jeon D, Lee G, Kim HN, Lee HR, Eom HH, Lee ZH, Kim OH, Park WY, Park SS, Ikegawa S,Yoo WJ, Choi IH, & Kim JW. (2012). A Single Recurrent Mutation in the 5'-UTR of IFITM5 Causes Osteogenesis Imperfecta Type V. Am J Hum Genet. 91:343-8.

Merner ND, Girard SL, Catoire H, Bourassa CV, Belzil VV, Rivière JB, Hince P, Levert A, Dionne-Laporte A, Spiegelman D, Noreau A, Diab S, Szuto A, Fournier H, Raelson J, Belouchi M, Panisset M, Cossette P, Dupré N, Bernard G, Chouinard S, Dion PA, & Rouleau GA. (2012). Exome Sequencing Identifies FUS Mutations as a Cause of Essential Tremor. Am J Hum Genet. 91, 313-9.

Rosewich H, Thiele H, Ohlenbusch A, Maschke U, Altmüller J, Frommolt P, Zirn B, Ebinger F, Siemes H, Nürnberg P, Brockmann K, & Gärtner J. (2012). Heterozygous de-novo mutations in ATP1A3 in patients with alternating hemiplegia of childhood: a whole-exome sequencing gene-identification study. Lancet Neurol. 11,764-73.

Heinzen EL, Swoboda KJ, Hitomi Y, Gurrieri F, Nicole S, de Vries B, et al. (2012). De novo mutations in ATP1A3 cause alternating hemiplegia of childhood. Nat Genet. 44, 1030-4.

Tsurusaki Y, Saitoh S, Tomizawa K, Sudo A, Asahina N, Shiraishi H, Ito JI, Tanaka H, Doi H, Saitsu H, Miyake N, & Matsumoto N. (2012). A DYNC1H1 mutation causes a dominant spinal muscular atrophy with lower extremity predominance. Neurogenetics. [Epub ahead of print]

Chiang PW, Wang J, Chen Y, Fu Q, Zhong J, Chen Y, Yi X, Wu R, Gan H, Shi Y, Chen Y, Barnett C, Wheaton D, Day M, Sutherland J, Heon E, Weleber RG, Gabriel LA, Cong P, Chuang K, Ye S, Sallum JM, & Qi M. (2012). Exome sequencing identifies NMNAT1 mutations as a cause of Leber congenital amaurosis. Nat Genet. 44,:972-4.

Koenekoop RK, Wang H, Majewski J, Wang X, Lopez I, Ren H, Chen Y, Li Y, Fishman GA, Genead M, Schwartzentruber J, Solanki N,Traboulsi EI, Cheng J, Logan CV, McKibbin M, Hayward BE, Parry DA, Johnson CA, Nageeb M; Finding of Rare Disease Genes (FORGE) Canada Consortium, Poulter JA, Mohamed MD, Jafri H, Rashid Y, Taylor GR, Keser V, Mardon G, Xu H, Inglehearn CF, Fu Q, Toomes C, & Chen R. (2012). Mutations in NMNAT1 cause Leber congenital amaurosis and identify a new disease pathway for retinal degeneration. Nat Genet. 44,1035-9.

Falk MJ, Zhang Q, Nakamaru-Ogiso E, Kannabiran C, Fonseca-Kelly Z, Chakarova C, Audo I, Mackay DS, Zeitz C, Borman AD, Staniszewska M, Shukla R, Palavalli L, Mohand-Said S, Waseem NH, Jalali S, Perin JC, Place E, Ostrovsky J, Xiao R, Bhattacharya SS, Consugar M, Webster AR, Sahel JA, Moore AT, Berson EL, Liu Q, Gai X, & Pierce EA. (2012). NMNAT1 mutations cause Leber congenital amaurosis. Nat Genet. 44, 1040-5.

Elo JM, Yadavalli SS, Euro L, Isohanni P, Götz A, Carroll CJ, Valanne L, Alkuraya FS, Uusimaa J, Paetau A, Caruso EM, Pihko H, Ibba M,Tyynismaa H, & Suomalainen A. (2012). Mitochondrial phenylalanyl-tRNA synthetase mutations underlie fatal infantile Alpers encephalopathy. Hum Mol Genet. [Epub ahead of print]

Wu CH, Fallini C, Ticozzi N, Keagle PJ, Sapp PC, Piotrowska K, Lowe P, Koppers M, McKenna-Yasek D, Baron DM, Kost JE, Gonzalez-Perez P, Fox AD, Adams J, Taroni F, Tiloca C, Leclerc AL, Chafe SC, Mangroo D, Moore MJ, Zitzewitz JA, Xu ZS, van den Berg LH, Glass JD, Siciliano G, Cirulli ET, Goldstein DB, Salachas F, Meininger V, Rossoll W, Ratti A, Gellera C, Bosco DA, Bassell GJ, Silani V, Drory VE, Brown RH Jr, &

Landers JE. (2012). Mutations in the profilin 1 gene cause familial amyotrophic lateral sclerosis. Nature. 488, 499-503.

Jones WD, Dafou  D, McEntagart  M, Woollard  WJ, Elmslie  FV, Holder-Espinasse  M, Irving  M, Saggar AK, Smithson S, Trembath RC,Deshpande C, Simpson MA. (2012) De Novo Mutations in MLL Cause Wiedemann-Steiner Syndrome. Am J Hum Genet. 91, 358-64.

Gardiner AR, Bhatia KP, Stamelou M, et al. (2012). PRRT2 gene mutations: From paroxysmal dyskinesia to episodic ataxia and hemiplegic migrane. Neurology, [Epub ahead of print].

Wang JL, Cao L, Li XH et al. (2011). Identification of PRRT2 as the causative gene of paroxysmal kinesigenic dyskinesias. Brain, 134:3493-3501.

Strom SP, Gao YQ, Martinez A, Ortube C, Chen Z, Nelson SF, Nusinowitz S, Farber DB, Gorin MB. (2012). Molecular diagnosis of putative stargardt disease probands by exome sequencing. BMC Med Genet. 13, 67.

Shamseldin HE, Swaid A, Alkuraya FS. (2012). Lifting the lid on unborn lethal Mendelian phenotypes through exome sequencing. Genet Med. doi: 10.1038/gim.2012.130. [Epub ahead of print]

Puffenberger EG, Jinks RN, Wang H, et al. (2012). A homozygous missense mutation in HERC2 assciated with global developmental delay and autism spectrum disorder. Hum. Mutat., 33:1639-46.

Pillay N, Plagnol V, Tarpey PS, et al. (2012). A common single-nucleotide variant in T is strongly associated with chordoma. Nature Genetics, 44:1185-7.

Rossi D, Trifonov V, Fangazio M, Bruscaggin A, Rasi S, Spina V, Monti S, Vaisitti T, Arruga F, Famà R, Ciardullo C, Greco M, Cresta S,Piranda D, Holmes A, Fabbri G, Messina M, Rinaldi A, Wang J, Agostinelli C, Piccaluga PP, Lucioni M, Tabbò F, Serra R, Franceschetti S,Deambrogi C, Daniele G, Gattei V, Marasca R, Facchetti F, Arcaini L, Inghirami G, Bertoni F, Pileri SA, Deaglio S, Foà R, Dalla-Favera R,Pasqualucci L, Rabadan R, Gaidano G. (2012). The coding genome of splenic marginal zone lymphoma: activation of NOTCH2 and other pathways regulating marginal zone development. J Exp Med. 209, 1537-51.

Andrade DM, Paton T, Turnbull J, Marshall CR, Scherer SW, Minassian BA. (2012). Mutation of the CLN6 Gene in Teenage-Onset Progressive Myoclonus Epilepsy. Pediatr Neurol. 47, 205-8.

Thomas S, Legendre M, Saunier S, Bessières B, Alby C, Bonnière M, Toutain A, Loeuillet L, Szymanska K, Jossic F, Gaillard D, Yacoubi MT, Mougou-Zerelli S, David A, Barthez MA, Ville Y, Bole-Feysot C, Nitschke P, Lyonnet S, Munnich A, Johnson CA, Encha-Razavi F,Cormier-Daire V, Thauvin-Robinet C, Vekemans M, Attié-Bitach T. (2012). TCTN3 Mutations Cause Mohr-Majewski Syndrome. Am J Hum Genet. 91, 372-8.

Avila-Fernandez A, Corton M, Nishiguchi KM, Muñoz-Sanz N, Benavides-Mori B, Blanco-Kelly F, Riveiro-Alvarez R, Garcia-Sandoval B, Rivolta C, Ayuso C. (2012). Identification of an RP1 Prevalent Founder Mutation and Related Phenotype in Spanish Patients with Early-Onset Autosomal Recessive Retinitis.Ophthalmology. [Epub ahead of print]

Ishiura H, Sako W, Yoshida M, Kawarai T, Tanabe O, Goto J, Takahashi Y, Date H, Mitsui J, Ahsan B, Ichikawa Y, Iwata A, Yoshino H, Izumi Y, Fujita K, Maeda K, Goto S, Koizumi H, Morigaki R, Ikemura M, Yamauchi N, Murayama S, Nicholson GA, Ito H, Sobue G, Nakagawa M, Kaji R, Tsuji S. (2012). The TRK-Fused Gene Is Mutated in Hereditary Motor and Sensory Neuropathy with Proximal Dominant Involvement. Am J Hum Genet. 91,:320-9.

Majczenko K, Davidson AE, Camelo-Piragua S, Agrawal PB, Manfready RA, Li X, Joshi S, Xu J, Peng W, Beggs AH, Li JZ, Burmeister M,Dowling JJ. (2012). Dominant Mutation of CCDC78 in a Unique Congenital Myopathy with Prominent Internal Nuclei and Atypical Cores. Am J Hum Genet. 91, 365-71.

Boileau C, Guo  DC, Hanna  N, Regalado  ES, Detaint  D, Gong  L, Varret  M, Prakash SK, Li  AH, d'Indy H, Braverman AC, Grandchamp B,Kwartler CS, Gouya L, Santos-Cortez RL, Abifadel M, Leal SM, Muti

C, Shendure J, Gross MS, Rieder MJ, Vahanian A, Nickerson DA,Michel JB; National Heart, Lung, and Blood Institute (NHLBI) Go Exome Sequencing Project, Jondeau G, Milewicz DM. (2012). TGFB2 mutations cause familial thoracic aortic aneurysms and dissections associated with mild systemic features of Marfan syndrome. Nat Genet. 44, 916-921.

Zanni G, Calì T, Kalscheuer VM, Ottolini D, Barresi S, Lebrun N, Montecchi-Palazzi L, Hu H, Chelly J, Bertini E, Brini M, Carafoli E. (2012). Mutation of plasma membrane Ca2+ ATPase isoform 3 in a family with X-linked congenital cerebellar ataxia impairs Ca2+ homeostasis. Proc Natl Acad Sci 109, 14514-9.

Takano K, Liu D, Tarpey P, Gallant E, Lam A, Witham S, Alexov E, Chaubey A, Stevenson RE, Schwartz CE, Board PG, Dulhunty AF. (2012). An X-linked channelopathy with cardiomegaly due to a CLIC2 mutation enhancing ryanodine receptor channel activity. Hum Mol Genet. [Epub ahead of print]

Prabhu S, Pe'er I. (2009). Overlapping pools for high-throughput targeted resequencing. Genome Research, 19:1254-1261.

Bi C, Wu J, Jiang T, Liu Q, Cai W, Yu P, Cai T, Zhao M, Jiang YH, Sun ZS. (2012). Mutations of ANK3 identified by exome sequencing are associated with Autism susceptibility. Hum Mutat. doi: 10.1002/humu.22174. [Epub ahead of print]

Dewan AT, Egan KB, Hellenbrand K, Sorrention K, Walsh KM, Bracken MB. (2012). Whole-exome sequencing of a pedigree segregating asthma. BMC Medical Genetics.13(1):95.

Tsurasaki Y, Kobayashi Y, Hisano M, Ito S, Doi H, Nakashima M, Saitsu H, Matsumoto N, Miyake N. (2012). The diagnostic utility of exome sequencing in Joubert syndrome and related disorders. J Hum Genet. doi: 10.1038/jhg.2012.117. [Epub ahead of print]

de Ligt J, Willemsen MH, van Bon BW, Kleefstra T, Yntema HG, Kroes T, Vulto-van Silfhout AT, Koolen DA, de Vries P, Gilissen C, Del Rosario M, Hoischen A, Scheffer H, de Vries BB, Brunner HG, Veltman JA, Vissers LE. (2012). Diagnostic exome sequencing in persons with severe intellectual disability. N Engl J Med. 367(20): 1921-9.

Heinzen EL, Depondt C, Cavalleri GL, Ruzzo EK, Walley NM, Need AC, Ge D, He M, Cirulli ET, Zhao Q, Cronin KD, Gumbs CE, Campbell CR, Hong LK, Maia JM, Shianna KV, McCormack M, Radtke RA, O'Conner GD, Mikati MA, Gallentine WB, Husain AM, Sinha SR,Chinthapalli K, Puranam RS, McNamara JO, Ottman R, Sisodiya SM, Delanty N, Goldstein DB. (2012). Exome sequencing followed by large-scale genotyping fails to identify single rare variants of large effect in idiopathic generalized epilepsy. Am J Hum Genet. 91, 293-302.

Need AC, McEvoy JP, Gennarelli M, Heinzen EL, Ge D, Maia JM, Shianna KV, He M, Cirulli ET, Gumbs CE, Zhao Q, Campbell CR, Hong L, Rosenquist P, Putkonen A, Hallikainen T, Repo-Tiihonen E, Tiihonen J, Levy DL, Meltzer HY, Goldstein DB. (2012). Exome sequencing followed by large-scale genotyping suggests a limited role for moderately rare risk factors of strong effect in schizophrenia. Am J Hum Genet. 91, 303-12.

Krauthammer M, Kong Y, Ha BH, Evans P, Bacchiocchi A, McCusker JP, Cheng E, Davis MJ, Goh G, Choi M, Ariyan S, Narayan D, Dutton-Regester K, Capatana A, Holman EC, Bosenberg M, Sznol M, Kluger HM, Brash DE, Stern DF, Materin MA, Lo RS, Mane S, Ma S, Kidd KK,Hayward NK, Lifton RP, Schlessinger J, Boggon TJ, Halaban R. (2012). Exome sequencing identifies recurrent somatic RAC1 mutations in melanoma. Nat Genet. 44, 1006-14.

Gonzalez-Aguilar A, Idbaih A, Boisselier B, Habbita N, Rossetto M, Laurenge A, Bruno A, Jouvet A, Polivka M, Adam C, Figarella-Branger D, Miquel C, Vital A, Ghesquieres H, Gressin R, Delwail V, Taillandier L, Chinot O, Soubeyran P, Gyan E, Choquet S, Houillier C,Soussain C, Tanguy ML, Marie Y, Mokhtari K, Hoang-Xuan K. (2012). Recurrent mutations of MYD88 and TBL1XR1 in primary central nervous system lymphomas. Clin Cancer Res. [Epub ahead of print]

Pugh TJ, Weeraratne SD, Archer TC, Pomeranz Krummel DA, Auclair D, Bochicchio J, Carneiro MO, Carter SL, Cibulskis K, Erlich RL, Greulich H, Lawrence MS, Lennon NJ, McKenna A, Meldrim J, Ramos AH, Ross MG, Russ C, Shefler E, Sivachenko A, Sogoloff B, Stojanov P, Tamayo P, Mesirov JP, Amani V, Teider N, Sengupta S, Francois JP, Northcott PA, Taylor MD, Yu F, Crabtree GR, Kautzman AG, Gabriel SB, Getz G, Jäger N, Jones DT, Lichter P, Pfister SM, Roberts TM, Meyerson M, Pomeroy SL, Cho YJ. (2012). Medulloblastoma exome sequencing uncovers subtype-specific somatic mutations. Nature. 488, 106-10.

Zhou B, Irwanto A, Guo YM, Bei JX, Wu Q, Chen G, Zhang TP, Lei JJ, Feng QS, Chen LZ, Liu J, Zhao YP. (2012). Exome sequencing and digital PCR analyses reveal novel mutated genes related to the metastasis of pancreatic ductal adenocarcinoma. Cancer Biol Ther. 13, 871-9.

Hanchard NA, Murdock DR, Magoulas PL, Bainbridge M, Muzny D, Wu Y, Wang M, McGuire AL, Lupski JR, Gibbs RA, Brown CW. (2012). Exploring the utility of Whole-Exome Sequencing as a diagnostic tool in a child with Atypical Episodic Muscle Weakness. Clin Genet. doi: 10.1111/j.1399-0004.2012.01951.x. [Epub ahead of print]

Futema M, Plagnol V, Whittall RA, et al. (2012). Use of targeted exome sequencing as a diagnostic tool for Familial Hypercholesterolaemia. J Med Genet. 49:644-649.

Borry P. (2009). Coming of age of personalized medicine: challenges ahead. Genome Med. 1:109.

Gurwitz G & Bregman-Eschet Y. (2009). Personal genomics services: whose genomes? Eur. J. Hum. Genet. 17:883-889.

Gibson G, Copenhaver GP. (2010). Consent and internet-enabled human genomics. PLoS Genet. 6(6), e1000965.

Cassa CA, Savage SK, Taylor PL, et al. (2012). Disclosing pathogenic genetic variants to research participants: quantifying an emerging ethical responsibility. Genome Res. 22(3):421-8.

Oliver JM, Slashinski MJ, Wang T, et al. (2012). Balancing the risks and benefits of genomic data sharing: genome research participants' perspectives. Public Health Genomics.15(2):106-14.

# Whole Genome Amplification: Technologies and Applications

Daniel W.H. Ho
*Department of Health Technology and Informatics*
*The Hong Kong Polytechnic University, Hong Kong SAR, China*

Shea Ping Yip
*Department of Health Technology and Informatics*
*The Hong Kong Polytechnic University, Hong Kong SAR, China*

# 1    Introduction

Genotyping of sequence variants is a routine data-generating procedure in many genetic studies. With the advancement in genotyping technologies, different genotyping platforms have emerged. From simple non-multiplexing assays, e.g. Sanger sequencing and restriction fraction length polymorphism (RFLP), to highly multiplexed array-based assays or even massive parallel next generation sequencing (NGS), scientists have access to a wide range of options for their needs.

No matter which platform is chosen, the common issues are the increasing number of genetic markers (most likely single nucleotide polymorphisms – SNPs) being genotyped and the huge amount of data being generated. With the availability of complete catalog of reference human genome information and NGS technology, an increasing number of genetic markers is being identified and examined. Studying these genetic markers involves the concomitant consumption of DNA samples, which therefore makes it impossible for massive testing in most cases.

Subject recruitment and sample collection are time-consuming and expensive processes in the multi-stage implementation pipeline of genetic studies. In most occasions, the precious DNA samples are in limited supply and therefore will not last long upon extensive use. This imposes severe constraints on such genetic studies, especially for those working on subjects who are no long available, specific tissues that can only be obtained in small quantities or forensic samples.

Various methods of whole genome amplification (WGA) have been developed. They vary in the fundamental principles and practical efficiency. Studies have been undertaken for comparing different WGA methods. Whole genome amplified DNA (wgaDNA) samples have been tested and applied in numerous applications of different genotyping platforms with a wide spectrum of multiplexing levels. They differ in the underlying chemistry and complexity of the assays. WGA can also be used with a great variety of sample sources with minimal requirement for the quality and quantity of the starting material. It is therefore possible to achieve balanced and accurate amplification of the genome through WGA of minute amounts of input DNA (e.g. the DNA from a few cells of an early embryo).

The emergence of WGA has profound influence on modern genetic studies. However, the benefit of this technology is not confined to scientists in the research community or those working on DNA samples. As a result of the facilitated testing services and studies of disease gene mapping that utilize wgaDNA samples as well as the improved understanding of many diseases, the whole society can take advantage of this valuable technology.

# 2    Common Methods for WGA

In the past, Epstein-Barr virus-transformed cell lines were commonly used to provide an unlimited source of DNA. Nevertheless, this method is labour-intensive, expensive and inapplicable to existing DNA samples (Lovmar & Syvanen, 2006). As a result, different technologies of WGA have been developed to scale up the limited DNA resources to meet the ever-growing demand.

The development of WGA dated back to the early 1990s. Early WGA methods were based on modified polymerase chain reaction (PCR). These PCR-based methods used two strategies to enable genome-wide amplification. One strategy used either random or degenerate primers to initiate primer extension throughout the genome: primer extension preamplification (PEP) and degenerate oligonucleotide primed polymerase chain reaction (DOP-PCR) (Zhang *et al.*, 1992; Telenius *et al.*, 1992). Another strategy employed a pair of universal primers annealing to adaptors ligated to sheared genomic DNA (gDNA) of appropriate size – OmniPlex (Kamberov *et al.*, 2002; Langmore, 2002). These methods require thermocyling and the use of *Taq* DNA polymerase or other similar enzymes, which lack 3'-5' proofreading activity and hence have higher error rates. Newer WGA methods still used random primers, but amplified gDNA isothermally without thermocycling – multiple displacement amplification MDA (Lizardi *et al.*, 1998). Isothermal amplification is catalyzed by phi29 DNA polymerase, whose strand displacement activity eliminates thermocycling so long as the gDNA is denatured in the initial phase. Another advantage of using phi29 DNA polymerase is a lower error rate because of its intrinsic 3'-5' proofreading activity.

In spite of the difference in carrying out the amplification process, their common ultimate goals are to faithfully amplify input gDNA with substantial genomic coverage, but minimal bias in generating a considerable amount of product. MDA is now the most widely used method for WGA and hence will be discussed first.

## 2.1   Multiple Displacement Amplification (MDA)

Originally developed for amplifying circular DNA templates of plasmid and bacteriophage, phi29 DNA polymerase was used to perform rolling circle amplification in the presence of exonuclease-resistant random primers (Lizardi *et al.*, 1998). This technology relies on the great processivity of phi29 DNA polymerase to carry out isothermal (30°C) strand displacement reaction for amplification of DNA strands (Figure 1).

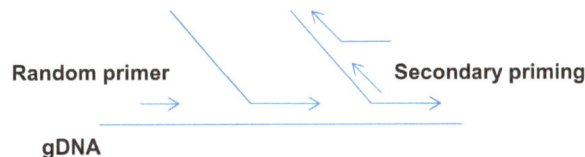

**Random primer**        **Secondary priming**

**gDNA**

**Figure 1:** In multiple displacement amplification, random primers bind to a genomic DNA (gDNA) template and are extended by phi29 DNA polymerase. When the phi29 DNA polymerase encounters a DNA strand in front of it, it displaces this strand and continues to extend the primer. Random primers can also bind the displaced DNA strands and are in turn extended by the DNA polymerase.

It was later applied by Dean *et al.* (2002) to gDNA. It was found that MDA could amplify the genome with high uniformity and that the bias in representation of different loci was relatively low (less than 3-fold in contrast to 4-6 orders of magnitude for other PCR-based WGA methods). The length of the generated DNA product was relatively long, more than 10 kb on average. The yield of an MDA reaction was found to be less dependent on the amount of input DNA. In contrast, since the reaction was self-limiting, the reaction conditions and the amount of reagents were the actual limiting factors for the final yield of product. The wgaDNA generated by MDA was also found to give satisfactory performance in a variety of applications including genotyping of SNPs, Southern blotting, RFLP and comparative genome hybridization (CGH). As few as less than 10 copies of human gDNA could generate WGA product of reasonable amount (20-30 μg). Moreover, crude whole blood and tissue culture cells could also be used directly for WGA by MDA method without the initial DNA purification.

Interestingly, MDA did not require denaturation by high temperature to generate single-stranded template from double-stranded input gDNA. Omission of the denaturation step was suggested to increase the specificity of the WGA reaction. It was postulated that DNA fragments generated from denaturation contributed to nonspecific priming of amplification artefacts (Dean *et al.*, 2002).

In a subsequent study (Bergen *et al.*, 2005b), the amount of input DNA for WGA by MDA was carefully studied, over a range of 1 to 200 ng, to assess its effect on genotyping performance (genotype completion and genotype concordance). There was a very mild deterioration in genotyping performance for wgaDNA produced from all gDNA input levels although the reduction was not statistically significant. Increased variation of allelic amplification was believed to primarily account for the reduction in genotyping performance of wgaDNA, resulting in loss of heterozygosity and increased undetermined genotypes. A minimal input of 10 ng of gDNA for MDA was suggested to obtain equivalent genotyping performance as gDNA for SNP genotyping. Over 100 ng of gDNA input were required for small tandem repeat (STR) genotyping. Another issue worth noting was that MDA would produce product even in the absence of input template. Therefore, there would be problems for negative control of MDA reaction.

## 2.2  OmniPlex Technology

This technology is based on a proprietary *in vitro* method (Kamberov *et al.*, 2002; Langmore, 2002) to reformat DNA templates into amplifiable molecule of controllable size (typically 0.5-6 kb) called "Plexisome". Plexisomes are created at the termini of DNA templates by a controlled nick-translation reaction (Figure 2).

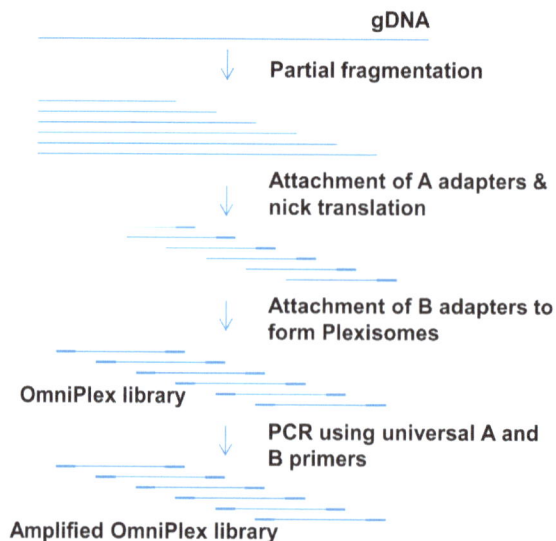

**Figure 2:** The OmniPlex technology produces a library of fragments which presumably constitutes the whole genome, and are each flanked by two adaptors.

Each terminus of DNA templates is ligated with a special oligonucleotide adapter having a synthetic nick. DNA polymerase with both 3' polymerase and 5' exonuclease activities adds new nucleotides to one side of the nick and removes existing nucleotides at the other. This process causes the nick to be translated towards the centre of the DNA template. The strand replacement reaction is highly synchronous while the nick-translation reaction is efficient, reproducible and sequence-independent. The product has uniform length determined by the length of polymerization process. After the nick-translation reaction is stopped, a second adapter is added to the 3' end of the nick-translated molecule to form Plexisome. The collection of Plexisomes generated from gDNA templates produces the OmniPlex library, which represents the genome.

The OmniPlex library can be used to amplify the entire genome as a family of overlapping molecules by PCR with universal primers complementary to the 2 flanking adapters of Plexisomes. WGA can be achieved through amplifying the entire genomic representation of Plexisomes. Alternatively, directed amplification can be performed using locus-specific primers.

According to the manufacturer, as little as 100 ng of starting material can be amplified up to 2000-fold. OmniPlex wgaDNA was found to accurately represent all the 79 tested loci with a maximal bias of only 4-fold. It was also found to maintain allelic representation in standard SNP assays (Buntaine *et al.*).

## 2.3    Primer Extension Preamplification (PEP) Using Random Oligonucleotide Primers

This method relies on the sensitivity of PCR to enable WGA even for a single haploid cell. With *Taq* DNA polymerase and a *random* mixture of 15-base oligo primers ($4^{15}$ of different sequences), multiple rounds of amplification are utilized to generate copies of the DNA templates present in the input sample (Figure 3) (Zhang *et al.*, 1992).

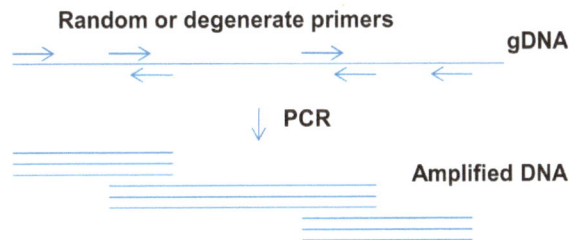

**Figure 3:** Short *random* primers are used to produce PCR fragments covering the whole genome in primer-extension preamplification (PEP) while *degenerate* primers are utilized to generate PCR fragments in degenerate oligonucleotide-primed PCR (DOP-PCR).

Similar to ordinary PCR, denaturation by high temperature is followed by annealing and extension. However, there are some major differences between PEP and ordinary PCR. First, relatively low annealing temperature of 37°C and extension temperature of 55°C are used. Second, the ramping rate between annealing and extension steps is relatively slow (10 seconds per degree). By doing so, the primers will non-specifically attach to DNA templates and amplify the genome. It was later refined as improved PEP (I-PEP) by using a high fidelity PCR system with proofreading activity and modified thermocycling procedures. This modified I-PEP method was shown to be superior to the original PEP and DOP-PCR. It allowed multiple reliable microsatellite analyses for detecting microsatellite instability, loss of heterozygosity and mutation even at the single cell level (Dietmaier *et al.*, 1999). Recently, I-PEP was successfully applied to amplifying bovine genome with minimal input DNA from single cells (Moghaddaszadeh-Ahrabi *et al.*, 2012).

### 2.4    Degenerate Oligonucleotide Primed PCR (DOP-PCR)

This is another method making use of PCR for WGA. Partially *degenerate* oligonucleotide primers bind to multiple sites throughout the genome (Figure 3). Together with an annealing step at low temperature, this degeneracy allows efficient priming for subsequent cycling of amplification (Telenius *et al.*, 1992). This technology can produce a substantial amount of wgaDNA even from a single cell (Wells *et al.*, 2002). However, the non-random amplification by DOP-PCR may produce misleading results in applications sensitive to genomic balance such as CGH. Similar to PEP, DOP-PCR generates relatively short wgaDNA products. In an improved protocol, DNA polymerase possessing 3'-5' exonuclease proofreading activity and increased annealing and extension times were incorporated (Kittler *et al.*, 2002). In addition to the use of proofreading polymerase, further modifications of using more degenerate primers and cycles of low annealing temperature were included. These improvements were reported to give longer amplification products and increased genome coverage. However, there was variation in the performance of different proofreading polymerases. This highlights the importance of appropriate choice of polymerase in carrying out the amplification by DOP-PCR (Bonnette *et al.*, 2009).

## 3    Potential problems of WGA

Associated with WGA are several major issues that can potentially cause misleading outcomes in analysis or diagnosis. The first issue is amplification bias, a situation in which sequences at different parts of the genome are not represented to the same extent in the WGA product. The second issue is preferential amplification, in which reduced amplification of one of the heterozygous alleles results in imbalance in allelic products. The extreme of preferential amplification is allelic dropout – random occurrence of failed amplification of an allele such that one allele will not be detected in a heterozygous sample. Obviously, the accuracy of the amplification process is critical to any downstream application of the WGA product. Besides, WGA reactions involve using random or degenerate primers to initiate amplification. This will easily result in amplification of contaminating DNA, in addition to the target DNA. The problem could lead to misleading results in downstream applications of the wgaDNA. Techniques for decontamination (Woyke *et al.*, 2011) and WGA on single cells (Rodrigue *et al.*, 2009) have been developed to minimize such problem. Last but not least, the efficiency of the WGA method must be high enough to generate sufficient amounts of wgaDNA from a tiny amount of input sample. If any of the above criteria cannot be fulfilled, the resulting WGA product is very likely to introduce undesirable uncertainty and error to the downstream applications. Such error can be catastrophic if the result is to be used for diagnostic purposes. These issues should therefore be considered seriously in order to ensure robustness and reproducibility of the assay outcome.

## 4    Comparison of WGA methods

Compared with the PCR-based WGA methods (DOP-PCR and PEP), MDA has been found to generate products that are less biased and of longer length and higher yield (Dean et al., 2002). WGA products from MDA also have high uniformity in genome coverage. In this regard, MDA can produce wgaDNA of superior quality than the counterparts from PCR-based methods.

OmniPlex technology represents a relatively new method for WGA. Based on a proprietary technology, it can potentially provide quality amplification of the genome. Detailed comparisons have been published for the genotyping performance of WGA products generated by MDA and OmniPlex (Barker *et al.*, 2004; Bergen *et al.*, 2005a; Park *et al.*, 2005; Pask *et al.*, 2004). Samples amplified by MDA show less variability and higher reliability than those amplified by OmniPlex (Park *et al.*, 2005). OmniPlex wgaDNA demonstrated more severe deterioration in genotyping performance than that by MDA (Bergen *et al.*, 2005a). Indeed, MDA method has been regarded as a major breakthrough in the application of WGA methods (Lovmar & Syvanen, 2006). Many studies have considered MDA to be the most reliable WGA method and the method of choice if WGA is going to be undertaken (Berthier-Schaad *et al.*, 2007; Gunderson *et al.*, 2005; Ho *et al.*, 2011; Paez *et al.*, 2004; Park *et al.*, 2005; Pinard *et al.*, 2006; Rodrigue *et al.*, 2009; Winkel *et al.*, 2011; Yilmaz & Singh, 2011). Table 1 summarizes and compares the characteristics of these methods.

| Method | MDA | OmniPlex | PEP | DOP-PCR |
|---|---|---|---|---|
| Product size | Relatively longer | Relatively shorter | Relatively shorter | Relatively shorter |
| PCR-based | No | Yes | Yes | Yes |
| Scalability of reaction | High | Limited | Limited | Limited |
| DNA yield | Relatively higher | Relatively lower | Relatively lower | Relatively lower |
| Amplification bias | Relatively lower | Relatively lower | Relatively higher | Relatively higher |

**Table 1**: Overview of WGA technologies

# 5  Applications of WGA products

## 5.1  Ordinary Applications

It has been shown that no excessive amplification bias could be found in WGA products for common methods of genetic analysis such as SNP genotyping, Southern blotting, RFLP analysis, DNA sequencing and quantitative PCR (Dean *et al.*, 2002). In another study of SNP genotyping, genotyping performance in terms of concordance between paired wgaDNA and gDNA samples was found to be satisfactory and comparable to the results of previous studies using a variety of genotyping methods (Berthier-Schaad *et al.*, 2007). Similar studies have also suggested that wgaDNA is suitable for TaqMan genotyping assay (Philips *et al.*, 2012) and high resolution melting curve analysis (van Eijk *et al.*, 2010; Winkel *et al.*, 2011).

## 5.2  Copy Number Analysis by Comparative Genomic Hybridization (CGH)

CGH and the more automated version with better resolution, array-CGH (aCGH), have been developed and applied to the study of copy number aberrations, e.g. deletions, duplications, amplifications or even aneuploidy in genomic DNA. However, the amount of sample available is sometimes a limiting factor for utilizing these strategies for genomic analysis. WGA is a possible solution, but unbiased amplification of different regions of the genome is essential for accurate detection of copy number changes.

Although one study (Dean *et al.*, 2002) has reported nearly complete genome coverage with high accuracy and low amplification bias, other studies have identified significant amplification bias between different genomic sequences (Bergen *et al.*, 2005b; Talseth-Palmer *et al.*, 2008). Nevertheless, as suggested, this limitation could be alleviated by using DNA samples generated by WGA for both case and control samples (Lage *et al.*, 2003).

In another study, wgaDNA from formalin-fixed paraffin-embedded (FFPE) samples was demonstrated to be technically suitable for aCGH, and dosage alterations of genes at a magnitude of at least 3 folds could be observed with high reproducibility for as few as 1000 cells as the starting material (Hirsch *et al.*, 2012). Previous studies have similarly suggested the ability to generate consistent chromosomal copy number profile from 1000 cells (Arriola *et al.*, 2007; Cardoso *et al.*, 2004; Hughes *et al.*, 2004) or even a single cell (Hellani *et al.*, 2004; Iwamoto *et al.*, 2007; Le Caignec *et al.*, 2006; Ling *et al.*, 2009). In conclusion, wgaDNA may be applicable to copy number analysis using CGH or aCGH, but caution must be taken about the potential amplification bias in producing inaccurate and non-reproducible indication of chromosomal abnormalities.

## 5.3    Genotyping of Short Tandem Repeats (STRs)

STRs are repetitive sequences of several (usually 2-5) base pairs throughout the genome. The slippage of STRs is a common phenomenon for PCR-based WGA methods (Zheng *et al.*, 2011). WGA was reported to increase or decrease STRs by a length of one repeat presumably by slippage (Wells et al., 1999). It was believed to be due to the low annealing temperatures of PCR-based WGA methods. This problem could be resolved by providing sufficient amount of DNA (Cheung & Nelson, 1996) or simply by using non-PCR-based MDA method for WGA.

In a study comparing genotyping performance of wgaDNA generated by MDA or OmniPlex methods in STR genotyping using AmpF*l*STR Identifier assay, wgaDNA demonstrated significantly lower genotype completion and concordance rates than gDNA (Bergen *et al.*, 2005a). As for different WGA methods, MDA protocol resulted in significantly higher genotype completion and concordance rates than OmniPlex technology. In terms of stutter peaks observed with amplitude of fluorescence signal strong enough to be called as alleles, OmniPlex product exhibited such phenomenon in several STR loci while stutter peaks for MDA wgaDNA had low peak amplitude resembling that of gDNA. For most of the discordant genotypes between gDNA and wgaDNA, homozygous genotypes were genotyped as heterozygotes or homozygotes of the other allele in wgaDNA. For most of the discordant genotypes appearing as heterozygous with gDNA, wgaDNA would be determined as homozygous for the shorter allele plus a second peak of correctly observed length but with amplitude below the peak height ratio required.

The same group also conducted another study assessing the effect of the amount of gDNA input on genotyping performance (Bergen *et al.*, 2005b). It was found that over 100 ng of gDNA was required to generate wgaDNA by MDA in order to obtain optimal STR genotyping performance by AmpF*l*STR Identifier assay equivalent to that of unamplified gDNA.

## 5.4    Medium-throughput Genotyping Assays

Many factors like the type of genetic polymorphisms tested can potentially affect the overall complexity of the assay. It is intuitive to think that the complexity of the assay increases with increasing level of multiplexing, which poses greater difficulty to the assay and reduces the genotyping performance (Ho *et al.*, 2011). It is therefore reasonable to postulate that genotyping performance deteriorates with increasing level of multiplexing for genotyping assays. In performing genetic association studies, medium-throughput genotyping assays are usually utilized for testing a moderate number of sequence variants for genes selected by a candidate-gene approach or for following up suggestive findings from initial studies. On the one hand, the number of markers to be tested for some candidate gene association studies exceeds the capacity of conventional non-multiplexing assays or it is not cost-effective to do so. On the other hand, the relatively high cost of the higher-end technology of genomewide array-based assays makes it intractable to be used. As a result, medium-throughput genotyping technologies have been developed to fill in the gap. The MassARRAY Sequenom assay (Ho *et al.*, 2011; Hollegaard *et al.,* 2009c) and the Illumina GoldenGate assay (Hansen *et al.*, 2007; Paynter *et al.*, 2006) have been tested on a custom panel of SNP markers and found to give satisfactory genotyping performance with wgaDNA samples.

## 5.5  High-throughput Genomewide Array-based Genotyping Assays

Affymetrix and Illumina are the two major platforms providing genomewide array-based assays. With the advancement of technologies, the number of SNP markers incorporated in a genotyping array has been increased dramatically. A number of studies have been undertaken to verify the validity of applying wgaDNA to high-throughput genotyping arrays with such a great number of markers.

In a study testing wgaDNA with Affymetrix 10K Mapping Array (Paez *et al.*, 2004), the genome representation was estimated to be 99.82% complete with high concordance between genotypes of wgaDNA and gDNA. Intriguingly, six regions of a maximum total size of 5.6 Mb consistently failed to be amplified. However, using the same genotyping array, such genotyping error was not detected in another study (Tzvetkov *et al.*, 2005). This reduced efficiency of WGA was suggested to be due to inter-reaction variations rather than special features of specific chromosomal loci. Moreover, no region of reduced amplification was detected, except for some SNPs located near telomeres. A similar study using Affymetrix 500K Mapping Array reported high genotype call rate for wgaDNA (Croft *et al.*, 2008). Therefore, amplification failure was more likely due to technical issues in processing the arrays.

For the Illumina platform, the high-density genotyping array Human610-Quad has been tested using wgaDNA from both MDA and OmniPlex methods (Hollegaard *et al.*, 2009a). The reported call rates were at least 99% and the discordance from genotypes of reference gDNA was minimal. This indicates that WGA provides a cost-effective alternative to collecting new samples. Indeed, in the sample manipulating procedures of Illumina (Gunderson *et al.*, 2005), WGA by MDA is used to generate a sufficient amount of DNA from source gDNA sample for subsequent hybridization. In a recent study using ovine gDNA and wgaDNA for Illumina arrays (Magee *et al.*, 2010), high genotype call rate was demonstrated and the concordance rate was also exceptionally high between the genotypes generated from wgaDNA and gDNA counterparts.

## 5.6  Next Generation Sequencing (NGS)

NGS technology represents a fast-growing and powerful tool in exploring multiple aspects of genomic data. It provides both qualitative and quantitative data of the genome, which can be applied to a great variety of studies such as genetic mapping, copy number analysis and expression profiling. The amount of input DNA is a potential limiting factor for performing assays including NGS.

A recent study evaluated products of different WGA methods for whole genome sequencing of 2 bacterial species by conducting sequence-based karyotyping for the amplified and control genomes, and examined high-resolution comparison of coverage bias (Pinard *et al.*, 2006). The genome coverage varied by bacterial genome and WGA technology. Unamplified samples achieved a coverage of 85% for *Halobacterium* species NRC-1 and 99% for *Campylobacter jejuni*. The coverage dropped substantially with amplified samples. The coverage for *Halobacterium* ranged from 50.1% (MDA) to 9.7% (DOP-PCR) while that for *Campylobacter jejuni* was more satisfactory for most of the amplified samples. Most amplified samples (MDA and PEP) covered over 90% of the genome, with the exception for DOP-PCR-amplified samples giving only 17%. It was believed that the relatively poor coverage for *Halobacterium* species might be due to the presence of 2 minichromosomes in addition to the main chromosome and the high frequency of repeat regions within them (13.4% repeat for *Halobacterium* species versus 2.7% repeat for *Campylobacter jejuni*). The repeat regions were disproportionally heavily sequenced relative to their frequency. Such bias in representation of regions could also be illustrated in read depth. As measured by reads per 100-base bin, the number of reads was disproportionately higher for minichromosomes relative to main chromosome for *Halobacterium* species. Read depth bias was similarly found in repeat regions. As shown by the distribution of reads per bin comparing unamplified and amplified samples, all WGA technologies induced significant bias. Nevertheless, MDA method generated the least bias and produced significantly higher yield of WGA product. Interestingly, there was a substantial difference in coverage for the two bacterial genomes even for unamplified samples.

With further advancement in NGS technologies, WGA is coupled with NGS for the analysis of even a single cell. Making use of WGA for single-cell genome sequencing, a recent study described a pipeline that combined single-cell isolation by cell sorting, amplification power of MDA and post-amplification normalization procedure (Rodrigue *et al.*, 2009). It was demonstrated to have improved sequencing efficiency and facilitated the assembly of genome sequences. As high as 99.6% genome recovery was observed with reference-guided assembly while 95% was seen with *de novo* assembly. Read depth was found to vary over the whole genome in all replicates, but no clear pattern could be concluded. However, this might somehow represent uneven amplification. Future development in single-cell genomics should therefore address this issue such that sequencing efficiency can be facilitated through lowering amplification bias. Overall speaking, evidence highlights the great potential of single-cell WGA for extensive use in genome sequencing by NGS technology. Since then, application of WGA to single-cell genome sequencing has been advocated (Yilmaz & Singh, 2011) and implemented (Navin *et al.*, 2011). Protocols are now available for copy number analysis of single cell using WGA and NGS (Baslan *et al.*, 2012).

## 5.7    Other Applications

Radiation hybrid (RH) mapping has been widely used in recent decades for constructing physical maps of genomes. RH maps of high resolution have been demonstrated to be useful in manipulating genome sequence assemblies and construction of such maps remains an active area of research in the near future (Karere *et al.*, 2010). There are several taxing issues in the process of constructing RH maps: the cell culture required for generating enough DNA for marker mapping, the inherent instability of RH clones, and the limited amount of DNA available from the same passage of cells. With the emergence of WGA technologies, the major constraint on DNA sample may potentially be resolved. Indeed, WGA has been used to amplify DNA from hybrid cell lines in RH map construction (Guyon *et al.*, 2010; Karere *et al.*, 2010; Senger *et al.*, 2006). These studies confirm the validity of applying WGA to RH mapping. With the use of WGA, analysis of early RH clone passages is made possible. This can limit the heterogeneity and hence the undesirable artefacts of RH maps.

## 5.8    A Summary of Applications of WGA

The tremendous amplification power of WGA enables the enormous scalability of the DNA sample stock. Constraint on DNA sample is no long a major limiting factor for some of the originally intractable tasks. However, users must be alert to potential problems when using wgaDNA samples because artefacts of WGA may lead to misleading results in some occasions.

# 6    Sample Sources of DNA for WGA

## 6.1    Ordinary tissues

WGA methods were originally applied to and evaluated using ordinary input DNA samples of guaranteed quality, including gDNA prepared from blood or cell lines, and sperm DNA (Table 2) (Dean *et al.*, 2002; Kamberov *et al.*, 2002; Telenius *et al.*, 1992; Zhang *et al.*, 1992). It is therefore believed that such input DNA samples possess certain level of quality with little degradation. These studies provide adequate experimental data for addressing the general concern of using commonly available DNA samples for WGA. Since then, WGA has been applied to a wide variety of other samples (Hirsch *et al.*, 2012; Moore *et al.*, 2007).

| Sources | Ordinary tissues | Special tissues |
|---|---|---|
| **Quantity and/or quality in the first collection/use** | Adequate | Inadequate |
| **Purpose to do WGA** | Provide DNA for extended use | Provide adequate DNA even for the first use |
| **Examples** | Blood cells, cell lines, any tissues of adequate amount, etc | Buccal swabs, dried blood spots, FFPE tissues, cells from early embryos, etc |

**Table 2**: Sample sources of DNA for WGA

## 6.2    Special tissues

WGA is particularly useful for special samples and tissues with limited DNA amounts (Table 2). In a study testing several sample sources of DNA, MDA was found to be efficient and reliable for DNA from whole blood and buccal swab, but not for DNA from dried blood spot or degraded and fragmented DNA (Park *et al.*, 2005). In another study assessing the genotyping performance of wgaDNA derived from gDNA obtained from mouthwash, buffy coat and lymphoblasts, differential performance was observed (Bergen *et al.*, 2005a). Higher yield was obtained from buffy coat samples based on WGA by OmniPlex method. Besides, buffy coat wgaDNA demonstrated higher completion rates of STR genotyping for all WGA methods. In terms of undetermined and discordant genotypes, mouthwash wgaDNA had poorer performance when compared with other counterparts. In contrast, another study demonstrated high call rate, replicate concordance and concordance with reference genotype for wgaDNA derived from gDNA obtained from whole blood, buccal samples, dried blood spot or even urine (urothelial cells) (Paynter *et al.*, 2006). This study also showed that both wgaDNA and gDNA could be used for highly multiplexed Illumina assays with minimal misclassification.

Neonatal dried blood spot (NDBS) is a popular sample source for isolating gDNA for WGA. In several recent studies (Hollegaard *et al.*, 2009a; Hollegaard *et al.*, 2009b; Hollegaard *et al.*, 2009c; Winkel *et al.*, 2011), NDBS was tested with MassARRAY Sequenom assay, Illumina BeadChip, high resolution melting (HRM) curve and sequencing analysis. All these studies provide evidence supporting that wgaDNA derived from NDBS samples is reliable for the above technologies and the period of storage for NDBS is not crucial. The use of NDBS can open up a rich resource for DNA sample as an alternative to ordinary whole blood. It also highlights the usefulness of many existing biobanks for contributing valuable archived samples for future studies.

FFPE sample is another frequently studied tissue for WGA application. In most cases, FFPE samples are obtained from biopsies so that the amount is usually limited. In addition, formalin fixation usually leads to fragmentation of the isolated gDNA. Therefore, this restricts the usage of FFPE samples. WGA methods provide a solution to this limitation of using FFPE samples. Studies have shown that wgaDNA from FFPE cancer samples were applicable to HRM analysis for somatic mutation detection and aCGH (Dietmaier *et al.*, 1999; Hirsch *et al.*, 2012; van Eijk *et al.*, 2010).

Preimplantation genetic screening (PGS) or diagnosis (PGD) is a procedure that is performed on embryos before implantation. It allows identification of genetic defects and is sometimes used in couple with *in vitro* fertilization. With very limited amount of DNA from a polar body of a fertilized oocyte or a blastomere of embryo biopsy, comprehensive genetic testing is not feasible. WGA provides a solution for studying biopsied embryo. From a single or a few blastomeres isolated from cleavage-stage embryos, microgram quantities of wgaDNA could be obtained for downstream diagnostic testing (Figure 4), though with some preferential amplification or allele dropout at heterozygous loci (Handyside *et al.*, 2004). Since then, WGA has been widely used for PGD with various applications (Zheng *et al.*, 2011).

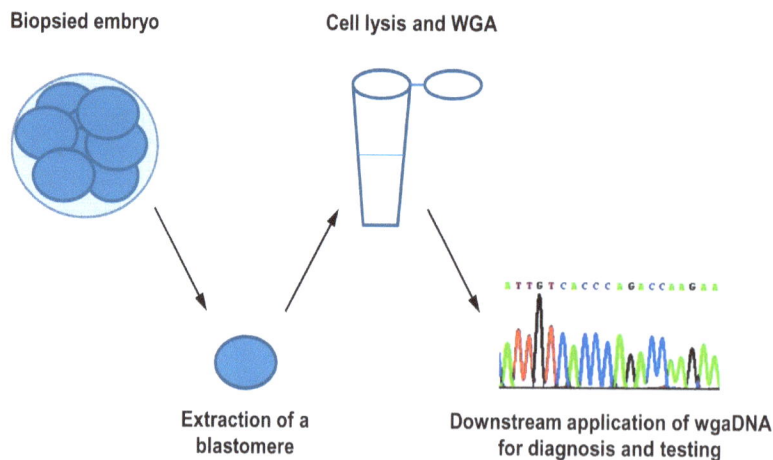

**Figure 4:** Application of WGA in preimplantation genetic diagnosis.

WGA product has been shown to be applicable in many cases. However, as evaluated by a study on the effect of electron-beam irradiation used to sterilize mail, wgaDNA derived from irradiated gDNA exhibited a marked reduction in the yield of WGA product, and genotyping completion and concordance rates. Increasing the amount of input irradiated gDNA improved the genotyping performance of wgaDNA, but the adverse effect of irradiation could not be completely eliminated (Bergen *et al.*, 2005c).

# 7    Quantification of WGA product

UV absorbance at 260nm, PicoGreen fluorescence and real-time PCR can be used to quantify the amount of DNA in a sample (Haque *et al.*, 2003). The PicoGreen method is used in many studies for determining the amount of wgaDNA (Bergen *et al.*, 2005c; Hollegaard *et al.*, 2009a; Paynter *et al.*, 2006; Talseth-

Palmer *et al.*, 2008; Winkel *et al.*, 2011). PicoGreen is a fluorochrome that selectively binds to double-stranded DNA (dsDNA). When it is bound to dsDNA, the fluorescence enhancement is exceptionally high with minimal background signal because unbound PicoGreen has essentially no fluorescence (Ahn *et al.*, 1996).

Some challenges are noteworthy when quantifying wgaDNA. First, there are residual WGA reagents that may influence the quantification by UV absorbance. Second, WGA methods have been reported to yield amplification artefacts even for no-template controls (Bergen *et al.*, 2005a; Bergen *et al.*, 2005b). The non-specific side products are indistinguishable from the authentic genomic amplification products by physical means. In these cases, exact quantification by real-time PCR is preferred.

In a study comparing existing methods for wgaDNA quantification (Hansen *et al.*, 2007), physical quantification methods (UV absorbance and PicoGreen fluorescence) indicated high level of WGA product even though no gDNA was added to the WGA reaction. This phenomenon was not detected using quantitative PCR. Moreover, when wgaDNA quantification methods were compared for genotyping quality in terms of genotype concordance between wgaDNA and corresponding unamplified gDNA samples (high-quality, moderate-quality and poor-quality groups), locus-specific quantitative PCR was found to be the only method reflective of this correlation (the higher the indicated amount of wgaDNA, the better the genotyping quality). When quantified by quantitative PCR, wgaDNA samples showed three distinctive concentration ranges for the three different quality groups. Other quantification methods under study demonstrated overlapping sample concentrations for the three quality groups, indicating the inability to distinguish between WGA products and amplification artefacts. Overall, quantitative PCR is the most reliable method for estimatiing the efficiency of WGA, and can determine the suitability of wgaDNA before being used for the actual genotyping process.

## 8    Effect of multiplexing level on genotyping performance of wgaDNA

Although several studies have tested the suitability of wgaDNA for high-throughput genotyping such as array-based genotyping assays (Berthier-Schaad *et al.*, 2007; Hollegaard *et al.*, 2009c), little has been done in clarifying the issue about whether wgaDNA would affect genotyping performance with respect to the multiplexing level of an assay. Indeed, different assays have different underlying reaction chemistries. Successful application of wgaDNA in high-throughput assays does not necessarily provide evidence to support that genotyping performance would not be adversely affected by an increasing level of multiplexing upon the use of wgaDNA. It is also intuitive to think that the complexity of the assay increases with increasing level of multiplexing, and this poses greater difficulty to the assay and adversely affects the genotyping performance.

In a recent study addressing this issue (Ho *et al.*, 2011), variable multiplexing ability of MassARRAY platform with iPLEX GOLD chemistry was employed to study the correlation between multiplexing level of assay and genotyping efficiency (in terms of genotype completion rate). Significant but weak correlation was detected between multiplexing level and genotyping efficiency in both gDNA and wgaDNA samples. This result suggested that genotyping efficiency decreased monotonically with increasing multiplexing level (i.e., complexity of assay). More importantly, with gDNA as the reference, the result also suggested that the correlation was not disrupted or exaggerated by the use of wgaDNA. This finding could be interpreted as follows: the use of wgaDNA did not impose additional adverse burden on genotyping efficiency although increasing multiplexing level was suggested to result in mild deterioration in genotyping efficiency. On the other hand, for genotyping accuracy, the genotype concordance rates were not found to be statistically different among different multiplexing levels and no significant correlation between genotype concordance rate and multiplexing level could be detected. As a whole, the genotyping performance of wgaDNA was found to be similar to that of gDNA with respect to different multiplexing levels.

## 9    Effect of Storage on Genotyping Performance of wgaDNA

As demonstrated by studies of amplifying DNA extracted from archived sample or FFPE sample, the freshness of the input gDNA is not a decisive factor for WGA. Nevertheless, the effect of the storage period of wgaDNA on genotyping performance has not been extensively studied.

In a recent study comparing genotyping performance of gDNA, freshly prepared wgaDNA and stored wgaDNA (frozen at -70°C for 18 months) (Ho *et al.*, 2011), significant difference in genotyping efficiency (genotype completion rate) for 174 SNPs could be detected among the three groups of samples. With further pairwise comparisons, the most remarkable difference in genotyping efficiency was found to be between gDNA (96.8%) and stored wgaDNA (93.0%). Difference could also be found between freshly prepared wgaDNA (96.2%) and stored wgaDNA (93.0%), but the magnitude was less obvious. On the other hand, no significant difference was identified between gDNA and freshly prepared wgaDNA. These findings suggested the inferior quality of stored wgaDNA.

Another aspect of genotyping performance is the genotyping accuracy in terms of concordance between sample groups. By pairwise comparison of genotypes obtained from the three sample groups, significant difference could be identified. This suggested the use of stored wgaDNA was likely to reduce genotyping accuracy. With unamplified gDNA as the reference, the genotype concordance rate reflects the variability or uncertainty in the genotyping accuracy. The lower the genotype concordance rate with gDNA is, the more uncertain it is for the genotyping result. As some degree of genotype discrepancies could be found between gDNA and freshly prepared wgaDNA, it implied that even the freshly prepared wgaDNA could introduce some degree of uncertainty to the genotypes as a result of WGA. With even worse genotype concordance between gDNA and stored wgaDNA, this indicated that the 18-month storage further deteriorated the performance by introducing further uncertainty.

Therefore, the overall findings demonstrated that genotyping performance of freshly prepared wgaDNA was similar to that of unamplified gDNA, but this was not true for stored wgaDNA. The storage period is thus a determining factor for genotyping performance of wgaDNA. Evidence substantiated the importance of using freshly prepared wgaDNA of warranted quality as a replacement for gDNA counterpart in obtaining satisfactory genotyping performance. In order to retain the freshness of wgaDNA samples, cautions must be taken to avoid repeated freezing-thawing cycles and better planning of experiments for minimizing the storage period of wgaDNA. It is desirable to carry out proper purification of WGA products because the ingredients of WGA reagents can trigger degradation of wgaDNA.

## 10    Other issues

Single cell genomics is a powerful and increasingly popular tool. However, commercially available WGA reagents are frequently contaminated with unwanted DNA, which will be amplified along with input DNA. This could lead to confounding result in analysis (Woyke *et al.*, 2011). Verified by shotgun sequencing of *E. coli* single amplified genomes, a recent study (Woyke *et al.*, 2011) showed that 60 min UV treatment or an accumulative dose of 11.4 J/cm$^2$ of the MDA reagents (including phi29 DNA polymerase and random hexamer primers) effectively eliminated DNA contaminants without observable negative effect on subsequent WGA. This method suggested a simple but effective solution to confounding factor for WGA on single cells.

# 11    Conclusions

Several methods of WGA have been developed to provide wgaDNA as a replacement for gDNA in genetic studies. These methods vary in their fundamental principles and practical efficiency. Up to now, wgaDNA samples have been tested and used in numerous applications. WGA can be applied to a wide range of sample sources with minimal requirement for the quality and quantity of the starting material. In summary, the emergence of WGA has profound impact on modern genetic studies. These technologies are beneficial to not only scientists in the research community, but also the whole society as a result of the facilitated studies of disease gene mapping and improved understanding of many diseases.

# References

Ahn, S. J., Costa, J., & Emanuel, J. R. (1996). PicoGreen quantitation of DNA: effective evaluation of samples pre- or post-PCR. Nucleic Acids Res, 24(13), 2623-2625.

Arriola, E., Lambros, M. B., Jones, C., Dexter, T., Mackay, A., Tan, D. S., Tamber, N., Fenwick, K., Ashworth, A., Dowsett, M., & Reis-Filho, J. S. (2007). Evaluation of Phi29-based whole-genome amplification for microarray-based comparative genomic hybridisation. Lab Invest, 87(1), 75-83.

Barker, D. L., Hansen, M. S., Faruqi, A. F., Giannola, D., Irsula, O. R., Lasken, R. S., Latterich, M., Makarov, V., Oliphant, A., Pinter, J. H., Shen, R., Sleptsova, I., Ziehler, W., & Lai, E. (2004). Two methods of whole-genome amplification enable accurate genotyping across a 2320-SNP linkage panel. Genome Res, 14(5), 901-907.

Baslan, T., Kendall, J., Rodgers, L., Cox, H., Riggs, M., Stepansky, A., Troge, J., Ravi, K., Esposito, D., Lakshmi, B., Wigler, M., Navin, N., & Hicks, J. (2012). Genome-wide copy number analysis of single cells. Nat Protoc, 7(6), 1024-1041.

Bergen, A. W., Haque, K. A., Qi, Y., Beerman, M. B., Garcia-Closas, M., Rothman, N., & Chanock, S. J. (2005a). Comparison of yield and genotyping performance of multiple displacement amplification and OmniPlex whole genome amplified DNA generated from multiple DNA sources. Hum Mutat, 26(3), 262-270.

Bergen, A. W., Qi, Y., Haque, K. A., Welch, R. A., & Chanock, S. J. (2005b). Effects of DNA mass on multiple displacement whole genome amplification and genotyping performance. BMC Biotechnol, 5, 24.

Bergen, A. W., Qi, Y., Haque, K. A., Welch, R. A., Garcia-Closas, M., Chanock, *et al.* (2005c). Effects of electron-beam irradiation on whole genome amplification. Cancer Epidemiol Biomarkers Prev, 14(4), 1016-1019.

Berthier-Schaad, Y., Kao, W. H., Coresh, J., Zhang, L., Ingersoll, R. G., Stephens, R., & Smith, M. W. (2007). Reliability of high-throughput genotyping of whole genome amplified DNA in SNP genotyping studies. Electrophoresis, 28(16), 2812-2817.

Bonnette, M. D., Pavlova, V. R., Rodier, D. N., Thompson, L. P., Boone, E. L., Brown, K. L., Meyer, K. M., Trevino, M. B., Champagne, J. R., & Cruz, T. D. (2009). dcDegenerate oligonucleotide primed-PCR for multilocus, genome-wide analysis from limited quantities of DNA. Diagn Mol Pathol, 18(3), 165-175.

Buntaine, B., Vassar, D., Brown, C., Mueller, E., & Kayser, K. GenomePlex Whole Genome Amplification: Sigma-Aldrich Biotechnology.

Cardoso, J., Molenaar, L., de Menezes, R. X., Rosenberg, C., Morreau, H., Moslein, G., Fodde, R., & Boer, J. M. (2004). Genomic profiling by DNA amplification of laser capture microdissected tissues and array CGH. Nucleic Acids Res, 32(19), e146.

Cheung, V. G., & Nelson, S. F. (1996). Whole genome amplification using a degenerate oligonucleotide primer allows hundreds of genotypes to be performed on less than one nanogram of genomic DNA. Proc Natl Acad Sci U S A, 93(25), 14676-14679.

Croft, D. T., Jr., Jordan, R. M., Patney, H. L., Shriver, C. D., Vernalis, M. N., Orchard, T. J., & Ellsworth, D. L. (2008). Performance of whole-genome amplified DNA isolated from serum and plasma on high-density single nucleotide polymorphism arrays. J Mol Diagn, 10(3), 249-257.

Dean, F. B., Hosono, S., Fang, L., Wu, X., Faruqi, A. F., Bray-Ward, P., Sun, Z., Zong, Q., Du, Y., Du, J., Driscoll, M., Song, W., Kingsmore, S. F., Egholm, M., & Lasken, R. S. (2002). Comprehensive human genome amplification using multiple displacement amplification. Proc Natl Acad Sci U S A, 99(8), 5261-5266.

Dietmaier, W., Hartmann, A., Wallinger, S., Heinmoller, E., Kerner, T., Endl, E., Jauch, K. W., Hofstadter, F., & Ruschoff, J. (1999). Multiple mutation analyses in single tumor cells with improved whole genome amplification. Am J Pathol, 154(1), 83-95.

Gunderson, K. L., Steemers, F. J., Lee, G., Mendoza, L. G., & Chee, M. S. (2005). A genome-wide scalable SNP genotyping assay using microarray technology. Nat Genet, 37(5), 549-554.

Guyon, R., Senger, F., Rakotomanga, M., Sadequi, N., Volckaert, F. A., Hitte, C., & Galibert, F. (2010). A radiation hybrid map of the European sea bass (Dicentrarchus labrax) based on 1581 markers: Synteny analysis with model fish genomes. Genomics, 96(4), 228-238.

Handyside, A. H., Robinson, M. D., Simpson, R. J., Omar, M. B., Shaw, M., Grudzinskas, J. G., & Rutherford, A. Isothermal whole genome amplification from single and small numbers of cells: a new era for preimplantation genetic diagnosis of inherited disease. Mol Hum Reprod, 10(10), 767-772.

Hansen, H. M., Wiemels, J. L., Wrensch, M., & Wiencke, J. K. (2007). DNA quantification of whole genome amplified samples for genotyping on a multiplexed bead array platform. Cancer Epidemiol Biomarkers Prev, 16(8), 1686-1690.

Haque, K. A., Pfeiffer, R. M., Beerman, M. B., Struewing, J. P., Chanock, S. J., & Bergen, A. W. (2003). Performance of high-throughput DNA quantification methods. BMC Biotechnol, 3, 20.

Hellani, A., Coskun, S., Benkhalifa, M., Tbakhi, A., Sakati, N., Al-Odaib, A., & Ozand, P. (2004). Multiple displacement amplification on single cell and possible PGD applications. Mol Hum Reprod, 10(11), 847-852.

Hirsch, D., Camps, J., Varma, S., Kemmerling, R., Stapleton, M., Ried, T., & Gaiser, T. (2012). A new whole genome amplification method for studying clonal evolution patterns in malignant colorectal polyps. Genes Chromosomes Cancer, 51(5), 490-500.

Ho, D. W., Yiu, W. C., Yap, M. K., Fung, W. Y., Ng, P. W., & Yip, S. P. (2011). Genotyping performance assessment of whole genome amplified DNA with respect to multiplexing level of assay and its period of storage. PLoS One, 6(10), e26119.

Hollegaard, M. V., Grauholm, J., Borglum, A., Nyegaard, M., Norgaard-Pedersen, B., Orntoft, T., Mortensen, P. B., Wiuf, C., Mors, O., Didriksen, M., Thorsen, P., & Hougaard, D. M. (2009a). Genome-wide scans using archived neonatal dried blood spot samples. BMC Genomics, 10, 297.

Hollegaard, M. V., Grove, J., Thorsen, P., Norgaard-Pedersen, B., & Hougaard, D. M. (2009b). High-throughput genotyping on archived dried blood spot samples. Genet Test Mol Biomarkers, 13(2), 173-179.

Hollegaard, M. V., Thorsen, P., Norgaard-Pedersen, B., & Hougaard, D. M. (2009c). Genotyping whole-genome-amplified DNA from 3- to 25-year-old neonatal dried blood spot samples with reference to fresh genomic DNA. Electrophoresis, 30(14), 2532-2535.

Hughes, S., Lim, G., Beheshti, B., Bayani, J., Marrano, P., Huang, A., & Squire, J. A. (2004). Use of whole genome amplification and comparative genomic hybridisation to detect chromosomal copy number alterations in cell line material and tumour tissue. Cytogenet Genome Res, 105(1), 18-24.

Iwamoto, K., Bundo, M., Ueda, J., Nakano, Y., Ukai, W., Hashimoto, E., Saito, T., & Kato, T. (2007). Detection of chromosomal structural alterations in single cells by SNP arrays: a systematic survey of amplification bias and optimized workflow. PLoS One, 2(12), e1306.

Kamberov, E., Sleptsova, I., Suchyta, S., Bruening, E., Zeihler, W., Nagel, J. S., Langmore, J., & Makarov, V. (2002). Use of in vitro OmniPlex Libraries for high-throughput comparative genomics and molecular haplotyping. Proceedings of SPIE, 4626, 340-351.

Karere, G. M., Lyons, L. A., & Froenicke, L. (2010). Enhancing radiation hybrid mapping through whole genome amplification. Hereditas, 147(2), 103-112.

Kittler, R., Stoneking, M., & Kayser, M. (2002). A whole genome amplification method to generate long fragments from low quantities of genomic DNA. Anal Biochem, 300(2), 237-244.

Lage, J. M., Leamon, J. H., Pejovic, T., Hamann, S., Lacey, M., Dillon, D., Segraves, R., Vossbrinck, B., Gonzalez, A., Pinkel, D., Albertson, D. G., Costa, J., & Lizardi, P. M. (2003). Whole genome analysis of genetic alterations in small DNA samples using hyperbranched strand displacement amplification and array-CGH. Genome Res, 13(2), 294-307.

Langmore, J. P. (2002). Rubicon Genomics, Inc. Pharmacogenomics, 3(4), 557-560.

Le Caignec, C., Spits, C., Sermon, K., De Rycke, M., Thienpont, B., Debrock, S., Staessen, C., Moreau, Y., Fryns, J. P., Van Steirteghem, A., Liebaers, I., & Vermeesch, J. R. (2006). Single-cell chromosomal imbalances detection by array CGH. Nucleic Acids Res, 34(9), e68.

Ling, J., Zhuang, G., Tazon-Vega, B., Zhang, C., Cao, B., Rosenwaks, Z., & Xu, K. (2009). Evaluation of genome coverage and fidelity of multiple displacement amplification from single cells by SNP array. Mol Hum Reprod, 15(11), 739-747.

Lizardi, P. M., Huang, X., Zhu, Z., Bray-Ward, P., Thomas, D. C., & Ward, D. C. (1998). Mutation detection and single-molecule counting using isothermal rolling-circle amplification. Nat Genet, 19(3), 225-232.

Lovmar, L., & Syvanen, A. C. (2006). Multiple displacement amplification to create a long-lasting source of DNA for genetic studies. Hum Mutat, 27(7), 603-614.

Magee, D. A., Park, S. D., Scraggs, E., Murphy, A. M., Doherty, M. L., Kijas, J. W., & MacHugh, D. E. (2010). Technical note: High fidelity of whole-genome amplified sheep (Ovis aries) deoxyribonucleic acid using a high-density single nucleotide polymorphism array-based genotyping platform. J Anim Sci, 88(10), 3183-3186.

Moghaddaszadeh-Ahrabi, S., Farajnia, S., Rahimi-Mianji, G., & Nejati-Javaremi, A. (2012). A short and simple improved-primer extension preamplification (I-PEP) procedure for whole genome amplification (WGA) of bovine cells. Anim Biotechnol, 23(1), 24-42.

Moore, L. E., Bergen, A. W., Haque, K. A., Qi, Y., Castle, P., Chanock, S. J., Egan, K., Newcomb, P., Titus-Ernstoff, L., Alguacil, J., Rothman, N., & Garcia-Closas, M. (2007). Whole genome amplification of buccal cytobrush DNA collected for molecular epidemiology studies. Biomarkers, 12(3), 303-312.

Navin, N., Kendall, J., Troge, J., Andrews, P., Rodgers, L., McIndoo, J., Cook, K., Stepansky, A., Levy, D., Esposito, D., Muthuswamy, L., Krasnitz, A., McCombie, W. R., Hicks, J., & Wigler, M. (2011). Tumour evolution inferred by single-cell sequencing. Nature, 472(7341), 90-94.

Paez, J. G., Lin, M., Beroukhim, R., Lee, J. C., Zhao, X., Richter, D. J., Gabriel, S., Herman, P., Sasaki, H., Altshuler, D., Li, C., Meyerson, M., & Sellers, W. R. (2004). Genome coverage and sequence fidelity of phi29 polymerase-based multiple strand displacement whole genome amplification. Nucleic Acids Res, 32(9), e71.

Park, J. W., Beaty, T. H., Boyce, P., Scott, A. F., & McIntosh, I. (2005). Comparing whole-genome amplification methods and sources of biological samples for single-nucleotide polymorphism genotyping. Clin Chem, 51(8), 1520-1523.

Pask, R., Rance, H. E., Barratt, B. J., Nutland, S., Smyth, D. J., Sebastian, M., Twells, R. C., Smith, A., Lam, A. C., Smink, L. J., Walker, N. M., & Todd, J. A. (2004). Investigating the utility of combining phi29 whole genome amplification and highly multiplexed single nucleotide polymorphism BeadArray genotyping. BMC Biotechnol, 4, 15.

Paynter, R. A., Skibola, D. R., Skibola, C. F., Buffler, P. A., Wiemels, J. L., & Smith, M. T. (2006). Accuracy of multiplexed Illumina platform-based single-nucleotide polymorphism genotyping compared between genomic and whole genome amplified DNA collected from multiple sources. Cancer Epidemiol Biomarkers Prev, 15(12), 2533-2536.

Philips, S., Rae, J. M., Oesterreich, S., Hayes, D. F., Stearns, V., Henry, N. L., Storniolo, A. M., Flockhart, D. A., & Skaar, T. C. (2012). Whole genome amplification of DNA for genotyping pharmacogenetics candidate genes. Front Pharmacol, 3, 54.

Pinard, R., de Winter, A., Sarkis, G. J., Gerstein, M. B., Tartaro, K. R., Plant, R. N., Egholm, M., Rothberg, J. M., & Leamon, J. H. (2006). Assessment of whole genome amplification-induced bias through high-throughput, massively parallel whole genome sequencing. BMC Genomics, 7, 216.

Rodrigue, S., Malmstrom, R. R., Berlin, A. M., Birren, B. W., Henn, M. R., & Chisholm, S. W. (2009). Whole genome amplification and de novo assembly of single bacterial cells. PLoS One, 4(9), e6864.

Senger, F., Priat, C., Hitte, C., Sarropoulou, E., Franch, R., Geisler, R., Bargelloni, L., Power, D., & Galibert, F. (2006). The first radiation hybrid map of a perch-like fish: the gilthead seabream (Sparus aurata L). Genomics, 87(6), 793-800.

Talseth-Palmer, B. A., Bowden, N. A., Hill, A., Meldrum, C., & Scott, R. J. (2008). Whole genome amplification and its impact on CGH array profiles. BMC Res Notes, 1, 56.

Telenius, H., Carter, N. P., Bebb, C. E., Nordenskjold, M., Ponder, B. A., & Tunnacliffe, A. (1992). Degenerate oligonucleotide-primed PCR: general amplification of target DNA by a single degenerate primer. Genomics, 13(3), 718-725.

Tzvetkov, M. V., Becker, C., Kulle, B., Nurnberg, P., Brockmoller, J., & Wojnowski, L. (2005). Genome-wide single-nucleotide polymorphism arrays demonstrate high fidelity of multiple displacement-based whole-genome amplification. Electrophoresis, 26(3), 710-715.

van Eijk, R., van Puijenbroek, M., Chhatta, A. R., Gupta, N., Vossen, R. H., Lips, E. H., Cleton-Jansen, A. M., Morreau, H., & van Wezel, T. (2010). Sensitive and specific KRAS somatic mutation analysis on whole-genome amplified DNA from archival tissues. J Mol Diagn, 12(1), 27-34.

Wells, D., Escudero, T., Levy, B., Hirschhorn, K., Delhanty, J. D., & Munne, S. (2002). First clinical application of comparative genomic hybridization and polar body testing for preimplantation genetic diagnosis of aneuploidy. Fertil Steril, 78(3), 543-549.

Wells, D., Sherlock, J. K., Handyside, A. H., & Delhanty, J. D. (1999). Detailed chromosomal and molecular genetic analysis of single cells by whole genome amplification and comparative genomic hybridisation. Nucleic Acids Res, 27(4), 1214-1218.

Winkel, B. G., Hollegaard, M. V., Olesen, M. S., Svendsen, J. H., Haunso, S., Hougaard, D. M., & Tfelt-Hansen, J. (2011). Whole-genome amplified DNA from stored dried blood spots is reliable in high resolution melting curve and sequencing analysis. BMC Med Genet, 12, 22.

Woyke, T., Sczyrba, A., Lee, J., Rinke, C., Tighe, D., Clingenpeel, S., Malmstrom, R., Stepanauskas, R., & Cheng, J. F. (2011). Decontamination of MDA reagents for single cell whole genome amplification. PLoS One, 6(10), e26161.

Yilmaz, S., & Singh, A. K. (2011). Single cell genome sequencing. Curr Opin Biotechnol, 23, 1-7.

Zhang, L., Cui, X., Schmitt, K., Hubert, R., Navidi, W., & Arnheim, N. (1992). Whole genome amplification from a single cell: implications for genetic analysis. Proc Natl Acad Sci U S A, 89(13), 5847-5851.

Zheng, Y. M., Wang, N., Li, L., & Jin, F. (2011). Whole genome amplification in preimplantation genetic diagnosis. J Zhejiang Univ Sci B, 12(1), 1-11.

# Whole Genome Microarray Gene Expression Profiling of Atherosclerosis Genes after Treatment with Captopril

Joshua Abd Alla
*Molecular Pharmacology*
*ETH Zürich, Switzerland*

Ursula Quitterer
*Molecular Pharmacology*
*ETH Zürich, Switzerland*

# 1   Introduction

Atherosclerotic vascular disease is the cause of severe cardiovascular diseases such as arterial hypertension, coronary artery disease, myocardial infarction, and cerebrovascular insult (Roger *et al.,* 2012). Since 1900, cardiovascular disease is the number one cause of death in industrialized countries. Meanwhile, 29% of all deaths worldwide are attributed to cardiovascular diseases (Mathers *et al.,* 2008). Although the therapy of cardiovascular diseases has improved, treatment options are still limited. And new targets for early diagnosis and treatment are urgently needed.

In recent years, it has become clear that major risk factors promote the development of atherosclerosis and cardiovascular disease, which can be controlled by life-style modification and/or drug therapy, e.g. hypercholesterolemia, hyperlipidemia, arterial hypertension, adiposity, diabetes mellitus, lack of exercise, smoking and stress (Berry *et al.,* 2012; Liu *et al.,* 2012). In addition, a multitude of genetic risk factors of atherosclerosis were identified (Austin *et al.,* 2004; Arnett *et al.,* 2007). Genetic risk factors have contributed much to the current understanding of the pathophysiology of atherosclerosis (Soutar & Naoumova, 2007). Notably, transgenic disease models are available which mimic gene defects of patients. A widely used model of atherosclerosis is the apolipoprotein E-deficient mouse (Plump *et al.,* 1992; Piedrahita *et al.,* 1992). Similar to patients, ApoE-deficient (ApoE$^{-/-}$) mice develop hypercholesterolemia and are prone to the development of atherosclerotic plaques (Plump *et al.,* 1992). To investigate pathomechanisms of atherosclerosis we applied the ApoE-deficient mouse model. As the target organ of atherosclerosis we isolated the aorta and determined the gene expression profile of atherosclerotic lesions by a whole genome microarray.

Whole genome gene expression profiling was also used in previous investigations to study pathomechanisms of atherosclerosis with ApoE$^{-/-}$ mice (Van Assche et al., 2011; Gräbner *et al.,* 2009). Those studies identified genes that were differentially regulated during the progression of atherosclerosis relative to non-transgenic control mice (Van Assche *et al.,* 2011; Gräbner *et al.,* 2009). Complementary to those studies, we demonstrate here the suitability of whole genome microarray analysis to directly assess the treatment effect of a widely used cardiovascular drug, the angiotensin-converting enzyme (ACE) inhibitor, captopril. The whole genome microarray technique identified genes, which were regulated during the treatment of atherosclerosis. Because ACE inhibition retards the development of atherosclerosis without affecting the plasma cholesterol level (AbdAlla *et al.,* 2004), our study identified pathomechanisms, which may be suitable to modify atherosclerosis progression independent of the risk factor cholesterol.

The experimental approach may be also relevant for patients with atherosclerosis because inhibition of the angiotensin II system by an ACE inhibitor (or an angiotensin II AT1 receptor antagonist) retards the progression of cardiovascular disease in patients (McMurray *et al.,* 2006). That notion is supported by the observation that the identified target gene, CCR9, was also highly expressed on artery biopsies of patients with coronary artery disease.

Taken together we describe here an integrated approach based on the method of whole genome microarray gene expression profiling to identify a potential new target for diagnosis and treatment of atherosclerosis.

## 2    Animal Model of Atherosclerosis and Patients

Inhibition of the angiotensin II system, either by (i) an inhibitor of the angiotensin-converting enzyme (ACE) or (ii) antagonist of the angiotensin II AT1 receptor, retards the development and progression of atherosclerosis in different animal models of atherosclerosis and patients (Hayek *et al.,* 1998; AbdAlla *et al.,* 2004; McMurray *et al.,* 2006). We used ApoE$^{-/-}$ mice to study the treatment effect of an angiotensin II inhibitor on the development of atherosclerosis. ApoE$^{-/-}$ mice are hypercholesterolemic and prone to atherosclerosis. ApoE$^{-/-}$ mice with C57BL/6J (B6) background and B6 controls were used at an age of 4 to 6 weeks. Mice were fed a diet containing 7% fat and 0.15% cholesterol (AIN93 diet). All mice had free access to food and water. To inhibit the ACE-dependent angiotensin II generation, one group of mice received captopril ($20 mg/kg/d$) supplied in drinking water. At an age of 7 to 8 months, mice were sacrificed and aortas were isolated. All animal experiments were performed in accordance with international guidelines for the care and use of animals, and approved by local committees on animal care and use (University of Zürich and Hamburg).

The investigation also used biopsy specimens of coronary arteries from patients with coronary artery atherosclerosis. Biopsies were taken during bypass surgery with the full informed consent of patients. The study conforms to the principles of the Declaration of Helsinki and was performed with approval from the local Ethics Committee (Ain Shams University, Cairo, Egypt).

## 3    The Technique of Whole Genome Microarray Gene Expression Profiling

A schematic diagram illustrates the applied technique of whole genome microarray gene expression profiling (Figure 1).

As illustrated in Figure 1, microarray gene expression analysis requires total RNA of the tissue of interest. For our study, we isolated the total RNA (containing single-stranded mRNA, rRNA and tRNA) from aortic tissue of three different groups of mice:

(i) B6 mice

(ii) untreated ApoE$^{-/-}$ mice, and

(iii) captopril-treated ApoE$^{-/-}$ mice.

The extracted mRNA is used to synthesize a cDNA by reverse transcription. The cDNA is transcribed into cRNA and biotin-labeled (Figure 2). The labeled, fragmented cRNA is finally hybridized onto the Affymetrix Array Chip (Affymetrix GeneChip® Mouse Genome 430 2.0 Array). Each spot of the array chip is coated with a short oligonucleotide, which is complementary to the RNA of a transcribed gene. The GeneChip® Mouse Genome 430 2.0 Array contains more than 45,000 probe sets and detects the whole genome. Scanning of the array chips was performed with the Affymetrix GeneChip Scanner 7G. The signals were processed with the Scanner Software GCOS (Affymetrix, v. 1.4) and normalized to a target value of 200.

For whole genome microarray gene expression profiling we used the Affymetrix GeneChip® Eukaryotic Target Labeling Assay for Expression Analysis - One-Cycle Target Labeling Method. With this method, the extracted mRNA is separated from rRNA and tRNA, amplified and labeled with biotin (Figure

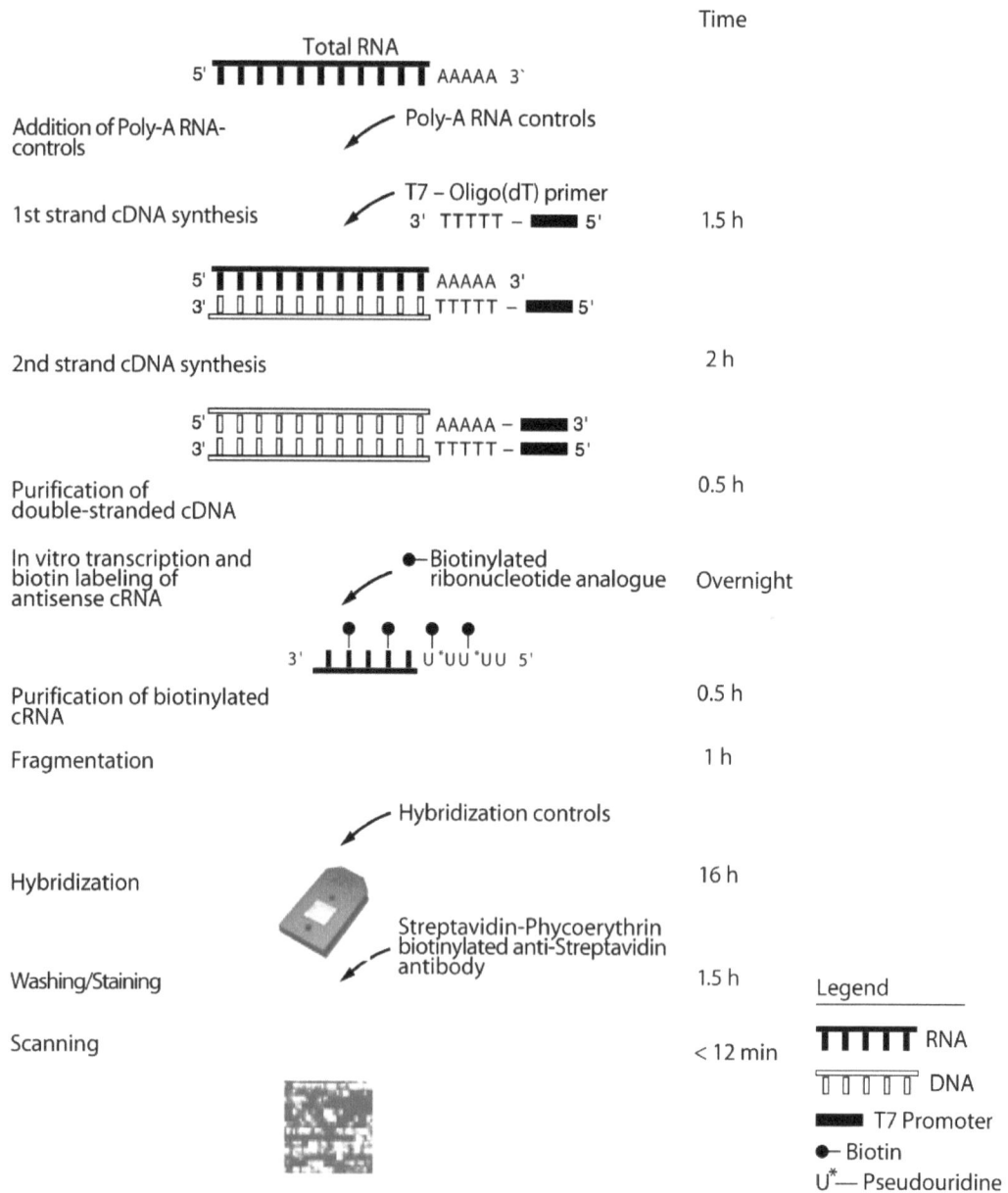

**Figure 1:** Overview of the technique of whole genome microarray gene expression profiling (adapted from the Affymetrix GeneChip Expression Analysis Technical Manual, Rev. 3).

1). Single-stranded mRNA is specifically reverse-transcribed into double-stranded cDNA, while rRNA and tRNA cannot be transcribed. The cDNA is used as a template to synthesize cRNA with the inclusion of biotinylated nucleotides. During this step, the cRNA is biotin-labeled and amplified (Figure 1).

## 3.1 Isolation of Total RNA for Whole Genome Microarray Gene Expression Profiling

### 3.1.1 Precautions to Reduce the Degradation of RNA by Ribonucleases

RNA integrity is crucial for whole genome microarray gene expression profiling. RNA is very sensitive to degradation by the ubiquitous ribonucleases (RNases). Because RNases exert an important role in the regulation of gene translation, all organisms and cells produce RNases. Therefore RNases are present ubiquitously in the environment. Moreover, RNases are extremely stable against denaturation and difficult to inactivate.

To prevent degradation of RNA, the contact between RNA and RNases was reduced to a minimum. The following precautions were taken.

- Use of RNase-free water, which was prepared by treatment with diethyl pyrocarbonate (DEPC; Sigma D5758): $2ml$ of DEPC were added to $2000ml$ $H_2O$, and the solution was stirred for 1 h at maximum speed. After immediate autoclaving, the DEPC-treated water was stored at $4°C$.

- Careful cleaning of all equipment and surfaces by RNase Away$^{TM}$ (Molecular BioProducts), followed by rinsing with RNase-free water to reduce contamination with RNases.

- Rapid extraction of RNA from the aortic tissue to minimize the degradation of RNA by endogenous RNases.

- Exclusive use of RNase-free, aerosol resistant (ART$^®$; Molecular BioProducts) pipette tips and reaction tubes.

- Use of reagents and chemicals of molecular grade, if available.

- Careful protection of hands with gloves, and avoidance of body contact with equipment and materials.

### 3.1.2 Isolation of Aortas

Aortas were isolated from anesthetized mice (anesthesia with ketamine/xylazine; $100mg/10mg/kg$ i.p.), after cardiac perfusion with sterile PBS. For RNA isolation, aortas were put on ice, dissected free of connective tissue under a dissecting microscope (Leica Microsystems), and immediately frozen in liquid nitrogen. The progression of atherosclerosis was determined with aortas from another group of mice. To this end, three aortas from each group were opened longitudinally, stained with the lipophilic dye, Oil Red O, and the area of Oil Red O-stained atherosclerotic plaques was quantified.

### 3.1.3 Extraction of Total RNA from Aortic Tissue

Total RNA was isolated from aortic tissue with the RNeasy$^®$ Mini (Midi) Kit according to the instructions of the manufacturer (Qiagen). Frozen aortic tissue was put in a mortar and homogenized under liquid nitrogen with a pestle. Pulverized aortic tissue was transferred to an Eppendorf reaction tube and lysis buffer (part of the Qiagen kit) was added. Then the tissue was homogenized using a syringe and a 20G needle. RNase-free

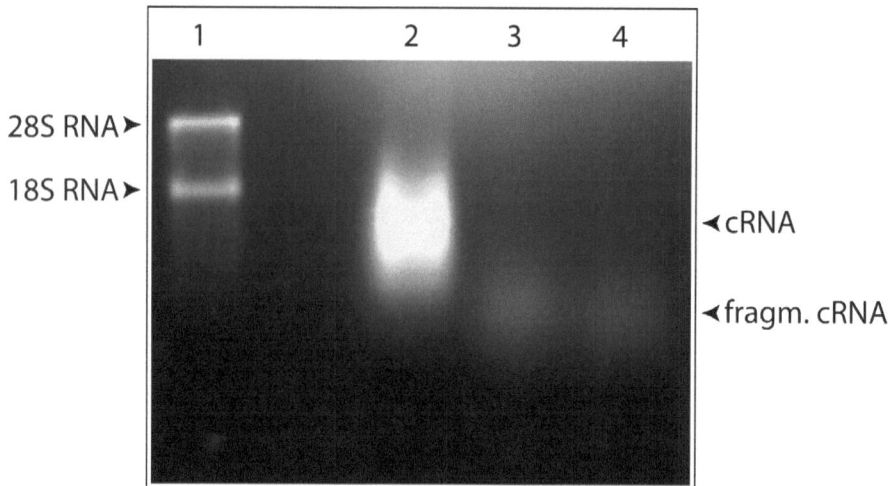

**Figure 2:** Denaturing formaldehyde agarose gel electrophoresis of total aortic RNA (lane 1), biotin-labeled cRNA (lane 2) and fragmented biotin-labeled cRNA (lanes 3,4).

water was added to the emulsion, followed by $35\mu l$ of proteinase K solution ($20mg/ml$ $H_2O$). Proteinase K digestion was performed for 25min at 55°C. After centrifugation (3 min $> 10000 \times g$), the supernatant was transferred into a new reaction tube, and the pellet was discarded. Ethanol 100% (0.5 volumes) was added to the supernatant, followed by 1 volume of Ethanol 70%. The resulting solution was loaded onto an RNeasy® spin column mini (midi) (Qiagen), which was put into a collection vial. The column was centrifuged at $> 8000 \times g$ for $15s$. The flow-through was discarded, and the column was washed once with washing buffer. Thereafter digestion of DNA was performed with $80\mu l$ of DNase I-solution (190 Kunitz units) loaded directly onto the column. After an incubation for 25 min at 20-30 °C, the column was washed with $350\mu l$ of washing buffer (part of the Qiagen kit). Next, the column was washed twice with $500\mu l$ of RPE-buffer (Qiagen kit) and centrifuged. After the second washing step, an additional centrifugation step for 2 min at $> 8,000 \times g$ was performed. To elute the RNA, the column was put into an RNase-free reaction tube, $30\mu l$ of RNase-free $H_2O$ were added to the column, and the RNA was eluted by centrifugation. The elution step was repeated a second time, and both eluates were pooled.

The RNA concentration was determined by spectrophotometry with an UV-spectrophotometer (Eppendorf) and RNase-free cuvettes. The RNA concentration was determined at $\lambda = 260nm$, i.e. the absorption maximum of RNA. Purity was assessed by the quotient of $A260/A280$, which detects protein contamination.

The purified RNA was stored at 80 °C in an RNase-free reaction tube until further use.

### 3.1.4   Control of RNA Integrity by Denaturing Formaldehyde Agarose Gel Electrophoresis

Formaldehyde agarose gel electrophoresis was used to determine the integrity of the isolated RNA (Figure 2).

The agarose gel ($100ml$) was prepared by mixing 1.2 g agarose (Agarose MP, Roche) with $10ml$ of 10 x formaldehyde gel buffer ($200mM$ MOPS, $50mM$ sodium acetate, $10mM$ EDTA, pH 7) and water (RNase-free) ad $100ml$. Agarose was dissolved by heating to 65°C. After cooling to 37°C, $1.8ml$ of formaldehyde solution (36.5%, $12.3M$) and $1\mu l$ of ethidium bromide solution ($10mg/ml$ in water) were added. The agarose gel was poured into a gel tray (in a fume hood), and set for 30 min. Before loading, the gel was equilibrated > 30 min in formaldehyde running buffer. Samples were prepared for gel loading by adding 1 volume of 5 × formaldehyde loading buffer (16$\mu l$ saturated bromophenol blue, 80$\mu l$ 50$mM$ EDTA-solution [pH 8], 720$\mu l$ 37% [12.3M] formaldehyde solution, 2$ml$ glycerine, 3084$\mu l$ formamide and 4$ml$ 10 × formaldehyde gel buffer with RNAse-free water ad 10$ml$) to 4 volumes of RNA sample. After mixing, RNA samples were denatured at 65°C for 5 min, cooled on ice and loaded onto the wells of the gel. After loading, the gel was run in 1 × formaldehyde running buffer at 5 – 7$V/cm$ until the bromophenol blue front had migrated ~ 2/3 of the way through the gel. The ethidium bromide-RNA complexes were visualized by UV light. Figure 2 shows a typical image of total RNA, cRNA and fragmented cRNA separated on a denaturing agarose gel. The bands of the 28S and 18S ribosomal RNA are clearly visible in intact total RNA (Figure 2, lane 1). Lane 2 shows biotin-labeled cRNA obtained after reverse transcription and transcription, and fragmented biotin-labeled cRNA is shown in lanes 3,4 (Figure 2).

### 3.1.5   Spectrophotometry of RNA by NanoDrop$^{TM}$ 1000 (Thermo Scientific)

The purity of total RNA, biotin-labeled cRNA and fragmented biotin-labeled cRNA was also controlled with a NanoDrop$^{TM}$ 1000 Spectrophotometer (Thermo Scientific).

To this end, 1$\mu l$ of the RNA solution was poured into the chamber of the NanoDrop$^{TM}$ 1000. The purity of the RNA is determined by measuring the absorption A at $\lambda = 260nm$ and $\lambda = 280nm$. Absorbance at 260$nm$ is due to RNA whereas contaminants such as proteins and phenol absorb at 280$nm$. The quotient of A260/A280 should be between 1.8 and 2.0. RNA is contaminated if the quotient is < 1.8. With additional measurements, the RNA concentration is determined in $ng/ml$, and absorption spectra are evaluated.

### 3.1.6   Control of RNA Integrity with the 2100 Bioanalyzer (Agilent)

The integrity of the total RNA isolated from murine aorta was also analyzed with the Agilent 2100 Bio-analyzer and a Nucleic Acid Assay Chip. The 2100 Bioanalyzer performs an automated microcapillary electrophoresis. Sample, gel and dye are localized in small chambers on the nucleic acid chip. The micro-gels are stored digitally and enable the control of RNA integrity and quality. The 2100 Bioanalyzer also performs a spectrophotometric analysis of RNA.

### 3.2   Synthesis of cDNA

### 3.2.1   First Strand cDNA Synthesis (Reverse Transcription)

To synthesize the first strand cDNA, the total RNA isolated from the aortic tissue was transferred into a reaction vial. Then *T7-Oligo(dT) Primer was added and water ad 12$\mu l$. After a 10 min incubation at 70°C, the reaction was cooled at 4°C on ice. During this step, annealing of the T7-Oligo(dT) Primer on the Poly-A tails of the mRNA molecules occurred. Then, the *5× First Strand Reaction Mix, *DTT-solution, and *dNTP were added to the tube followed by a short incubation at 42°C. In the next step, *SuperScript II, an RNA-dependent T7-DNA-Polymerase, was added. During an incubation at 42°C, for 1h, the polymerase synthesized the first cDNA strand complementary to the mRNA. The reaction was stopped by cooling to 4°C. As a result, cDNA-RNA hybrids were generated by reverse transcription. (*Part of Affymetrix GeneChip One-Cycle Target Labeling System, or the Invitrogen SuperScript One-Cycle cDNA Kit).

### 3.2.2   Second Strand cDNA Synthesis

For second strand cDNA synthesis, a reaction mixture was pipetted into a reaction tube containing *RNase H, *E.coli DNA ligase and *E.coli DNA Polymerase I, *5× Second Strand Reaction Mix, *dNTP and *RNase-free water. RNase H fragments residual tRNA and rRNA, as well as the mRNA strand of the cDNA-RNA hybrid molecules. The E.coli DNA Polymerase I synthesizes the second cDNA strand complementary to the first cDNA strand, and the E.coli DNA ligase ligates the cDNA fragments. After 2h of incubation at 20°C, T4 DNA Polymerase is added. The T4 DNA Polymerase complements the synthesis of the complementary strands. This is achieved by 5 minutes of incubation at 20°C. The reaction is stopped by the addition of an EDTA solution, which complexes free divalent metal ions required for the enzyme activity. As a result of the above-described experimental steps, double stranded cDNA was synthesized. *(\*Part of Affymetrix GeneChip One-Cycle Target Labeling System, or the Invitrogen SuperScript ® One-Cycle cDNA Kit).*

### 3.3   Extraction of cDNA

The Qiagen "cDNA-Extraction-Set" was used for extraction of the double-stranded cDNA from the reaction mix (The "cDNA extraction set" is an integral part of the Affymetrix Sample Cleanup Module). To extract the cDNA, the solution containing double-stranded cDNA was transferred to a new reaction tube, and *cDNA-Binding-Buffer was added, which contains a pH indicator. The pH was adjusted (if necessary) by $10\mu l$ of $3M$ sodium acetate pH 5.0. Thereafter, the cDNA was loaded onto the *cDNA Cleanup Spin Column by centrifugation. The cDNA bound to the silica-matrix and was washed with $750\mu l$ of *cDNA-Wash-Buffer by centrifugation ($>8000 \times g$). The flow-through was discarded. After the washing step, residual buffer was removed from the column by an additional centrifugation at maximum speed. For the elution, the column was placed into a new reaction tube, $14\mu l$ of *cDNA Elution Buffer were added directly onto the membrane of the column. After 1 min of incubation, the column was centrifuged at maximum speed for 1 min. The recovered eluate contains the purified double-stranded cDNA. *(\*Part of the Affymetrix Sample Cleanup Module).*

### 3.4   Synthesis of Biotin-Labeled cRNA

For transcription of cDNA into cRNA (IVT, in vitro transcription) and introduction of biotin-labeled bases, the total amount of cDNA (from step 3.3) was transferred into a new reaction tube. After addition of *10 × IVT Labeling Buffer, *IVT Labeling NTP-Mix, *IVT Labeling Enzyme Mix and RNase-free water ad $40\mu l$, the reaction mixture was incubated for 16 $h$ at 37°C in an incubator. During that incubation, the DNA-dependent RNA polymerase transcribes (with the use of biotin-labeled nucleotide triphosphates) the cDNA into biotin-labeled cRNA. *(\*Part of the Affymetrix GeneChip® IVT Labelling kit).*

### 3.5   Clean-Up of Biotin-Labeled cRNA

The cRNA was isolated from the reaction mixture by another column chromatography step. *RNase-free Water, *IVT cRNA Binding Buffer and Ethanol (100%) were added into the reaction tube, which contained the cRNA. After mixing, the cRNA-containing solution was loaded onto an *IVT cRNA Cleanup Spin Column by centrifugation (15s, $> 8000 \times g$). Thereafter, the column was washed with *IVT cRNA Washing Buffer (supplemented with ethanol 100%), followed by ethanol (80%). Residual ethanol was removed by a second centrifugation step (5 min, maximum speed). Elution of the cRNA was performed with *RNase-free Water. The elution step was repeated, and both eluates were combined. The concentration of the isolated cRNA was determined by spectrophotometry. Microcapillary electrophoresis and denaturing formaldehyde agarose gel electrophoresis were used to determine cRNA integrity and DNA contaminants (cf. 3.1.4. and 3.1.6).

As an alternative, steps 3.2 – 3.5 can be also performed with the Affymetrix GeneChip® 3′IVT Express Kit. *(Part of the Affymetrix Sample Cleanup Module)*

## 3.6    Fragmentation of Biotin-Labeled cRNA

The biotin-labeled cRNA needs to be fragmented prior to hybridization with the oligonucleotides on the GeneChip®. For fragmentation, the required amount of cRNA was mixed with *5× Fragmentation Buffer (with *RNase-free water ad 40μl) in a reaction tube and incubated at 94 °C (Thermal Cycler). After 35 min, the fragmentation was stopped on ice. Denaturing formaldehyde agarose gel electrophoresis was used to control the fragmentation reaction (cf. Figure 2) and microcapillary electrophoresis. *(Part of the Affymetrix Sample Cleanup Module).*

## 3.7    Hybridization of Biotin-Labeled cRNA with the GeneChip

For hybridization of the biotin-labeled, fragmented cRNA with the GeneChip®, the following Hybridization Cocktail was prepared:

- 15μg biotin-labeled, fragmented cRNA

- 5μl Control Oligonucleotide B2

- 15μl 20× Eukaryotic Hybridization Controls

- 3μl Herring Sperm DNA (10mg/ml)

- 3μl BSA (50mg/ml)

- 150μl 2× Hybridization buffer

- 30μl DMSO with RNase-free water ad 300μl

The Hybridization Cocktail was incubated for 5 min at 99°C followed by an incubation at 45°C for 5 min. Prior to the hybridization, the cocktail was centrifuged for 5 min at maximum speed, to remove insoluble material.

The GeneChip (Affymetrix GeneChip Mouse Genome 430 2.0 Array) was warmed to room temperature and equilibrated with 200μl of Pre-Hybridization Mix for 10 min at 45°C (under rotation). Thereafter the hybridization buffer was removed, and the hybridization was initiated by incubation of the gene chip with 200 μl of Hybridization Cocktail in a Hybridization Oven 640.

After the hybridization for 16 h at 45°C, the Hybridization Cocktail was removed, and non-stringent wash buffer (Buffer A) was loaded onto the chip. The array chip was placed into the Affymetrix Fluidics Station 450, and computer-controlled washing and staining steps were performed with Wash buffer A at 30°C followed by Wash buffer B at 50°C.

- Wash buffer A (Non-stringent wash buffer) 6 x SSPE, 0.01% Tween 20

- Wash buffer B (Stringent wash buffer) 100 mM MES, 0.1 M [Na+], 0.01% Tween-20

Thereafter, the incubation with the Streptavidin-Phycoerythrin-Conjugate (SAPE-solution) was performed at 35°C for 5 min. Streptavidin is a protein from Streptomyces avidinii, which has 4 binding sites for biotin. With the biotin-binding sites, streptavidin binds specifically to the biotin-labeled cRNA-oligonucleotide-hybrids. Phycoerythrin is synthesized by cyanobacteria and blue algae and contains a chromophoric group.

After an additional washing step with Wash buffer A, bound Streptavidin-Phycoerythrin was labeled in the next step with the antibody solution for 35 min at 35°C followed by another incubation with SAPE-solution for 5 min at 35°C, and an additional washing step. After the labeling reaction, the final wash buffer remained on the chip.

## 3.8   Scanning of the Microarray GeneChip

For the scanning, all air bubbles in the wash buffer were removed, which would disturb the scanning process. Chip scanning was performed with the Affymetrix GeneChip Scanner 7G, with a laser excitation wavelength of $570nm$. Fluorescence intensity of each probe set was determined. Fluorescence intensity is correlated with the amount of bound fluorescent Phycoerythrin-Streptavidin interacting with the biotin-labeled cRNA hybridized to the oligonucleotides on the gene-chip. Since the amount of cRNA is directly proportional to the mRNA expression level of a given gene, fluorescent intensity of a given probe set is an indicator of the relative gene expression level.

## 3.9   Microarray Data Collection

Data recording was performed with the operating software of the array chip scanner Affymetrix GCOS (Version 1.4). The initial data evaluation of GCOS-normalized data (target value 200) was made with the Multiexperiment Viewer MeV v.4.0.

Gene ontology (GO) analyses of microarrray data were performed with GCOS/RMA-processed data using GeneSpring GX software (Agilent). Genes with significantly different expression between two groups were identified with the unpaired Student's t-test. A $P$-value of $< 0.05$ was considered significant, if not otherwise stated.

For one GeneChip®, the RNA of three different animals was pooled. And for each group, two different microarray GeneChips were analyzed. Results shown were reproduced in three independent series of experiments. The chosen group size is sufficient because the animal model of ApoE$^{-/-}$ mice is a genetically homogeneous transgenic line with genetic background of the inbred B6 mouse strain.

All microarray data were submitted to NCBI GEO database and are available under the accession number GSE19286.

# 4    Application of Whole Genome Microarray Gene Expression Profiling to Analyze Atherosclerosis Treatment with Captopril

We applied the technique of whole genome microarray gene expression profiling to study pathomechanisms of atherosclerosis. Atherosclerosis-prone ApoE$^{-/-}$ mice were used to investigate the treatment effect of the ACE inhibitor, captopril, on the development of atherosclerosis and atherosclerotic plaques. Due to massive hypercholesterolemia, ApoE$^{-/-}$ mice develop atherosclerotic plaques in the aorta. Three groups of mice were analyzed: (i) non-treated ApoE$^{-/-}$ mice, (ii) ApoE$^{-/-}$ mice treated for 7 months with captopril, and (iii) age-matched non-transgenic healthy B6 mice (C57BL/6J). At the age of 8 months, aortas were isolated after terminal anesthesia with ketamine/xylazine and cardiac perfusion with PBS.

The aortic root is the prominent region of the aorta, which is prone to the development of atherosclerotic plaques and lesions. Hematoxylin-eosin (H&E)-stained sections of the aortic root were prepared to analyze the drug effect of captopril on the progression of atherosclerosis (Figure 3A). Aortic root sections showed a high atherosclerotic plaque load in the untreated aortas of ApoE$^{-/-}$ mice compared to those of captopril-treated ApoE$^{-/-}$ mice (Figure 3A). Quantitative evaluation showed that the atherosclerotic plaque load in the aortic root was 79±9% lower in the captopril-treated group compared to that of untreated ApoE$^{-/-}$ mice (Figure 3B). The strongly delayed development of atherosclerotic lesions in captopril-treated ApoE$^{-/-}$ mice confirmed the anti-atherosclerotic effect of the ACE inhibitor captopril (Hayek *et al.*, 1998; AbdAlla *et al.*, 2004).

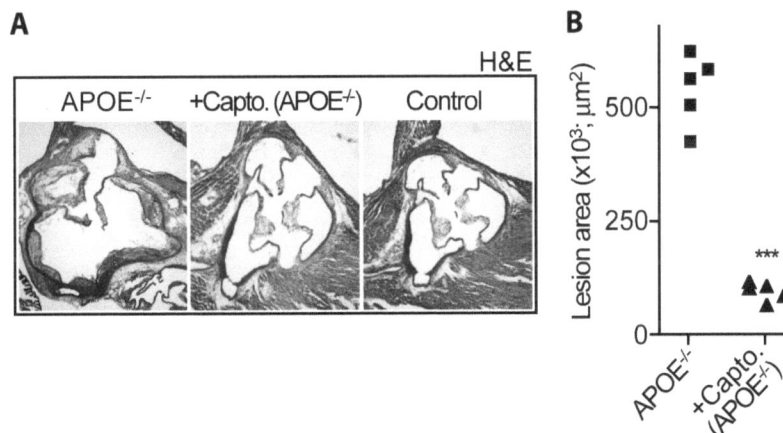

**Figure 3:** The ACE inhibitor captopril reduced the formation of atherosclerotic plaques in the aorta of ApoE$^{-/-}$ mice (adapted from Abd Alla *et al.*, 2010).

Prior to aortic RNA isolation, the treatment effect of captopril was further controlled (Figure 4). Aortas from three groups of mice were opened longitudinally with micro-scissors, fixed with formaldehyde and atherosclerotic plaques were stained with oil red O. The macroscopic assessment confirmed the high plaque load of aortas from non-treated ApoE$^{-/-}$ mice relative to captopril-treated ApoE$^{-/-}$ mice (Figure 4). The macroscopic analysis confirmed the absence of atherosclerotic plaques in non-transgenic B6 mice (Figure 4).

For whole genome microarray gene expression profiling, aortic RNA from three mice per group was

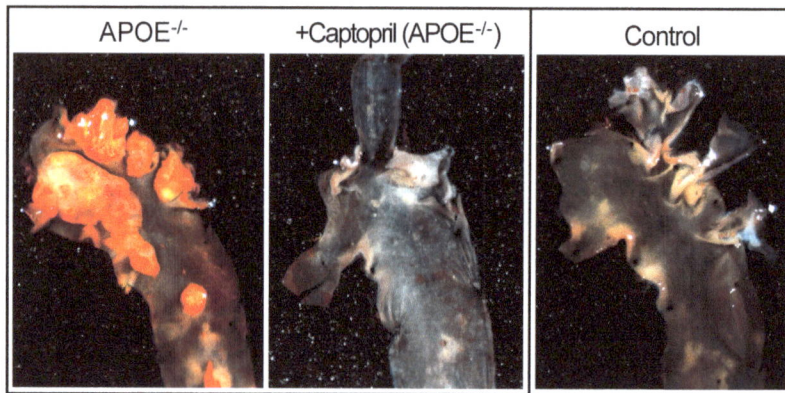

**Figure 4:** Oil red O staining of longitudinally opened aortas isolated from an untreated ApoE$^{-/-}$ mouse (left), a captopril-treated ApoE$^{-/-}$ mouse (middle) and a healthy non-transgenic B6 control mouse (right), (adapted from Abd Alla *et al.,* 2010).

pooled for one gene chip. Aortic RNA was isolated with the RNeasy® Mini (Midi) Kit (Qiagen) after tissue homogenization, transcribed into cDNA by reverse transcription and finally transcribed into cRNA and biotin-labeled (cf. section 3). Integrity and purity of total RNA and biotin-labeled cRNA were controlled by formaldehyde agarose gel electrophoresis, microcapillary electrophoresis and *NanoDrop*™ analysis.

After fragmentation, the biotin-labeled cRNAs were hybridized to Affymetrix GenChip Mouse genome MG430 2.0 Arrays, which contain more than 45 000 probe sets covering the whole mouse genome.

# 5    GO Analysis of Microarray Data Revealed Major Atherosclerosis-Promoting Actions of the Angiotensin II System

Information about the whole genome microarray gene expression analysis on the anti-atherosclerotic treatment effect of captopril is publicly available. Following MIAME guidelines (miminum information about a microarray experiment, Brazma *et al.,* 2001), the unprocessed dataset was submitted to the international data repository NCBI GEO database (accession number GSE 19286).

The dataset was also selected by NCBI as a GEO profile with presentation on 2256 web pages (20 probe sets/page):

- `http://www.ncbi.nlm.nih.gov/sites/GDSbrowser?acc=GDS3683`

- `http://www.ncbi.nlm.nih.gov/geoprofiles?term=GDS3683[ACCN]`

Gene chip scanning revealed that data from three different groups of mice showed uniform quality. Quality criteria were the comparable number of probe sets with Call present, and the $3'/5'$ ratio of probe sets detecting so-called house-keeping genes, for instance GAPDH or beta-actin. After data normalization, significantly different probe sets between groups were identified. Statistical data evaluation was done with the unpaired Student's t-test. To increase the stringency of the data evaluation, only probe sets with a P-value $\leq 0.01$ were included in subsequent data analysis. After the statistical test, datasets were subjected to data filtering. Probe sets were identified, which showed ≥ 2-fold difference between two groups (Figure 5).

The Venn diagram of the filtered data illustrates that inhibition of atherosclerosis progression by captopril in ApoE$^{-/-}$ mice significantly changed the expression of 582 probe sets (Figure 5). For comparison, the number of significantly different probe sets was 1131 between ApoE$^{-/-}$ and non-transgenic B6 mice without atherosclerotic plaques (Figure 5). Interestingly, 266 probe sets (i.e. 45.7%) of significantly altered probe sets were normalized by captopril treatment towards B6 control level (Figure 5).

Commonly regulated probe sets were subjected to gene ontology (GO) analysis because the captopril-induced normalization of probe sets towards B6 control level may indicate its involvement in atherosclerotic lesion development. GO analysis was performed with the GeneSpring GX software (Agilent) by using the category "Biological processes" (Figure 5). The subcategory "Cell differentiation" showed that captopril had normalized two major processes, i.e. the process of leucocyte differentiation and smooth muscle cell differentiation (Figure 5).

The result of the GO analysis is of interest because it is complementary to previous studies, which had demonstrated that the pro-atherogenic action of angiotensin II could be attributed to two major components:

(i) Enhancement of the aortic recruitment and differentiation into foam cells of circulating leucocytes/monocytes/macrophages (Fukuda & Sata, 2008; Keidar, 1998; AbdAlla et al., 2004).

(ii) Stimulation of the transformation of smooth muscle cells from a contractile to a synthetic phenotype (Schmidt-Ott, et al., 2000; Eto et al., 2008).

Thus, whole genome microarray gene expression analysis of atherosclerosis treatment with the angiotensin-converting enzyme inhibitor captopril identified major atherosclerosis-promoting actions of the angiotensin II system.

# 6    Whole Genome Microarray Gene Expression Profiling Provided Evidence that Captopril Reduces the Aortic Recruitment of Pro-Atherogenic Immune Cells

The GO analysis identified the category leucocyte differentiation as a major process, which was normalized by captopril treatment towards control level (Figure 5). We took a closer look on that category to gain further insight into the mechanism of captopril-mediated inhibition of atherosclerosis development. That approach is supported by previous studies, which have shown effects of angiotensin II and angiotensin II inhibitors on aortic immune cell migration (AbdAlla et al., 2004; Guzik et al., 2007).

To decipher the whole spectrum of captopril/angiotensin II-sensitive immune cells recruited to the atherosclerotic aorta, stringent data filtering was performed according to the following criteria:

1. Significantly different signal intensity between captopril-treated and non-treated ApoE$^{-/-}$ mice (*, $P < 0.05$)

2. A more than 50% decrease in signal intensity of captopril-treated relative to non-treated ApoE$^{-/-}$ mice

3. Membrane localization according to GO analysis

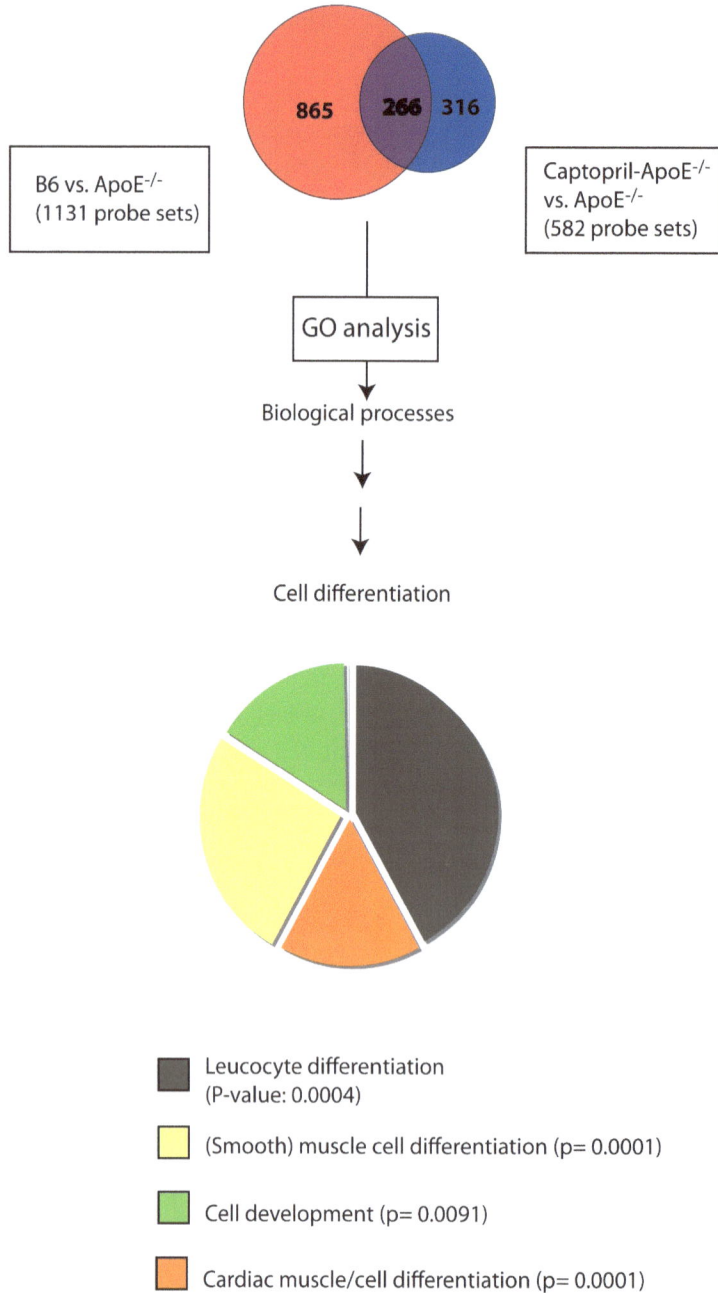

**Figure 5:** The Venn diagram (upper panel) illustrates the identification of commonly regulated probe sets between aortic tissue of healthy B6 control mice and captopril-treated ApoE$^{-/-}$ mice. The identified probe sets were subjected to GO analysis (lower panel).

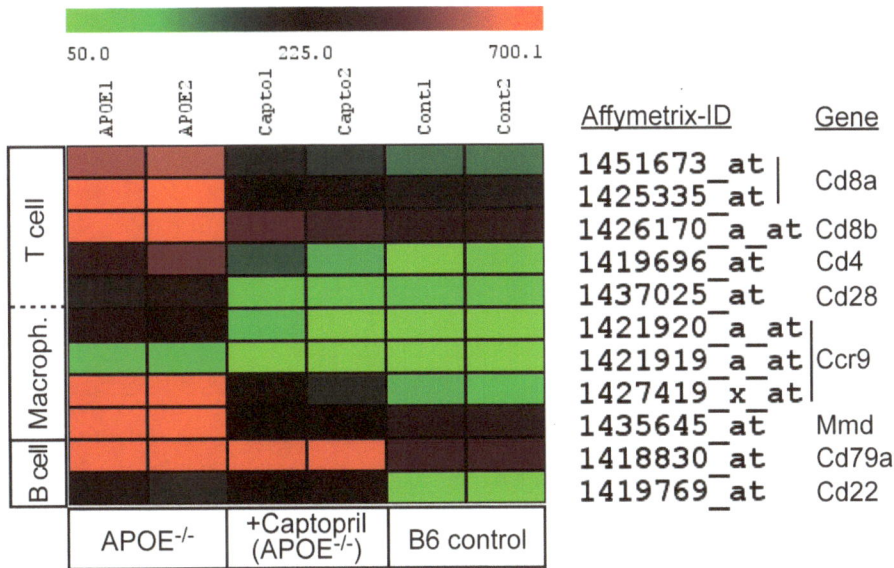

**Figure 6:** Heat map of probe sets detecting T-cell- and macrophage- specific membrane proteins in aortic tissue of ApoE$^{-/-}$ mice, which were normalized by captopril treatment towards B6 control level. As a control, captopril did not significantly change the expression of B cell-specific membrane proteins (adapted from Abd Alla *et al.,* 2010).

## 4. Immune cell specificity.

With the data filtering approach, 9 different probe sets were identified of immune cell-specific membrane proteins, which were normalized by captopril. A heat map was created to visualize the identified probe sets with their gene names and signal intensities among different groups (Figure 6).

The heat map illustrates that captopril had significantly reduced the signal intensity of probe sets detecting major T-cell-specific genes, e.g. Cd8a, Cd8b, Cd4 and Cd28 relative to non-treated ApoE$^{-/-}$ mice. Moreover, the expression of three Ccr9-specific probe sets was also significantly smaller in aortic tissue from captopril-treated ApoE$^{-/-}$ mice relative to non-treated ApoE$^{-/-}$ mice with atherosclerotic plaques (Figure 6). Ccr9 is not only expressed on T-cells but also on monocytes/macrophages (Vicari *et al.,* 1997; Wurbel *et al.,* 2000). Apart from Ccr9, we also identified Mmd (monocyte to macrophage-specific protein) as another macrophage-specific gene, which was down-regulated by captopril. Taken together these observations strongly indicate that captopril had reduced the aortic recruitment of pro-atherogenic T-cells and macrophages into the atherosclerosis-prone aorta.

In contrast to T-cells and macrophages, captopril did not significantly reduce the signal intensity of probe sets detecting B-cell-specific genes, Cd79a, Cd22 (Figure 6). This observation is significant because B-cells are considered atheroprotective (Caligiuri *et al.,* 2002). Thus, captopril may sustain the aortic presence of atheroprotective B-cells while decreasing the pro-atherogenic T-cells and macrophages. As a control, expression of all markers detecting T-cells, macrophages and B-cells was low in aortic tissue from B6 non-transgenic control mice confirming the absence of pro-inflammatory immune cells in the healthy aorta (Figure 6).

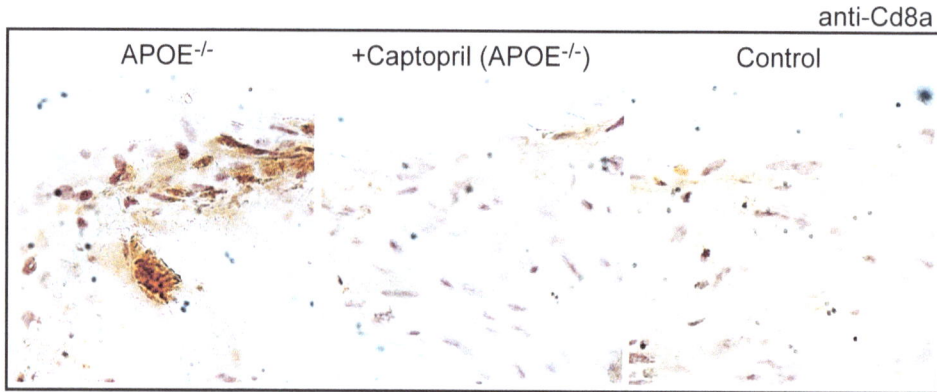

**Figure 7:** Immunohistological detection of Cd8a-positive T-cells in the aortic tissue of an ApoE$^{-/-}$ mouse, a captopril-treated ApoE$^{-/-}$ mouse and a non-transgenic healthy B6 control mouse. The density of Cd8a-positive immune cells was significantly lower in aortic tissue of the captopril-treated ApoE$^{-/-}$ mouse (adapted from Abd Alla *et al.*, 2010).

# 7    Validation of Microarray Data by Immunhistology and Immunoblotting

To validate the microarray data, the effect of captopril on aortic T-cell recruitment was analyzed by immunohistology. The immunohistological detection of Cd8a showed a strong staining of Cd8a-positive cells in the aorta of an untreated ApoE$^{-/-}$ mouse relative to the captopril-treated ApoE$^{-/-}$ aorta and the non-transgenic B6 aorta, respectively (Figure 7). Thus, immunohistology confirmed microarray data on the captopril-mediated inhibition of the aortic recruitment of Cd8a-positive T-cells.

In addition to T-cell-specific markers, the microarray data revealed that captopril treatment led to a strongly reduced expression of a potential novel target of proinflammatory immune cells, i.e. the chemokine receptor, Ccr9, (Figure 8A). Immunoblot detection of Ccr9 confirmed the microarray data showing that captopril had strongly decreased the amount of Ccr9 protein in the aortic tissue from ApoE$^{-/-}$ mice (Figure 8B, lane 4 vs. 3). For comparison, the Ccr9 protein was not detectable in aortic tissue from non-transgenic B6 control mice (Figure 8B, lane 5).

The presence of Ccr9 was also analyzed with Ccr9-specific antibodies by immunohistology, to localize Ccr9 in the atherosclerotic aorta. Immunohistological detection of Ccr9 showed a strong staining of Ccr9-positive cells in the atherosclerotic plaque of an untreated ApoE$^{-/-}$ mouse whereas Ccr9 was virtually absent in the aortic section of the captopril-treated ApoE$^{-/-}$ mouse (Figure 8C). As a control, the aorta of the healthy B6 mouse was also negative for Ccr9 (Figure 8C).

Localization of Ccr9-positive cells in the atherosclerotic aorta was further investigated by immunohistology at a higher magnification. The analysis revealed Ccr9-positive cells, which - while attaching to the HE-stained atherosclerotic aortic intima - apparently prepared their migration into the aortic tissue (Figure 9). Taken together, immunohistology and immunoblotting confirmed microarray data on the captopril-mediated inhibition of pro-atherogenic immune cell recruitment into the aorta. Immunohistology analysis also revealed Ccr9-positive immune cells attaching to the atherosclerotic aortic intima from the side of the aortic lumen.

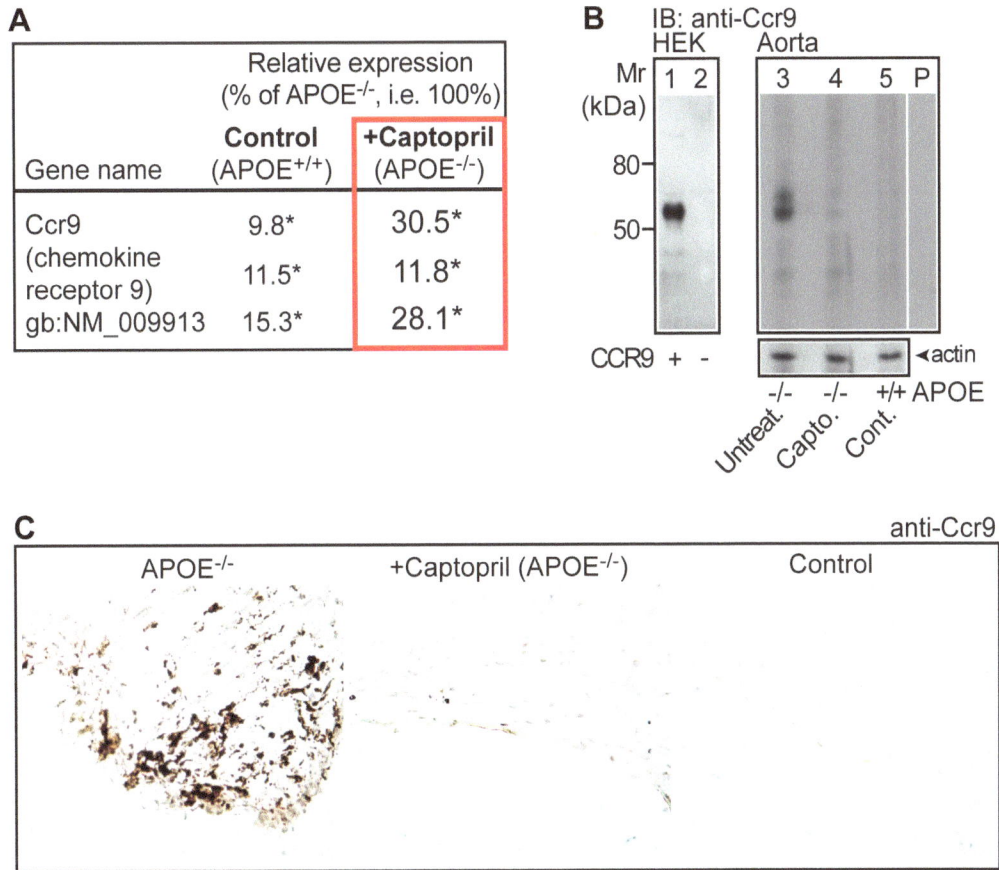

**Figure 8:** A: Microarray data showed down regulation of Ccr9 expression in aortic tissue of ApoE$^{-/-}$ mice. B: Immunoblot detection of Ccr9 in aortic tissue confirmed the microarray data. C: Immunohistological detection of Ccr9 on aortic root sections of an ApoE$^{-/-}$ mouse, a captopril-treated ApoE$^{-/-}$ mouse and a non-transgenic healthy B6 control mouse (adapted from Abd Alla *et al.*, 2010).

# 8   Identification of the Ccr9-Ccl25 Axis as a Novel Pro-Atherogenic Factor on Plaque-Forming Foam Cells

The CC-chemokine ligand 25, Ccl25, is the specific ligand for Ccr9 and attracts Ccr9-positive cells (Vicari *et al.,* 1997; Wurbel *et al.,* 2000). In addition to Ccr9, the microarray gene expression analysis also demonstrated a strongly increased expression of Ccl25 in the aortic tissue of untreated ApoE$^{-/-}$ mice relative to non-transgenic B6 control mice. The increased expression of Ccl25 was normalized by captopril treatment (Figure 10A). Immunoblotting confirmed the microarray data showing a significantly lower level of Ccl25 protein in aortic tissue of captopril-treated ApoE$^{-/-}$ mice (Figure 10B).

To analyze the cellular localization of the Ccr9-specific ligand, Ccl25, in the aortic tissue, we performed immunofluorescence histology analysis with aortic root sections from an untreated ApoE$^{-/-}$ mouse.

The immunofluorescence localization experiment revealed multinucleated cells in the atherosclerotic

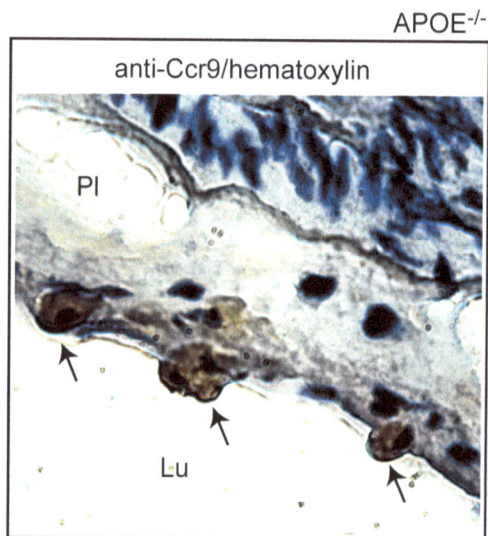

**Figure 9:** Immunohistological detection of Ccr9-positive cells docking to the aortic intima (with atherosclerotic plaque, Pl) from the side of the aortic lumen (Lu) of an ApoE$^{-/-}$ mouse. The aortic root section was counterstained with hematoxylin (adapted from Abd Alla *et al.,* 2010).

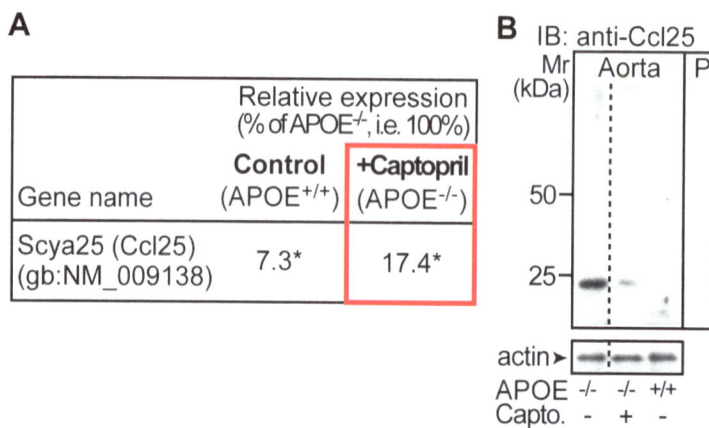

**Figure 10:** A: Microarray data revealed down-regulation of the expression of the Ccr9-specific ligand, Ccl25, in aortic tissue of captopril-treated ApoE$^{-/-}$ mice. B: The immunoblot detection of Ccl25 confirmed the microarray data (adapted from Abd Alla *et al.,* 2010).

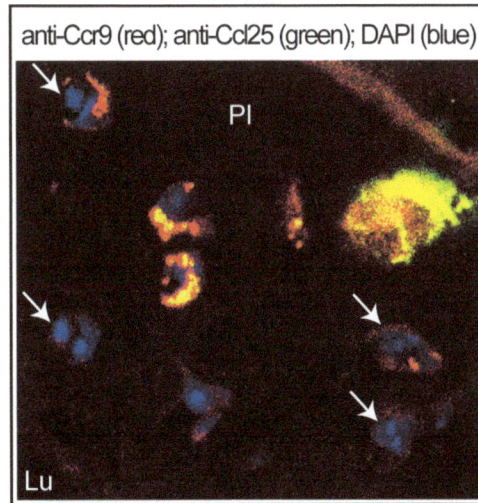

anti-Ccr9 (red); anti-Ccl25 (green); DAPI (blue)

Pl

Lu

**Figure 11:** Immunofluorescence histology analysis revealed co-localization of Ccr9 with the Ccr9-specific ligand, Ccl25, on an aortic root section (with atherosclerotic plaque, Pl) of an ApoE[-/-] mouse (adapted from Abd Alla et al., 2010).

aorta of an ApoE[-/-] mouse, which were positive for Ccr9 (Figure 11). Ccr9 co-localized with plaque-resident cells, which were also positive for the Ccr9-specific ligand, Ccl25 (Figure 11). The cells appeared as fused, multinucleated and degenerated macrophages displaying all characteristics of foam cells, which are a major constituent of atherosclerotic plaques. Thus, plaque-forming foam cells are Ccr9-positive and co-localize with its specific chemoattractant, Ccl25.

# 9    Inhibition of Ccr9 by RNA Interference Confirmed the Microarray Gene Expression Analysis and Revealed the Atherosclerosis-Promoting Action of Ccr9

The co-localization of Ccr9 and its specific ligand, Ccl25, on foam cells strongly suggested an involvement of Ccr9 in the initiation/progression of atherosclerotic plaques. To assess the relationship between the aortic recruitment of circulating Ccr9-positive cells and atherosclerosis development, the expression of Ccr9 was down-regulated in vivo, in ApoE[-/-] mice, by bone marrow transplantation of hematopoietic progenitors (isolated from ApoE[-/-] mice) transduced with a lentivirus targeting Ccr9 by RNA interference (RNAi).

Four months after transplantation of lentivirus-transduced hematopoietic progenitor cells, ApoE[-/-] mice showed a significantly reduced protein level of Ccr9 on circulating mononuclear cells (Figure 12A). Concomitantly, the development of atherosclerotic lesions was significantly reduced as determined by oil red O staining of longitudinally opened aortas (Figure 12B, C). This experiment provided strong evidence for an involvement of circulating Ccr9-positive cells in the development of atherosclerotic plaques of ApoE[-/-] mice.

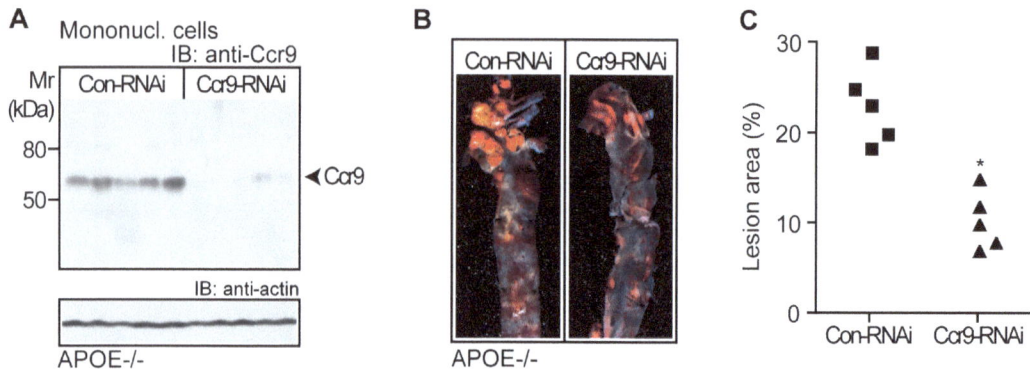

**Figure 12:** A: Immunoblot detection revealed down regulation of the Ccr9 protein level on membranes of circulating mononuclear cells isolated from ApoE$^{-/-}$ mice with lentiviral-mediated RNAi inhibition of Ccr9 in hematopoietic progenitors. B: Representative image of an oil red O-stained aorta isolated from an ApoE$^{-/-}$ mouse with lentiviral-mediated inhibition of Ccr9 in hematopoietic progenitors relative to the aorta of an ApoE$^{-/-}$ mouse transduced with a control lentivirus (Con-RNAi). C: Quantitative evaluation of the atherosclerotic lesion area was performed by quantitative image analysis of the oil red O-stained aortic lesion area (adapted from Abd Alla *et al.,* 2010).

## 10    The Identified Target, CCR9, was Localized on Atherosclerotic Lesions of Patients with Coronary Artery Disease

We analyzed the presence of CCR9 on biopsy specimens of human coronary arteries isolated from patients with coronary artery disease. Biopsies were taken during bypass surgery. Longitudinal sections were stained with oil red O to visualize atherosclerotic plaques (Figure 13, upper panels). Oil red O staining detected the atherosclerotic plaque area in the coronary artery of a patient with coronary artery disease (Figure 13, upper left vs. right). Immunohistological localization of CCR9 demonstrated that coronary artery segments with atherosclerotic lesions showed a strong infiltrate of CCR9-positive cells (Figure 13, lower left). As a control, coronary artery biopsy specimens without atherosclerotic lesions - as controlled by the absence of oil red O-positive lesions - showed significantly less CCR9 staining (Figure 13, upper and lower right).

Taken together, whole genome microarray gene expression profiling was successfully applied to study the drug treatment effect of a widely used cardiovascular drug, i.e. the ACE inhibitor captopril. A major result of the whole genome microarray gene expression study was the identification of a potential new target protein, which could be involved in the formation of atherosclerotic plaques.

## References

Abd Alla J., Langer A., Elzahwy S. S., Arman-Kalcek G., Streichert T., & Quitterer U. (2010). Angiotensin-converting enzyme inhibition down-regulates the pro-atherogenic chemokine receptor 9 (CCR9)-chemokine ligand 25 (CCL25) axis. Journal of Biological Chemistry, 285, 23496-23505.

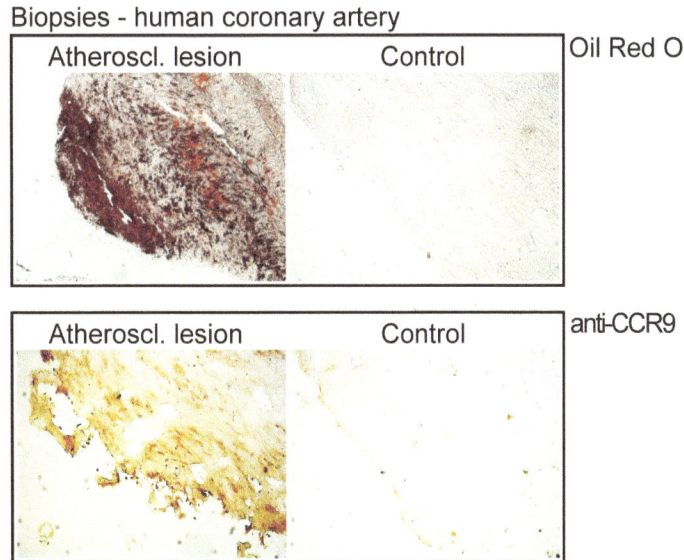

**Figure 13:** Infiltrates of CCR9-positive cells in the atherosclerotic lesion of a patient with coronary artery disease (adapted from Abd Alla *et al.,* 2010).

AbdAlla S., Lother H., Langer A., el Faramawy Y., & Quitterer U. (2004). Factor XIIIA transglutaminase crosslinks AT1 receptor dimers at the onset of atherosclerosis. Cell, 119, 343-354.

Arnett D. K., Baird A. E., Barkley R. A., Basson C. T., Boerwinkle E., Ganesh S. K., Herrington D. M., Hong Y., Jaquish C., McDermott D. A., & O'Donnell C. J.; American Heart Association Council on Epidemiology and Prevention; American Heart Association Stroke Council; Functional Genomics and Translational Biology Interdisciplinary Working Group (2007). Relevance of genetics and genomics for prevention and treatment of cardiovascular disease: a scientific statement from the American Heart Association Council on Epidemiology and Prevention, the Stroke Council, and the Functional Genomics and Translational Biology Interdisciplinary Working Group. Circulation, 115, 2878-2901.

Austin M. A., Hutter C. M., Zimmern R. L., & Humphries S. E. (2004). Genetic causes of monogenic heterozygous familial hypercholesterolemia: a HuGE prevalence review. American Journal of Epidemiology, 160, 407-420.

Berry J. D., Dyer A., Cai X., Garside D. B., Ning H., Thomas A., Greenland P., Van Horn L., Tracy R. P., & Lloyd-Jones D. M. 2012. Lifetime risks of cardiovascular disease. New England Journal of Medicine, 366, 321-329.

Brazma, A., Hingamp, P., Quackenbush, J., Sherlock, G., Spellman, P., Stoeckert, C., Aach, J., Ansorge, W., Ball, C.A., Causton, H.C., Gaasterland T., Glenisson P., Holstege F. C., Kim I. F., Markowitz V., Matese J. C., Parkinson H., Robinson A., Sarkans U., Schulze-Kremer S., Stewart J., Taylor R., Vilo J., & Vingron M. (2001). Minimum information about a microarray experiment (MIAME) - towards standards for microarray data. Nature Genetics, 29, 365-371.

Caligiuri G., Nicoletti A., Poirier B., & Hansson, G. K. (2002). Protective immunity against atherosclerosis carried by B cells of hypercholesterolemic mice. Journal of Clinical Investigation, 109, 745-753.

Eto H., Miyata M., Shirasawa T., Akasaki Y., Hamada N., Nagaki A., Orihara K., Biro S., & Tei C. (2008). The long-term effect of angiotensin II type 1a receptor deficiency on hypercholesterolemia-induced atherosclerosis. Hypertension Research, 31, 1631-1642.

Fukuda D. & Sata M. (2008). Role of bone marrow renin-angiotensin system in the pathogenesis of atherosclerosis. Pharmacology & Therapeutics, 118, 268-276.

GrŁbner R., Ltzer K., Dpping S., Hildner M., Radke D., Beer M., Spanbroek R., Lippert B., Reardon C. A., Getz G. S., Fu Y. X., Hehlgans T., Mebius R. E., van der Wall M., Kruspe D., Englert C., Lovas A., Hu D., Randolph G. J., Weih F., & Habenicht A. J. (2009). Lymphotoxin beta receptor signaling promotes tertiary lymphoid organogenesis in the aorta adventitia of aged ApoE-/- mice. Journal of Experimental Medicine, 206, 233-248.

Guzik T. J., Hoch N. E., Brown K. A., McCann L. A., Rahman A., Dikalov S., Goronzy J., Weyand C., & Harrison D. G. (2007). Role of the T cell in the genesis of angiotensin II induced hypertension and vascular dysfunction. Journal of Experimental Medicine, 204, 2449-2460.

Hayek T., Attias J., Schmith J., Breslow J. L., & Keidar S. (1998). Antiatherosclerotic and antioxidative effects of captopril in apolipoprotein E-deficient mice. Journal of Cardiovascular Pharmacolology, 31, 540-544.

Keidar S. (1998). Angiotensin, LDL peroxidation and atherosclerosis. Life Sciences, 63, 1-11.

Liu K., Daviglus M. L., Loria C. M., Colangelo L. A., Spring B., Moller A. C., & Lloyd-Jones D. M. (2012). Healthy lifestyle through young adulthood and the presence of low cardiovascular disease risk profile in middle age: the Coronary Artery Risk Development in (Young) Adults (CARDIA) study. Circulation, 125, 996-1004.

Lusis A. J., Mar R., & Pajukanta P. (2004). Genetics of atherosclerosis. Annual Review of Genomics and Human Genetics, 5, 189-218.

Mathers C. D., Bernard C., Iburg K. M., Inoue M., Ma Fat, D., Shibuya K., Stein C., Tomijima N., & Xu H. (2008). WHO: Global Burden of Disease: data sources, methods and results. [online] http://www.who.int/healthinfo/global_burden_disease/en/index.html  https://apps.who.int/infobase/Mortality.aspx?l=&Group1=RBTCntyByRg&DDLCntyByRg=AMR&DDLCntyName=1002&DDLYear=2004&TextBoxImgName=go

McMurray J., Solomon S., Pieper K., Reed S., Rouleau J., Velazquez E., White H., Howlett J., Swedberg K., Maggioni, A., Kber L., Van de Werf F., Califf R., & Pfeffer M. (2006). The effect of valsartan, captopril, or both on atherosclerotic events after acute myocardial infarction: an analysis of the Valsartan in Acute Myocardial Infarction Trial (VALIANT). Journal of the American College of Cardiology, 47, 726-733.

Piedrahita J. A., Zhang S. H., Hagaman J. R., Oliver P. M., & Maeda N. (1992). Generation of mice carrying a mutant apolipoprotein E gene inactivated by gene targeting in embryonic stem cells. Proceedings of the National Academy of Sciences of the United States of America, 89, 4471-4475.

Plump A. S., Smith J. D., Hayek T., Aalto-SetŁlŁ K., Walsh A., Verstuyft J. G., Rubin E. M., & Breslow J. L. (1992). Severe hypercholesterolemia and atherosclerosis in apolipoprotein E-deficient mice created by homologous recombination in ES cells. Cell, 71, 343-353.

Roger V. L., Go A. S., Lloyd-Jones D. M., Benjamin E. J., Berry J. D., Borden W. B., Bravata D. M., Dai S., Ford E. S., Fox C. S., Fullerton H. J., Gillespie C., Hailpern S. M., Heit J. A., Howard V. J., Kissela B. M., Kittner S. J., Lackland D. T., Lichtman J. H., Lisabeth L. D., Makuc D. M., Marcus G. M., Marelli A., Matchar D. B., Moy C. S., Mozaffarian D., Mussolino M. E., Nichol G., Paynter N. P., Soliman E. Z., Sorlie P. D., Sotoodehnia N., Turan T. N., Virani S. S., Wong N. D., Woo D., & Turner M. B.; American Heart Association Statistics Committee and Stroke Statistics Subcommittee (2012). Heart disease and stroke statistics–2012 update: a report from the American Heart Association. Circulation, 125, e2-220.

Schmidt-Ott K. M., Kagiyama, S., & Phillips, M.I. (2000). The multiple actions of angiotensin II in atherosclerosis. Regulatory Peptides, 93, 65-77.

Soutar A. K. & Naoumova R. P. (2007). Mechanisms of disease: genetic causes of familial hypercholesterolemia. Nature Clinical Practice Cardiovascular Medicine, 4, 214-225.

Van Assche T., Hendrickx J., Crauwels H. M., Guns P. J., Martinet W., Fransen P., Raes M., & Bult H. (2011). Transcription profiles of aortic smooth muscle cells from atherosclerosis-prone and resistant regions in young apolipoprotein E-deficient mice before plaque development. Journal of Vascular Research, 48, 31-42.

Vicari A. P., Figueroa D. J., Hedrick J. A., Foster J. S., Singh K. P., Menon, S., Copeland, N. G., Gilbert, D. J., Jenkins, N. A., Bacon K. B., & Zlotnik, A. (1997). TECK: a novel CC chemokine specifically expressed by thymic dendritic cells and potentially involved in T cell development. Immunity, 7, 291-301.

Wurbel M. A., Philippe J. M., Nguyen C., Victorero G., Freeman T., Wooding P., Miazek A., Mattei M. G., Malissen M., Jordan B. R., Malissen B., Carrier A., & Naquet P. (2000). The chemokine TECK is expressed by thymic and intestinal epithelial cells and attracts double- and single-positive thymocytes expressing the TECK receptor CCR9. European Journal of Immunology, 30, 262-271.

# Utilization of Large-insert Libraries to Genome Analysis of Genetically Uncharacterized Organisms

Yuji Yasukochi
*Insect Genome Research Unit*
*National Institute of Agrobiological Sciences, Japan*

# 1   Introduction

Whole genome approaches are highly effective for characterizing model organisms; however, "clone by clone" approaches using large-insert genomic libraries are still useful for genetically uncharacterized organisms lacking reference genome sequences. Although recent progress in next generation sequencing (NGS) technologies has been remarkable, the cost of *de novo* sequencing of higher eukaryote genomes is too expensive for the small research community, especially for analyzing genetically heterogeneous species. In addition, in genetically uncharacterized species the need for high-quality sequence is limited to specific genomic regions since widely conserved mechanisms tend to be analyzed using species with rich genetic resources which usually have precise and relatively complete genome sequences. Consequently, it is expected that most determined sequences are not effectively utilized even if whole genome sequencing of relatively uncharacterized species is possible. Therefore, it is crucially important to minimize the genomic region to be sequenced in-depth and to do it at minimum cost. Large-insert libraries are powerful tools for this purpose. This section is a brief overview of BACs and fosmids, currently the most common large-insert vectors.

## 1.1   History of Large-insert Genomic Libraries

Until the 1980s, genomic libraries were tentatively constructed for screening with lambda phage vectors (up to 23kb). Most "negative" clones were then discarded after clones harboring the targeted sequences were, fortunately, isolated and stored. Construction and screening of genomic libraries were often limiting factors for the complete success of experiments. Furthermore, library screening and preparation of phage DNA are laborious compared with plasmid vectors. It was evident that such an inefficient and poorly reproducible system could not support analyses of higher eukaryotes with large and complicated genomes. Thus, many efforts were made to improve insert size and stable maintenance of inserts. Later, the cosmid was developed by insertion of *cos* sequences required for in vitro packaging of lambda phage into plasmid vectors (Collins & Hohn, 1978). Once transected into *Escherichia coli* cells, cosmids can be treated in the same manner as plasmids. Approximately 40kb foreign fragments can be cloned into a cosmid. However, a cosmid is a multi-copy vector and inserts are sometimes unstably maintained, presumably because of recombination via repetitive sequences or the toxic effects of genes located on them.

The yeast artificial chromosome (YAC) was then developed (Burke *et al.,* 1987) and widely used in early genome projects. The remarkable ability of YACs to clone large foreign fragments (100kb – 1Mb) enabled coverage over the whole genome with a limited number of contiguous clones (contigs) (e.g., Cai *et al.,* 1994). However, increased difficulty in library construction and low transformation efficiency made it impossible to discard negative clones after screening, and the current strategy for usage of large-insert genomic libraries was established. That is, all clones are stored without screening and repeated screening of permanently stocked libraries is performed by colony hybridization (Brownstein *et al.,* 1989) or PCR-based methods (Green & Olson, 1990).

In spite of the great advantage in cloning huge genomic fragments, YACs have several disadvantages. One is a relatively high occurrence of chimerism, co-localization of non-contiguous fragments in a single clone, which leads to incorrect genome assembly. In addition, YAC-DNA cannot be easily separated from host genomic DNA since a YAC has a yeast centromere, telomere and an autonomously replicating sequence and behaves just like the host chromosomes. This makes it necessary to recover DNA from YAC-specific bands on agarose gels fractionated by pulsed-field gel electrophoresis for subcloning and se-

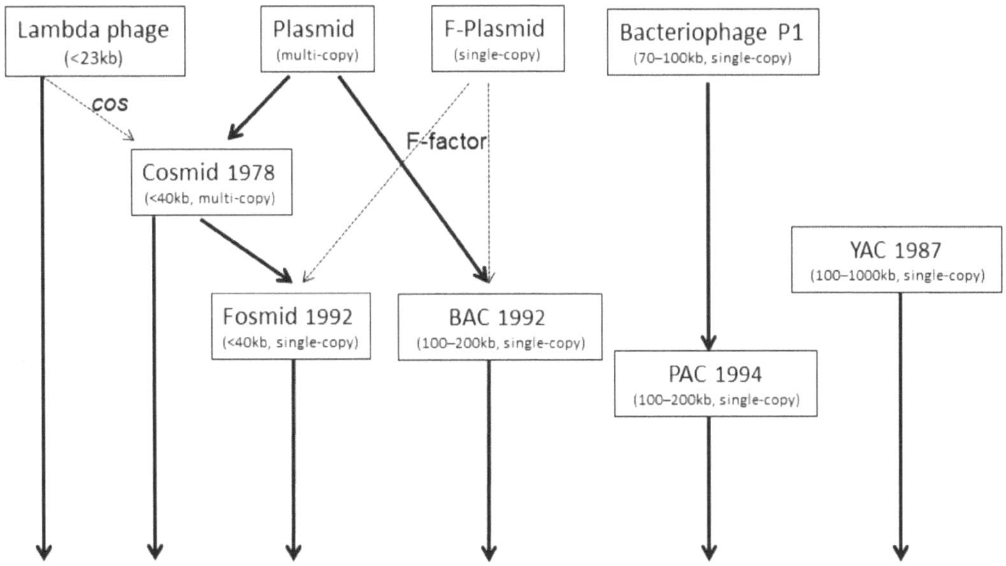

**Figure 1:** Schematic representation of improvements of large-insert vectors.

quencing of inserts. Furthermore, many researchers were not so familiar with genetic manipulation of yeast as *E. coli*.

In 1992, two vector systems, bacterial artificial chromosomes (BAC) and fosmids, were developed, which are commonly based on the *E. coli* F factor (Shizuya et al., 1992; Kim *et al.,* 1992). The F factor includes the *parA* and *parB* genes that stably maintain BACs and fosmids at one to two copies per *E. coli* cell, which reduces the potential risk of recombination and internal deletions of inserts. In addition, BACs and fosmids exist as supercoiled circular plasmids in *E. coli*, and can be isolated by a commonly used alkaline lysis method at a low risk of host DNA contamination. An attempt to develop a similarly effective system was made by modification of the bacteriophage P1, resulting in the P1-derived artificial chromosome (PAC) which gained the ability to clone larger inserts but lost the ability of phage-mediated introduction into *E. coli* cells (Ioannou *et al.,* 1994).

BACs immediately became widespread as an essential resource for construction of a minimum tiling path for the "clone by clone" sequencing approach, although the average insert size of BAC libraries (100 – 200kb) was generally shorter than that of YAC libraries. Fosmids have *cos* sequences used for in vitro packaging into lambda phage particles, which limits the maximum cloning capacity to approximately 40kb. On the other hand, the phage-mediated virulence transformation efficiency of fosmids is significantly higher than BACs, which are introduced into *E. coli* cells by electroporation. Thus, the technical difficulty of constructing fosmid libraries is relatively lower than for BACs. Essential features of BACs and fosmids are compared below (see section 1.2).

During the 1990s, a whole genome shotgun sequencing (WGS) approach was gradually adopted for analysis of organisms having a large genome size (Fleischmann et al., 1995; Adams *et al.,* 2000), and paired-end sequencing of NGS is now drastically reducing the time and cost required for the WGS strategy. However, large-insert libraries still play important roles in genome analysis (see section 1.3).

## 1.2    BAC or Fosmid?

BAC and fosmid libraries are the most commonly used long-insert libraries. The most important difference between them is that the maximum cloning capacity of fosmids is physically limited by the size of the lambda phage particle. In general, the average insert size of a BAC is 3 – 5 times as large as that of a fosmid, which greatly diminishes the number of stored or screened clones required for the same genome coverage. Reducing the number of stored clones saves the cost and labor for picking, replication and transportation of libraries, as well as valuable space in deep freezers. An increase in the number of clones also leads to an increase in the cost of library screening. In addition, due to its longer insert size, a BAC contig can be easily extended by chromosome walking compared with a fosmid. Therefore, BACs are particularly useful for sequence determination of the relatively long region necessary for map-based cloning or characterization of complex duplicated or extremely long genes.

Nevertheless, BAC libraries are usually constructed by partial digestion of high molecular weight DNA with a restriction enzyme, and coverage at a specific chromosomal point is considerably influenced by the distribution of the restriction sites. This disadvantage can be reduced by construction of multiple libraries using different restriction enzymes, although the cost required for library construction increases. In contrast, fosmid libraries are constructed by physical shearing of high molecular weight DNA which are expected to cover a whole genome more evenly. Thus, fosmids are valuable for filling gaps between BAC contigs, making it better to construct two or more BAC and fosmid libraries rather than multiple BAC libraries alone.

If already constructed libraries are available from genomic resource centers such as Children's Hospital Oakland Research Institute (bacpac.chori.org/) and the Clemson University Genome Institute (www.genome.clemson.edu/services), the cost required for distribution is usually inexpensive. If not, custom library construction is needed. However, it might be troublesome to find a skillful constructor. Now, it is impractical for most researchers to master the technique of BAC library construction by themselves, since there are many commercial or non-profit organizations which undertake the task at a reasonable cost. From common starting materials, most constructors are able to construct excellent BAC libraries without failure since they have already accumulated significant experience. In contrast, it is more challenging to construct BAC libraries from organisms for which the method of DNA preparation is not yet established. The quality of BAC libraries, typically represented by average insert size, critically depends on preparation of high molecular weight DNA, and shorter DNA cannot fully utilize the advantage of BACs for the maximum cloning capacity. In these cases, construction of fosmid libraries should be considered as a better option.

The insert size of a fosmid is sufficient for analyzing genomic structure around genes of medium or small size. For this purpose, fosmids are superior to BACs to ensure sufficient sequence depth and coverage under the same sequencing conditions, which lessen additional labor necessary to fill gaps and correct uncertain reads. In addition, a significantly higher yield is achieved in the preparation of fosmid-DNA compared with BAC-DNA, especially for copy-control vectors whose copy-number per cell can be induced up to 50. The higher yield of DNA improves the success rate of direct sequencing and reduces the scale of DNA preparation, which saves additional cost and labor. Shorter inserts are also helpful to subclone DNA fragments of interest into other vectors. Therefore, it is worthwhile to consider carefully whether BACs are really the best option.

| Features of organisms | Effective | Less effective |
|---|---|---|
| Genome size | large | small |
| Reference genome | absence | presence |
| Genetic distance from reference genome | distant | close |
| Repetitive sequences | abundant | rare |
| Intraspecific variations | abundant | rare |
| Body size | small | large |
| Culture/reproduction | difficult | easy |
| Linkage analysis | difficult | easy |
| Ploidy | polyploid | diploid |

**Table 1:** Table 1: Relative utility of large-insert libraries.

## 1.3    Roles of Large-insert Libraries in Current Genome Analysis

In earlier genome projects, construction of large-insert libraries was one of the critical processes which should be performed first. The next step was to construct minimal tiling paths which took at least several years before starting sequence determination. Now, several WGS runs using NGS enable us to generate draft sequences of higher eukaryotes immediately, inevitably altering the need for large-insert libraries. Nevertheless, a continuing important role of large-insert libraries in genome assembly is to order sequence scaffolds determined by NGS.

Sequencing of large-insert clones from both ends of inserts efficiently connects scaffolds separated by long gaps, which is difficult using paired-end sequencing of NGS. Paired-end libraries with longer intervals tend to contain shorter fragments than expected, and it is impossible to estimate intervals experimentally. Large-insert libraries are also useful to assign sequence scaffolds onto chromosomes. Fluorescence *in situ* hybridization (FISH) analysis using large-insert clones as probes is a powerful tool to identify chromosomal position which is capable of confirming genome assembly and genetic linkage analysis.

In addition, large-insert libraries still play a central role in map-based cloning. For example, for the detection of genetic differences underlying phenotypic changes, it is necessary to determine the complete sequence of genomic regions responsible for the phenotypes. It is critically important to perform an extensive search to find candidate genes, and it is not rare that the range of the responsible region exceeds several hundreds of kilobases. A BAC contig is essential for this purpose.

Finally, large-insert clones are clearly superior to paired-end libraries for NGS in that they can be used directly for further analysis by subcloning into other vectors.

## 1.4    Relative Utility of Large-insert Libraries Compared with WGS Sequencing and Linkage Analysis

Recently, the cost needed for genome-wide NGS has been reducing, whereas the initial cost required for construction of genomic libraries has remained constant regardless of the scale of analysis. Therefore, the trade-off between the benefit and cost of large-insert libraries should be considered carefully. Table 1 summarizes the relative utility of large-insert libraries to analyze organisms with contrasting features.

Needless to say, sufficient sequence depth can be easily accomplished for WGS sequencing of organisms with relatively small genomes at only the cost required for library construction and a whole-genome approach is an attractive option even if only a bit of the whole genome information is needed to assess the potential utility of the rest of the determined sequences in the future. Similarly, a limited scale of sequencing is informative if the genome sequence of a closely related species is precisely determined. Conversely, large-insert libraries are useful for organisms of considerably large genome size without any reference genome sequence.

Repetitive sequences which are abundant in large eukaryote genomes often interfere with genome assembly. Intra-specific variations also confound genome assembly, which is troublesome, especially for species lacking inbred lines selected for multiple generations. Very small body size makes this problem more serious since template DNA used for NGS is derived from multiple genetically heterogeneous individuals. In contrast, the sequence identity of DNA from a single large-insert clone is helpful to assure accurate assembly of continuous and long sequences.

Metagenomics is another promising field for large-insert libraries. Metagenomic libraries are constructed from DNA extracted from a mixture of multiple organisms collected from environmental samples such as soil, water or sediment (Rondon *et al.,* 2000). Although NGS is quite effective for gene discovery of viable but non-culturable microorganisms, large-insert libraries have a distinct advantage to identify large-scale structural organization of such microorganisms, especially for those of low abundance in a population.

The feasibility of linkage analysis is also an important factor, since the role of linkage analysis in genome assembly overlaps considerably with that of physical mapping using large-insert libraries (e.g., minimal tiling path, FISH analysis). Fine-scale linkage analysis is generally difficult for organisms of very small body size, few progeny per single mating, long generation time, or lack or excess of polymorphisms. The relationship between genetic and physical distances varies significantly depending on genomic regions. Physical mapping is more effective than linkage analysis to order sequence scaffolds located in cold spots where meiotic recombination rarely occurs.

Large-insert libraries are critical tools for genome analysis of polyploid organisms widely present among major crops. Similar sequences derived from different homoeologous chromosomes cause confusions in both genome assembly and linkage analysis. Longer and continuous sequences determined from large-insert clones are a robust solution for the problem. Combined with flow cytometry technology, it is possible to construct libraries specific for a portion of a particular chromosome (e.g., Sehgal *et al.,* 2012).

For identification of novel phenotypes caused by a single gene mutation, a whole-genome approach is evidently inefficient to analyze slight genetic differences between newly generated and parental strains. Combined with linkage analysis, large-insert libraries are helpful to focus on specific genomic region responsible for the phenotype and save time, cost and labor.

## 2    Utilization of Large-insert Libraries used in Lepidopteran Genetics and Genomics

Lepidoptera is an insect order consisting of more than 150,000 named species of butterflies and moths. Butterflies attract attention by their diverse and fascinating wing patterns, while herbivorous caterpillars have aroused the hostility of farmers from ancient times. In addition, silk taken from moth cocoons has been one of the most luxurious textile fibers. Based on both practical and intellectual interest, Lepidoptera comprise a major section of entomology and lepidopteran genetics began soon after the re-discovery of Mendelian inheritance, mainly based on the domesticated silkworm, *Bombyx mori*. However, it is only one of several species which are now genetically characterized.

The body-size of evolved Lepidoptera is relatively large for an insect and several hundred progeny are generated from a single pair mating of many species, which facilitates detailed linkage analysis using PCR-based methods. Since *B. mori* has been domesticated for thousands of years and lost the capability of flight and escape, it is an ideal experimental animal by nature (For review, Banno *et al.*, 2010). During the history of more than a century, many spontaneous and artificially induced mutants have been isolated and stored as genetic resources (e.g. http://www.shigen.nig.ac.jp/silkwormbase/index.jsp). Genome sequencing of *B. mori* was completed in 2008 (International silkworm genome consortium 2008), and more than 30 genes causing mutant phenotypes have been identified by map-based cloning.

We have constructed several BAC and fosmid libraries from moths (Wu *et al.*, 1999; Yoshido *et al.*, 2011; Kamimura *et al.*, 2012) and established a high-throughput PCR-based screening system for isolating clones of interest from these and other libraries (Yasukochi *et al.*, 2011a). Fluorescence in situ hybridization (FISH) probes are another application of large-insert clones which enables mapping of sequence scaffolds onto chromosomes (Yoshido *et al.*, 2005a). This technique is also useful for comparing genetically uncharacterized species with model sequenced species, which facilitates genetic analysis in uncharacterized species (Yasukochi *et al.*, 2009; Yoshido *et al.*, 2011). BAC libraries are also useful to analyze large gene clusters such as Hox and odorant receptors (Yasukochi *et al.*, 2004; Yasukochi *et al.*, 2011b). In this section, I describe utilization of lepidopteran large-insert libraries mainly based on our own work.

## 2.1   Genome Assembly

WGS of the *B. mori* genome was performed by Sanger sequencing before NGS was commonly utilized. Thus, coverage of sequence reads is not so high and end sequences of both BAC and fosmid clones played a critical role for scaffolding of sequence contigs (International silkworm genome consortium 2008). Conversely, end sequences were used for assignment of BAC and fosmid clones onto genomic sequences and chromosomes, which are available via a genome database, Kaikobase (Shimomura *et al.*, 2009). However, this approach is now too expensive and labor-intensive, and newer genome projects will stress more a combination of several NGS sequencing runs under different conditions (Zhan *et al.*, 2011). Recently, a detailed genome sequence of a nymphalid butterfly, *Heliconius melpomene*, was reported, in which BAC end sequences were used for assembly verification of sequence scaffolds determined by NGS (*Heliconius* Genome Consortium, 2012).

As described below, gene order and chromosome organization are generally well conserved among the lepidopteran species examined so far, and precise genome assembly of a limited number of species is not necessarily a top priority. Considering the great diversity of Lepidoptera, it is more important to sequence as many species as possible for understanding molecular mechanisms underlying similar and different phenotypes by direct and comparative analysis. In line with these aims, a community of entomologist recently announced the launch of the "i5k" initiative, to sequence the genomes of 5000 species of insects and other arthropods (Robinson *et al.*, 2011). Easy access to genome sequences of a wide variety of species will greatly accelerate functional analysis in arthropods, and large-insert libraries will play an essential role in narrowing down the genomic region to be analyzed.

## 2.2    Comparative Genomics

In general, differences in the gene order between two species increase in proportion to the time after their divergence by accumulation of chromosomal rearrangements and translocations of genes. However, the extent of conservation varies depending on the taxonomic group. We speculated that the gene order is well-conserved among lepidopteran species since most of their chromosome numbers are 28–31. In particular, the haploid karyotype of the common ancestor is likely to be n=31 since more than half of many independent lineages carry this chromosome number (Robinson, 1971). Therefore, we intended to construct a synteny map covering a wide range of lepidopteran species.

First, an integrated map of *B. mori* was constructed, on which 523 BAC contigs including 342 genes and 85 expressed sequence tags (ESTs) were localized (Yasukochi *et al.*, 2006). During the process, we confirmed significant synteny and conserved gene order between *B. mori* and *H. melpomene* in four linkage groups (Yasukochi *et al.*, 2006). In the next step, it was necessary to add analyzed species. One option was to construct a detailed linkage map for each one. However, for this aim it is necessary to map multiple (preferably 4 or more) highly conserved single-copy genes for each chromosome for comparison of karyotypes, since paralogs of multi-copy genes and small-scale chromosomal translocation prevent correct assignment of orthologous chromosomes. Although we established an effective method to generate polymorphic genetic markers by partial sequencing of BAC clones harboring targeted genes (Yasukochi *et al.*, 2006), it was still hard to detect polymorphisms from nearly one hundred conserved genes.

Therefore, we selected FISH analysis to compare genomes using BAC clones as probes (BAC-FISH) (Figure 2). BAC-FISH mapping does not require polymorphism in the genes examined, the use of numerous sibs from matings or multiple genetically homogeneous strains, which are essential for genetic linkage analysis. Therefore, a relatively small number of heterogeneous insects collected from wild populations can be analyzed directly (Yasukochi *et al.*, 2009). Moreover, BAC-FISH is highly robust to intra- and interspecific sequence variation and BAC probes may not necessarily be derived from the examined species (Yasukochi *et al.*, 2009).

The availability of EST data and already constructed libraries influences the cost and time required for BAC-FISH mapping. We selected four moths, the tobacco horn worm, *Manduca sexta*, the tobacco budworm, *Heliothis virescens*, the European corn borer, *Ostrinia nubilalis*, and the diamondback moth, *Plutella xylostella*, as species to be analyzed immediately in this respect. We first constructed a BAC-FISH karyotype identifying all 28 chromosomes of *M. sexta* by mapping 124 loci using the corresponding BAC clones containing orthologous single-copy genes (Yasukochi *et al.*, 2009). *B. mori* and *M. sexta* have identical haploid chromosome numbers of $n = 28$; nevertheless, one-to-one correspondence was observed only for 25 chromosomes despite highly conserved gene order, indicating that at least three chromosome fusion events occurred independently in the the the two lineages (Yasukochi *et al.*, 2009).

We then isolated 108 – 184 BAC clones representing 101 – 182 conserved genes from the remaining three moths, which are not closely related to each other, but share a putative ancestral haploid karyotype of $n = 31$ (Yasukochi *et al.*, 2011a). Isolated clones are used for FISH analysis in the same strategy (Sahara *et al.*, manuscript in preparation). Recently, construction of a dense linkage map of *P. xylostella* based on restriction-site associated DNA (RAD) sequencing was reported, and an orthologous relationship between two *P. xylostella* and one *B. mori* chromosome was identified for *B. mori* chromosomes 11, 23 and 24 (Baxter *et al.*, 2011) (Figure 3). Our unpublished results for karyotypes of *O. nubilalis* and *Helicoverpa armigera* probed with *H. virescens* BAC clones support these results, strongly suggesting that $n = 31$ is the

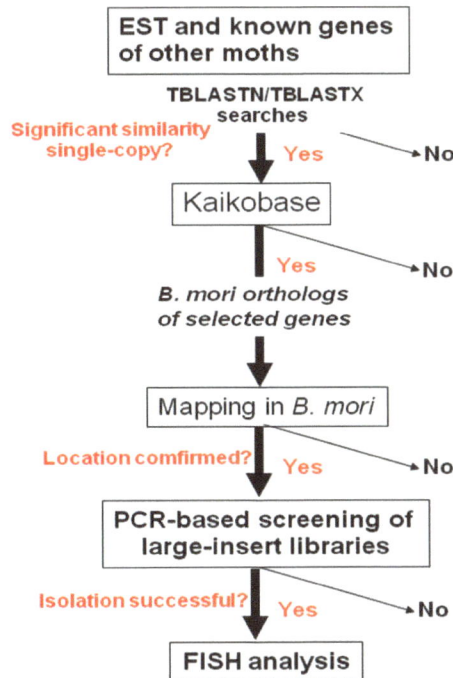

**Figure 2:** Strategy of comparative FISH analysis. Known genes and ESTs of other moths were used as queries against a B. *mori* genome database, Kaikobase (Shimomura *et al.,* 2009). Genes and ESTs showing significant similarity to putative single-copy B. *mori* genome sequences were selected and checked for localization of their B. *mori* orthologs. For location of confirmed genes, BAC or fosmid libraries were screened and isolated clones were used as BAC probes in FISH analysis.

ancestral karyotype. In addition, RAD sequencing of *H. melpomene* with a haploid chromosome number of 21 also showed that all the chromosomes are composed of 31 units (*Heliconius* Genome Consortium, 2012) (Figure 3).

We also attempted to use fosmids in place of BACs as FISH probes to reduce the cost of library construction (Yoshido *et al.,* 2011; Kamimura *et al.,* 2012). A wild silkmoth, *Samia cynthia*, is unusual in that geographic subspecies have different chromosome numbers, ranging from $2n = 25 - 28$, due to variable sex chromosome constitution (Yoshido *et al.,* 2005b). FISH analysis was necessary to reveal the relationship between highly different karyotypes of *S. cynthia* and *B. mori*; however, no BAC libraries of *S. cynthia* or related species were available. Thus, we constructed an *S. cynthia* fosmid library. Using 64 fosmid probes that generated stable signals by adjusting experimental conditions, a low-number karyotype of *S. cynthia* was revealed to be the result of chromosome fusions (Yoshido *et al.,* 2011) (Figure 3). It is of great interest that putative chromosome fusions occurred independently in each lineage and chromosome fission events rarely occurred in Lepidoptera, suggesting the utility of karyotyping to determine phylogenetic relationships among related species having variable chromosome numbers.

Large-insert libraries can also be utilized for sequence comparison of a relatively large region to analyze micro-synteny (Papa *et al.,* 2008; d'Alençon *et al.,* 2010); however, the use of NGS is now more

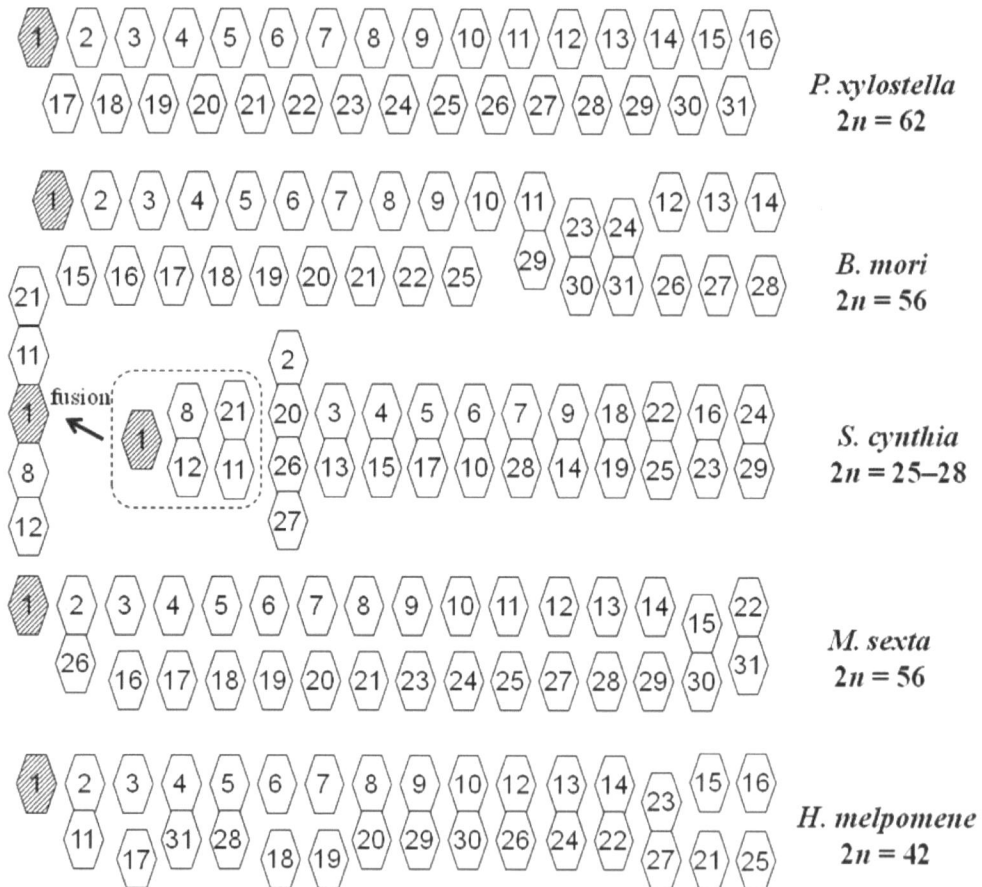

**Figure 3:** Proposed model of karyotypes of lepidopteran species on the assumption that *P. xylostella* has the ancestral karyotype based on Baxter et al. 2011, Yasukochi et al. 2009, Yoshido et al. 2011 and *Heliconius* genome consortium 2012. Hexagons represent 31 ancestral chromosome units. Note that chromosome fusions were likely to occur independently in each lineage. It is not identified to which chromosomes the ancestral units 30 and 31 are fused in S. *cynthia*. Shaded hexagons represent the Z (sex) chromosome, and recent chromosome fusions generated a novel enlarged Z chromosome in a subspecies of S. *cynthia*.

advantageous for this purpose (Zhan *et al.*, 2011; *Heliconius* Genome Consortium, 2012). Compared with recent great progress in genome sequencing, genotyping is still a laborious and time-consuming effort. NGS is also applicable to genotyping (for a recent review, see Davey *et al.*, 2011), and RAD sequencing reduces the labor and cost per locus in large-scale analyses as reported in *P. xylostella* and *H. melpomene* (Baxter *et al.*, 2011; *Heliconius* Genome Consortium, 2012). However, the cost required for these analyses is not so low and may be somewhat excessive for many purposes including the need for sufficient informatic support. In addition, it is difficult to focus on a specific chromosomal region using high throughput NGS methods. FISH analysis using large-insert libraries, though technically exacting and requiring access to sufficient meiotic or mitotic tissue, is particularly suitable for comparative genomics covering a wide variety of less characterized genomes.

## 2.3    Map-based Cloning

During the first one hundred years of silkworm genetics before the release of the genome sequence, only eight genes were identified to be associated with mutant phenotypes (Yasukochi *et al.*, 2008). Now, map-based cloning of *B. mori* genes responsible for a mutant phenotype is so frequently reported that it is difficult to sum up exact number of identified genes. BAC and fosmid libraries play a critical role in these studies. However, most mutations so far examined are recessive and caused by loss of function.

Typically, map-based cloning in *B. mori* is first performed by detailed linkage analysis to narrow the responsible region, followed by filling gaps in the reference genome sequence of the region using BAC and fosmid clones. Then, candidate genes are picked up from the sequences and expression and genomic structure of the genes are analyzed in mutants and compared with wild-type. It is difficult to analyze a gain of function mutation because large-insert libraries for genome sequencing are usually constructed from wild-type silkworms and additional work must be done to determine the genome structure of mutants. Therefore, construction of large-insert libraries from mutants is a crucial factor to characterize dominant mutations. Utilization of mutants harboring multiple dominant phenotypes for library construction promises to reduce the cost and labor per locus.

Map-based cloning in other lepidopteran species without a reference genome is still difficult (Baxter *et al.*, 2010; Gahan *et al.*, 2010); however, an increase in the number of sequenced genomes is anticipated in the near future and will facilitate such projects.

## 2.4    Analysis of Clustered Genes

Analysis of clustered genes is an important application for large-insert libraries. Determination of precise sequence is important for understanding duplication and inactivation processes, as well as transcriptional control. We reported construction of BAC contigs covering the Hox genes of *B. mori* (Yasukochi *et al.*, 2004). The Hox genes determine developmental fate along the anterior-posterior (A-P) axis of the embryo and are located along the chromosome in the same order as their functional domains along the A-P axis, which is well conserved among a wide range of animals. We first showed that the Hox gene cluster of *B. mori* is much longer than in other insects and the *labial* gene is located separately on the same chromosome as that of other insects (Yasukochi *et al.*, 2004). This structure was recently shown to be conserved in *H. melpomene* (*Heliconius* Genome Consortium, 2012), suggesting translocation of the *labial* gene occurred early during the diversification of Lepidoptera.

Evolution of genes responsible for sex pheromone communication in moths is an attractive model for investigating the relationship between the divergence of genes and mechanisms of speciation. A promising strategy is to compare the sequences of odorant receptor (OR) genes between closely related species that use different female sex pheromone compounds. We isolated *O. nubilalis* BAC clones containing OR genes for FISH analysis and sequence determination, and found at least seven OR genes were in tandem arrays on the Z chromosome (Yasukochi *et al.*, 2011b). In addition, a 181-bp direct repeat sequence encompassing exon 7 and intron 7 was conserved among four of them, suggesting the possibility that gene duplication was caused by unequal crossovers via the repeat. The chromosomal region where the cluster was located, determined by FISH analysis, was orthologous to *BmOr1*, a sex pheromone receptor gene of *B. mori* (Yasukochi *et al.*, 2011b).

We have constructed fosmid libraries from *O. furnacalis* and *O. latipennis*, and sequence determination of the genes is now underway (Yasukochi *et al.*, unpublished results). In this case, we selected fosmids instead of BACs due to the reduced cost of library construction and ease of sequence determination. This strategy is effective to concentrate on slight differences between mutant and wild-type or among closely related species/subspecies when a BAC library is already constructed for a wild-type or model species.

### 2.5   PCR-based Screening

Genomic libraries without an efficient screening system are like a book lacking an index. End sequencing is the most stable but expensive way for anchoring clones to the reference genome sequence. However, a decreased tendency to perform end-sequencing for genome assembly makes library screening more important. I previously described a method for PCR-based screening of BAC libraries (Yasukochi, 2002). *In situ* hybridization using high-density replica (HDR) filters is another method to screen libraries. However, preparation of HDR filters is substantially impossible for ordinary laboratories without special equipment and unsuitable for custom libraries. PCR-based screening can be carried out using standard thermal cyclers without any special skills, and stepwise changes in the scale of screening using a pooling strategy reduces time and labor. In addition, PCR-based screening can be easily performed for gene sequences downloaded from public databases, whereas DNA probes for *in situ* hybridization either have to be obtained from the original investigators or prepared independently (Yasukochi *et al.*, 2011a). Therefore, I strongly recommend PCR-based screening especially for fosmid libraries.

## 3   Conclusion

In spite of the current widespread use of NGS, large-insert libraries have irreplaceable roles in genome analysis as described above. It seems undeniable that utilization of large-insert libraries needs considerable cost, experience and patience to establish experimental systems, especially for uncharacterized organisms. However, it enables a tried-and-true approach for analyzing complex phenotypes without definitive clues about the underlying genes or mechanism.

## Acknowledgement

I am grateful to M. R. Goldsmith for ciritical reading of the manuscript.

# References

Adams, M. D., Celniker, S. E., Holt, R. A., Evans, C. A., Gocayne, J. D., et al. (2000). The genome sequence of *Drosophila melanogaster*. Science, 287, 2185–2195.

Banno, Y., Shimada, T., Kajiura, Z., & Sezutsu, H. (2010). The silkworm-an attractive BioResource supplied by Japan. Exp Anim., 59, 139–146.

Baxter, S. W., Chen, M., Dawson, A., Zhao, J.-Z., Vogel, H., Shelton, A. M., Heckel, D. G., & Jiggins, C. D. (2010) Misspliced transcripts of nicotinic acetylcholine receptor a6 are associated with field evolved Spinosad resistance in *Plutella xylostella* (L.). PLoS Genet, 6, e1000802.

Baxter, S. W., Davey,J. W., Johnston, J. S., Shelton, A. M., Heckel, D. G., Jiggins, C. D.,& Blaxter, M. L. (2011). Linkage mapping and comparative genomics using next-generation RAD sequencing of a non-model organism. PLoS ONE 6, e19315.

Brownstein, B. H., Silverman, G. A., Little, R. D., Burke, D. T., Korsmeyer, S. J., Schlessinger, D. & Olson, M. V. (1989). Isolation of single-copy human genes from a library of yeast artificial chromosome clones. Science, 244, 1348–1351.

Burke, D. T., Carle, G. F., & Olson, M. V. (1987). Cloning of large-segments of exogenous DNA into yeast by means of artificial chromosome vectors. Science, 236, 806–812.

Cai, H., Kiefel, P., Yee, J., & Duncan, I. (1994). A yeast artificial chromosome clone map of the *Drosophila* genome. Genetics, 136, 1385–1401.

Collins, J. & Hohn, B. (1978). Cosmids: A type of plasmid gene-cloning vector that is packageable *in vitro* in bacteriophage λ heads Proc. Nadl. Acad. Sci. USA, 75, 4242–4246.

d'Alençon, E., Sezutsu, H., Legeai, F., Permal, E., Bernard-Samain, S., Gimenez, S., Gagneur, Z., et al., (2010). Extensive synteny conservation of holocentric chromosomes in Lepidoptera despite high rates of local genome rearrangements. Proc. Nadl. Acad. Sci. U.S.A., 107, 7680–7685.

Davey, J. W., Hohenlohe, P. A., Etter, P. D., Boone, J. Q., Catchen, J. M. & Blaxter, M. L. (2011). Genome-wide genetic marker discovery and genotyping using next-generation sequencing. Nature Rev. Genet., 12, 499–510.

Gahan, L. J., Pauchet, Y., Vogel, H., & Heckel, D. G. (2010). An ABC transporter mutation is correlated with insect resistance to *Bacillus thuringiensis* Cry1Ac toxin. PLoS Genet., 6, e1001248.

Green, E. D. & Olson, M. V. (1990). Systematic screening of yeast artificial-chromosome libraries by use of the polymerase chain reaction. Proc. Nadl. Acad. Sci. USA, 87, 1213–1217.

*Heliconius* Genome Consortium (2012). Butterfly genome reveals promiscuous exchange of mimicry adaptations among species. Nature, 487, 94–98.

International Silkworm Genome Consortium. (2008). The genome of a lepidopteran model insect, the silkworm *Bombyx mori*. Insect Biochem. Mol. Biol. 38, 1036–1045.

Ioannou, P. A., Amemiya, C. T., Garnes, J., Kroisel, P. M., Shizuya, H., Chen, C, Batzer, M. A. & de Jong, P. J. (1994). A new bacteriophage P1-derived vector for the propagation of large human DNA fragments. Nature genetics, 6, 84–89.

Kamimura, M., Tateishi, K., Tanaka-Okuyama, M., Okabe, T., Shibata, F., Sahara, K. & Yasukochi, Y. (2012). EST sequencing and fosmid library construction in a non-model moth, *Mamestra brassicae*, for comparative mapping. Genome, 55 , 775–781.

Kim, U-J., Shizuya, H., de-Jong, P. J., Birren, B., & Simon, M. I. (1992). Stable propagation of cosmid sized human DNA inserts in an F factor based vector. Nucl. Acids Res., 20, 1083–1085.

Papa, R., Morrison, C. M., Walters, J. R., Counterman, B. A., Chen. R., et al. (2008). Highly conserved gene order and numerous novel repetitive elements in genomic regions linked to wing pattern variation in *Heliconius* butterflies. BMC Genomics, 9, 345.

Robinson, G. E., Hackett, K. J., Purcell-Miramontes, M., Brown, S. J., Evans, J. D., Goldsmith, M. R., Lawson, D., Okamuro, J., Robertson, H.M. & Schneider, D. J. (2011). Creating a buzz about insect genomes. Science, 331, 1386.

Robinson, R. (1971). "Lepidoptera Genetics," Pergamon Press, Oxford

Rondon, M.R., August, P.R., Bettermann, A.D., Brady, S.F., Grossman, T.H., Liles, M.R., Loiacono, K.A., Lynch, B.A., MacNeil, I.A., Minor, C., Tiong, C.L., Gilman, M., Osburne, M.S., Clardy, J., Handelsman, J., & Goodman, R.M., (2000) Cloning the soil metagenome: a strategy for accessing the genetic and functional diversity of uncultured microorganisms. Appl. Environ. Microbiol., 66, 2541–2547.

Sehgal, S. K., Li, W., Rabinowicz, P. D., Chan, A..Šimková H., Doležel, J., & Gill, B. S. (2012). Chromosome arm-specific BAC end sequences permit comparative analysis of homoeologous chromosomes and genomes of polyploid wheat. BMC Plant Biol., 12, 64.

Shimomura, M., Minami, H., Suetsugu, Y., Ohyanagi, H., Satoh, C., Antonio, B., Nagamura, Y., Kadono-Okuda, K., Kajiwara, H., Sezutsu, H., Nagaraju, J., Goldsmith, M.R., Xia, Q., Yamamoto, K. & Mita, K. (2009). KAIKObase: an integrated silkworm genome database and data mining tool. BMC Genomics, 10, 486.

Shizuya, H., Birren, B., Kim, U. J., Mancino, V., Slepak, T., Tachiiri, Y., & Simon M (1992). Cloning and stable maintenance of 300-kilobase-pair fragments of human DNA in *Escherichia coli* using an F-factor-based vector. Proc. Natl. Acad. Sci. USA 89, 8794–8797.

Yasukochi, Y. (2002). PCR-based screening for bacterial artificial chromosome libraries. Methods in Mol Biol 192, 401–420.

Yasukochi, Y., Ashakumary, L., Wu, C., Yoshido, A., Nohata, J., Mita, K., & Sahara, K. (2004). Organization of the Hox gene cluster of the silkworm, Bombyx mori: A split of the Hox cluster in a non-Drosophila insect. Dev. Genes Evol, 214, 606–614.

Yasukochi, Y., Fujii, H., & Goldsmith, M. R. (2008) Lepidoptera: Silkworm, *Bombyx mori* In Genome Mapping in Animals Volume: Insects, edited by Chitta Kole and Wayne Hunter, 43–57.

Yasukochi, Y., Tanaka-Okuyama, M., Shibata, F., Yoshido, A., Marec, F., Wu, C., Zhang, H., Goldsmith, M.R., & Sahara, K. (2009). Extensive conserved synteny of genes between the karyotypes of *Manduca sexta* and *Bombyx mori* revealed by BAC-FISH mapping. PLoS ONE 4, e7465.

Yasukochi, Y., Tanaka-Okuyama, M., Kamimura, M., Nakano, R., Naito, Y., Ishikawa, Y., & Sahara, K. (2011a). Isolation of BAC clones containing conserved genes from libraries of three distantly related moths: a useful resource for comparative genomics of Lepidoptera. J Biomed. Biotechnol. 2011, 165894.

Yasukochi, Y., Miura, N., Nakano, R., Sahara, K., &. Ishikawa, Y. (2011b). Sex-linked pheromone receptor genes of the European corn borer, *Ostrinia nubilalis*, are in tandem arrays. PLoS ONE 6, e18843.

Yoshido, A., Yasukochi, Y., & Sahara, K. (2005a). The *Bombyx mori* karyotype and the assignment of linkage groups. Genetics 170, 675–685.

Yoshido, A., Marec, F., Sahara, K., (2005b). Resolution of sex chromosome constitution by genomic *in situ* hybridization and fluorescence *in situ* hybridization with (TTAGG) n telomeric probe in some species of Lepidoptera. Chromosoma 114,193–202.

Yoshido, A., Yasukochi, Y., & Sahara, K. (2011). *Samia cynthia* versus *Bombyx mori*: comparative gene mapping between a species with a low-number karyotype and the model species of Lepidoptera. Insect Biochem. Mol. Biol. 41, 370–377.

Wu, C., Asakawa, S., Shimizu, N., Kawasaki, S., & Yasukochi, Y. (1999). Construction and characterization of bacterial artificial chromosome libraries from the silkworm, *Bombyx mori*. Mol. Gen. Genet. 261, 698–706.

Zhan, S., Merlin, C., Boore, J.L., & Reppert, S.M. (2011). The monarch butterfly genome yields insights into long-distance migration. Cell 147, 1171–1185.

# Application of a Real-Time qPCR Methodology to Identify Microorganisms as Indicators of Biogas Production During Anaerobic Digestion

Deborah Traversi
*Department of Public Health and Microbiology*
*University of the Study of Turin, Italy*

Valeria Romanazzi
*Department of Public Health and Microbiology*
*University of the Study of Turin, Italy*

Giorgio Gilli
*Department of Public Health and Microbiology*
*University of the Study of Turin, Italy*

# 1    Biologic Methane Production

Two serious environmental and public health problems characterise our society today. The first problem is to reduce and treat produced waste, especially in high-density demographic areas, and the second is to answer the energetic request of limiting the use of conventional fuels (Das Neves *et al.*, 2009). In urban communities, these goals have no clear resolution, but renewable energy sources are most likely one of the key strategies (Balat & Balat, 2009). The anaerobic digestion (AD) process of organic waste combines the removal of organic pollutants and the reduction of organic waste volumes and concurrently produces energy conservation in the form of biogas production (Rozzi & Remigi, 2004). AD is intrinsically a sequential complex chemical and biochemical process, and many factors (e.g., microbiological, operational, and chemical) can affect its performance. The great complexity of AD may lead to many serious problems (such as instability, long retention times, low efficiency, and highly polluted supernatant) that prevent this technique from being widely used and commercialised (Batstone *et al.*, 2006; Mata-Alvarez *et al.*, 2011). The primary aim of AD is to transform most of the organic content into biogas. This process takes place in anaerobic digesters where sludge is stored for a mean hydraulic retention time, generally ranging between approximately 15 and 30 days at a temperature of $25 - 35$°C (mesophilic conditions) or higher than 35°C (thermophilic conditions). These temperatures are ideal for a particular set of anaerobic bacteria. These microorganisms, living in the absence or in a very little amount of oxygen or other oxidants (reductive conditions; (Diaz *et al.*, 2011b), can use organic matter for their fermentative metabolic processes. The main end products of fermentation are methane and carbon dioxide as well as other components and organic compounds in trace; this mixture is called biogas. The overall conversion process of complex organic matter into biogas can be divided into the following four steps: 1) hydrolysis; 2) acidification; 3) acetogenesis; 4) methanogenesis. In the hydrolysis process, macromolecules such as proteins, polysaccharides and fats that compose the cellular mass of the excess sludge are converted into molecules with smaller atomic masses that are soluble in water, such as peptides, saccharides and fatty acids. Hydrolysis can be a relatively slow process, and in general it limits the rate of the overall AD process. This happens particularly when hydrolysis occurs without a specific pre-treatment of complex materials such as lignocelluloses. The second step of the AD process is acidogenesis or acidification, a process that results in the conversion of the hydrolysed products into simple molecules with a low molecular weight, including fatty acids, alcohols, aldehydes and gases such as $CO_2$, $H_2$ and $NH_3$. In the third step, acetogenesis, the products of the acidification are converted into acetic acid, hydrogen, and carbon dioxide by acetogenic bacteria. The first three steps of AD are often grouped together as acid fermentation. During acid fermentation, no organic material is removed from the liquid phase; the organic material is instead transformed into a substrate form that is suitable for the subsequent process of methanogenesis. In the final step of the AD process, the products of the acid fermentation (mainly acetic acid) are converted into $CO_2$ and $CH_4$. Generally, digesters are not directly heated, but sludges inside them are continuously re-circulated and mixed with fresh sludge from the pre-thickening process. This mixture is heated by hot water from the cogeneration section, resulting in electrical and thermal power produced in the internal combustion engines as a result of the biogas. Produced biogas commonly is re-circulated at the bottom of digesters to provide a good internal mixing. AD of the organic fraction of various wastes, such as water treatment sludge and municipal solid waste, is a strategic process for several reasons, including organic waste stabilisation before disposal, energy recovery (both electric and thermal), reducing the mass of the waste materials and producing a stabilised sludge with excellent rheological properties, as well as a substantial improvement in the hygienic quality of the digested sludge due to the efficient reduction of pathogens (Amani *et al.*, 2011). The nature of the raw materials and the operational conditions used during AD determine the chemical composition of the biogas. Raw biogas consists mainly of $CH_4$. And trace amounts of other components such as water ($H_2O$, $5-10\%$), hydrogen sulphide ($H_2S$, $0.005-2\%$), mercaptans ($0-0.02\%$), siloxanes ($0-0.02\%$), halogenated hydrocarbons (VOC,$< 0.6\%$), ammonia ($NH_3$, $<1\%$), oxygen ($O_2$, $0-1\%$), carbon monoxide (CO, $<0.6\%$) and nitrogen ($N_2$, $0-2\%$) can be present and might be inconvenient when not removed. The treatment of biogas generally aims to be a cleaning process, in which the harmful trace components are removed, and an upgrading process, in which CO2 is removed to adjust the calorific value. After transformation, the final product is referred to as biomethane, typically containing $95-97\%$ $CH_4$ and $1-3\%$ $CO_2$ (Ryckebosch *et al.*, 2011). Biomethane can be used as an alternative for natural gas for various applications, including automotive energy vectors and fuel cell technologies.

## 2    Involved Microbe Communities

Different groups of anaerobic microorganisms with specific growth conditions, physiological properties, and metabolic activities are involved in the AD process. Interactions of anaerobic microorganisms are incredibly complicated, and the effective performance of AD strongly depends on the balance of these relationships. The syntrophic interaction of acetogens and methanogens is an important relationship in AD because methanogenesis follows acetogenesis (Liu & Whitman, 2008). The syntrophic reaction can naturally occur only with the continuous removal of the products by the methanogens. Thermodynamically, two reactions (i.e., the methyl transfer to CoM and the reduction of the heterodisulfide) are exergonic and involved in energy conservation (De Vrieze et al., 2012). Moreover, operational and chemical factors affect the anaerobes in certain ways. It is believed that there are many ambiguous points in AD that are not yet known. Therefore, controlling and monitoring each of the microbiological, operational, and chemical parameters may enhance AD performance. Wet AD can address numerous organic wastes, such as wastewater sludge, pre-treated organic household waste, food processing wastes, agro-zootechnic waste, working refuse, and selected crops (Bouallagui *et al.*, 2005; Schievano *et al.*, 2009). Biogas production is the consequence of a series of metabolic interactions among bacterial and archaeal microorganisms (Ward et al., 2008). At the end of these interactions, methanogenic Archaea produce mainly $CH_4$ and $CO_2$ by converting $H_2$, formate and acetate. A particular ecosystem is present in an anaerobic reactor, where several groups of microorganisms work interactively to convert complex organic matter into biogas during the fourth stage. From a microbiologic point of view, the first group of microorganisms secretes enzymes that hydrolyse polymers to monomers, so particulate materials are converted into dissolved materials by the action of exoenzymes excreted by hydrolytic fermentative bacteria, such as Bacillus and Pseudomonas (Whitman et al., 2006). This group includes both obligate and facultative anaerobes, which may be present in concentrations of up to $10^8-10^9$ cells/ml of sewage sludge digesters. They remove the small amounts of $O_2$ present and create anaerobic conditions. During the acidogenic phase, the action of diverse fermentative bacteria groups is observed. The groups usually belong to the Clostridiaceae and Bacteroidaceae families. These bacteria hydrolyse and ferment the organic materials, e.g., cellulose, starch, proteins, sugars, and lipids, and produce organic acids, $CO_2$ and $H_2$. These bacteria are species that often form spores that can survive in an adverse environment. Acetogenic bacteria then convert these monomers to $H_2$ and volatile fatty acids. Only a few articles have been published on the characterisation of the first group of bacteria described above, and the other prominent bacterial phylotypes detected are related to several Firmicutes, two Bacteroidetes and a Synergistetes with well-known hydrolytic and fermentative activities and produce acetate as the main product. The bacteria among these families include *Aminobacterium colombiense*, which ferments amino acids to acetate and propionate; *Alkaliflexus imshenetskii*, which ferments carbohydrates to propionate; *Sedimentibacter saalensis*, which ferments amino acids to acetic and butyric acids; C. *clariflavum*, which hydrolyses cellulose and ferments cellobiose to acetate and lactate; *Clostridium disporicum*, which is a starch that hydrolyses bacterium that ferments sugars to acids; and *Moorella perchloratireducens*, which ferments monosaccharides to acetate (Bertin *et al.*, 2012). The final phase of biogas production is carried out by aceticlastic methanogens, mainly *Methanosarcina* with a high acetate level ($> 10^{-3}M$) and *Methanosaeta* with a lower acetate level, and hydrogenotrophic methanogens.

## 2.1    Methanogens

Methanogenesis is considered, after a good hydrolysis, the rate-limiting step. Moreover, this phase is most vulnerable to temperature or pH variations and toxic chemicals (Liu *et al.*, 2008). Low methanogen activity occurs to conduct accumulation of $H_2$ and short chain fatty acids with a consequent decrease of the pH; enhancing methanogenesis is thus a major route for improving the performance of anaerobic digesters. There are three substantial substrates useful to methanogens: $CO_2$, methyl-group containing compounds and acetate. Methanogens acquire energy from exergonic biochemist reactions (from $-31,0$ to $-135,6$ kJ/mol $CH_4$; (Whitman *et al.*, 2006). Acetate is a major intermediary in the anaerobic food chain, and as much as two-thirds of the biologically generated methane is produced from this molecule (Liu *et al.*, 2008). There are many novel coenzymes that are associated with methane synthesis, most of which are also involved in bacteria biosynthetic reactions.

Among these novel coenzymes are methanofuran, tetrahydromethanopterin, 7-mercaptoheptanoyl-threonine phosphate, methyl coenzyme M and coenzyme F430. The first three previously mentioned coenzymes are also expressed in bacteria (Liu *et al.*, 2008). Although every pathway starts out differently, they all end with the same step, i.e., the reaction of methyl-coenzyme M (HS-CoM) with a second thiol coenzyme (coenzyme B, HS-CoB), forming methane and the mixed disulphide of coenzyme M and coenzyme B. This reaction is catalysed by methyl-coenzyme M reductase (Mcr), making Mcr the key enzyme in methanogenesis (Friedrich, 2005; Luton *et al.*, 2002). In its active site, this enzyme contains a unique prosthetic group, which is a nickel (Ni) porphinoid called coenzyme F430 (Hedderich& Whitman, 2006). The trace elements present in the digester, such as Ni, Co and Se, are of great importance because these are cofactors for enzymes that influence the growth and metabolism of the anaerobic microbial community. Because HS-CoM has been found in all of the examined methanogens, it has been proposed as a sensitive biomarker for quantitative and qualitative identification in different anaerobic environments. Despite their key role as the terminal oxidisers in a complex microbial community, very little is known about the methanogen community structure. Most likely, only a fraction of the methanogens in nature have been described, and most of the species descriptions are based on the examination of few strains, so the phenotypic characterisation is far from complete.

A microbiologic understanding of the process is most likely able to reveal a biological indicator as the effect or a sufferance indicator, as well as the stability or accumulation indicators of the digestion. The former respond (relatively) quickly and in an observable or measurable manner to physical or chemical stress, ensuring from the above characterisation of stress and strain resistance that effect indicators should be low-resistance systems with low adaptive potential. Stability indicators, in contrast, must dispose of a fairly high amount of strain resistance, which enables them to incorporate for a considerable time without injury, depending on the uptake-excretion ratio and potentially toxic substances. Generally microorganisms are very sensitive to environmental variations, and determination methods are generally not expensive. Biological indicators are thus being developed in various fields to diagnose environmental stressors (Franzle, 2006).

Methanogens are classified into five orders (i.e., Methanobacteriales, Methanococcales, Methanomicrobiales, Methanosarcinales, Methanopyrales) and further divided into 10 families and 31 genera. Anaerobic digesters are a typical habitat, especially for the following genera: *Methanobacterium*, *Methanothermobacter*, *Methanomicrobium*, *Methanoculleus*, *Methanofollis*, *Methanospirillum*, *Methanocorpusculum*, *Methanosarcina* and *Metanosaeta* (Liu *et al.*, 2008). The genera frequently isolated are *Methanobacterium*, *Methanospirillum* and *Methanobrevibacter*.

One of the major drawbacks of AD, however, is the sensitivity of the methanogenic consortium to different environmental factors. An abrupt change in pH, an increase in salt or organic matter concentration, an alteration of the loading rate or the introduction of a toxic compound often causes system failure (Wijekoon *et al.*, 2011). Overloading is a frequent problem in AD because it leads to the accumulation of fatty acids, which are no longer efficiently removed by the methanogens. This problem is a result of their low growth rates, compared to the acidogenic and acetogenic bacteria, which cause the acetogenic bacteria and methanogens to uncouple. Overloading thus causes an accumulation of fatty acids to concentrations that may have a toxic effect on the methanogens (Ma *et al.*, 2008). It also lowers the pH to suboptimal values because the optimal pH range for methanogens lies between 6.8 and 7.5 (Appels *et al.*, 2008). For these reasons, AD in continuously stirred tank reactors commonly operates at organic loading rates below their optimum capacity to avoid overloading and at sludge retention times in the order of 20 days or more to avoid the washout of the methanogens (Appels *et al.*, 2008). It has, however, been reported that *Methanosarcina spp.* have high growth rates (i.e., doubling growth on the order of $1.0 - 1.2$ days) and are tolerant to sudden changes in pH of approximately $0.8 - 1.0$ units, caused by overloading, compared to the other methanogens, which have doubling times of a minimum of $4 - 6$ days and tend to be affected by a pH shock of 0.5 units or even less (De Vrieze *et al.*, 2012). Compared to *Methanosaeta spp*, *Methanosarcina spp.* are able to use both the acetoclastic and hydrogenotrophic methanogenesis pathways, making them more tolerant to specific inhibitors of the acetoclastic pathway, such as fluoroacetate and methyl fluoride (Liu *et al.*, 2011). Additionally, *Methanosarcina spp* are tolerant to levels of ammonium up to $7,000mg$ of total ammonia nitrogen per litre. *Methanosarcina spp.* are therefore able to achieve stable growth at low retention times (even as low as 4 days), high organic loading rates and high levels of ammonium (Schnurer & Nordberg, 2008). Conversely, both acetotrophic and hydrogenotrophic methanogens are essential for methanogenesis conclusion. At a low concentration of acetate, Methanosaeta spp. dominate, while a prevalent Methanosarcina spp. role can be observed in presence of toxic agents and during thermophilic digestion (Demirel & Scherer, 2008). Due to these considerations, during co-digestion with a high concentration of the acetate system, *Methanosarcina spp.* could be proposed as stability biomarkers of the methanogenesis, while other taxa such as *Metanosaeta spp.* could be proposed as sufferance biomarkers of the process.

## 2.2    The Role of the Syntrophic Acetogenic Bacteria, Syntrophic Acetate Oxidising Bacteria and Methanotrophs

AD is susceptible to different forms of disruption because of the delicate balance between the different microbial consortia in the AD process, of which the methanogens are most vulnerable. *Methanosarcina spp.*, as just discussed, differ from other methanogens, as they are often tolerant against different stressors. Their interaction with the syntrophic acetogenic bacteria (SAB) is the key to a good biomethanisation. The SAB consist mostly of Clostridium spp. at both mesophilic and thermophilic conditions (Schnurer *et al.*, 1996). Conversely, the four most common forms of stress are ammonium toxicity, overcharging the loading rate and its related problems, high salt concentrations and temperature variation. High ammonium concentrations and elevated acetate levels seem to suppress the growth of *Methanosaeta spp.* and thus enhance the syntrophic acetate oxidising (SAO) bacteria. However, *Methanosarcina* is also able to tolerate these enhanced concentrations and is both acetoclastic and hydrogenotrophic. The coupled growth of syntrophic acetate oxidising bacteria and *Methanosarcina spp.* into nanowires seems to be able to enhance reactor stability (De Vrieze *et al.*, 2012). The SAO bacteria in mesophilic conditions are mainly *Clostridium ultunense* and *Syntrophaceticus schinkii* (Nettmann *et al.*, 2010).

Another aspect of the anaerobic reactor microbiome to consider is the anaerobic methanotrophic Archaea (MO). These microorganisms were detected in organic waste, such as wastewater treatment sludge, though their physiology remains unknown (Meulepas *et al.*, 2010). In general, methanotrophic taxa are able to metabolise methane as their only source of carbon and energy, and they can grow both aerobically and anaerobically. Experiments with the bioreactor biomass in its early phase have shown that these microorganisms are very poorly represented compared with the methanogens (Ettwig *et al.*, 2008; Knittel & Boetius, 2009). Moreover, other microbial population analyses of biogas reactors, in meso- and thermophilic conditions, did not detect a sequence affiliation to methane-oxidising archaea (Bauer *et al.*, 2008). However, the presence of anaerobic methanotrophic archaea in the bio-digester cannot be excluded and should be further investigated. A recent study investigated the diversity of methanotrophs in a biogas reactor running on cattle dung using a sequence analysis of the functional gene, i.e., the particulate methane monooxygenase (subunit A; *pmoA*), and concluded that in biogas plants there is a methanotrophic diversity but that the abundance is most likely very limited (Rastogi *et al.*, 2009).

## 2.3    Sulphate Reducing Bacteria

In anaerobic reactors, both sulphate reduction and methanogenesis can be regarded as the final steps in the substrate degradation process because sulphate reducers are capable of utilising many of the intermediates formed during methanogenesis. Hydrogen and acetate are the key precursors to methane formation during normal anaerobic wastewater treatment. In anaerobic reactors, Sulphate-Reducing Bacteria (SRB) and methanogens coexist and are considered competitors for these available substrates in anaerobic wastewater treatment systems. This is a problem for two reasons: first, the production of hydrogen sulphide affects the biogas quality, thus limiting its utilisation, and second, this metabolic approach subtracts the suitable substrates for methanogen work. The influent $COD/SO_4^{2-}$ ratio should be one of the most important factors affecting the outcome of substrate competition between sulphate reducers and methanogens. More specifically, a $COD/SO_4^{2-}$ ratio higher than 3 (*g/g*) supports an environment for methanogen growth, whereas a ratio lower than 3 (*g/g*) promotes sulphate reducers growth (Chou *et al.*, 2011).

SRBs that use sulphate as a terminal electron acceptor constitute a unique physiological group of microorganisms that couple anaerobic electron transport to ATP synthesis, resulting in the production of hydrogen sulphide (Muyzer & Stams, 2008). These bacteria can use a large variety of compounds as electron donors and to mediate electron flow, but they have many proteins with redox active groups. These features are all strongly involved in the dissimilatory sulphate reduction pathway for the central metabolism of SRBs. Among SRBs, more than 220 species of 60 genera of SRB have been described. SRBs belong to seven phylogenetic lineages, five within Bacteria (i.e., Deltaproteobacteria, Nitrospirae, Clostridia, Thermodesulfobiaceae, Thermodesulfobacteria) and two within Archaea (i.e., Euryarchaeota and Crenarchaeota) (Muyzer *et al.*, 2008).

Regarding sulphur and sulphate reduction, the group of sulphidogenic bacteria ($H_2S$ producers) includes microorganisms capable of producing hydrogen sulphide by breaking down organic substances containing sulphur and using sulphate, elemental sulphur, and sometimes thiosulfate or sulphite as final electron acceptors. From an environmental biotechnology perspective, those bacteria are the most important organisms involved in the dissimilatory reduction of sulphate and elemental sulphur; some of these genera (*Desulfovibrio* and *Desulfotomaculum*) have been well known for a long time. Among sulphidogenic bacteria, SRB have a key role in the sulphur cycle. They use sulphate as a terminal electron acceptor in the degradation of organic matter, which results in the production of hydrogen sulphide ($H_2S$).

Sulphur reduction was described for the first time in *Desulfomonas acetoxidans*, an anaerobic and mesophilic bacterium that can reduce elemental sulphur to hydrogen sulphide using acetate as an electron donor. More general bacteria belonged to genus of *Desulfuromonas*, and many hyperthermophilic Archaea are capable of sulphur reduction.

Conversely, the utilisation of sulphur-oxidising microorganisms able to oxidise hydrogen sulphide when oxygen is present as an electron acceptor could be an important modification to minimise the output of hydrogen sulphide. The development of microorganisms responsible for sulphide oxidation depends on the oxygen content available to perform the oxidation. The micro-oxygenation of the bio-digester could thus be an alternative approach to reduce the quantity of hydrogen sulphide that results from the living environment supporting sulphur-oxidising bacteria (Diaz *et al.*, 2011a; Jenicek *et al.*, 2010). In aerobic conditions and with a neutral pH, $HS^-$ is rapidly and spontaneously oxidised; moreover, most of the sulphur-bacteria are aerobic. Due to the rapidity of this spontaneous reaction, the bacterial sulphur oxidation is performed only when $H_2S$ arises from deeply anoxic zones towards oxic areas. Chemolithotrophic sulphur-oxidising bacteria (e.g., *Thiobacillus spp* or *Beggiatoa spp.*) aerobically oxidise the sulphide and sulphur. These aerobic transformations were recently exploited in the desulfurisation process of the biogas production using biotrickling filters to enhance the conversion from biogas after its production to biomethane (Fortuny *et al.*, 2011).

In anaerobic environments, phototrophic sulphur bacteria (e.g., Chlorobium spp.) perform sulphide and sulphur oxidation to elemental sulphur (4°) and $SO_4^{2-}$. Other transformations, which are carried out by specialised groups of microorganisms, result in sulphur disproportionation (*Desulfovibrio sulfodismutans*) or organic sulphur compounds, such as dimethylsulphoxide (DMSO), which can be transformed into dimethylsulphide (DMS) and vice versa by several groups of microorganisms.

The most extensive biochemical and physiological research have been done with SRB members of the genus *Desulfovibrio*, which are the most easily and rapidly cultured sulfate reducers. SRBs fall into three major branches: the σ-subclass of Proteobacteria with more than twenty-five genera (to which the genera *Desulfovibrio* belongs), the Gram-positive bacteria with the genera *Desulfotomaculum* and *Desulfosporosinus*, and branches formed by *Thermodesulfobacterium* and *Thermodesulfovibrio* (Rabus *et al.*,

2006).

The SRB possess a number of unique biochemical and physiological characteristics such as the requirement for ATP to reduce sulphate, the cytoplasmic localization of key enzymes involved in the pathway of respiratory sulfate reduction (Kremer *et al.*, 1988), the periplasmic localization of some hydrogenases (Fauque *et al.*, 1988) and the abundance of multihemic c-type cytochromes. Because all enzymatic steps leading from sulfate to sulfide occur in the cytoplasm or in association with the inner side of the cytoplasmic membrane, sulfate has to be transported into the cell. Sulfate uptake in SRBs is driven by an ion-gradient (Rabus et al., 2006).

As mentioned above, SRBs constitute a heterogeneous group, including members of several phyla and domains; the use of specific SRB probes should thus be considered. Three key enzymes mediate the dissimilatory process in all of the recognised sulphate-reducing prokaryotes (SRP). After ATP sulfurylase (Sat) activates the chemically inert sulphate to adenosine-5'-phosphosulfate (APS), the second enzyme, APS reductase (Apr), converts APS to AMP and sulphite, which is finally reduced to sulphide by the activity of the sulphite reductase (Dsr; (Meyer & Kuever, 2007a; Meyer & Kuever, 2007b).

The *dsr* gene, which encodes dissimilatory sulphate reductase (i.e., the key enzyme in dissimilatory sulphate reduction) can be used as a phylogenetic marker to identify SRBs in wastewater samples (Klein *et al.*, 2001; Wagner *et al.*, 1998). Specifically, the *dsr* gene sequence encodes for the alpha and beta subunits of the gene. Because of this specificity, these genes can be found in all known sulphate-reducing prokaryotes (Zverlov *et al.*, 2005). In addition, the entire coding region of the dissimilatory APS reductase (aprBA) can be used as a target (Fritz *et al.*, 2000). Both subunits of the APS AB reductase are highly conserved, and these genes have been proposed as useful phylogenetic markers for SRBs. The literature suggests many types of different sequences that can be used to identify these two different genes through the Real-Time PCR method (Ben-Dov *et al.*, 2007; Dar *et al.*, 2007; Foti *et al.*, 2007; Loy *et al.*, 2004; Loy *et al.*, 2002; Meyer *et al.*, 2007a; Meyer *et al.*, 2007b; Minz *et al.*, 1999; Wagner *et al.*, 1998).

## 3    Bio-molecular Detection Methods

Methanogens and other anaerobe populations are difficult to study through culture-based methods, although methanogenesis represents the critical step in biogas production in anaerobic reactors (Liu *et al.*, 2008). The possibility of growing this type of microorganism in vitro is not very common. This predicament is mainly due to the necessity of strict anaerobic conditions, compelling researchers to develop various biomolecular methods to identify methanogen sub-populations, such as ribosomal RNA sequence analysis (Whitman *et al.*, 2006). Quantitative Real-Time Polymerase Chain Reaction (qRT-PCR) is an alternative technique capable of determining the copy number of a particular gene present in the DNA extracted from an environmental sample (Smith & Osborn, 2009). Various approaches can be applied to environmental samples to study the microbe communities with or without a cultivation step. In the last few years, a metagenomics approach has been developed because, in principle, this approach can access 100% of the genetic resources of an environment sample. However, metagenomics requires greater attention to sampling, and assessing the sample diversity using various means is necessary to ensure that the sample is representative. Extracting the appropriate nucleic acids from the sample is another step that can be challenging in a metagenomics project. The DNA from samples can then either be sequenced or assessed for the functions it encodes. The sequence can sometimes be assembled into complete genomes of community members, but it can also be analysed in other ways. The more recent, bead-based pyrosequencing allows direct sequencing of PCR products without the cloning step (Edwards *et al.*, 2006; Xu, 2010). Currently, using this type of biomolecular approach is favourable, as illustrated in Figure 1. Few studies have used PCR for a quantitative examination of methanogen communities, and most of these studies have exclusively targeted a constitutive gene, i.e., *16S rRNA* (Freitag & Prosser, 2009; Rizzi *et al.*, 2006). However, in the last few years, methods based on a functional gene, i.e., *mcrA*, and its diversity have been proposed as screening methods (Freitag *et al.*, 2009). The analysis of *mcrA* can be used in conjunction with or independently of the 16S rRNA gene, and it minimises potential problems with non-specific amplification (Steinberg & Regan, 2008). Mcr is exclusive to methanogens, with the exception of methane-oxidising Archaea (Knittel *et al.*, 2009; Whitman *et al.*, 2006), and specific primers have been developed for the Mcr α-subunit gene sequence *(mcrA)*((Franke-Whittle *et al.*, 2009; Luton *et al.*, 2002; Steinberg *et al.*, 2008). TaqMan probes were also designed to target nine different phylogenetic groups of methanogens in qRT-PCR assays. Members of the *Methanosaeta* (*msa* probe), *Methanosarcina* (*msar* probe), and Methanocorpusculaceae (*mcp* probe) and MCR2b clusters (*mcr2b* probe) were detected in environmental samples (Steinberg & Regan, 2009; Traversi *et al.*, 2011).

Most of the known methane-oxidising Archaea have the key enzyme methane monooxygenase. One of the two forms of this enzyme is the particulate methane monooxygenase. The gene coding for the alpha subunit of pMMO (*pmoA*) is widely used as a biological marker to study methanotrophic bacteria. A recent study targeted the *mcrA* and *pmoA* genes to examine the relationship between biogeochemical process rates and microbial functional activity (Freitag *et al.*, 2010). Regarding the equilibrium condition that promotes a good methanisation, SAO has a role, as previously described (section 2.2). SAO bacteria can be quantified using the formyltetrahydrofolate synthetase (*fhs*) gene, which can be used an ecological biomarker for syntrophic acetate oxidation, although this enzyme also catalyses the formation of acetate from $H_2$ and $CO_2$ (Hori *et al.*, 2011; Xu *et al.*, 2009). Sulphate reduction is associated with a set of unique proteins. Some of these proteins are also present in sulphur-oxidising organisms, whereas others are shared with anaerobes such as methanogens. *Deltaproteobacteria*, mostly *Desulfovibrio spp* (Matias et al., 2005; Rabus *et al.*, 2004), but previous analyses have indicated that the composition of energy metabolism proteins could vary significantly between different SRB (Junier *et al.*, 2010; Pereira *et al.*, 2011; Rabus *et al.*, 2004). Although there are very few published data on sulphate-reducing bacteria during AD, a recent study used a qRT-PCR analysis of *dsrAB*, a gene that codes for the α subunit of dissimilatory sulphite reductase. The SRBs concentrations ranged between $10^4 - 10^7$ cells for each gram of volatile solids, at least four orders less than methanogen concentrations (Merlino *et al.*, 2012). On the whole, the qRT-PCR method seems to be suitable for microbiologic evaluation during AD (Merlino *et al.*, 2012; Traversi *et al.*, 2012). Therefore qRT-PCR is an advantageous tool for identifying the indicators that are able to predict sufferance condition to avoid biogas loss and improve biogas quality.

# 4    Prevalent Microbe Communities during Methanogenesis

A literature review on the quantification of the microbe communities during AD shows a relevant number of cells that is greater than $10^16$ per ml. This population consists mainly of bacteria and methanogens (~ $10^8$ cells/mL) (Amani *et al.*, 2010). Recent research has focused on the precise characterisation of the consortia with the final objective to link microbial community structure to function. Toward this aim, molecular techniques, such as denaturing gradient gel electrophoresis (DGGE) and correlated molecular analysis parameters, are valuable tools (Marzorati *et al.*, 2008). The bacterial sequences generated from the anaerobic digester were distributed among three major phyla: Firmicutes (> 80%); Actinobacteria (~10%); Bacteroidetes (~3%), along with other phyla at minor predominance (Garcia-Pena *et al.*, 2011). There was a high variability observable in the composition of the microbe communities. However, with respect to the bacterial profiles, the archaeal community patterns differed among diverse reactors but showed a minor diversity (Lerm *et al.*, 2012). The morphology and structure of the granules in the feedings have been studied, and different families of bacteria and methanogens were found to be present on the surface and in the dark centre (Nizami & Murphy, 2011). Recent classification of metagenome reads during anaerobic digestion identified Clostridium as most prevalent bacteria in the hydrolysis phase, indicating a predominant role for plant material digestion. *Methanosarcina* and *Methanothermobacter* were revealed as most prevalent methanogenic Archaea.

However, the metagenome analysis unveiled a large number of reads with unidentified microbial origin, indicating that the anaerobic degradation process may also be conducted by species currently unknown (Rademacher *et al.*, 2012).

Figure 2 shows the prevalent methanogens during the anaerobic co-digestion of organic fractions of municipal solid waste (OFMSW) and wastewater sludge. In this type of reactor, the Methanomicrobiales are generally prevalent. The most abundant is Methanosarcina with nearly $10^7$ gene copies/l. Between the most prevalent and the other detected methanogen families, there is nearly a 3-fold log difference in abundance. *Methanosaeta* and *Methanocorpuscolaceae* are present nearly at the same level. Both the *Methanosarcina* and *Methanosaeta* concentrations are significantly correlated with the biogas production rate ($0.744p < 0.01$ and $0.641p < 0.05$) (Traversi *et al.*, 2011). The acetoclastic Methanosaetaceae was more sensitive than hydrogenotrophic Methanobacteriales and Methanomicrobiales to the effects of toxins. Quantication of the syntrophic acetate oxidising bacteria is required to gain better insight into the dominating pathway of acetate degradation. SAO bacteria can be quantified using the formyltetrahydrofolate synthetase (*fhs*) gene, which can be an ecological biomarker for syntrophic acetate oxidation, although this enzyme also catalyses the formation of acetate from $H_2$ and $CO_2$ (Hori *et al.*, 2011; Xu *et al.*, 2009). As reflected by the increase in *fhs* gene copy numbers ($\sim 10^7 - 10^8$/ml), reductive homoacetogenesis from $H_2/CO_2$ was also stimulated by selective inhibition of methanogenesis with, for example, 2-bromoethanesulfonate (Xu *et al.*, 2010).

Methanotrophs can be present in the digester, and this possibility can affect the methanogens determination, depending on the functional gene *mcrA*. However, the level of these microorganisms in an anaerobic condition is much lower than the level of methanogens. Furthermore, concerning biogas quality, to control the presence of sulphur compounds in the biogas, various bio-molecular based methods can be adopted. Different studies describe the SRB communities in diverse environmental sample, including an anaerobic reactor, as summarised in Table 1. Generally, we describe the use of functional genes as targets. This presents some advantages, including fewer copies of the gene in each cell than there are copies of the constitutive genes and a higher GC content.

In Table 2, some biomolecular tools of the anaerobic reactors are described, such as indicators of ratios between different communities in the microbial flora. For each proposed ratio, a hypothetical benchmark is high-flyer theorised. The proposed integrative tools, with some clearly still in the development phase, can help judge the anaerobic reactor microbiomes overall performance as an anaerobic digester and enhance the biogas quality. However, using qRT-PCR methods in applied microbiology can be affected by an over- or undervaluation in relation to the chosen gene target and reaction efficiency.

| Sample type | Gene target | SRB quantification – principal findings | References |
|---|---|---|---|
| Industrial wastewater | dsrAB and aps A | SRB displayed a higher abundance during the summer (~ $10^7 - 10^8$ targets /mL) and lower during the winter (~ $10^4 - 10^5$ targets/mL) | (Ben-Dov *et al.*, 2007) |
| Saline and hypersaline soda lakes | dsr | Ranged from $10^5 - 10^8$ cell/ml of sediment in different lakes. The results demonstrated the existence of active SRB halophilic communities with a high diversity in soda lakes. | (Foti *et al.*, 2007) |
| Marine sediments of Black Sea | mcrA, dsr, aprA, cbbl (for RuBiSco enzyme complex) as functional genes, 16S RNA and 18S RNA as constitutive genes | apr A=$10^9$ copies/ml. Similar quantification between 16S RNA and functional genes | (Schippers *et al.*, 2012) |
| Marine sediments Per and Black Sea | dsrA, aprA | The dsr A and apr A copy numbers decreased from $10^7 - 10^8$ copies/g at the sediment surface to less than $10^5$ copies/g below 0.6 mbsf. | (Blazejak & Schippers, 2011) |
| Water samples from oil-water separation tanks from oil fields | dsrB and 16S RNA | Samples have a numbers of sulfate reducers approximately in the range of $10^5 - 10^6$ copies/mL of dsr B gene. The 16S RNA gene copies were in the magnitude of $10^6 - 10^7$ copies/mL of production. | (Agrawal *et al.*, 2009) |
| Industrial wastewater evaporation ponds | dsrA | $10^6 - 10^8$ targets/ml during the summer, $10^3 - 10^5$ targets/ml during the spring-autumn. | (Ben-Dov *et al.*, 2009) |
| Faecal samples | aps, 16S RNA | The sulphate reducing bacterial gene APS reductase was detected at densities ranging from 0,0083% ($10^7$ genes/g) to 5,5681% ($10^9$ genes/g) of the total microbial population among adults. | (Stewart *et al.*, 2006) |
| Sediment of the Sein estuary | dsrAB | Maximal values were observed in June, with a peak of $6630 \pm 1061$ dsr AB genes per ng of DNA | (Leloup *et al.*, 2005) |

**Table 1:** Literature reporting the quantification of SRB from different sample types, through molecular biology methods (qRT-PCR, DGGE).

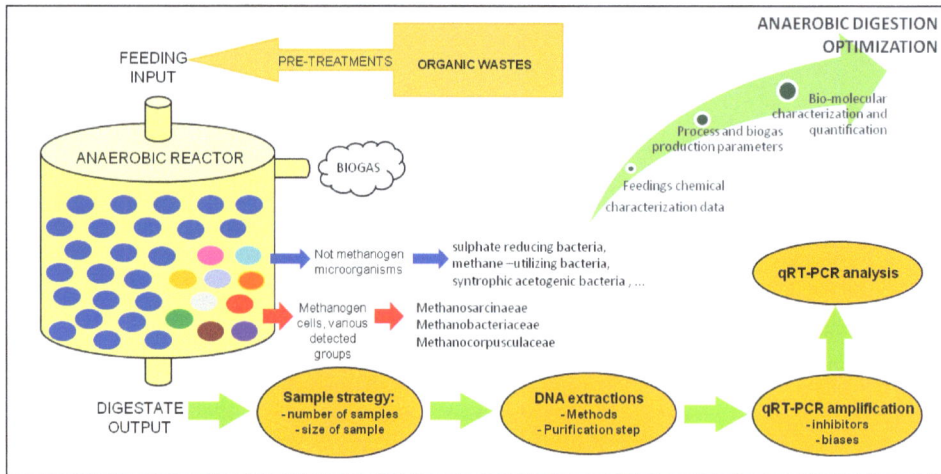

**Figure 1:** A pilot or full-scale digester is necessary for the study model. The input material has to be well known; the material generally consists of selected and pre-treated organic waste. In the anaerobic reactor, a selection of the microorganisms takes place. The key microorganisms influencing the biogas quantity and quality are methanogens and non-methanogens. The yellow ovals consist of a schematic representation of the steps required to quantify microorganisms using quantitative PCR in an AD system and other key considerations. In the grey square is summarised the objective of this biomolecular approach, which is to correlate feeding properties, process descriptions and biogas production with bio-molecular quantification to attain AD optimisation.

| Microbiologic ratio | Target gene in qPCR | Hypothetical |
|---|---|---|
| Total methanogens/Total microbial flora | *mcrA*/16sRNA | >0.001 |
| Methanosarcina /Total methanogens | *probemsar*/*mcrA* | >0.1 |
| Methanosaeta/Total methanogens | *probemsa*/*mcrA* | <0.01 |
| Methanosaeta /Methanosarcina | *probemsa*/*probemsar* | <0.1 |
| | | |
| Total SRB/Total microbial flora | *dsrAB*/16sRNA | <0.000001 |
| Total SRB/Total methanogens | *dsrAB*/*mcrA* | ¡0.001 |
| | | |
| Total SAO/Total microbial flora | *fhs*/16sRNA | ≥ 0.0001 |
| Total MO/Total microbial flora | *pmoA*/16sRNA | <0.0000001 |
| | | |
| Total SAO/Total methanogens | *fhs*/*mcrA* | ≥ 0.01 |
| Total MO/Total methanogens | *pmoAmcrA* | <0.0001 |

**Table 2:** Integrative tools for monitoring the microbiome of methanogenic bioreactors

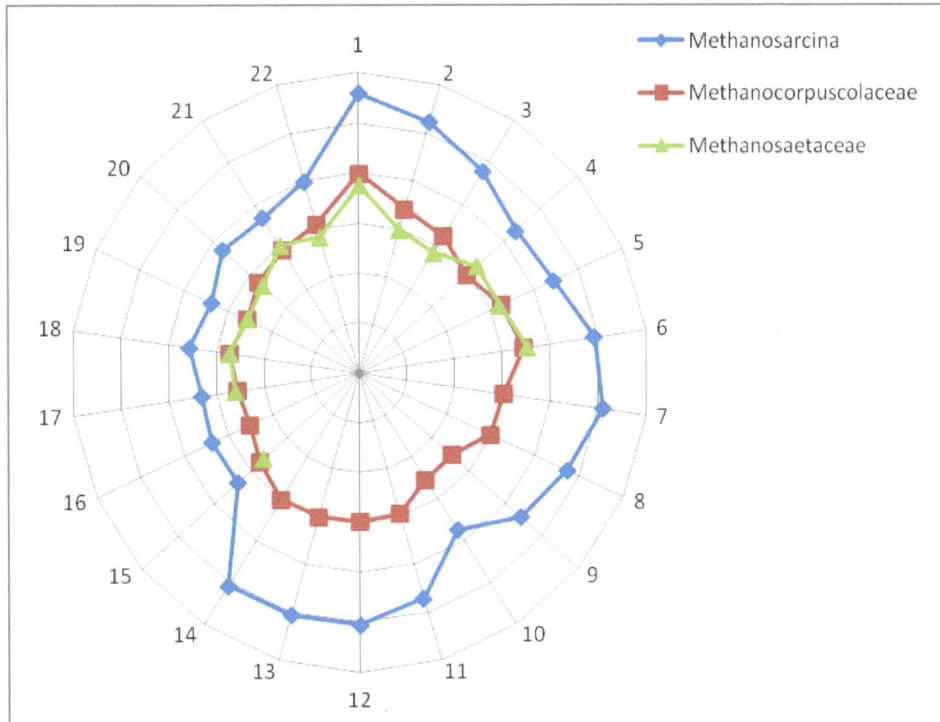

**Figure 2:** Methanogen taxa prevalence, expressed as 1/threshold cycle, in an anaerobic digester feeding with urban solid organic waste and wastewater treatment sludge. The areas in the colored lines are proportional to microorganism abundance in the same digester during the digestion.

# 5    Conclusion

AD can be considered one of the most important techniques to convert organic waste streams into renewable energy in the form of methane. AD is a widely used technique because it is able to carry out biogas production and organic waste stabilisation. It has several other advantages, including a low cell yield, a high organic loading rate, limited nutrient demand and low costs of operation and maintenance of the reactor system. The quality of the produced biogas is affected by the microorganism interactions in the digester. Monitoring the microbial community, especially the methanogen communities and SRB and SOB communities, in the anaerobic digester is therefore of crucial importance to promote optimal operational control. The methanogenic communities can be monitored using real-time PCR to determine various microbial parameters. For example, the ratio between *Methanosaeta* and *Methanosarcina* can be monitored within the archaeal community because it has been suggested that quantifying the total Archaea only is insufficient for operational stability. The quantification of other microorganisms such as the SOB, SRB and MO will be required to gain better insight into digestion control. SOB may help reveal the dominating pathway of acetate degradation, SRB quantification may help control the presence of sulphur compounds in the biogas, and MO can be used as indicator of methanotroph reactions in the reactor. The biomolecular approach seems to be a useful and illuminating strategy for AD improvement; however, several technical and methodological aspects of qRT-PCR application to the anaerobic microbiome have to be improved and standardised.

# References

References Agrawal A., Vanbroekhoven K. and Lal B. (2009). Diversity of culturable sulfidogenic bacteria in two oil-water separation tanks in the north-eastern oil fields of India. Anaerobe 16:12-8.

Amani T., Nosrati M. and Mousavi S. M. (2011). Using enriched cultures for elevation of anaerobic syntrophic interactions between acetogens and methanogens in a high-load continuous digester. Bioresour Technol 102:3716-23.

Amani T., Nosrati M. and Sreekrishnan T. R. (2010). Anaerobic digestion from the viewpoint of microbiological, chemical, and operational aspects - a review. Environmental Reviews 18:255-278.

Appels L., Baeyens J., Degreve J. and Dewil R. (2008). Principles and potential of the anaerobic digestion of waste-activated sludge. Progress in Energy and Combustion Science 34:755-781.

Balat M. & Balat H. (2009). Biogas as a Renewable Energy SourceA Review. Energy Sources Part a-Recovery Utilization and Environmental Effects 31:1280-1293.

Batstone D. J., Keller J. and Steyer J. P. (2006). A review of ADM1 extensions, applications, and analysis: 2002-2005. Water Sci Technol 54:1-10.

Bauer C., Korthals M., Gronauer A. and Lebuhn M. (2008). Methanogens in biogas production from renewable resources - a novel molecular population analysis approach. Water Science and Technology 58:1433-1439.

Ben-Dov E., Brenner A. and Kushmaro A. (2007). Quantification of sulfate-reducing bacteria in industrial wastewater, by real-time polymerase chain reaction (PCR) using dsrA and apsA genes. Microb Ecol 54:439-51.

Ben-Dov E., Kushmaro A. and Brenner A. (2009). Long-term surveillance of sulfate-reducing bacteria in highly saline industrial wastewater evaporation ponds. Saline Systems 5:2.

Bertin L., Bettini C., Zanaroli G., Frascari D. and Fava F. (2012). A continuous-flow approach for the development of an anaerobic consortium capable of an effective biomethanization of a mechanically sorted organic fraction of municipal solid waste as the sole substrate. Water Res 46:413-24.

Blazejak A. & Schippers A. (2011). Real-Time PCR Quantification and Diversity Analysis of the Functional Genes aprA and dsrA of Sulfate-Reducing Prokaryotes in Marine Sediments of the Peru Continental Margin and the Black Sea. Front Microbiol 2:253.

Bouallagui H., Touhami Y., Cheikh R. B. and Hamdi M. (2005). Bioreactor performance in anaerobic digestion of fruit and vegetable wastes. Process Biochemistry 40:989-995.

Chou H. H., Huang J. S., Chen S. K. and Lee M. C. (2011). Process kinetics of an expanded granular sludge bed reactor treating sulfate-containing wastewater. Chemical Engineering Journal 170:233-240.

Dar S. A., Yao L., van Dongen U., Kuenen J. G. and Muyzer G. (2007). Analysis of diversity and activity of sulfate-reducing bacterial communities in sulfidogenic bioreactors using 16S rRNA and dsrB genes as molecular markers. Appl Environ Microbiol 73:594-604.

Das Neves L. C. M., Converti A. and Penna T. C. V. (2009). Biogas Production: New Trends for Alternative Energy Sources in Rural and Urban Zones. Chemical Engineering & Technology 32:1147-1153.

De Vrieze J., Hennebel T., Boon N. and Verstraete W. (2012). Methanosarcina: The rediscovered methanogen for heavy duty biomethanation. Bioresour Technol 112:1-9.

Demirel B. & Scherer P. (2008). The roles of acetotrophic and hydrogenotrophic methanogens during anaerobic conversion of biomass to methane: a review. Rev Environ Sci Biotechnol 7:173-190.

Diaz I., Donoso-Bravo A. and Fdz-Polanco M. (2011a). Effect of microaerobic conditions on the degradation kinetics of cellulose. Bioresour Technol 102:10139-42.

Diaz I., Perez S. I., Ferrero E. M. and Fdz-Polanco M. (2011b). Effect of oxygen dosing point and mixing on the microaerobic removal of hydrogen sulphide in sludge digesters. Bioresource Technology 102:3768-3775.

Edwards R. A., Rodriguez-Brito B., Wegley L., Haynes M., Breitbart M., Peterson D. M., Saar M. O., Alexander S., Alexander E. C., Jr. and Rohwer F. (2006). Using pyrosequencing to shed light on deep mine microbial ecology. BMC Genomics 7:57.

Ettwig K. F., Shima S., van de Pas-Schoonen K. T., Kahnt J., Medema M. H., op den Camp H. J. M., Jetten M. S. M. and Strous M. (2008). Denitrifying bacteria anaerobically oxidize methane in the absence of Archaea. Environmental Microbiology 10:3164-3173.

Fauque G., Peck H. D., Jr., Moura J. J., Huynh B. H., Berlier Y., DerVartanian D. V., Teixeira M., Przybyla A. E., Lespinat P. A., Moura I. and et al. (1988). The three classes of hydrogenases from sulfate-reducing bacteria of the genus Desulfovibrio. FEMS Microbiol Rev 4:299-344.

Fortuny M., Gamisans X., Deshusses M. A., Lafuente J., Casas C. and Gabriel D. (2011). Operational aspects of the desulfurization process of energy gases mimics in biotrickling filters. Water Research 45:5665-5674.

Foti M., Sorokin D. Y., Lomans B., Mussman M., Zacharova E. E., Pimenov N. V., Kuenen J. G. and Muyzer G. (2007). Diversity, activity, and abundance of sulfate-reducing bacteria in saline and hypersaline soda lakes. Appl Environ Microbiol 73:2093-100.

Franke-Whittle I. H., Goberna M. and Insam H. (2009). Design and testing of real-time PCR primers for the quantification of Methanoculleus, Methanosarcina, Methanothermobacter, and a group of uncultured methanogens. Can J Microbiol 55:611-6.

Franzle O. (2006). Complex bioindication and environmental stress assessment. Ecological Indicators 6:114-136.

Freitag T. E. & Prosser J. I. (2009). Correlation of methane production and functional gene transcriptional activity in a peat soil. Appl Environ Microbiol 75:6679-87.

Freitag T. E., Toet S., Ineson P. and Prosser J. I. (2010). Links between methane flux and transcriptional activities of methanogens and methane oxidizers in a blanket peat bog. FEMS Microbiol Ecol 73:157-65.

Friedrich M. W. (2005). Methyl-coenzyme M reductase genes: unique functional markers for methanogenic and anaerobic methane-oxidizing Archaea. Methods Enzymol 397:428-42.

Fritz G., Buchert T., Huber H., Stetter K. O. and Kroneck P. M. (2000). Adenylylsulfate reductases from archaea and bacteria are 1:1 alphabeta-heterodimeric iron-sulfur flavoenzymes–high similarity of molecular properties emphasizes their central role in sulfur metabolism. FEBS Lett 473:63-6.

Garcia-Pena E. I., Parameswaran P., Kang D. W., Canul-Chan M. and Krajmalnik-Brown R. (2011). Anaerobic digestion and co-digestion processes of vegetable and fruit residues: process and microbial ecology. Bioresour Technol 102:9447-55.

Hedderich R. & Whitman W. B. (2006).Physiology and Biochemistry of the mathane-producing Archeae in (1050-1079).

Hori T., Sasaki D., Haruta S., Shigematsu T., Ueno Y., Ishii M. and Lgarashi Y. (2011). Detection of active, potentially acetate-oxidizing syntrophs in an anaerobic digester by flux measurement and formyltetrahydrofolate synthetase (FTHFS) expression profiling. Microbiology-Sgm 157:1980-1989.

Jenicek P., Koubova J., Bindzar J. and Zabranska J. (2010). Advantages of anaerobic digestion of sludge in microaerobic conditions. Water Sci Technol 62:427-34.

Junier P., Junier T., Podell S., Sims D. R., Detter J. C., Lykidis A., Han C. S., Wigginton N. S., Gaasterland T. and Bernier-Latmani R. (2010). The genome of the Gram-positive metal- and sulfate-reducing bacterium Desulfotomaculum reducens strain MI-1. Environ Microbiol 12:2738-54.

Klein M., Friedrich M., Roger A. J., Hugenholtz P., Fishbain S., Abicht H., Blackall L. L., Stahl D. A. and Wagner M. (2001). Multiple lateral transfers of dissimilatory sulfite reductase genes between major lineages of sulfate-reducing prokaryotes. Journal of Bacteriology 183:6028-6035.

Knittel K. & Boetius A. (2009). Anaerobic Oxidation of Methane: Progress with an Unknown Process. Annual Review of Microbiology 63:311-334.

Kremer D. R., Veenhuis M., Fauque G., Peck H. D., Legall J., Lampreia J., Moura J. J. G. and Hansen T. A. (1988). Immunocytochemical Localization of Aps Reductase and Bisulfite Reductase in 3 Desulfovibrio Species. Archives of Microbiology 150:296-301.

Leloup J., Petit F., Boust D., Deloffre J., Bally G., Clarisse O. and Quillet L. (2005). Dynamics of sulfate-reducing microorganisms (dsrAB genes) in two contrasting mudflats of the Seine estuary (France). Microb Ecol 50:307-14.

Lerm S., Kleybocker A., Miethling-Graff R., Alawi M., Kasina M., Liebrich M. and Wurdemann H. (2012). Archaeal community composition affects the function of anaerobic co-digesters in response to organic overload. Waste Manag 32:389-99.

Liu C., Li L., Ma J. K., Wu G. and Yang J. L. (2011). [Analysis of methanogenic community of anaerobic granular sludge based on mcrA gene]. Huan Jing Ke Xue 32:1114-9.

Liu Y. C. & Whitman W. B. (2008). Metabolic, phylogenetic, and ecological diversity of the methanogenic archaea. Incredible Anaerobes: From Physiology to Genomics to Fuels 1125:171-189.

Loy A., Kusel K., Lehner A., Drake H. L. and Wagner M. (2004). Microarray and functional gene analyses of sulfate-reducing prokaryotes in low-sulfate, acidic fens reveal cooccurrence of recognized genera and novel lineages. Appl Environ Microbiol 70:6998-7009.

Loy A., Lehner A., Lee N., Adamczyk J., Meier H., Ernst J., Schleifer K. H. and Wagner M. (2002). Oligonucleotide microarray for 16S rRNA gene-based detection of all recognized lineages of sulfate-reducing prokaryotes in the environment. Appl Environ Microbiol 68:5064-81.

Luton P. E., Wayne J. M., Sharp R. J. and Riley P. W. (2002). The mcrA gene as an alternative to 16S rRNA in the phylogenetic analysis of methanogen populations in landfill. Microbiology 148:3521-30.

Ma J., Van Wambeke M., Carballa M. and Verstraete W. (2008). Improvement of the anaerobic treatment of potato processing wastewater in a UASB reactor by co-digestion with glycerol. Biotechnol Lett 30:861-7.

Marzorati M., Wittebolle L., Boon N., Daffonchio D. and Verstraete W. (2008). How to get more out of molecular fingerprints: practical tools for microbial ecology. Environ Microbiol 10:1571-81.

Mata-Alvarez J., Dosta J., Mace S. and Astals S. (2011). Codigestion of solid wastes: A review of its uses and perspectives including modeling. Critical Reviews in Biotechnology 31:99-111.

Matias P. M., Pereira I. A., Soares C. M. and Carrondo M. A. (2005). Sulphate respiration from hydrogen in Desulfovibrio bacteria: a structural biology overview. Prog Biophys Mol Biol 89:292-329.

Merlino G., Rizzi A., Villa F., Sorlini C., Brambilla M., Navarotto P., Bertazzoni B., Zagni M., Araldi F. and Daffonchio D. (2012). Shifts of microbial community structure during anaerobic digestion of agro-industrial energetic crops and food industry byproducts. Journal of Chemical Technology and Biotechnology 87:1302-1311.

Meulepas R. J., Jagersma C. G., Zhang Y., Petrillo M., Cai H., Buisman C. J., Stams A. J. and Lens P. N. (2010). Trace methane oxidation and the methane dependency of sulfate reduction in anaerobic granular sludge. FEMS Microbiol Ecol 72:261-71.

Meyer B. & Kuever J. (2007a). Molecular analysis of the distribution and phylogeny of dissimilatory adenosine-5'-phosphosulfate reductase-encoding genes (aprBA) among sulfur-oxidizing prokaryotes. Microbiology 153:3478-98.

Meyer B. & Kuever J. (2007b). Phylogeny of the alpha and beta subunits of the dissimilatory adenosine-5'-phosphosulfate (APS) reductase from sulfate-reducing prokaryotes–origin and evolution of the dissimilatory sulfate-reduction pathway. Microbiology 153:2026-44.

Minz D., Flax J. L., Green S. J., Muyzer G., Cohen Y., Wagner M., Rittmann B. E. and Stahl D. A. (1999). Diversity of sulfate-reducing bacteria in oxic and anoxic regions of a microbial mat characterized by comparative analysis of dissimilatory sulfite reductase genes. Appl Environ Microbiol 65:4666-71.

Muyzer G. & Stams A. J. (2008). The ecology and biotechnology of sulphate-reducing bacteria. Nat Rev Microbiol 6:441-54.

Nettmann E., Bergmann I., Pramschufer S., Mundt K., Plogsties V., Herrmann C. and Klocke M. (2010). Polyphasic analyses of methanogenic archaeal communities in agricultural biogas plants. Appl Environ Microbiol 76:2540-8.

Nizami A. S. & Murphy J. D. (2011). Optimizing the Operation of a Two-Phase Anaerobic Digestion System Digesting Grass Silage. Environmental Science & Technology 45:7561-7569.

Pereira I. A., Ramos A. R., Grein F., Marques M. C., da Silva S. M. and Venceslau S. S. (2011). A comparative genomic analysis of energy metabolism in sulfate reducing bacteria and archaea. Front Microbiol 2:69.

Rabus R., Hansen, T., and Widdel, F. (2006).Dissimilatory sulfate- and sulfur-reducing prokaryotes in Prokaryotes.M. Dworkin, Falkow, S., Rosenberg, E., Schleifer, K.H., and Stackebrandt, E.. Springer New York (659 - 768).

Rabus R., Ruepp A., Frickey T., Rattei T., Fartmann B., Stark M., Bauer M., Zibat A., Lombardot T., Becker I., Amann J., Gellner K., Teeling H., Leuschner W. D., Glockner F. O., Lupas A. N., Amann R. and Klenk H. P. (2004). The genome of Desulfotalea psychrophila, a sulfate-reducing bacterium from permanently cold Arctic sediments. Environ Microbiol 6:887-902.

Rademacher A., Zakrzewski M., Schluter A., Schonberg M., Szczepanowski R., Goesmann A., Puhler A. and Klocke M. (2012). Characterization of microbial biofilms in a thermophilic biogas system by high-throughput metagenome sequencing. FEMS Microbiol Ecol 79:785-99.

Rastogi G., Ranade D. R., Yeole T. Y., Gupta A. K., Patole M. S. and Shouche Y. S. (2009). Novel methanotroph diversity evidenced by molecular characterization of particulate methane monooxygenase A (pmoA) genes in a biogas reactor. Microbiol Res 164:536-44.

Rizzi A., Zucchi M., Borin S., Marzorati M., Sorlini C. and Daffonchio D. (2006). Response of methanogen populations to organic load increase during anaerobic digestion of olive mill wastewater. Journal of Chemical Technology and Biotechnology 81:1556-1562.

Rozzi A. & Remigi E. (2004). Methods of assessing microbial activity and inhibition under anaerobic contitions: a literature review. Reviews in Environemntal Science and Bio/Technology 3:93-115.

Ryckebosch E., Drouillon M. and Veruaeren H. (2011). Techniques for transformation of biogas to biomethane. Biomass & Bioenergy 35:1633-1645.

Schievano A., D'Imporzano G. and Adani F. (2009). Substituting energy crops with organic wastes and agro-industrial residues for biogas production. J Environ Manage 90:2537-41.

Schippers A., Kock D., Hoft C., Koweker G. and Siegert M. (2012). Quantification of Microbial Communities in Subsurface Marine Sediments of the Black Sea and off Namibia. Front Microbiol 3:16.

Schnurer A. & Nordberg A. (2008). Ammonia, a selective agent for methane production by syntrophic acetate oxidation at mesophilic temperature. Water Science and Technology 57:735-740.

Schnurer A., Schink B. and Svensson B. H. (1996). Clostridium ultunense sp. nov., a mesophilic bacterium oxidizing acetate in syntrophic association with a hydrogenotrophic methanogenic bacterium. Int J Syst Bacteriol 46:1145-52.

Smith C. J. & Osborn A. M. (2009). Advantages and limitations of quantitative PCR (Q-PCR)-based approaches in microbial ecology. FEMS Microbiol Ecol 67:6-20.

Steinberg L. M. & Regan J. M. (2008). Phylogenetic comparison of the methanogenic communities from an acidic, oligotrophic fen and an anaerobic digester treating municipal wastewater sludge. Appl Environ Microbiol 74:6663-71.

Steinberg L. M. & Regan J. M. (2009). mcrA-targeted real-time quantitative PCR method to examine methanogen communities. Appl Environ Microbiol 75:4435-42.

Stewart J. A., Chadwick V. S. and Murray A. (2006). Carriage, quantification, and predominance of methanogens and sulfate-reducing bacteria in faecal samples. Lett Appl Microbiol 43:58-63.

Traversi D., Villa S., Acri M., Pietrangeli B., Degan R. and Gilli G. (2011). The role of different methanogen groups evaluated by Real-Time qPCR as high-efficiency bioindicators of wet anaerobic co-digestion of organic waste. AMB Express 1:28.

Traversi D., Villa S., Acri M., Pietrangeli B., Degan R. and Gilli G. (2012). The role of different methanogen groups evaluated by Real-Time qPCR as high-efficiency bioindicators of wet anaerobic co-digestion of organic waste. AMB Express 1:28.

Wagner M., Roger A. J., Flax J. L., Brusseau G. A. and Stahl D. A. (1998). Phylogeny of dissimilatory sulfite reductases supports an early origin of sulfate respiration. J Bacteriol 180:2975-82.

Ward A. J., Hobbs P. J., Holliman P. J. and Jones D. L. (2008). Optimisation of the anaerobic digestion of agricultural resources. Bioresour Technol 99:7928-40.

Whitman W. B., Bowen T. L. and Boone D. R. (2006). The Methanogenic Bacteria. Prokaryotes 3:165-207.

Wijekoon K. C., Visvanathan C. and Abeynayaka A. (2011). Effect of organic loading rate on VFA production, organic matter removal and microbial activity of a two-stage thermophilic anaerobic membrane bioreactor. Bioresour Technol, 102:5353-60.

Xu J. (2010).Metagenomics and ecosystems biology: conceptual frameworks, tools and methods in Metagenomics.D. Marco, Caister Academic Press Norfolk (UK) (1 - 13).

Xu K., Liu H. and Chen J. (2010). Effect of classic methanogenic inhibitors on the quantity and diversity of archaeal community and the reductive homoacetogenic activity during the process of anaerobic sludge digestion. Bioresour Technol, 101:2600-7.

Xu K. W., Liu H., Du G. C. and Chen J. (2009). Real-time PCR assays targeting formyltetrahydrofolate synthetase gene to enumerate acetogens in natural and engineered environments. Anaerobe, 15:204-213.

Zverlov V., Klein M., Lucker S., Friedrich M. W., Kellermann J., Stahl D. A., Loy A. and Wagner M. (2005). Lateral gene transfer of dissimilatory (bi)sulfite reductase revisited. J Bacteriol, 187:2203-8.

# Quantitative Analysis of DNA Transposon-mediated Gene Delivery: the *Sleeping Beauty* System as an Example

Orsolya Kolacsek
*Institute of Molecular Pharmacology, RCNS*
*Hungarian Academy of Sciences, Hungary*

Zsuzsanna Izsvák
*Mobile DNA Group*
*Max-Delbrück Center for Molecular Medicine, Germany*

Zoltán Ivics
*Division of Medical Biotechnology*
*Paul Ehrlich Institute, Germany*

Balázs Sarkadi
*Membrane Research Group of HAS*
*Semmelweis University and National Blood Center, Hungary*

Tamás I. Orbán
*Institute of Molecular Pharmacology, RCNS*
*Hungarian Academy of Sciences, Hungary*

# 1    Introduction – DNA Transposons as Genetic Tools

Transposons are special genetic elements that are capable of moving from one DNA locus to another. They were discovered in maize by Barbara McClintock in the 1940s, and these ground-breaking experiments later earned her the Nobel Prize in 1983. Transposons can be classified based on their replication intermediate (Class I retrotransposons and Class II DNA transposons), on their replication manner (replicative versus non-replicative transposons), or on their ability to disperse independently (autonomous versus non-autonomous elements) (Burns and Boeke, 2012). Once considered to be selfish units of replication, they are now believed to also represent inevitable driving forces for evolution, proven by their presence in all genomes examined so far (Kazazian, 2004; Hedges & Batzer, 2005; Feschotte & Pritham, 2007). The human genome is not an exception, as approximately 45% of our genetic material is made up of transposons (Biemont & Vieira, 2006; Mills *et al.*, 2006; Wicker *et al.*, 2007; Goodier & Kazazian, 2008; Solyom & Kazazian, 2012). The majority of the human transposons belong to the Class I retrotransposons (or RNA transposons) which move around by the replicative "copy and paste" mechanism. These contain currently active mobile elements which by all means played a significant role in human evolution (Mills *et al.*, 2007; Shen *et al.*, 2011). Moreover, LINE-1 retrotransposons were recently proven to be responsible for certain types of somatic mozaicisms present in vertebrate neurons (Singer *et al.*, 2010). Class II DNA transposons, however, make up a significantly smaller proportion (~3%) of the human genome. This moderate fraction might be attributable to the fact that the majority of them spread by the non-replicative "cut and paste" mechanism. In addition, none of the DNA transposons have been shown to be active in the human genome (Feschotte & Pritham, 2007; Collier & Largaespada, 2007; Izsvak *et al.*, 2010; Solyom & Kazazian, 2012).

Transposons as genetic tools have been widely used in invertebrate model organisms (*Drosophila* species or *Caenorhabditis elegans*), mainly exploiting active DNA transposons of the particular species. The most prominent examples are the P-elements which were used as proof of principle for the two component transposon gene delivery system in *Drosophila melanogaster* (Rubin & Spradling, 1982; Spradling & Rubin, 1982). For vertebrates, however, applications were limited to retrotransposons for a long time, with the obvious disadvantages of higher mutational rate (due to the reverse transcription process) and the long term genetic instability of the modified cells because of the potential remobilization of the integrated transgene (Uren *et al.*, 2005; Ostertag *et al.*, 2007). A significant breakthrough in vertebrate genetics was the creation of an artificial Tc1/Mariner-type transposon, the *Sleeping Beauty* (SB) system, which was the first DNA transposon proven to be active in vertebrates, including human cells (Ivics *et al.*, 1997). Its simple structure (Figure 1) made it easy to modify and to establish a controllable system by separating the transposase from its targets (the originally flanking terminal repeat sequences), thereby allowing the controlled delivery of any gene of interest into the genome (Izsvak *et al.*, 2000). However, the efficiency of the originally resurrected SB variant was still significantly lower than the widely used viral vectors so its potential seemed to be behind those other genetic vehicles, especially in human applications.

The success of "awakening" a new active DNA transposon initiated a wave of research aiming at establishing efficient novel transposon systems applicable in human cells. Apart from other reconstructed species (such as the *Frog Prince* from *Rana pipiens*, Miskey *et al.,* 2003), an active DNA transposon (*Tol2*) was discovered in medaka fish and successfully applied in various vertebrate species (Balciunas *et al.*, 2006). Moreover, a transposon from another insect species (*Trichoplusia ni*) called *piggyBac* (PB) was shown to be highly active in human cells (Ding *et al.*, 2005). In the meantime, hyperactive versions of the previously used DNA transposons were also established (Zayed *et al.*, 2004; Baus *et al.*, 2005; Pledger & Coates, 2005), opening the possibility of efficient non-viral gene delivery applications. The most promising of all was the 100 times more active form of SB (SB100x), providing a highly effective alternative to the existing viral gene delivery methods (Mates *et al.*, 2009).

In a recent study, the most hyperactive versions of three transposon systems (SB, PB and *Tol2*) were systematically tested and compared in terms of delivery efficiency, copy number and integration profile of the transgene (Grabundzija *et al.*, 2010). It was revealed that SB and PB are the most efficient gene delivery vehicles and, although transposition efficiency is known to decrease with the cargo size (Izsvak *et al.*, 2010), they are able to carry and integrate inserts of ≥10 kb, outweighing the packaging capacity of the most efficient viral vectors. It was also shown that in conditions where the amount of DNA transposon is limiting (modeling most gene therapy applications), SB is superior even to PB. Moreover, the integration profile of SB seems to be the most favorable one: in fact, it is the closest to random on the genomic level among all tested viral- and transposon-based systems so far (Vigdal *et al.*, 2002; Liu *et al.*, 2005; Yant *et al.*, 2005; Grabundzija *et al.*, 2010), providing the lowest risk for insertional mutagenesis and making the SB system particularly suitable for gene therapy applications. In addition, as opposed to PB, no potential endogenous elements resembling SB are present in the human genome (Ivics *et al.*, 1997; Ivics *et al.*, 2004) which is an important safety issue that further supported the initiation of a clinical trial experiment using this transposon system (Williams, 2008).

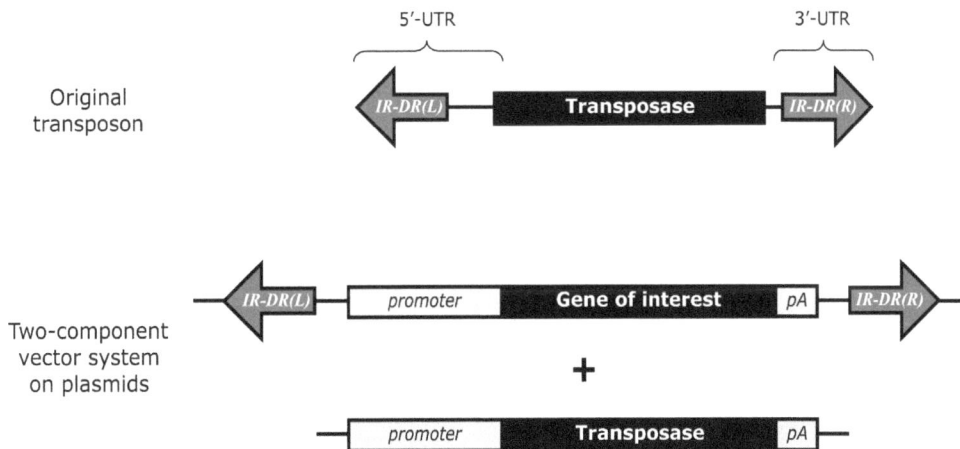

**Figure 1:** The structure of the *Sleeping Beauty* transposon system. In the natural transposon, the transposase gene is flanked by untranslated regions (UTRs) that include the terminal Inverted Repeat Direct Repeat regions (IRDR-L and IRDR-R), containing binding sites for the transposase. When used as a gene delivery vector system, the transposase coding region is replaced by a gene of interest within the transposable element that is maintained in a plasmid. This non-autonomous transposon can be mobilized if the transposase is supplied in trans by expression from a separate plasmid vector containing a suitable promoter. Co-transfection of the two components into candidate cells provides the platform for transposition from the donor plasmid to the cellular genome.

Considering all aspects, however, other efficient transposon systems with integration preferences into transcriptionally active regions (such as the PB system, Wilson *et al.*, 2007) might be more suitable when performing "traditional" forward genetic screens (Collier & Largaespada, 2005; Chew *et al.*, 2011; Guo *et al.*, 2011). Also, as the PB transposase is able to "tracelessly" remove the integrated transgene from the genome, it might be a method of choice when such a feature is desirable, exemplified by the removal of the reprogramming cassette after generating induced pluripotent stem cells from fibroblasts (Kaji *et al.*, 2009; Woltjen *et al.*, 2009). Nevertheless, there are still various aspects of the transposon-based technology that should be rigorously tested. Such issues include the potential silencing of the transgene which is often the drawback of viral vectors (Ellis, 2005), especially in the case of embryonic stem cells which are particularly prone to silence viral promoters (Meilinger *et al.*, 2009; Rowe *et al.*, 2010). So far, the already applied DNA transposon sequences did not seem to face this problem as in the case of SB the effect of silencing was shown to depend on the cargo sequence, and not on the transposon vector (Garrison *et al.*, 2007; Zhu *et al.*, 2010).

According to gene therapy guidelines or mutagenesis protocols, one of the most important issues is the exact and fast determination of transgene copy numbers (Bian & Belmont, 2010; Sivalingam *et al.*, 2010; Huang *et al.*, 2010). Various methods are available to perform this, including "traditional" blotting techniques (Southern blotting/dot blotting), or several polymerase chain reaction (PCR)-based techniques (Wicks *et al.*, 2000; Devon *et al.*, 1995). These usually involve the application of radioactively or fluorescently labeled probes, or – depending on the nature of the transgene – utilize the inherent signal originating from the transgene itself (such as quantifying GFP fluorescence, Moeller *et al.*, 2003). Apart from often requiring hazardous chemicals or being laborious, the general problem of these methods is that they are usually set up for a specific transgene, and changing the gene of interest will require optimizing the applied parameters of the method once again. Using the SB system in our laboratory, we aimed to develop an accurate and fast method to quantify transposon copy numbers that is applicable to any SB-based gene delivery experiments without *a priori* optimization of the protocol. We worked out a real-time PCR technique which is independent of the transgene sequence, hence we named it a "transgene independent" quantitative PCR technology (Kolacsek *et al.*, 2011). Apart from being sensitive, accurate and fast, this approach also offers a powerful non-radioactive technique as an alternative against other canonical methodologies.

In this chapter, using the SB transposon system as a prominent example, we address quantitative issues regarding the transposon-based gene delivery methods. We focus in detail on a transgene-independent qPCR method recently developed in our laboratory, providing more information in depth on the theoretical background and the technical aspects of this methodology published earlier (Kolacsek *et al.*, 2011). Additionally, we also cover a technique of measuring transposase activity at the excision phase of the reaction which allows comparative analysis of different transposase variants, different transposon systems or different conditions of application. We believe that these quantitative aspects of transposase activity are of great importance especially in light of the applicability of the DNA transposons for gene therapy purposes.

## 2    Selecting and Separating Transgenic Clones after Transposition

### 2.1    Selection Methodology

The basis of generating stable transgenic clones is to apply the most efficient but the least harmful gene delivery into the chosen cell types. The SB transposon is the method of choice in this respect as it offers a stable transgene integration technology with the least mutagenic potential among all available gene delivery techniques (see Section 1 above). Nevertheless, the bottleneck of this technology is that it involves the transfection of DNA into the host cells which might have low efficiency rates for certain cell types, such as embryonic stem cells. It is therefore necessary to apply an efficient and preferably non-invasive selection protocol to establish homogenous transgene expressing cells following transfection and transposition. Selection methods may sometimes be carried out utilizing the expression of the transgene but very often it is inescapable to use an additional marker gene even at the expense of having a larger genetic cargo, thereby lower delivery efficiency.

In applications where the cell source is not limiting, various chemical selection methods such as antibiotic selection can be applied to enrich for transgene expressing cells (Figure 2). However, depending on the cell type, this method might significantly disturb cell physiology, therefore other approaches are necessary to be applied. For example, the advantage of using fluorescent markers is that the transfected cells can be separated by Fluorescent Activated Cell Sorting (FACS) analysis (Figure 3), although some cell types may not tolerate such physical stress and this method could also decrease cell viability. The aim is to optimize the transfection/selection procedure for the particular cell type reaching the highest possible gene delivery efficiency with the lowest possible cell mortality rate.

## 2.2 Separating uniform clones

Some transgenic applications (e.g. transgenic animals) require genetically uniform cell populations, which can be precisely characterized from various aspects, including copy number and integration sites. These features can contribute to the transgenic phenotype to a large extent. To develop a "reliable" designated method for copy number determination, our goal was to detect the lowest (1) stable copy per cell, and to clearly differentiate cells differing in copy numbers by one (e.g. cells carrying 2 copies from those with 1 or 3 copies). In other words, with this method we wanted to detect the copy number as corpuscular units in the cells. This was an important reason why we aimed at working with genetically uniform clones that carry the same transgenic cassette in different copy numbers.

The simplest way for cloning is the threshold limit dilution of heterogeneous transgenic cell population, previously selected by the transgene or the marker gene expression. In this method, a serial dilution of the cells is spread in a 96-well cell culture plate and those wells are considered to represent one clone where only one colony can be seen by microscopy; those cell clones are then further maintained and utilized. However, this method cannot be applied to all cell types, such as human embryonic stem cells which naturally grow only in clumps. In such cases, other manual methods may be applied, including FACS selection or using cloning rings.

## 2.3 Isolation of a Single Copy Insertion Serving as a Calibration Unit

The major difficulty to start a particular copy number measurement project is the lack of reference samples with known copy numbers, also known as calibrators. If such samples determined by other techniques are not available, the first step is to isolate clones carrying 1 copy of the transgene.

Applying the hyperactive SB transposases often results in high copy numbers and working with such high efficiency transposon delivery may provide only small number of cells carrying 1 copy of the transgene. An obvious 1 copy clone source is the random integration of plasmids that most of the cases results in 1 transgenic copy. These integrations will contain the majority or the whole plasmid sequence, due to a random breakage of the transfected transposon vector. This can be achieved by transfecting the transposon donor plasmid either with the inactive mutant transposase variant or without the transposase expressing helper plasmid. Random integration is very ineffective, occurs usually in less than 1% of the transfected cells, but they can be selected out and can be cloned as well. This transfection serves as transposition control (Figure 2) resulting in traces of random integrations contrary to the active transposition, which has much higher integration efficiency, and it could provide us an excellent source of one copy clones.

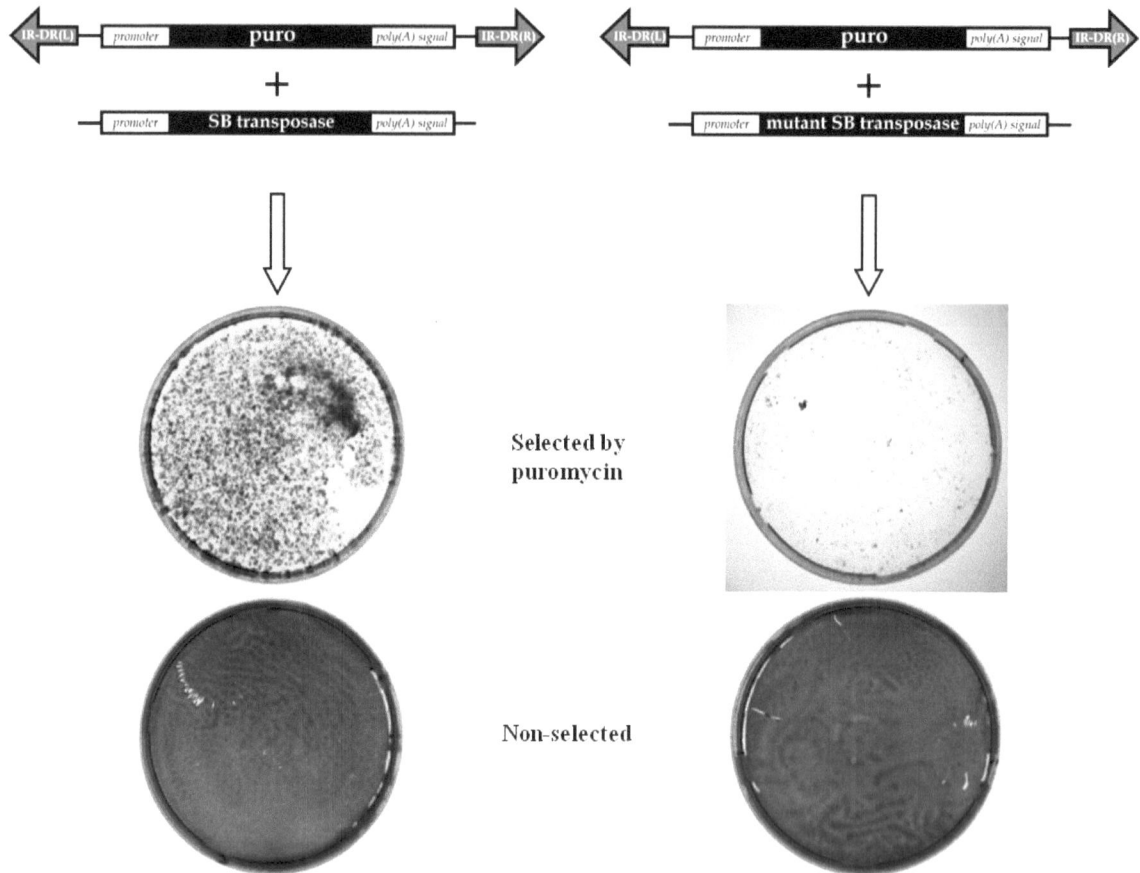

**Figure 2:** A typical experiments using SB tranposons: establishing transgenic HEK-293 cells expressing a puromycin resistance gene (puro). 2 days posttransfection, cells were passed into puromycin containing medium and selected for 10 days; living cells were visualized by Giemsa-staining following selection. The efficiency of transposition is obvious when comparing the selected cells after co-transfection with the transposase expressing helper plasmid (left) to the control experiment with the mutant transposase (right), the latter one indicating random integration events. As a negative control, non-selected cells are also shown in both experimental setups.

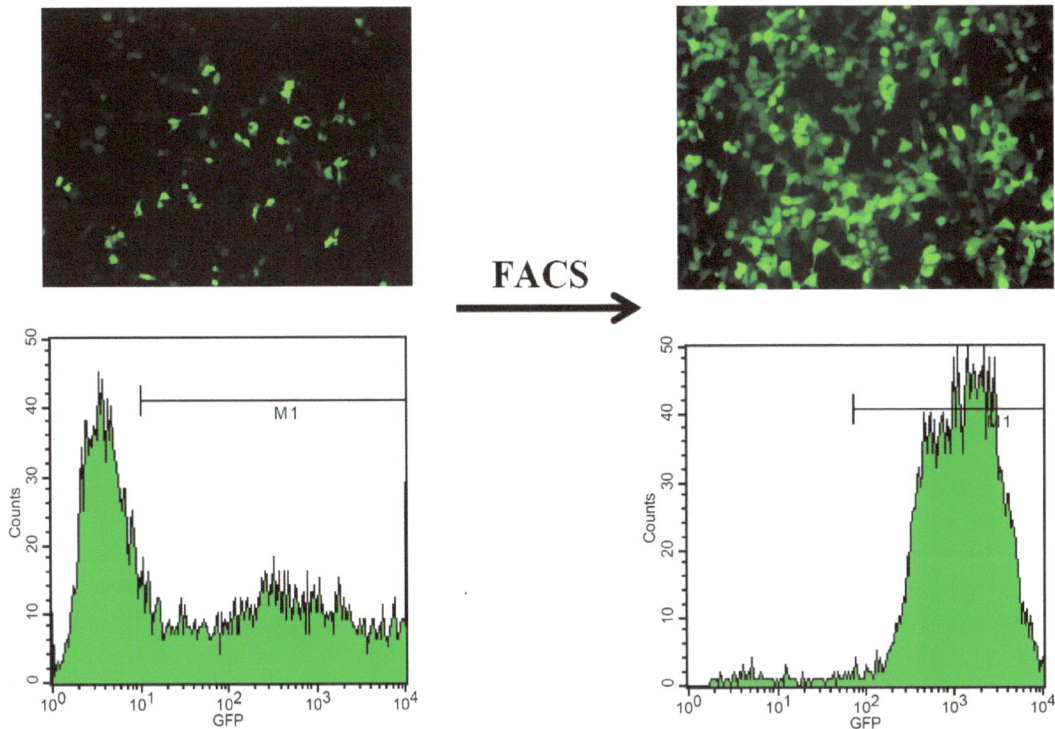

**Figure 3:** Transgene selection after transposition using GFP expression. The expression cassette is delivered into HEK-293 cells by the SB transposon system resulting in a heterogeneous cell population (left panels). Transgenic cells were selected by FACS experiment (right panels). Fluorescence microscopy images of x200 magnification and FACS histograms of GFP intensities can be seen. Cell numbers (Counts) are shown as a function of fluorescence intensity plotted in a logarithmic scale. M1: marker indicating GFP expressing cells.

# 3   Real-time PCR for Sequence Quantification

The polymerase chain reaction (PCR) is a technique for the in vitro amplification of specific DNA sequences by the simultaneous primer extension of complementary strands of DNA (Kleppe *et al.*, 1971; Mullis & Falona, 1987). It was a major development in molecular biology because it has simplified existing technologies and enabled a rapid development of new techniques which otherwise would not have been possible. PCR theoretically amplifies DNA exponentially, doubling the number of double stranded sequences present in each amplification cycle. After the logarithmic (log) phase of the reaction, the amount of the PCR product reaches the plateau phase (Figure 4). The amount of the product is proportional to the starting sequence copy number during the log phase, providing the basis for reliable quantitative comparisons.

In traditional (endpoint) PCR, detection and quantification of the amplified sequence are performed at the end of the reaction after the last PCR cycle, and involve post-PCR analysis such as gel electrophoresis, signal detection or image analysis. However, this allows only semi-quantitative analysis

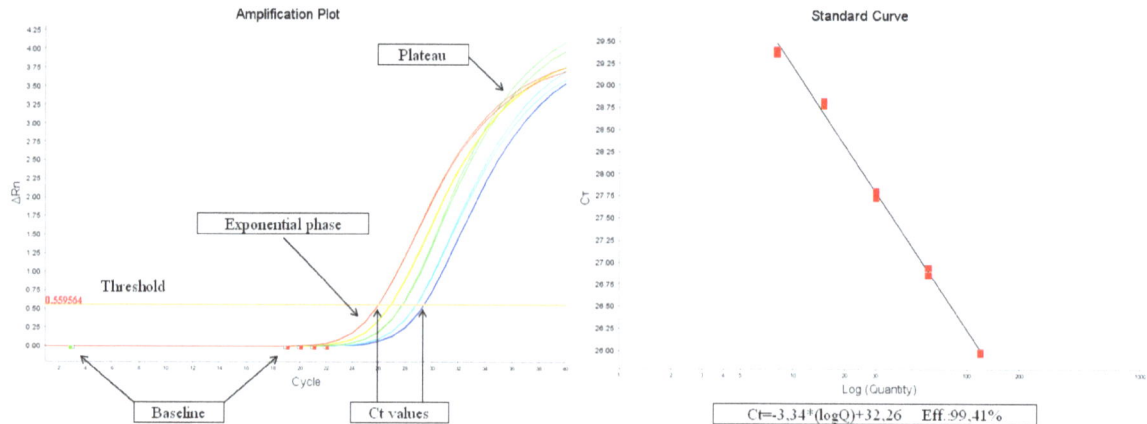

**Figure 4:** Example of a real-time PCR experiment determining the efficiency of the GFP TaqMan® assay using a standard curve of dilution points. Twofold dilutions were prepared from gDNA of pooled transgenic clones with the same copy number. Measurements were performed on a StepOnePlus™ Real-Time PCR platform (Applied Biosystems, Foster City, CA). Data were analyzed with the StepOne™ Software v2.1. Amplification plot (left panel) shows the increase of fluorescence signal as a function of cycle numbers (baseline fluorescence is subtracted, hence ΔRn; different colors represent different dilution reactions). Typical parameters of the reaction are indicated. The right panel shows the standard curve derived from the experiment, showing Ct values as a function of gDNA input (expressed in logarithm of DNA quantity in nanograms). The line of best fit is calculated by linear regression using the standard points; the equation is also shown from which efficiency of the reaction is calculated.

carried out in samples collected at multiple points throughout the amplification process, thus ensuring the analysis before the plateau is reached. This approach is usually combined with analysis of dilution series of the samples, it also requires known standards and provides a detection range of usually only tenfold difference (Chelly *et al.*, 1988; Wang *et al.*, 1989). In real-time quantitative PCR (qPCR), the amount of PCR product is measured at each cycle by the use of fluorescent dyes (Higuchi *et al.*, 1992; Livak *et al.*, 1995). This ability to monitor the reaction during its exponential phase enables the user to determine the initial amount of target with great precision. Apart from being simple and fast, the powerful benefit of qPCR is the increased dynamic range of comparisons.

The most popular fluorescent detection technologies are double-stranded DNA (dsDNA) binding agents, e.g. SYBR® Green, and fluorescent probes (Livak *et al.*, 1995; Wittwer *et al.*, 1997; Morrison *et al.*, 1998). SYBR® Green signal is measured at the end of each extension step and the intensity depends on the amount of dsDNA that is present. This technology is simple because the dye can be added to any kind of sequence amplification, but lacks specificity because it will also bind to PCR artifacts, e.g. primer-dimers. Good primer design and quality of starting materials are critical to avoid nonspecific products. Specificity of the reaction could be assessed using a melting curve measured at the end of the reaction (Figure 5). Melting curve determines the melting point (Tm) characteristic to the specific PCR product which assures differentiation of valid qPCR reactions from PCR artifacts (Ririe *et al.*, 1997). Those melting curves showing multiple peaks or one peak with rather different Tm than of the main product result from nonspecific PCR products indicating invalid reactions with false Ct values.

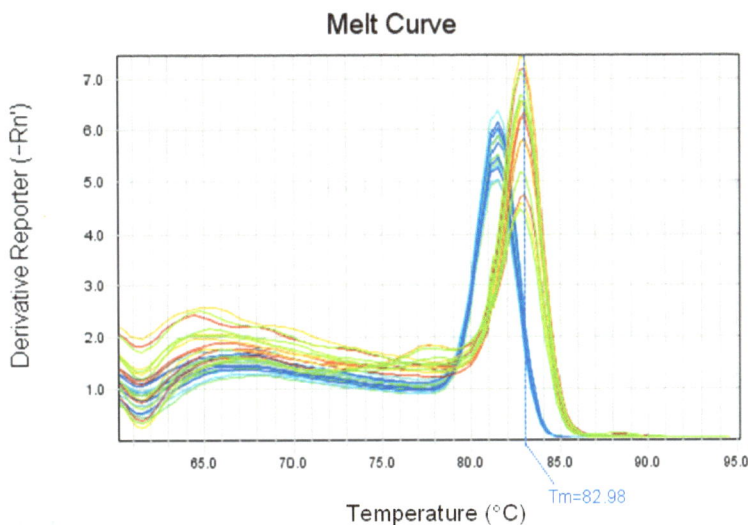

**Figure 5:** Representative melting curve analysis of a SYBR® Green qPCR experiment. Derivative of the fluorescence signal of the reporter (Rn') is shown as a function of the temperature. Two sequences (a target and an endogenous control) were amplified in various wells of this plate, therefore two melting peaks are visible; the melting temperature of the target is indicated. Different colors represent different reaction wells of the plate.

Fluorescent oligonucleotide probes (e.g. TaqMan® probes) are designed to hybridize to the sequence amplified by the primers. At the annealing step of each cycle, the probe will bind to the target sequence, and will be subsequently cleaved by the 5' nuclease activity of the polymerase during the extension phase. A dual labeled probe with a reporter dye at the 5' end and a quencher dye at the 3' end of the oligonucleotide will generate a fluorescent signal when the probe is degraded which is detected at the end of the extension phase (Livak *et al.*, 1995; Heid *et al.*, 1996). Probe-based systems provide highly specific detection of DNA, however, dual-labeling and complex design make them more expensive.

In qPCR, the cycle number in which the signal appears at the beginning of the log phase is considered to be inversely correlated to the amount of starting template, as a higher amount will result in sooner amplification. Threshold is the level of signal that reflects a statistically significant increase over the baseline fluorescent signal (Figure 4). In most cases, the real-time PCR software automatically sets the threshold at least 10 times the standard deviation of the fluorescence value of the baseline. However, the positioning of the threshold can be set manually at any point in the exponential phase of PCR. Threshold cycle (Ct) is the cycle number determined by the software at which the amplification plot crosses the threshold. Passive reference dyes (usually added to the qPCR master mixes) are frequently used in qPCR to normalize the fluorescent signal of reporter dyes (Rn). This allows the correction of fluctuations in fluorescence that is non-PCR-based, e.g. changes from well to well in reagent concentration or volume, or in instrument scanning (Figure 4).

Validation of the qPCR assay is generally carried out by the analysis of the slopes from standard curves. A standard curve is generated by plotting the results of a dilution series of the template against the Ct for each dilution (Figure 4). In theory, if the reaction is 100% efficient, the PCR duplicates the template in each cycle, and in the log scale of template amount, the slope will be $-3.32$ $(1/[\lg(x)-\lg(2x)] =$

–3.32). The reaction efficiency is related to assay sensitivity, which can be calculated from the slope (Real Time PCR Handbook, http://tools.invitrogen.com/content.cfm?pageid=12257):

$$\text{Efficiency} = 10^{(-1/\text{slope})} - 1.$$

The template used to generate the standard curve should match – as closely as possible – that is being used for the experiment (e.g. the same total RNA or DNA sample). The dilution range or dynamic range should span the concentration range expected for the unknown samples. The simplest way to ensure this is pooling the unknown samples (such as gDNAs from transgenic clones), and using it as a standard. The acceptable range of the efficiency, which most scientists agree on is between 90% – 110%. If efficiency is higher than 100%, it can reflect an inhibitory effect. In this case, scaling down the starting material usually helps by lowering the concentration of the suspected inhibitor. The desirable window of 90 to 110% defines the range of input template quantities that may be measured in a particular qPCR.

In the following three sections, we describe three different approaches which could be applied to determine transgene copy numbers of transgenic clones using a real-time PCR-based strategy.

# 4    Determining Transgene Copy Numbers of Transgenic Clones

## 4.1    First Approach: Verifying Presumably One Copy Clones with Absolute Quantification using the Marker Sequence

We generated SB transgenic clones carrying a GFP expressing cassette separating them by FACS analysis. Few clones were prepared also from random integration experiments, being obvious sources of 1 copy integrations as mentioned formerly. Since random integrations can be derived from breakage of the plasmid at any point, the presence of fluorescence in these clones assures the presence of the GFP transcription unit, so the GFP sequence can be reliably used for the copy number analysis. Therefore, specific TaqMan® assays were designed for the two terminal Inverted Repeat Direct Repeat (IRDR) motifs of the SB transposon (left and right, IRDR-L and IRDR-R), as well as for the GFP sequence. Sequences of primers and probes can be found in our previous publication (Kolacsek *et al.*, 2011).

In the absence of a reference clone with known copy number, we have to compare the absolute Ct values to known plasmid dilutions containing the transposon sequence. The recommended amount of gDNA input is in the range of 10 to 40 ng (we used 30 ng) but other input size of the starting material can also be accepted if in previous pilot experiments, the efficiency at that point was shown to be in the desired range. For calculations of the required plasmid dilutions, first we need to know how many genome copies are present in the 30ng gDNA input. The average molecular weight of a DNA base pair is 618g/mol, so using the Avogadro's number of $6.02 \times 10^{23}$ entities/mol, the molecular weight of a single haploid genome is $(3 \times 10^9$ bp/genome $\times$ 618 g/mol) / $6.02 \times 10^{23} = 3.08$ pg. Therefore, 30ng gDNA contains 30000 pg / 2 × 3.08 = 4870 copy of diploid cell genome and so a one copy clone must contain 4870 copy of the transgene. (Genome weight of other species can be found in the genome size database at www.genomesize.com.) Since we used a plasmid of 5800 bp in length, for the signal equivalent to the single copy clone, we needed approximately 4870 × (5800 bp × 618 g/mol) / $6.02 \times 10^{23} = 0.029$ pg of plasmid input. Considering a plasmid with concentration of 100 ng/µl, at least a $3.45 \times 10^6$-fold dilution is required to be in the similar range. The equivalent plasmid amount was put in the middle of our standard curve and two neighboring points of twofold dilutions were taken for the standard curve (Figure 6). With this setup applying the GFP TaqMan® assay, 5317 ± 195 copy was calculated for a randomly integrated GFP expressing clone, slightly differing from the desired 4870, estimating the copy number as $(5317 \pm 195) / 4870 = 1.09 \pm 0.04$.

In absolute quantification, each template must have sufficient purity and the input amount needs to be precisely quantified. The accuracy of the assay is directly related to the quality of the standard curve. Several dilution steps preceding each assay have to be performed with special attention, however, no matter how much care is taken, real-time PCR sensitivity amplifies minute human errors. In addition, the plasmid template used to generate the standard curve might not be an ideal specimen as it might not really represent the complex properties of the unknown samples. Due to such difficulties, absolute quantification seemed inconvenient for our routine transposon applications. Nevertheless, once we have successfully selected one copy clones, we could use them as reference samples for comparative analysis.

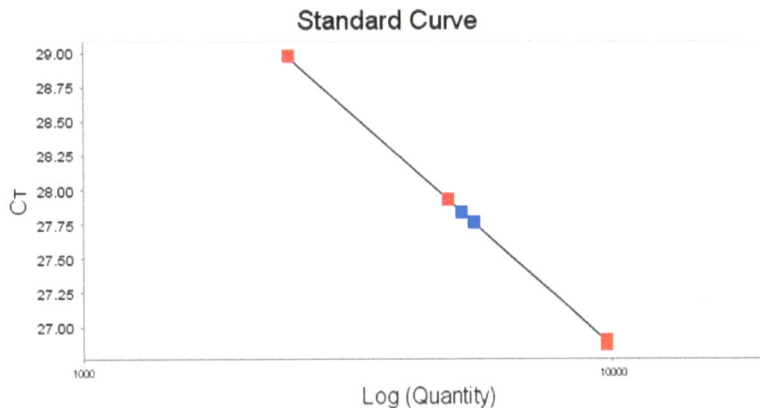

**Figure 6:** Absolute quantification of a presumably one copy clone using the GFP TaqMan® assay: comparison of the Ct values to known plasmid dilutions. Ct values are shown as a function of the quantity. Standard curve points of plasmid dilutions around the expected quantity are shown in red, whereas Ct values measured for the clone were put on this curve and are shown in blue. Quantity is illustrated as plasmid copy number input. The interpolated copy number for this clone was around 5300. See more informations and calculations in the text.

## 4.2   Second Approach: Comparative Quantification using One Copy Calibrator Samples

The alternative to identify a potential calibrator clone is to screen for the lowest transgene or marker gene expression. We have analyzed GFP expressing HEK-293 clones by FACS, and measured different green fluorescent intensities (Figure 7). The fluorescence intensities of the selected clones were compared to that of a one copy clone previously identified by absolute quantification. The GFP intensity of this latter one was similar to most of the lowest level expressing clones confirming that these clones are suitable for reference samples with one copy integration for subsequent analysis. Although expression level can be affected by its insertion site, we may say that one copy clones have significantly and uniformly lower GFP intensity than the few copy ones, but other transgene expressions may show wider differences.

Comparative qPCR quantification, while still technically challenging, does not require the same level of stringency. In this approach, the assay for target sequence is compared to a reference sample (a calibrator), and instead of precise copy number determination, it focuses on relative fold changes. In our application the copy number can be calculated based on the relative quantity of a single copy insertion. The method is based on the assumption that the threshold number of the sample and reference molecules

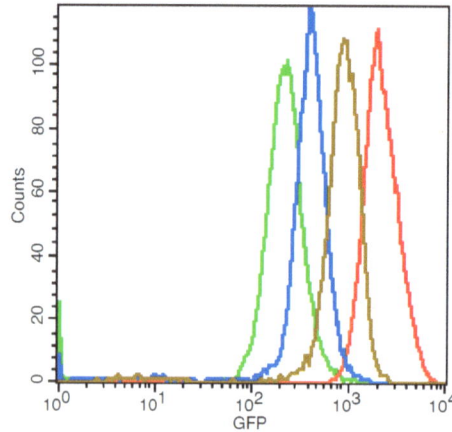

**Figure 7:** FACS histograms of representative HEK-293 clones expressing GFP as a transgene. Differences in GFP intensities correlate with GFP copy numbers.

is equal (Livak, 1997):

$$R_{Ct\ Sample} = R_{Ct\ Reference}$$

where RCt stands for the number of molecules at the threshold cycle. With the theoretical 100% efficiency, PCR duplicates the target in each cycle:

$$R_{Ct\ Sample} = R_{0\ Sample} \times 2^{Ct\ Sample}$$

$$R_{Ct\ Reference} = R_{0\ Reference} \times 2^{Ct\ Reference}$$

where R0 Sample and R0 Reference are the initial number of molecules of the sample and reference, respectively. The fold difference can therefore be calculated as:

$$R_{0\ Sample} / R_{0\ Reference} = 2^{-\Delta Ct},$$

where:

$$\Delta Ct = Ct_{Sample} - Ct_{Reference}$$

However, when the efficiency is not 100% but it is reproducibly identical, efficiency correction should be incorporated into the ΔCt method.

$$\text{Fold difference:}\ (1 + E)^{-\Delta Ct}.$$

For each novel assay, it is advisable to determine the efficiency values using the standard curve methodology discussed previously. As formerly mentioned, the most suitable specimen for such standard curve analysis is pooled gDNA of transgenic clones, because it has similar complexity to the unknown samples being analyzed. For comparison, the interpolated values from the standard curves can be used. A concrete example for the copy number calculation is as follows: the derived amount of the unknown sample is 24,99±0,15ng, whereas that of the single copy reference sample is 6.37 ± 0.18ng, so:

Fold difference – unknown/reference: (24.99 ± 0.15ng)/(6.37 ± 0.18ng)

Relative quantity (RQ) = 3.93      RQ Min = 3.80   RQ Max = 4.06

The upper example is still based on comparison of the absolute values of target Ct, however, a single Ct does not always reflect the expected number because of specimen discrepancies. Abandoning absolute quantification did not eliminate the deviations arising from differences in sample quality of the compared clones. Although the input of the template is always standardized, Ct deviations can still be attributable to certain errors, such as DNA concentration measurements. Normalization to an endogenous control sequence can overcome this problem. The control sequence should be similar in abundance to the target sequence and it must be present at a consistent level among all samples being compared. As an endogenous control for the human genome, the RPPH1 gene (the H1 RNA subunit of the RNaseP enzyme complex) was chosen which is a widely-accepted one copy gene of the haploid human genome. As mentioned earlier, without knowing the efficiency values, standard curves of both sequences have to be applied (Figure 8).

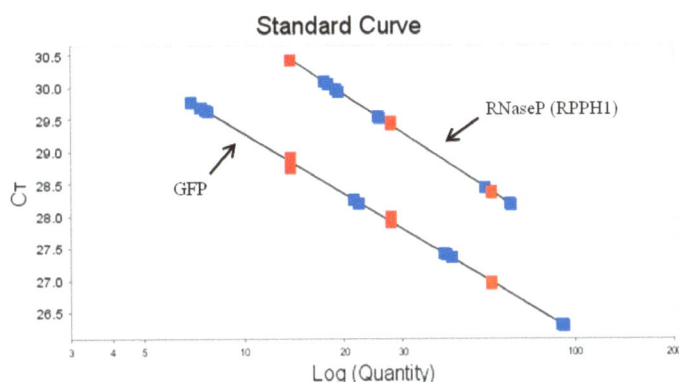

**Figure 8:** Example of a relative standard curve experiment. Standard curves for GFP and RNaseP (RPPH1) TaqMan® assay can be seen. Dilutions were made from pooled gDNA of unknown clones analyzed in the measurement; quantity is expressed in nanograms of gDNA input. Regression lines calculated from the measurement points of the two assays are parallel to each other, indicating very similar efficiency values. Red points represent points of the standard curves, whereas blue ones represent measurements of examined clones. See more informations and calculations in the text.

A relative standard curve experiment is based on sequential comparisons. First, both the target and the endogenous control are interpolated separately from the respective standard curves. Specimen comparisons showed formerly can be carried out only after normalizations to the endogenous control, for example:

*Normalizations – Target/EndCont:*

Sample → (54.23 ± 2.60ng) / (42.34 ± 0.82ng)

Reference → (6.13 ± 0.70ng)/(19.43 ± 0.25ng)

*Fold difference – Sample/Reference:*

Relative quantity (RQ) = 4.07      RQ Min = 3.76      RQ Max = 4.35

Alternatively, comparative analysis could be based on the real efficiency values:

*Fold difference – Difference in the target/Difference in the endogenous control:*

$$(1 + E_{Target})^{-\Delta Ct\ Target} / (1 + E_{EndCont})^{-\Delta Ct\ EndCont}$$

where:

$$\Delta Ct_{Target} = Ct_{Target\ Sample} - Ct_{Target\ Reference}$$

$$\Delta Ct_{EndCont} = Ct_{EndCont\ Sample} - Ct_{EndCont\ Reference}$$

However, if efficiencies of both the target and the endogenous control are proven to be close to identical, the $\Delta\Delta Ct$ method could be chosen:

$$\text{Fold difference:}\ (1 + E)^{-\Delta\Delta Ct}$$

where:

$$\Delta\Delta Ct = \Delta Ct_{Target} - \Delta Ct_{EndCont}$$

Ideally, efficiencies of both the target and the endogenous control are close to 100%.

$$\text{Fold difference:}\ 2^{-\Delta\Delta Ct}$$

The main requirement for the $\Delta\Delta Ct$ method is that the efficiencies of the assays are identical. The deviation of the two efficiencies can be determined by plotting the $\Delta Ct$-s from the standard curves points, and if the slope of this so called relative efficiency plot (Figure 9) is in the range of < 0.1, then it is acceptable to employ the $\Delta\Delta Ct$ method. Another way to test the applicability is analyzing the relative standard curve experiment data with the $\Delta\Delta Ct$ method. Similar outcome of the two methods will show the acceptability of the comparative Ct method, and in such cases, standard curves can be leaved behind. As the GFP sequence worked well in combination with the RPPH1 endogenous control, we continued to examine if assays designed for SB transposon sequences can also be utilized for copy number determination with similar methodology.

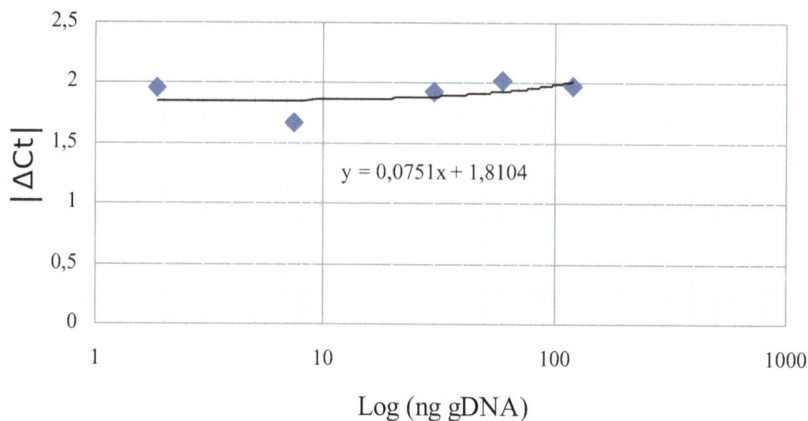

**Figure 9:** Relative efficiency plot comparing TaqMan® assays of IRDR-L and RNaseP (RPPH1). Dilution series were prepared from pools of gDNA containing one copy of SB transposon. Absolute values of $\Delta Ct$ (target minus endogenous control) from the standard curve points were plotted against gDNA quantities and the equation of the regression line calculated from the measurement points is shown. A line with a slope of very small value (close to 0) indicates identical efficiencies of the two assays across all input concentrations.

### 4.3   Third Approach: Comparative Quantification using the SB IRDR Sequence Independently of the Transgene

As the SB transposon system is generally applied in our laboratory, we aimed at developing a real-time PCR-based technique that is transgene-independent, specific for the transposon regions, and therefore widely applicable. As for most transposon flanking sequences, the two IRDR regions are repeat-rich DNA sequences which make PCR primer design relatively difficult. Moreover, the left and the right IR-DRs are very similar to each other which further narrows the possibility to design specific assays for them. Nevertheless, we could still develop specific TaqMan® assays for each: neither of the IRDR-L nor the IRDR-R probe set gives signals in the exclusive presence of the other template.

Next we tested both assays designed for the transposon sequences, whether these fit to the GFP copy numbers. As formerly mentioned, random integrations can be the result from the breakage of the plasmid at any points, therefore randomly integrated one copy clones are not reliable candidates for reference samples when utilizing transposon sequences. Only after validating the one copy candidates cloned from the active transposition experiments with the GFP assay, were these clones used as reference samples with the transposon specific assays. The results based on GFP and the IRDR-L were in agreement with each other (Figure 10) and most standard curve analysis showed similar result with the comparative Ct method indicating that we could directly use the ΔΔCt method. In addition, technical errors could be further decreased using a pool of gDNA samples with known copy number as a reference. Here we show the calculation with the row Ct values by the example of G2C2 clone in Figure 10 with Cts resulted in IRDR-L assay. Ct mean values are calculated as the mean of Cts of 3 simultaneous PCR reactions:

$$Ct_{\text{Mean IRDR-L}} \text{ of G2C2: } 31.065$$

$$Ct_{\text{Mean RNaseP}} \text{ of G2C2: } 30.951$$

$$Ct_{\text{Mean IRDR-L}} \text{ of one copy clone pool: } 31.457$$

$$Ct_{\text{Mean RNaseP}} \text{ of one copy clone pool: } 29.773$$

Calculations of $\Delta Ct - s$:

$$\Delta Ct_{\text{IRDR-L}} = 31.065\text{-}31.457 = -0.392$$

$$\Delta Ct_{\text{RNaseP}} = 30.951\text{-}29.773 = 1.178$$

Calculation of $\Delta\Delta Ct$: $\Delta\Delta Ct = -0.392 - 1.178 = -1.57$

Relative quantity: $RQ = 2^{-\Delta\Delta Ct} = 2^{1.57} = 2.969$ (3 copies)

These experiments therefore supported the use of the IRDR-L repeat specific assay for transposon copy number determination as it gave the same results as the assay specific for the carried internal transgene (GFP). However similar application of IRDR-R TaqMan® assay for the previously analyzed clones was unreliable to determine the exact copy number and the assay usually showed lower efficiency than the GFP and the IRDR-L. So initially we concluded that we have to leave out the specific but less efficient assay for the IRDR-R region (Kolacsek et al., 2011).

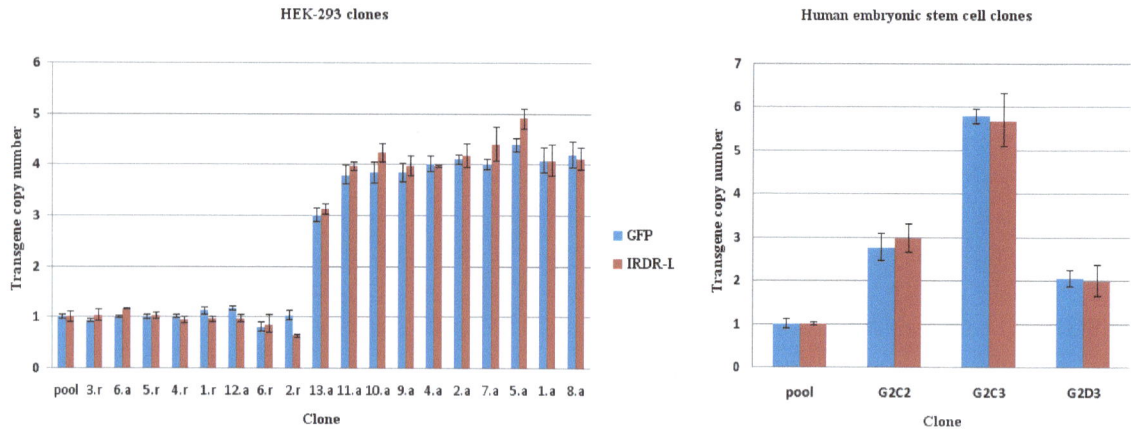

**Figure 10:** Copy numbers determined by the GFP or the IRDR-L TaqMan® assays in different clones of HEK-293 (left panel) and human embryonic stem cells (right panel). Results of the transgene independent, SB transposon specific IRDR-L assay correlated well with the GFP-based copy numbers. Pool: a mixture of equal amounts of one copy clones. Figure partially adopted from Kolacsek et al., Mobile DNA (2011), 2(1):5, published by BioMed Central.

Concerning SB transposon mutants and variants, "symmetrical" SB transposons with two IRDR-L (but not with two IRDR-R) flanking sequences were shown to be functional (Izsvak *et al.*, 2002). The assay for the left transposon sequence is also applicable for such constructs with a correction factor of 0.5. Searching for such mutant transposon clones, we used the IRDR-R assay to determine the presence of the right terminal repeat sequence. During this presence-absence examination studies, we could achieve higher sensitivity of the IRDR-R TaqMan® with elevating the input range of the gDNA. However, the sensitivity and the reliability of IRDR-R was still below to that of the IRDR-L assay, and only lower copy number clones showed reliable measurements (Figure 11). In addition, we still have to emphasize here that sample quality has a deep impact on reproducibility of all assays.

As a major general recommendation, we routinely analyze more parts of the inserted transgene sequence (e.g. IRDR-L and GFP regions or IRDR-L and IRDR-R regions). It is also advisable using at least two separate single copy clones as reference samples and two few copy (3 – 4) clones as controls in all analyses. The application of more than one reference clone makes it possible to choose the most appropriate one with which low copy control clones give the best precise round copy numbers. In fact, the use of the few (3 – 4) copy clones as references is helpful to approximate extreme copies (> 15) more precisely.

# 5    Validation of Transgene-independent qPCR Copy Number Quantification

To compare our transgene-independent quantification approach with other techniques, we measured copy numbers of clones that were generated from different cell types by transposons containing various transgene sequences. Such clones were ideal for comparison due to the different transgene sequence and because copy numbers in those cases were also determined either by the Southern/dot blotting techniques,

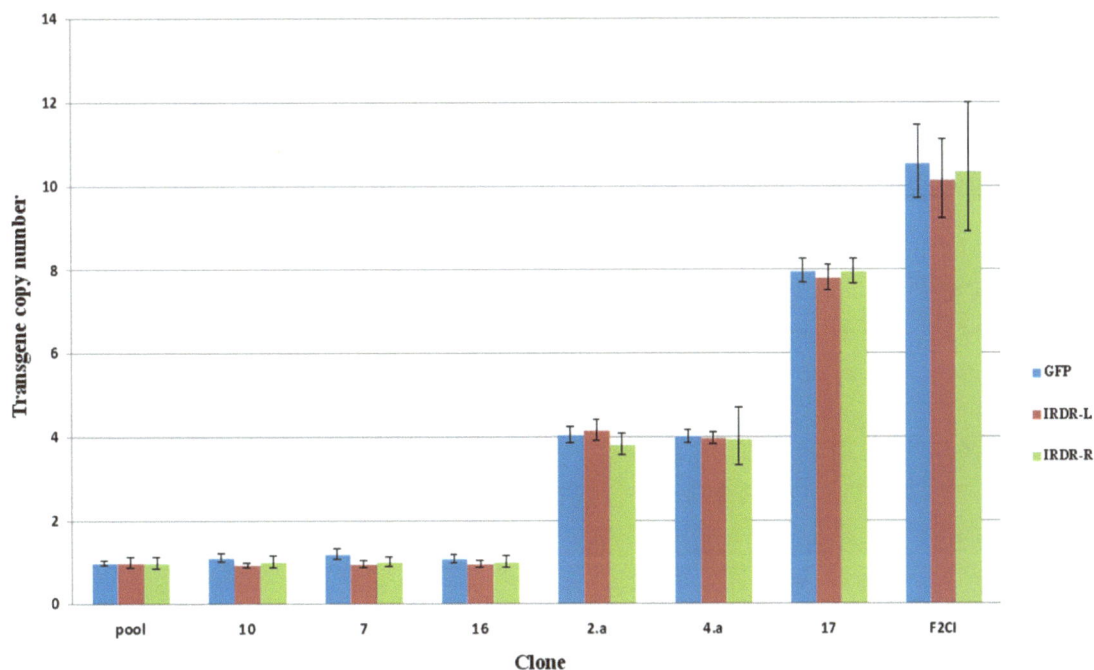

**Figure 11:** Comparison of transposon copy number determinations based on three different TaqMan® assays. Using higher amount of input gDNA (90ng) resulted in reliable correlation of the IRDR-R assay with the copy numbers determined by the GFP and IRDR-L specific qPCR measurements.

or by the transposon display method, or by estimations from transgene integration assays (Splinkerette PCR/Inverse PCR). Using the IRDR-L assay with the $\Delta\Delta$Ct methodology, copy numbers were estimated ranging from 1 to 50 copies in various clones (Table 1 and 2). The measured transposon copies were almost always the same by the qPCR as by the canonical methods. As canonical methods – with the exception of dot blot – utilize restriction enzyme sites flanking the integration point, which may be sensitive to sequence environment, therefore all integrated copies may not be reliably detected by the canonical methods. Perhaps this is why copy numbers were underestimated in some of the cases comparing to our qPCR method. For higher (> 5) copy-number clones, our method was also accurate, with occasional low relative-error margins ($\leq$ 9%). The slight differences in these cases could be due to the inaccuracy of the standard methods for this range. In addition, it has been suggested that precise values of very high copy numbers are more reliably measured by dot blot rather than transposon display method.

By the above described experiments, the newly developed transgene independent method for determining SB transposon copy numbers could be validated since (i) it provided the same results as the assays specific for the carried transgene sequence and (ii) it could also reliably replace widely used canonical radioactive techniques. The TaqMan® assay designed for the IRDR-L region of the transposon provides the basis for transgene independence as it is present in all SB constructs (Kolacsek *et al.*, 2011).

| Clone | Canonical methods | Copy numbers | |
|---|---|---|---|
| | | by canonical methods | by qPCR IRDR-L |
| 2/1 | Transposon display/Southern blotting | 8 – 10 | 8 |
| 2/2 | Transposon display/Southern blotting | 3 | 4 |
| 2/3 | Transposon display/Southern blotting | 10 – 12 | 10 |
| 2/9 | Transposon display/Southern blotting | 1 | 1 |
| 1 | Transposon display/Southern blotting | 12 – 13 | 13 |
| 4 | Dot blot | 52 | 50 |
| 5 | Transposon display/Southern blotting | 15 | 15 |
| 6 | Transposon display/Southern blotting | 12 | 11 |
| 7 | Transposon display/Southern blotting | 1 | 1 |
| 8 | Transposon display/Southern blotting | 2 | 2 |
| 9 | Transposon display/Southern blotting | 1 | 1 |
| A3 | Splinkerette PCR/Inverse PCR | 2 | 2 |
| A4 | Splinkerette PCR/Inverse PCR | 4 | 4 |
| A5 | Splinkerette PCR/Inverse PCR | 4 | 4,5 |
| A6 | Splinkerette PCR/Inverse PCR | 2 | 2 |
| B1 | Splinkerette PCR/Inverse PCR | 1 | 2 |
| B2 | Splinkerette PCR/Inverse PCR | 2 | 2 |
| B3 | Splinkerette PCR/Inverse PCR | 3 | 3 |
| B5 | Splinkerette PCR/Inverse PCR | 2 | 2 |
| C3 | Splinkerette PCR/Inverse PCR | 1 | 2 |
| C5 | Splinkerette PCR/Inverse PCR | 2 | 2 |
| 3 | Splinkerette PCR/Inverse PCR | 1 | 1 |
| 16 | Splinkerette PCR/Inverse PCR | 1 | 1 |
| 3.a | Splinkerette PCR/Inverse PCR | 1 | 1 |
| 6.a | Splinkerette PCR/Inverse PCR | 1 | 1 |
| 12.a | Splinkerette PCR/Inverse PCR | 1 | 1 |

**Table 1:** Comparing the IRDR-L qPCR-based method with other canonical techniques for transposon copy number determination. Additional data is added to the table adopted from Kolacsek et al., Mobile DNA (2011), 2(1):5, published by BioMed Central.

| Clone | Copy by qPCR | Sequence | Ref.seq. | Chrom. pos. | Nt.pos. of ref.seq. | Region | Seq. orient. | Method |
|---|---|---|---|---|---|---|---|---|
| C3 | 2 | TTCCTTGTTACTCCTTCAAAATGCT TAcagttgaagt | NT_007592.15 | Hs 6p22 | 51406968 | intergenic | Left | splinkerette pGEM |
| C5 | 2 | CAGTTTATTATTATTGTCATTGTA TAcagttgaagt | NT_167198.1 | Hs Xq28 | 2288320 | GABRA3 intron3 | L | splinkerette pGEM |
| | | CAGATCCTGATAAATGTTAGTTAC TAcagttgaagt | NT_030059.13 | Hs 10q21 | 4645679 | PRKG1 intron7 | L | inverse PCR pGEM |
| 3 | 1 | TTCCTCCCTGGACTTTAGGACATA TAcagttgaagt | NT_034772.6 | Hs 5q22 | 6866220 | intergenic | L | splinkerette |
| | | AGGAAGTATACACTCACCCTGTGA TAcagttgaagt | NT_034772.6 | Hs 5q22 | 6866220 | | Right | splinkerette |
| 16 | 1 | GACACAGCTGATTTTGAAGTCAGA TAcagttgaagt | NT_016354.19 | Hs 4q28 | 65845752 | SCOC intron1 | L | splinkerette |
| | | GAAGACTACCCTATCACTGTATTA TAcagttgaagt | NT_016354.19 | Hs 4q28 | 65845752 | | R | splinkerette |
| 3.a | 1 | TAGCACAATGAGTACTTTATCACA TAcagttgaagt | NT_032977.9 | Hs 1p31 | 82218216 | intergenic | L | inverse PCR pGEM |
| 6.a | 1 | AATACATGGAAGGTAGAACAGATC TAcagttgaagt | NT_032977.9 | Hs 1p31 | 88638434 | intergenic | L | splinkerette |
| | | TAAATTATACATGTCTGTTAAAGCA TAcagttgaagt | NT_032977.9 | Hs 1p31 | 88638434 | | R | splinkerette |
| 12.a | 1 | TCTGGAAAGCCACATTCGGGAACT TAcagttgaagt | NT_025028.14 | Hs 18q21 | 21860434 | intergenic | L | splinkerette |

**Table 2:** Examples of *bona fide* SB transposon integration sites in clones of human cell lines where transposon copy numbers were determined previously. L or R indicates whether the particular transposon integration site was determined from the direction of the left or the right terminal repeat region of SB. The 'TA' sequence (shown in red) next to the transposon terminal repeats provides evidence that these integrations are the results of *bona fide* transposition, as this dinucleotide marks the SB target sequence that is duplicated during the reaction. Hs=Homo sapiens.

# 6   Quantitative Excision PCR

In our laboratory, we have successfully applied different DNA transposon systems for various in vitro cell culture applications, including studies on directed tissue differentiation from embryonic stem cells and modeling *ex vivo* introduction of therapeutic transgenes into patient cells. Controlling the delivery efficiency is a crucial task for these applications which is usually characterized by testing the transgenic rate of transfectants. However these test methods are time consuming and not applicable in all of the cases, so we have developed a qPCR method to characterize transposition activity. This quantification is extremely useful when optimizing for conditions of a given delivery system, or comparing the efficiency of different transposon systems or variants of a particular transposase enzyme.

There are two major steps involved in transposition, the excision of the transposon from the donor site and the integration of the transposon into the target site. These steps are proven to be coupled since excision frequency of different transposon mutants from a donor plasmid was correlated to overall transposition efficiency (Liu *et al.*, 2004). Excision events can be detected by a PCR reaction with primers flanking the transposon sequence at the donor site (Figure 12). Following excision, the donor plasmid will be circularized by the double-strand DNA break repair mechanism of the cell, and only these excised and repaired plasmids will serve as a template for exponential amplification, because the transposon content is usually large enough not to be amplified from the original uncut sequence. Excision PCR can be carried out on samples taken on the second/third day after transfection, and both isolated plasmids, as well as cell lysates can be used as input material (we generally use isolated plasmids as input.) A semi quantitative version of this excision PCR has been applied by Liu *et al.* (2004) to describe the excision step of SB transposition.

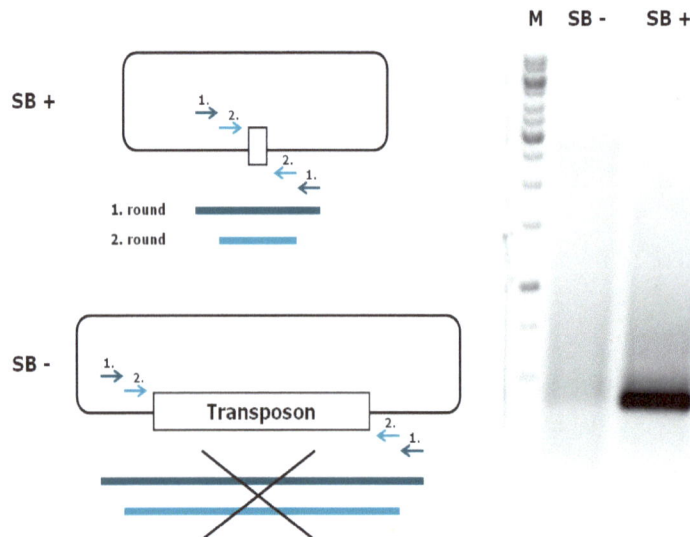

**Figure 12:** Principle of the excision PCR using transposon containing donor plasmids. This is a nested PCR technique using two sets of primers specific to the transposon flanking sequences, and amplifying the products in two consecutive rounds of PCR. In case of transposition (SB+), there is a distinct product that can be visualized by agarose gel electrophoresis (right panel). In the absence of transposition (SB-), the PCR cannot amplify the target sequence due to its large size. For more details, see the text.

Due to the error-prone double-stranded break repair mechanism, the joining of the donor ends is remarkably imprecise, therefore real-time quantification of excision based on a TaqMan® probe with stringent sequence requirement could not be considered, and hence we adopted the SYBR® Green technology for this application. In some cases, since very small portion of the amount of transposon donor plasmids undergo excision, to increase the traceability, more than one round of nested PCR is necessary to quantify the excision reaction. For this reason, we apply a 10 – 13 cycle pre-amplification (first round of PCR), and after a thousand-fold dilution we measure the real-time round (second round of PCR) with nested primers using SYBR® Green. Amplification from another segment of the plasmid backbone (in our case, the ampicillin resistance gene sequence) could serve as a normalization control. Due to its large excess, ampicillin sequence is not pre-amplified but it is permanently present in our samples during all processes until the second round of excision PCR, so it can be correctly measured in all samples. Although the primers we routinely use are specific to the backbone of our transposon plasmid constructs which can differ among SB users, our primers might be useful for those who apply constructs with the same origin (Table 3). PCR efficiencies for the target and the control sequence were measured by serial dilutions of pooled samples and the $\Delta\Delta Ct$ method was proved to be reliable for comparison of excision efficiencies.

| | name | sequence 5′ → 3′ |
|---|---|---|
| 1 | exc.1 for | GCGAAAGGGGGATGTGCTGCAAGG |
| 2 | exc.1 rev | TCTTTCCTGCGTTATCCCCTGATTC |
| 3 | exc.2 for | CGATTAAGTTGGGTAACGCCAGGG |
| 4 | exc.2 rev | CAGCTGGCACGACAGGTTTCCCG |
| 5 | amp. for | TTTGCTCACCCAGAAACGC |
| 6 | amp. rev | AGTTGGCCGCAGTGTTATCAC |

**Table 3:** Sequences of primers used for the quantitative excision PCR. Primers with .1 extension are used for the first round, whereas others with .2 extension are used for the second round of the nested PCR; amp primers anneal to the sequence of the ampicillin resistance gene.

An excellent validation of our quantification method developed for measuring the transposition activity was to compare different SB transposase versions resulted from gradual improvement of the activity (Mates *et al.*, 2009). Relative quantification of excision efficiency of SB11x, SB32x and SB100x is correlated to their expected activity in HEK-293 and in HeLa cells as well (Figure 13).

Normalization to the plasmid backbone sequence makes this relative quantification technique independent of the transfection efficiency. This provides the basis for comparing various transposon delivery experiments, including different transposon systems (e.g. SB or PB), different transposase or transposon variants, different host cell types, or different experimental settings. Applying this quantitative technique could therefore be a reliable and fast screening approach for different transposon systems and gene delivery conditions before any applications with the desired transgene.

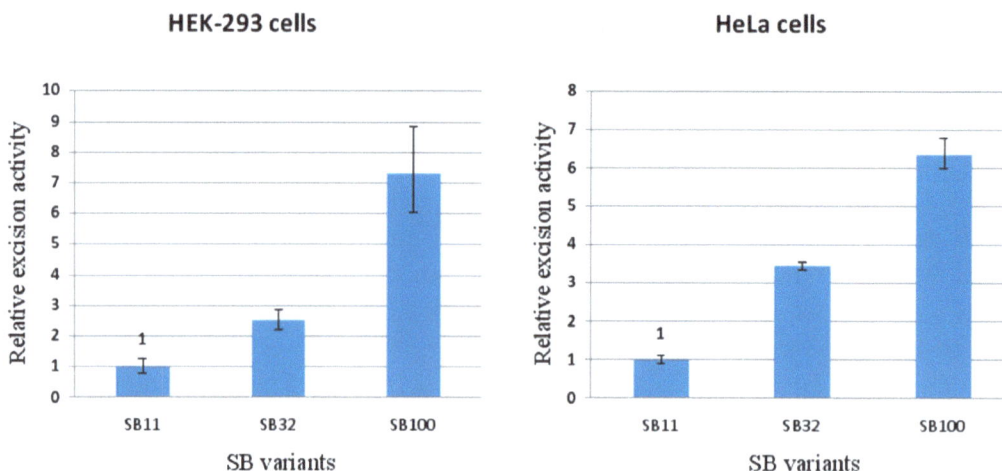

**Figure 13:** Relative excision efficiencies of SB transposase variants in different cell lines measured by real-time qPCR. Normalizing the excision PCR to the amount of the ampicillin sequence by specific PCR, here we quantify the excision events among all transfected transposon donor plasmids.

# 7    Related Works

As it was used for quantitative aspects of transposon-based gene delivery experiments, real-time PCR measurements are widely used and have become integral part of the methodology for gene delivery and gene therapy applications. On the other hand, careful design of the experiments or choosing suitable methodology are often missing from such studies, weakening the conclusion of the results. For example, Bian & Belmont (2010) have made absolute quantification of transgenic multi-copy insertions derived from linearized plasmid transfection, although they did not carry out any normalization of the input material. Huang *et al.* (2010) have detected random integration level with absolute quantification normalizing to the RNaseP one copy sequence. They used "empty" gDNA to mix with the target sequence containing plasmid for the standard curve samples; however, normalizing the absolute quantification with external template incorporates additional variability in the measurement. In the meantime, well-designed studies provide excellent new examples of combining existing technologies. Charrier *et al.* (2011) have applied an elegant solution for absolute quantification to determine lentiviral vector copy numbers with normalization to endogenous albumin. Standard curves were made from the same plasmid containing both the target and the endogenous control sequence, resulting in the smallest possible variability in their measurement. Ballester *et al.* (2004) determined copy number of transgenic mice carrying goat lactoglobulin gene using relative quantification with the comparative Ct method. The unique design of the measurement was the application of goat gDNA as a reference sample and the choice of glucagon sequence as an endogenous control, the latter one being strongly conserved between the two species.

Concerning SB transposon applications, a recent paper described a simultaneous analysis of excision activity of *Sleeping Beauty* and the resulting transgene copy number (Jin *et al.*, 2011). Excision was analyzed at days 1 to 3 after electroporation using the $\Delta\Delta$Ct method with a TaqMan® assay where the probe was specific to one of the transposon flanking regions. They also normalized to a plasmid backbone sequence, thus similarly to our qPCR studies, their quantification is independent of the electrotransfer efficiency. However, as the repair of the plasmid after excision is an error-prone process (see Section 7), using a strict TaqMan® probe sequence may not detect all excision products. They also determined the average copy number in transgenic cell population after four weeks of selection. They used an absolute quantification approach using dilution series of a one copy clone gDNA as a standard which is in fact an alternative to relative standard curve method using one copy as a reference.

# 8   Conclusions

Transposon-based technology is an emerging new method of choice for gene delivery and for gene therapy applications. Compared to viral vectors, transposon systems offer several advantages. Apart from being less expensive in terms of the required safety facilities, for several DNA transposons, the integration profile of the delivered transgene is more close to random, showing no preferences for coding regions, therefore making its application less susceptible for insertional mutagenesis. SB seems to be the safest delivery technique for two reasons: 1) its transgene integration profile is the closest to random among all known gene delivery vehicles; 2) SB was resurrected from an ancient non-functional fish mobile element, therefore no potential transposons are present in vertebrate species, including the human genome, that can remobilize the integrated transgene. Based on these characteristics, the SB system is the most suitable for cell and gene therapy applications, even if compared to other transposon vehicles.

Our work contributed to the quantification of transposon delivery in two important aspects. We have developed sensitive and reliable real-time PCR-based methods to measure (i) the first step of the transposition and (ii) the resulting copy number of the delivery. Quantitative excision PCR is extremely useful to control and to optimize transposon mediated gene delivery, whereas copy number determination is essential to characterize transgenic cells. Comparing our copy number method with widely used canonical methods, it was proved to be just as accurate as those, also offering a faster and non-radioactive approach at the same time. However, the real advantage of this method is the transgene-independence which makes it applicable for any scientists working with SB transposon constructs.

In this chapter, we gave a detailed protocol for designing quantitative measurements of integrated DNA sequences such as transposons, and show examples for developing reliable quantitative assays specific to any sequence. In general, however, this description may also serve as a stepwise guide providing a strategy for similar quantification purposes.

# Acknowledgements

Tamás I. Orbán is a recipient of the János Bolyai Scholarship of the Hungarian Academy of Sciences. Research in our laboratory was supported by grants from OTKA (NK83533), STEMKILL (OM00108/2008), and KMOP-1.1.2-07/1-2008-0003.

# References

Balciunas, D., Wangensteen, K. J., Wilber, A., Bell, J., Geurts, A., Sivasubbu, S., Wang, X., Hackett, P. B., Largaespada, D. A., McIvor, R. S., & Ekker, S. C. (2006). Harnessing a high cargo-capacity transposon for genetic applications in vertebrates. PLoS Genetics, 2(11), e169.

Ballester, M., Castello, A., Ibanez, E., Sanchez, A., & Folch, J. M. (2004). Real-time quantitative PCR-based system for determining transgene copy number in transgenic animals. Biotechniques, 37(4), 610-613.

Baus, J., Liu, L., Heggestad, A. D., Sanz, S., & Fletcher, B. S. (2005). Hyperactive transposase mutants of the Sleeping Beauty transposon. Molecular Therapy, 12(6), 1148-1156.

Bian, Q. & Belmont, A. S. (2010). BAC TG-EMBED: one-step method for high-level, copynumber-dependent, position-independent transgene expression. Nucleic Acids Research, 38(11), e127.

Biemont, C. & Vieira, C. (2006). Genetics: junk DNA as an evolutionary force. Nature, 443(7111), 521-524.

Burns, K. H. & Boeke, J. D. (2012). Human transposon tectonics. Cell, 149(4), 740-752.

Charrier, S., Ferrand, M., Zerbato, M., Pre´cigout, G., Viornery, A., Bucher-Laurent, S., Benkhelifa-Ziyyat, S., Merten, O. W., Perea, J., & Galy, A. (2011). Quantification of lentiviral vector copy numbers in individual hematopoietic colony-forming cells shows vector dose-dependent effects on the frequency and level of transduction. Gene Therapy, 18(5), 479-487.

Chelly, J., Kaplan, J. C., Maire, P., Gautron, S., & Kahn, A. (1988). Transcription of the dystrophin gene in human muscle and non-muscle tissue. Nature, 333(6176), 858-860.

Chew, S. K., Rad, R., Futreal, P. A., Bradley, A., & Liu, P. (2011). Genetic screens using the piggyBac transposon. Methods, 53(4), 366-371.

Collier, L. S. & Largaespada, D. A. (2005). Hopping around the tumor genome: transposons for cancer gene discovery. Cancer Research, 65(21), 9607-9610.

Collier, L. S. & Largaespada, D. A. (2007). Transposable elements and the dynamic somatic genome. Genome Biology, 8 Suppl 1, S5.

Devon, R. S., Porteous, D. J., & Brookes, A. J. (1995). Splinkerettes—improved vectorettes for greater efficiency in PCR walking. Nucleic Acids Research, 23(9), 1644-1645.

Ding, S., Wu, X., Li, G., Han, M., Zhuang, Y., & Xu, T. (2005). Efficient transposition of the piggyBac (PB) transposon in mammalian cells and mice. Cell, 122(3), 473-483.

Ellis, J. (2005). Silencing and variegation of gammaretrovirus and lentivirus vectors. Human Gene Therapy, 16(11), 1241-1246.

Feschotte, C. & Pritham, E. J. (2007). DNA transposons and the evolution of eukaryotic genomes. Annual Reviews of Genetics, 41, 331-368.

Garrison, B. S., Yant, S. R., Mikkelsen, J. G., & Kay, M. A. (2007). Postintegrative gene silencing within the Sleeping Beauty transposition system. Molecular and Cellular Biology, 27(24), 8824-8833.

Goodier, J. L. & Kazazian, H. H., Jr. (2008). Retrotransposons revisited: the restraint and rehabilitation of parasites. Cell, 135(1), 23-35.

Grabundzija, I., Irgang, M., Mates, L., Belay, E., Matrai, J., Gogol-Doring, A., Kawakami, K., Chen, W., Ruiz, P., Chuah, M. K., VandenDriessche, T., Izsvak, Z., & Ivics, Z. (2010). Comparative analysis of transposable element vector systems in human cells. Molecular Therapy, 18(6), 1200-1209.

Guo, G., Huang, Y., Humphreys, P., Wang, X., & Smith, A. (2011). A PiggyBac-based recessive screening method to identify pluripotency regulators. PLoS One, 6(4), e18189.

Hedges, D. J. & Batzer, M. A. (2005). From the margins of the genome: mobile elements shape primate evolution. Bioessays, 27(8), 785-794.

Heid, C. A., Stevens, J., Livak, K. J., & Williams, P. M. (1996). Real time quantitative PCR. Genome Research, 6(10), 986-994.

Higuchi, R., Dollinger, G., Walsh, P. S., & Griffith, R. (1992). Simultaneous amplification and detection of specific DNA sequences. Biotechnology, 10(4), 413-417.

Huang, X., Haley, K., Wong, M,, Guo, H., Lu, C., Wilber, A., & Zhou, X. (2010). Unexpectedly high copy number of random integration but low frequency of persistent expression of the Sleeping Beauty transposase after trans delivery in primary human T cells. Human Gene Therapy, 21(11), 1577-1590.

Ivics, Z., Hackett, P. B., Plasterk, R. H., & Izsvak, Z. (1997). Molcular reconstruction of Sleeping Beauty, a Tc1-like transposon from fish, and its transposition in human cells. Cell, 91(4), 501-510.

Ivics, Z. & Izsvak, Z. (2004). Transposable elements for transgenesis and insertional mutagenesis in vertebrates: a contemporary review of experimental strategies. Methods in Molecular Biology, 260, 255-276.

Izsvak, Z., Ivics, Z., & Plasterk, R. H. (2000). Sleeping Beauty, a wide host-range transposon vector for genetic transformation in vertebrates. Journal of Molecular Biology, 302(1), 93-102.

Izsvak, Z., Khare, D., Behlke, J., Heinemann, U., Plasterk, R. H., & Ivics, Z. (2002). Involvement of a bifunctional, paired-like DNA-binding domain and a transpositional enhancer in Sleeping Beauty transposition. The Journal of Biological Chemistry, 277(37), 34581-34588.

Izsvak, Z., Hackett, P. B., Cooper, L. J., & Ivics, Z. (2010). Translating Sleeping Beauty transposition into cellular therapies: victories and challenges. Bioessays, 32(9), 756-767.

Jin, Z., Maiti, S., Huls, H., Singh, H., Olivares, S., Mates, L., Izsvak, Z., Ivics, Z., Lee, D. A., Champlin, R. E., & Cooper, L. J. N. (2011). The hyperactive Sleeping Beauty transposase SB100X improves the genetic modification of T cells to express a chimeric antigen receptor. Gene Therapy, 18(9), 849-856.

Kaji, K., Norrby, K., Paca, A., Mileikovsky, M., Mohseni, P., & Woltjen K. (2009). Virus-free induction of pluripotency and subsequent excision of reprogramming factors. Nature, 458(7239), 771-775.

Kazazian, H. H., Jr. (2004). Mobile elements: drivers of genome evolution. Science, 303(5664), 1626-1632.

Kleppe, K., Ohstuka, E., Kleppe, R., Molineux. L., & Khorana, H. G. (1971). Studies on polynucleotides. XCVI. Repair replications of short synthetic DNA's as catalyzed by DNA polymerases. Journal of Molecular Biology, 56(2), 341-361.

Kolacsek, O., Krízsik, V., Schamberger, A., Erdei, Z., Apáti, A., Várady, G., Mátés, L., Izsvák, Z., Ivics, Z., Sarkadi, B., & Orbán, T. I. (2011). Reliable transgene-independent method for determining Sleeping Beauty transposon copy numbers. Mobile DNA, 2(1), 5.

Liu, G., Aronovich, E. L., Cui, Z., Whitley, C. B., & Hackett, P. B. (2004). Excision of Sleeping Beauty transposons: parameters and applications to gene therapy. The Journal of Gene Medicine, 6(5), 574-583.

Liu, G., Geurts, A. M., Yae, K., Srinivasan, A. R., Fahrenkrug, S. C., Largaespada, D. A., Takeda, J., Horie, K., Olson, W. K., & Hackett, P. B. (2005). Target-site preferences of Sleeping Beauty transposons. Journal of Molecular Biology, 346(1), 161-173.

Livak, K. J, Flood, S. J., Marmaro, J., Giusti, W., & Deetz, K. (1995). Oligonucleotides with fluorescent dyes at opposite ends provide a quenched probe system useful for detecting PCR product and nucleic acid hybridization. Genome Research, 4(6), 357-362.

Livak, K. J. (1997). ABI Prism 7700 Sequence Detection System, User Bulletin #2. Applied Biosystems.

Mates, L., Chuah, M. K., Belay, E., Jerchow, B., Manoj, N., Acosta-Sanchez, A., Grzela, D. P., Schmitt, A., Becker, K., Matrai, J., Ma, L., Samara-Kuko, E., Gysemans, C., Pryputniewicz, D., Miskey, C., Fletcher, B., Vandendriessche, T., Ivics, Z., & Izsvak, Z. (2009). Molecular evolution of a novel hyperactive Sleeping Beauty transposase enables robust stable gene transfer in vertebrates. Nature Genetics, 41(6), 753-761.

Meilinger, D., Fellinger, K., Bultmann, S., Rothbauer, U., Bonapace, I. M., Klinkert, W. E., Spada, F. & Leonhardt, H. (2009). Np95 interacts with de novo DNA methyltransferases, Dnmt3a and Dnmt3b, and mediates epigenetic silencing of the viral CMV promoter in embryonic stem cells. EMBO Reports, 10(11), 1259-1264.

Mills, R. E., Bennett, E. A., Iskow, R. C., Luttig, C. T., Tsui, C., Pittard, W. S., & Devine, S. E. (2006). Recently mobilized transposons in the human and chimpanzee genomes. The American Journal of Human Genetics, 78(4), 671-679.

Mills, R. E., Bennett, E. A., Iskow, R. C., & Devine, S. E. (2007). Which transposable elements are active in the human genome? Trends in Genetics, 23(4), 183-191.

Miskey, C., Izsvak, Z., Plasterk, R. H., & Ivics, Z. (2003). The Frog Prince: a reconstructed transposon from Rana pipiens with high transpositional activity in vertebrate cells. Nucleic Acids Research, 31(23), 6873-6881.

Moeller, F., Nielsen, F. C., & Nielsen, L. B. (2003). New tools for quantifying and visualizing adoptively transferred cells in recipient mice. Journal of Immunological Methods, 282(1-2), 73-82.

Morrison, T. B., Weis, J. J., & Wittwer, C. T. (1998) Quantification of low-copy transcripts by continuous SYBR Green I monitoring during amplification. Biotechniques, 24(6), 954-962.

Mullis, K. & Faloona, F. (1987). Specific synthesis of DNA in vitro via a polymerase-catalyzed chain reaction. Methods in Enzymology, 155, 335-350.

Ostertag, E. M., Madison, B. B., & Kano, H. (2007). Mutagenesis in rodents using the L1 retrotransposon. Genome Biology, 8 Suppl 1, S16.

Pledger, D. W. & Coates, C. J. (2005). Mutant Mos1 mariner transposons are hyperactive in Aedes aegypti. Insect Biochemistry and Molecular Biology, 35(10), 1199-1207.

Ririe, K. M., Rasmussen, R. P., & Wittwer, C. T. (1997) Product differentiation by analysis of DNA melting curves during the polymerase chain reaction. Analytical Biochemistry, 245(2), 154-160.

Rowe, H. M., Jakobsson, J., Mesnard, D., Rougemont, J., Reynard, S., Aktas, T., Maillard, P. V., Layard-Liesching, H., Verp, S., Marquis, J., Spitz, F., Constam, D. B., & Trono, D. (2010). KAP1 controls endogenous retroviruses in embryonic stem cells. Nature, 463(7278), 237-240.

Rubin, G. M. & Spradling, A. C. (1982). Genetic transformation of Drosophila with transposable element vectors. Science, 218(4570), 348-53.

Shen, S., Lin, L., Cai, J. J., Jiang, P., Kenkel, E. J., Stroik, M. R., Sato, S., Davidson, B. L., & Xing, Y. (2011). Widespread establishment and regulatory impact of Alu exons in human genes. Proceedings of the National Academy of Sciences of the United States of America, 108(7), 2837-42.

Singer, T., McConnell, M. J., Marchetto, M. C., Coufal, N. G., & Gage, F. H. (2010) LINE-1 retrotransposons: mediators of somatic variation in neuronal genomes? Trends in Neurosciences, 33(8), 345-54.

Sivalingam, J., Krishnan, S., Ng, W. H., Lee, S. S., Phan, T. T., & Kon, O. L. (2010). Biosafety assessment of site-directed transgene integration in human umbilical cord-lining cells. Molecular Therapy, 18(7), 1346-1356.

Solyom, S. & Kazazian, H. H. Jr. (2012) Mobile elements in the human genome: implications for disease. Genome Medicine, 4(2), 12.

Spradling, A. C. & Rubin, G. M. (1982). Transposition of cloned P elements into Drosophila germ line chromosomes. Science, 218(4570), 341-7.

Uren, A. G., Kool, J., Berns, A., & van Lohuizen, M. (2005). Retroviral insertional mutagenesis: past, present and future. Oncogene, 24(52), 7656-7672.

Vigdal, T. J., Kaufman, C. D., Izsvak, Z., Voytas, D. F., & Ivics, Z. (2002). Common physical properties of DNA affecting target site selection of sleeping beauty and other Tc1/mariner transposable elements. Journal of Molecular Biology, 323(3), 441-452.

Wang, A. M., Doyle, M. V., & Mark, D. F. (1989). Quantitation of mRNA by the polymerase chain reaction. Proceedings of the National Academy of Sciences of the United States of America, 86(24), 9717-9721.

Wicker, T., Sabot, F., Hua-Van, A., Bennetzen, J. L., Capy, P., Chalhoub, B., Flavell, A., Leroy, P., Morgante, M., Panaud, O., Paux, E., SanMiguel, P., & Schulman, A. H. (2007). A unified classification system for eukaryotic transposable elements. Nature Reviews Genetics, 8(12), 973-982.

Wicks, S. R., de Vries, C. J., van Luenen, H. G., & Plasterk, R. H. (2000). CHE-3, a cytosolic dynein heavy chain, is required for sensory cilia structure and function in Caenorhabditis elegans. Developmental Biology, 221(2), 295-307.

Williams, D. A. (2008). Sleeping beauty vector system moves toward human trials in the United States. Molecular Therapy, 16(9), 1515-1516.

Wilson, M. H., Coates, C. J., & George, A. L., Jr. (2007). PiggyBac transposon mediated gene transfer in human cells. Molecular Therapy, 15(1), 139-145.

Wittwer, C. T., Herrmann, M. G., Moss, A. A., & Rasmussen, R. P. (1997). Continuous fluorescence monitoring of rapid cycle DNA amplification. Biotechniques, 22(1), 130-138.

Woltjen, K., Michael, I. P., Mohseni, P., Desai, R., Mileikovsky, M., Hämäläinen, R., Cowling, R., Wang, W., Liu, P., Gertsenstein, M., Kaji, K., Sung, H. K., & Nagy, A. (2009) piggyBac transposition reprograms fibroblasts to induced pluripotent stem cells. Nature, 458(7239), 766-70.

Yant, S. R., Wu, X., Huang, Y., Garrison, B., Burgess, S. M., & Kay, M. A. (2005). High-resolution genome-wide mapping of transposon integration in mammals. Molecular and Cellular Biology, 25(6), 2085-2094.

Zayed, H., Izsvak, Z., Walisko, O., & Ivics, Z. (2004). Development of hyperactive sleeping beauty transposon vectors by mutational analysis. Molecular Therapy, 9(2), 292-304.

Zhu, J., Park, C. W., Sjeklocha, L., Kren, B. T., & Steer, C. J. (2010). High-level genomic integration, epigenetic changes, and expression of sleeping beauty transgene. Biochemistry, 49(7), 1507-1521.

# Prediction of Protein Function based on Machine Learning Methods: An Overview

Kiran Kadam, Sangeeta Sawant, Urmila Kulkarni-Kale
*Bioinformatics Centre*
*University of Pune, Pune, India*

Valadi K. Jayaraman
*Center for Development of Advanced Computing (C-DAC)*
*University of Pune Campus, Pune, India*
*Shiv Nadar University, Chithera (Gautam Budh Nagar), India*

# 1   Introduction

Proteins represent the most important class of biomolecules in living organisms. They carry out majority of the cellular processes and act as structural constituents, catalysis agents, signaling molecules and molecular machines of every biological system (Eisenberg *et al.*, 2000). Understanding of protein function is, thus, very essential for studying any biological process. In addition to experimental approaches and methods, several bioinformatics approaches have been developed and are being used to assign and predict functions on the basis of sequences and structures of proteins. Availability of overwhelming amount of genomic data from a large number of genome sequencing projects has further intensified the need for function prediction. Attempts are being made to experimentally solve structures of a large number of proteins under the structural genomics initiatives (Terwilliger *et al.*, 2009). Computational methods have been developed to expand the structural repertoire of proteins by predicting structures of homologous proteins. As a result, sequences and structures of a very large number of proteins are becoming available but their functions are not known. While classical experimental approaches have proved to be extremely useful, there are practical limitations to take them to genome scale (Saghatelian & Cravatt, 2005). Due to the obstacles faced by the experimental approaches, computational analysis for prediction of protein function has become absolutely necessary. Biological functions of proteins are described at various levels of biocomplexity such as biochemical, cellular, physiological and phenotypic levels. Gene Ontology (GO) terms provide a basis for precise description and understanding of various levels of protein function (Ashburner *et al.*, 2000). It is imperative to understand that it is the molecular or biochemical function of a protein that is illustrated using sequence and/or structure data and hence *in silico* approaches help to predict molecular function of a protein (Friedberg, 2006). The current status of sequence- and structure-based approaches for protein function prediction is briefly explained below. These methods have been extensively reviewed elsewhere (Sleator, 2012).

## 1.1   Sequence-Based Approaches for Prediction of Protein Function

The amino acid sequence of a protein is known as the primary structure of a protein and it is the most fundamental form of information available about the protein. It plays the most critical role in determining various characteristics of the protein such as its structure, function and sub-cellular localization. Because of this, amino acid sequence has tremendous potential to be used extensively for functional annotation of proteins (Bork & Koonin, 1998).

In any function prediction method, sequence to function approach is very common and is based on homology. There are mainly two strategies used for this kind of approach. First strategy includes methods based on global and local sequence alignments (Needleman & Wunsch, 1970; Smith & Waterman, 1981; Altschul *et al.*, 1990; Pearson, 1996; Sturrock & Collins, 1993) and second includes methods based on sequence motifs (Bairoch *et al.*, 1995; Henikoff & Henikoff, 1994; Attwood *et al.*, 1994). Identification of protein function by alignment-based sequence similarity search using BLAST (Altschul *et al.*, 1990) or FASTA (Pearson & Lipman, 1988) to find similar proteins in public domain databases is the most popular approach. The annotations of significant hits are used for prediction of protein function. However, it has been found that proteins that have diverged from a common ancestral gene may have the same function but no detectable sequence similarity (Benner *et al.*, 2000). Methods based on sequence profiles such as PSI-BLAST (Altschul *et al.*, 1997) have been developed which provide high sensitivity for detecting remote homologs. Sequence motifs and patterns are also used for detection of close and distant homologues. This approach yields a much higher sensitivity as well as specificity of function prediction as compared to alignment-based methods since many functional motifs and patterns have been identified for a large number of protein families. In spite of this, sequence similarity-based approaches may not be always adequate for function identification of novel proteins.

## 1.2    Structure-Based Approaches for Prediction of Protein Function

Computational methods utilizing three-dimensional (3D) structures of proteins can be employed when sequence-based function prediction cannot be achieved with high confidence level. This is due to the fact that protein structures are more conserved than sequences during evolution. Various aspects of structural data such as the overall fold, active site residues and their conformation, interactions with ligands and other biomolecules can provide insights into functions of proteins. Consequently, various categories of methods are available for structure-based function prediction. The methods that utilize the fold information depend on global and local structural alignments algorithms (Holm & Sander, 1993; Madej *et al.,* 1995; Orengo & Taylor, 1996; Harrison *et al.,* 2003). Global and local conformational similarities between proteins indicate functional similarities and are useful for inferring functions of novel proteins. Several methods have been developed to identify surface pockets and cavities in protein structures as well, that help in identification of potential active/binding sites and amino acid residues therein (Capra *et al.,* 2009; Najmanovich *et al.,* 2008; Gold & Jackson, 2006; Chang *et al.,* 2006; Wass *et al.,* 2010). This approach is especially useful for prediction of enzymatic functions. Detection of similar local geometries of functionally important residues implies similar functions even in distantly related proteins (Torrance *et al.,* 2005). Availability of co-crystal structures of protein-ligand, protein-protein and protein-DNA/RNA complexes have enabled characterization of detailed atomic interactions. Analyses of these structures have provided valuable insights into the principles that govern intermolecular interactions that are important for the functions of proteins and have led to development of approaches for prediction of function (Kinoshita *et al.,* 2008). Further, the applications of techniques for molecular dynamics and docking simulations have opened the vistas in understanding of molecular motions and interactions involved in function. Simulations also offer rich data to understand the detailed atomic-level mechanisms of function (Glazer *et al.,* 2009; Dodson *et al.,* 2008; Pierri *et al.,* 2010; Favia & Nobeli, 2011; Chang *et al.,* 2005). A combination of various structure-based approaches viz. structural alignments, active site identification, simulations and characterization of molecular interactions provide a useful methodology towards function prediction. Availability of high-resolution structural data of the target proteins or their homologues, however, remains the major limitation of this methodology.

## 1.3    Machine Learning-Based Approaches for Prediction of Protein Function

Until recently, sequence and structure-based methods that utilize homology relationships among proteins have dominated the scene in prediction of functions. However, these methods suffer from limitations of availability of adequate data of homologous proteins. They also fail when homology relationships cannot bc cstablished for target proteins (Whisstock & Lesk, 2003). Even though sequence similarity is correlated to functional similarity, exceptions are observed on both ends of the similarity scale (Galperin *et al.,* 1998; Rost, 2002). Protein function prediction based on the structure has been restricted in scope because of the availability of limited number of structures and folds in the databases. All of these factors have contributed to the development of approaches for computational function prediction, which can utilize several other important features in sequences and structures along with similarity measures.

Among these, machine learning-based approaches have been found particularly useful in predicting various functional aspects in proteins. The major advantage of these methods is their ability to map the problem of function prediction to the problem of generating classification models (Tan *et al.*, 2005). Machine learning based methods utilize protein sequence and/or structure data, represented by transformed and more meaningful information in the form of feature vectors. It has been shown that using machine learning classifiers, it is possible to predict the function of hypothetical proteins based on features of amino acid sequences of well characterized proteins, without using homology information (Han *et al.*, 2006). Similarly, more and more machine learning based methods are being developed which use 3D structure and function data of well characterized proteins to predict functions of unknown proteins (Al-Shahib *et al.*, 2007). The efficacy of these methods has been demonstrated through several recent studies and it is therefore important that bioinformatics researchers are aware of and have a basic understanding of these methods. In the succeeding sections of the chapter, various machine learning methods are described and their applications for the purpose of prediction of protein function are reviewed.

## 2   Machine Learning Algorithms

The essence of machine learning algorithms lies in development of models from the existing data and subsequently, classification and/or prediction using novel data. Methods based on machine learning algorithms are grouped into two classes; namely, supervised and unsupervised. In supervised learning, predefined class labels are available for all the training examples. This labeled training data is used to build a model, which is used to predict the class of new input data. In unsupervised learning, predefined class labels for the training examples are not available. The basic aim of unsupervised methods is to discover the patterns hidden in the input data and group (cluster) the data appropriately.

Methods based on machine learning algorithms have been used extensively for various applications in the field of biology (Tarca et al., 2007). These methods have been utilized in diverse domains like genomics, proteomics and systems biology (Larrañaga et al., 2006). Specifically, supervised machine learning approaches have found immense importance in numerous bioinformatics prediction methods. A brief review of methodologies for prediction of protein function with special emphasis on machine learning methods is available (Zhao et al., 2008). The aim of the present article is to provide an overview of the machine learning algorithms as well as application methods based on these algorithms.

**Artificial Neural Network (ANN)**

This algorithm is based on the concept of biological neurons. In biological systems, learning process is based on the minor adjustments to the synaptic connections between neurons, while in ANNs, the learning process is carried out by interconnections between the processing elements that constitute the network topology. Typically ANN consists of 3 layers, viz. input layer, hidden layer and output layer. ANN trains a hidden-layer-containing network and uses its connected structures for pattern recognition and classification (Wang & Larder, 2003; Drăghici & Potter, 2003). In the bioinformatics applications of ANNs, many different types of architectures are employed. Perceptron and multi-layer perceptron (MLP) are the simplest type of architectures. Radial Basis function networks and Kohonen self-organizing maps have also been found to be very useful architectures.

The major steps involved in an ANN algorithm are as follows:

- Generation of training and test datasets by processing of the available data

- Encoding of the data into digital format using various encoding systems (e.g. binary system)

- Design and development of ANN architecture consisting of 3 layers for prediction

- Training the ANN by using appropriate parameters and input data

- Selection of ANN model that gives the valid output

- Validation of ANN model using test dataset for estimation of efficacy for prediction

Major advantage of ANN is its ability to process and analyze large complex datasets, containing non-linear relationships. The method has other benefits like being able to handle noisy data and the capability of generalization. An apparent limitation of the method is the time taken for processing complex datasets (Lancashire *et al.*, 2009). In bioinformatics, ANNs have been extensively used for the tasks like gene prediction (Xu & Uberbacher, 1997), signal peptide prediction (Nielsen *et al.*, 1997), protein secondary structure prediction (Chae *et al.*, 2010) and sequence feature analysis (Blekas *et al.*, 2005).

## Hidden Markov Models (HMM)

Hidden Markov Models (HMMs) are very popular machine learning approaches in bioinformatics. These are probabilistic models which are generally applicable to time series or linear sequences. They can be used to describe the evolution of observable events that depend on internal factors, which are not directly observable. The observed event is referred to as a 'symbol' and the invisible factor underlying the observation is called as a 'state' (Yoon, 2009). An HMM consists of several states, connected by means of the transition probabilities, thus forming a Markov process. Each of these states has an observable symbol attached to it. An HMM consists of a visible process of observable events and a hidden process of internal states moving in tandem. The aim is to find the optimal path through the states, which maximizes the probability of occurrence of the observed sequence (of symbols).

The major steps associated in the algorithm for generation of HMM are as follows:

- Development of an HMM architecture using various states to represent the given set of features

- Assignment of hidden states to the features and construction of HMM model

- Training the HMM either using supervised or unsupervised technique so that the model sufficiently fits the problem under study

- Derivation of emission probabilities that govern the distribution of the observed symbols i.e. the probability that a symbol will be observed given that the HMM is in a particular state

- Decoding of the HMM for the prediction of hidden states from the data

- The major benefit associated with HMMs is their ease of use, requirement of smaller datasets and precise understanding of the process. Among the main drawbacks of HMMs is their greater computational cost. HMMs are the most effective method for biological sequence analysis and therefore they are routinely applied for multiple sequence alignments (Finn *et al.*, 2011), gene finding (Lukashin *et al.*, 1998) as well as protein secondary structure and function prediction (Majoros *et al.*, 2005; De Fonzo *et al.*, 2007).

**Support Vector Machine (SVM)**

SVM is a supervised methodology rigorously based on the statistical learning theory (Vapnik, 1995). For linearly separable examples, SVM constructs a maximum margin hyperplane separating the data points into two different classes. This hyperplane acts as a decision surface between the two classes. For nonlinearly separable data, SVM first transforms the data into a higher dimensional feature space and subsequently employs a linear maximum margin hyperplane. This may introduce a computational intractability requiring a transformation to high dimensional space. SVM handles this by defining appropriate kernel functions by virtue of which the computations can be carried out in the original space itself. Three popular kernel functions are Linear, Polynomial and Radial Basis Function (RBF). In bioinformatics, many domain specific kernel functions are also available like graph kernel and string kernel. The concept can be extended to multiclass classification. Two popular multiclass classification methods are employed viz., one against all and one against one.

The general steps involved in the SVM algorithm are as follows:

- Construction of a feature vector representing the positive and negative dataset: This feature vector consists of the properties of the input data like amino acid and/or dipeptide composition, physico-chemical properties etc.

- Choice of an appropriate kernel function suitable for the prediction task using the classifier training

- Training of SVM classifier by selecting optimum kernel parameters so as to achieve highest accuracy

- Selection of model with the best performance to perform predictions

- Application of selected model for performing predictions on the unknown input data set

SVM is the most robust classifier, and has the best generalization ability on the unseen data as compared to other methods. It is the most commonly used machine learning method in bioinformatics and computational biology. It has been employed for secondary structure prediction, fold recognition, binding site prediction as well as for gene finding (Yang, 2004; Tong et al., 2008; Kadam et al., 2012).

**k-nearest-neighbor (KNN) Classifiers**

KNN classifiers are based on finding the $k$ nearest examples in a reference set, and taking a majority vote among the classes of these $k$ examples (Johnson & Wichern, 1982) to assign a class to the query. Decision boundaries for assigning classes are implicitly derived in KNN.

Following are the important steps involved in development of KNN classifier.

- Construction of a feature set and a distance metric to compute distances between features

- Determination of the number of nearest neighbors (parameter k) for the training set

- Calculation of the Euclidian distances (or any other distance measure like Mahalanobis distance) between the query-instance and all the training samples

- Sorting of distances and determination of nearest neighbors based on the $k^{th}$ minimum distance

- Prediction of class label for new/unknown instance using the class label of nearest neighbors

The most prominent advantage of KNN method is its high efficiency on larger datasets and robustness when processing noisy data. The disadvantage of KNN is the high computation cost, which often reduces its speed. In bioinformatics, KNN has been employed successfully for performing various protein function prediction tasks (Huang & Yanda, 2004; Shen *et al*, 2006).

## Decision Tree (DT)

Decision tree refers to a branch-test-based classifier (Quinlan, 1993). Construction of decision trees involves analysis of a set of training examples for which the class labels are known. This information is then used to classify new and unseen examples. Every branch corresponds to a group of classes and a leaf denotes a specific class. A decision node specifies a test on a single attribute value, with one branch and its subsequent classes as possible outcomes.

The major steps involved in the DT algorithm are as follows:

- Preparation of training dataset in the appropriate form for the classifier by feature extraction from the input data

- Construction of a decision tree by placing the instances in training set at an initial node

- Division of the instances into two distinct classes (child nodes) based on chosen test value

- Recursive application of the last step until fulfillment of termination (pre-pruning) condition

- Pruning of the resultant tree and its application to perform predictions

DTs are very simple classifiers and hence have better interpretability than other machine learning methods (Kingsford & Salzberg, 2008). They have been widely used in bioinformatics for prediction of genetic interactions and similar applications (Wong *et al.*, 2004; Che *et al.*, 2011).

## Random Forests (RF)

Random Forests (RF) is an ensemble of randomly constructed independent classification and decision trees (Breiman, 2001). It normally exhibits substantial performance improvements over single-tree classifiers such as CART (Breiman *et al,* 1984) and C4.5 (Quinlan, 1993). Randomness may be introduced into the RF algorithm in two ways.

1. Bootstrapping: A bootstrap set is constructed from the original training data set using random sampling with replacement to generate each tree.

2. Node splitting: It is carried out by selecting a subset of attributes. While splitting a node, if there are M input attributes, then a number 'm', where $m \ll M$, is specified such that at each node, m attributes are selected at random and the best split on these are considered. A good value of 'm', which is selected as default by many implementations, considers 'm' as sqrt (M) for classification (Liaw & Wiener, 2002).

The classification tree is thus induced using the 'in bag' data based on the CART algorithm. Later, an out-of-bag (OOB) data, formed after leaving out the in-bag samples from the original data is used for cross validation.

The major steps of the RF algorithm are as follows:

- Employment of the CART algorithm on the data to grow random classification trees

- Use of a bootstrap data known as the in-bag set to train the CART algorithm

- Node splitting based on the best condition over a random subset of 'm' attributes

- Use of a majority voting strategy to decide class affiliation of each OOB sample

- A Variable Importance (VI) ranking, which can be used later to retrain the RF using a smaller subset of the most important variables

- Resistance to over-fitting of data

RF and its variants have been applied to solve a variety of bioinformatics problems, such as gene expression classification, analysis of mass spectroscopy data from protein expression, sequence annotation and prediction of protein-protein interactions (Qi, 2012).

**Ensemble Classifiers**

In ensemble classifiers, individual decisions of a set of classifiers are combined either by weighted or unweighted voting for classification of new instances. These are also known as multi-classifier systems. Ensemble classifiers are more effective for prediction tasks due to the fact that they use a combination of classifiers and can capture features that cannot be captured from any single model alone. Ensemble methods have been applied in different bioinformatics problems due to high prediction accuracy (Yang *et al.*, 2010). Table 1 briefly summarizes the important advantages and limitations of major machine learning algorithms.

| Algorithm | Advantages | Limitations |
|---|---|---|
| Artificial Neural Networks (ANN) | • Good approximation of nonlinear relationships<br>• Capacity to handle noisy data | • Greater computational burden<br>• Prone to over-fitting |
| Hidden Markov Models (HMM) | • Precise understanding of the background process<br>• Powerful and easy to use | • Computationally intensive<br>• Relatively slower than other methods<br>• Prone to over-fitting |
| Support Vector Machine (SVM) | • Provide the best generalization ability<br>• Robustness to the noisy datasets<br>• Less susceptible to over-fitting | • Computationally expensive in some cases such as in case of nonlinearly separable data |
| k- nearest neighbor (KNN) | • Simple and easy to learn<br>• Effective when training data is large<br>• Training is very fast | • Computational complexity<br>• Inconsistent performance when number of attributes increases |
| Decision Tree (DT) | • Able to handle both continuous and discrete attributes<br>• Better interpretability<br>• Good results for redundant attributes | • Error-prone in case of data with large number of classes<br>• Sensitive to small variations in the data |
| Random Forest (RF) | • High accuracy and speed<br>• Less prone to over-fitting<br>• Ability to evaluate each attribute for prediction | • Tendency to over-fitting when data is noisy |
| Ensemble classifiers | • Greater efficiency of prediction<br>• Better utilization of the data | • Greater computational complexity |

**Table 1:** Major machine learning algorithms with their advantages and limitations.

**A generalized protocol for bioinformatics applications based on machine learning algorithms**

Every machine learning algorithm has some uniqueness with respect to the model of learning and parameter optimization. But there are some common steps involved like preparation of datasets, feature selection methods and performance evaluation approaches. These steps are discussed in the succeeding sections. Figure 1 illustrates a schematic representation of the general protocol for classification/prediction using a machine learning approach.

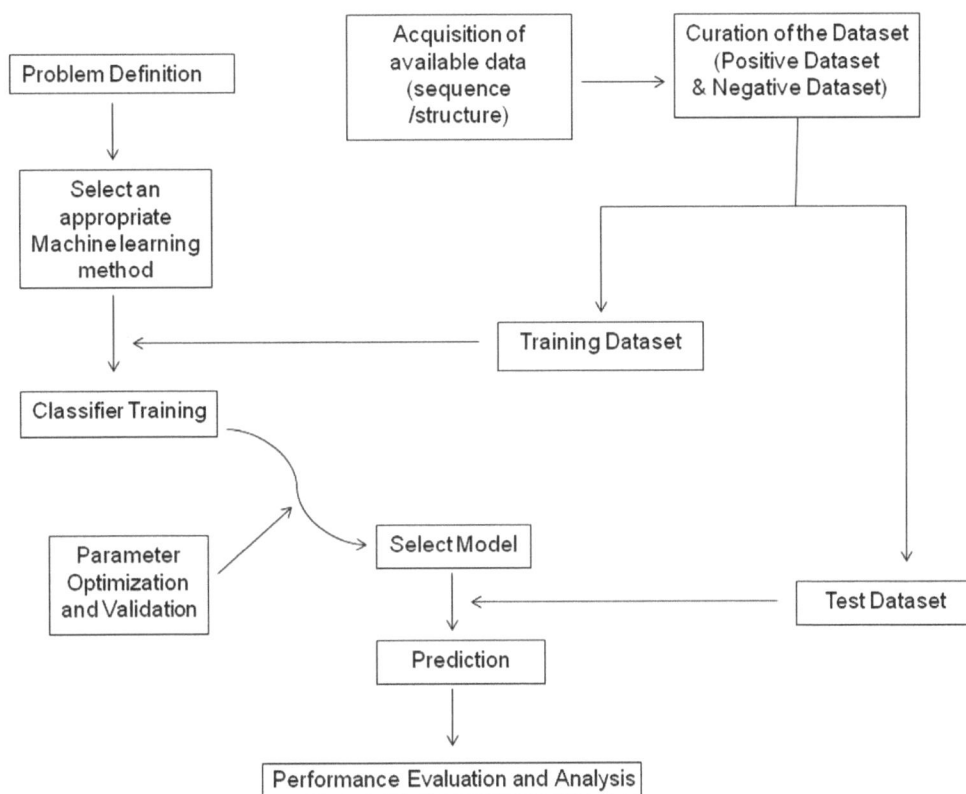

**Figure 1:** Schematic representation of prediction methodology by a machine learning approach.

## 2.1    Preparation of Datasets

Successful applications of the machine learning methods demand identification of discriminatory features, which is dependent on the quality of datasets used for training. Thus, selection and/or curation of discriminative datasets for training, testing and validation determine practical effectiveness of the method.

It is necessary to use non-redundant datasets for generating predictive models, irrespective of the type of machine learning algorithm as well as the type of input data being used. This is due to the fact that redundancy in the data leads to bias in the statistical analysis, which might result in overestimation of predictive performance (Nielsen *et al.*, 1996). Curation of the data to remove repetitive features is an essential pre-requisite. The criteria used for generating non-redundant datasets, however, should not be too rigorous as it can cause omission of valuable information from the dataset.

For an efficient classification algorithm, well-defined annotation classes and training dataset containing positive and negative data for each class are very critical. The positive dataset should represent the members of a particular annotation class whereas the negative dataset should represent non-members. The number of instances for each class should be balanced, as some classifiers like SVM tend to produce reduced accuracies for imbalanced datasets. Appropriate representation of the informative experimental data available and its conversion into datasets relevant to machine learning denotes the critical step of generating an efficient classifier (Juncker *et al.*, 2009).

## 2.2   Feature Extractions and Selection

In most of the machine learning classifiers, the input is represented by parameters that provide information for prediction. These parameters, denoted as features or attributes, are present in large numbers. Many of these features are redundant in nature and are not needed for efficient prediction of labels. The dimensionality of the original data can be reduced by feature extraction and feature selection methods (Jain *et al.*, 2000).

**Feature Extraction:**

It involves the production of a new set of features from the original features in the data, through the application of a mapping method. Well-known unsupervised feature extraction methods include Principal Component Analysis (PCA) and spectral clustering. PCA finds a linear projection of high dimensional data into a lower dimensional subspace, which leads to the maximization of the variance and minimization of the least square reconstruction error. Because of this, PCA has been found very effective for performing feature extraction (Li *et al.*, 2008). It has also been used extensively in the studies involving analysis of spectral data, with considerable efficiency (Grill & Rush, 2008).

**Feature Selection:**

Feature selection (also known as subset selection, attribute selection or variable selection) is the process of choosing a small subset of features that is sufficient to predict the target classes accurately. There are numerous advantages of applying feature selection techniques in prediction methods. The most notable are, i) to avoid over-fitting and improve prediction performance of the model generated; (ii) to reduce the computational complexity of learning and prediction algorithms; (iii) to provide faster and cost-effective models; and (iv) to gain a deeper insight into the underlying processes that generated the data (Saeys *et al.*, 2007). Considering these benefits that feature selection techniques offer, they have been widely applied in development of prediction methods. Based on the context of classification (prediction), feature selection techniques are grouped into three categories.

### 2.2.1   Filter Methods

In filter method, a predictive subset of features is determined based on simple statistics (scores) calculated from the empirical distribution/s. These scores represent relevance of the particular feature and hence filter method denotes intrinsic properties of the data to be classified. The most prominent advantage of filter method is its non-dependence on the classification algorithm. It is a simple and fast method that can also be applied to high dimensional datasets. Prominent examples of filter approach include Information gain, Chi-square test, Correlation based feature selection (CFS) and Mutual Information based feature selection (Saeys *et al.*, 2007).

### 2.2.2   Wrapper Methods

These methods employ a search through the available feature space to identify a subset of features. They use the estimated accuracy from an induction algorithm as the measure of efficiency for this purpose. Thus, in these methods, different subsets of features are generated and evaluated. The evaluation of a particular subset is coupled to the classification algorithm, making this approach algorithm specific. These methods have the advantage of utilizing feature dependencies and taking into account the interdependencies of feature subset search and final model selection. Algorithms based on the wrapper approach include Sequential Forward selection and SVM-RFE feature selection. Similarly, Genetic Algorithm is also found very efficient for performing feature selection with respect to size of the feature set and performance of the feature selection algorithm (Li *et al.*, 2004).

### 2.2.3   Embedded Methods

Like wrapper methods, embedded methods are specific to the given algorithm. In contrast to filter and wrapper approaches, the learning part and the feature selection part cannot be separated in embedded methods. These methods are computationally less intensive than wrapper methods. They make better use of all the available data as splitting of the data into training and validation datasets is not required. Feature selection using the decision trees and weight vector of SVM is an example of embedded approach (Guyon *et al*, 2002).

### 2.3   Performance Evaluation (Estimation of Accuracy)

For any statistical prediction method, it is of paramount importance to determine the efficacy of the method. Cross validation tests, along with benchmark datasets are employed for this purpose (Chou, 2011). Three cross-validation methods that are commonly used to estimate the prediction efficiency are briefly described below.

### 2.3.1   Independent Dataset Test

In the independent dataset test, instances in the test dataset are selected such that the examples used in the training of the classifier are not included. This ensures that there is no inherent memory bias in making predictions. Application of this test produces reliable estimate of accuracy only when the test dataset is adequately large. In case of insufficient data, the construction of independent dataset becomes inconsistent and variable results are obtained.

### 2.3.2   The Sub-sampling (n-fold Cross Validation) Test

In the n-fold cross validation, original dataset is divided into *n* subsamples. Out of these *n* subsamples, one is used as a test dataset while other *n-1* subsamples are used as training dataset. The cross validation process is carried out *n* times, with each of the *n* subsamples used once as a test dataset. For the sub-sampling test, 5-fold, 7-fold or 10-fold cross-validation is commonly applied. The most apparent advantage of this procedure is the requirement of less computational time. In any sub-sampling method, only a particular fraction of all the subsample selections is considered. Due to this, inconsistencies like biased predictions are observed when this method is applied to same datasets or same predictors. In cases where the available test dataset is small, this method can be utilized since it is known to produce reliable results.

### 2.3.3   The Jackknife Test

In the jackknife test, each instance is considered as a test data one by one; while remaining instances are used for training the predictor. This facilitates use of each instance in the input data set for training as well as testing and the memory bias, if any, is avoided. Due to the consistent results obtained for a particular predictor, the problem of arbitrariness observed in case of independent test datasets and subsampling is not encountered in this case. The jackknife test, therefore, has been widely used to estimate efficiencies of different classifiers.

### 2.4   A Case Study: Prediction of Antigens and Non-antigens from Sequence

Prediction and identification of the antigenic proteins of pathogens is one of the most important steps in design and development of vaccines using reverse vaccinology approach (Rappuoli, 2001; Kulkarni-Kale *et al.,* 2012). In this section, a case study of prediction of antigenic and non-antigenic proteins is presented using SVM as a classification and prediction method. Figure 2 shows protocol of the method as a flow chart. Compositional features viz. single amino acid and dipeptide frequencies are used for training and testing purposes.

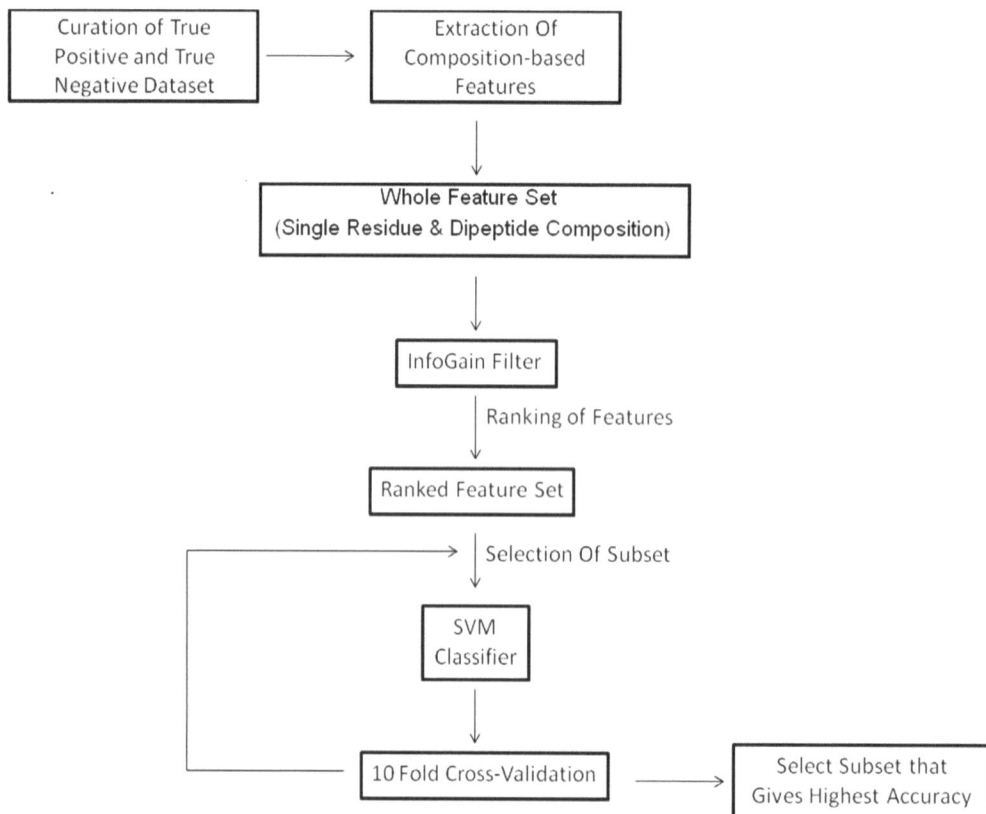

**Figure 2:** Flow chart depicting methodology of simple classifier generation for predicting antigens and non-antigens.

### 2.4.1 Dataset

The protein sequence dataset for this study is taken from the work of Doytchinova (Doytchinova & Flower, 2007). This training dataset comprises of 75 sequence instances each, of antigens (true positives) and non-antigens (true negatives). The antigenic protein sequences are known bacterial proteins that are used to design candidate vaccines. The sequences of non-antigenic proteins (negative dataset) are taken from the same bacterial species, which are used to derive the positive dataset of antigens.

### 2.4.2 Feature Extraction

For every sequence in the true positive and true negative datasets, single amino acid and dipeptide frequencies are calculated and are used as features. Amino acid composition is represented by 20 features while 400 features denote dipeptide composition. The feature vector is constructed for SVM-based prediction, with total of 420 features for each protein sequence.

### 2.4.3 Feature Selection

Feature selection is carried out using Waikato Environment for Knowledge Analysis (WEKA) software package (Hall *et al.*, 2009), to find the feature subset that gives the best results. Information Gain (InfoGain) is used as an attribute evaluator. InfoGain acts as a filter and it assigns a specific rank to each feature based on its effectiveness in classification.

### 2.4.4 Classification Method

SVM is employed for the classification purpose using LIBSVM (version 3.0) software package (Chang & Lin, 2011). Three kernel functions viz. Linear, Polynomial and Radial Basis Function (RBF) are used and 10 fold cross-validation is done to determine prediction accuracy, for the whole feature set as well as for subsets of selected features.

### 2.4.5 Validation

The RBF kernel is observed to provide the best cross-validation accuracies. The results obtained for all the feature subsets are listed in Table 2. The feature subset comprising of 20 features is observed to give maximum cross-validation accuracy of 83.33%. Both single amino acid and dipeptide composition features are found to contribute to this feature set. Thus a very compact and efficient SVM classifier is generated for prediction of antigens and non-antigens using combination of single amino acid and dipeptide compositions.

| Feature Set | Kernel | Gamma[*] | Cost[#] | Cross-validation Accuracy |
|---|---|---|---|---|
| 420 features (whole feature set) | RBF | 1e-05 | 100 | 80% |
| 37 ranked features selected by InfoGain | RBF | 0.5 | 0.31 | 81.33% |
| 20 top ranked features selected by InfoGain | RBF | 0.31 | 128 | 83.33% |
| 10 top ranked features selected by InfoGain | RBF | 0.5 | 0.5 | 82.66% |

[*]Gamma: Kernel parameter that regulates the nonlinearity of the classifier
[#]Cost: Kernel parameter that deals with over-fitting of the classifier

**Table 2**: Cross-validation results for different feature sets.

# 3     Machine Learning Approaches Using Sequence-based Features

Information present in the amino acid sequences of proteins has been very useful for prediction of protein function by machine learning methods (Han *et al.*, 2006). In this section, a detailed account of sequence-based machine learning methods is presented. These methods utilize the sequence information in different forms of features like amino acid and dipeptide frequencies (compositional features), sequence order information in the form of pseudo amino acid composition (Chou, 2001), position specific scoring matrix (PSSM) and/or profiles and functional domain compositions. The individual informative features and their combinations have been utilized very successfully for different function prediction applications like prediction of structural class, prediction of protein subcellular localization, prediction of protein-protein interactions and many others. A brief summary of the methods that have been developed for these applications is given below.

## 3.1     Compositional Features

Compositional features of proteins refer to the features derived directly from the amino acid sequence of the protein. Compositional features of proteins are mainly derived in the form of either single amino acid residues frequencies (monopeptide composition) or as frequencies of pairs of consecutive amino acid residues (dipeptide composition). Monopeptide composition is expressed as a vector of 20 numerical attributes, in which each numerical attribute is the occurrence of a specific amino acid residue (Yang, 2004). Similarly, dipeptide composition is represented as a vector of 400 numerical attributes (Fang *et al.*, 2008).

It has been shown that the structural class and overall fold of a protein are determined by its amino acid composition (Chou & Zhang, 1995). Compositional features have been, therefore, routinely used to predict structural classes of proteins using ANN (Rost & Sander, 1994; Chandonia & Karplus, 1995) and SVM (Cai *et al.*, 2002) based methods. Amino acid compositional features have been shown to be characteristic features for subcellular localization of proteins (Cedano *et al.*, 1997). Consequently, these features have been used in combination with machine learning algorithms to predict subcellular localization of novel/hypothetical proteins. The methods employed for this purpose include KNN (Nakai & Horton, 1999; Huang & Yanda, 2004) and SVM (Hua & Sun, 2001; Yu *et al.*, 2006a; Park & Kanehisa, 2003). SVM based methods have also been developed for prediction of subcellular localization of proteins from specific organisms such as prokaryotes (Bhasin *et al.*, 2005), Gram-negative bacteria (Yu *et al.*, 2004), plants (Tamura & Akutsu, 2007), and humans (Garg *et al.*, 2005).

Amino acid composition combined with ANN and SVM based classifiers have been successfully applied for prediction of DNA-binding residues (Wang & Brown, 2006a; Ofran *et al.*, 2007; Hwang *et al.*, 2007). Cai and Lin have presented a detailed account of SVM-based methods for predicting rRNA-, mRNA-, and DNA-binding proteins from amino acid sequence (Cai & Lin, 2003). A web server, ProteDNA (http://protedna.csbb.ntu.edu.tw/) is available to predict DNA-binding residues in transcription factors using SVM (Chu *et al.*, 2009). Prediction of RNA-binding sites using amino acid sequence has also been performed (Terribilini *et al.*, 2006). BindN (http://bioinformatics.ksu.edu/bindn/) is an efficient web-based tool for prediction of both DNA and RNA binding proteins (Wang & Brown, 2006b).

Prediction of protein-protein interactions has emerged as an important problem in recent bioinformatics research. SVM has been efficiently used for this task (Shen *et al.*, 2007; Yu *et al.*, 2010). Chang and co-workers utilized accessible surface area of amino acids derived from sequence-based predictions, to develop a novel and efficient method for inferring protein-protein interactions using kernel density estimation algorithm (Chang *et al.*, 2010).

Bhasin *et al.* used single amino acid and dipeptide composition for accurate classification of nuclear receptors (Bhasin & Raghava, 2004a) and only dipeptide composition for predicting G-protein coupled receptors (Bhasin & Raghava, 2004b). CTKPred (http://bioinfo.tsinghua.edu.cn/~huangni/CTKPred/) is an SVM-based online prediction server for the prediction and classification of cytokine superfamilies, which is based on the dipeptide composition (Huang *et al.*, 2005).

Prediction of secretory proteins is performed successfully using amino acid composition and similarity search (Garg & Raghava, 2008). ANN-based method is employed for prediction of novel archaeal enzymes using properties of sequences (Jensen *et al.*, 2002). An RF-based method for predicting protein motions from amino acid sequences has also been developed (Hirose *et al,* 2010). PrDOS (http://prdos.hgc.jp) is a server that predicts the disordered regions of a protein using SVM from its amino acid sequence (Ishida & Kinoshita, 2007).

## 3.2  Pseudo Amino Acid Composition

The pseudo amino acid (PseAA) composition is a unique way to represent a protein sequence in a discrete model without losing its sequence-order information completely. The PseAA composition of a given protein is denoted by a set of more than 20 discrete factors, where the first 20 factors represent the components of its conventional amino acid composition while the additional factors incorporate its sequence order information via various modes (Chou, 1999; Chou, 2001). This unique representation is generated by sequence correlation factors, which implicitly incorporate the effect of sequence order of the proteins. These correlation factors are discrete numbers that are derived from physico-chemical properties between amino acid pairs of the type (i, i+1), (i, i+2) and (i, i+3). The physicochemical properties incorporate the local sequence order effects that are independent of size, contiguity, and global order of the sequence. The PseAA composition greatly enhances the efficiency of protein function prediction and hence has been widely applied for functional annotation of variety of proteins.

SVM has been extensively utilized in prediction of protein structural class using the PseAA composition (Chen *et al.*, 2006a; Ding *et al.*, 2007; Chen *et al.*, 2006b), while fuzzy K nearest neighbors (FKNN) classifier is adopted as the prediction engine developed by Zhang and co-workers (Zhang *et al.*, 2008).

SVM has also been used for predicting subcellular localization (Shi *et al.*, 2007; Li & Li, 2008) using pseudo amino acid composition. A similar approach has been also applied specifically for prediction of subcellular localizations of proteins involved in apoptosis (Chen & Li, 2007). For prediction of subcellular localization of gram-negative bacterial proteins, a KNN based method (Wang & Yang, 2010) as well as a method based on multiple SVMs is available (Wang *et al.*, 2005). In a recent approach, Ma & Gu (2010) used the Elman Recurrent Neural Network (RNN) classifier to accurately predict subcellular localization of proteins. RNN is an enhanced ANN model in which an extra context layer is present, which makes the classifier more adaptable to time-varying properties of the network itself.

Membrane proteins are attractive targets for basic research and drug design. These proteins are grouped into five types viz. (i) type-1 (ii) type-2 (iii) multipass (iv) lipid chain-anchored and (v) GPI-anchored membrane proteins. Owing to the importance of these proteins as potential drug targets, it has become imperative to develop computational methods for prediction of the types of membrane proteins. Classifiers based on KNN (Shen *et al,* 2006) and weighted SVM (Wang *et al,* 2004) have been developed to predict types of membrane proteins.

Enzymes represent one of the most important biomolecules as they act as catalysts in almost all the cellular processes. Identification of a functional class of a newly found enzyme is very important for determining its biochemical function. SVM is the algorithm of choice for this purpose and it has been used with Discrete Wavelet Transform (Qiu *et al.*, 2010) and with amphiphilic pseudo-amino acid composition (Zhou *et al.*, 2007) and is known to yield high accuracy of predictions.

### 3.3    PSSM Profiles

The position-specific scoring matrix (PSSM) is a very useful quantitative representation of multiple sequence alignments (Henikoff, 1996). It facilitates integration of evolutionary information to predict protein function. PSSM profiles of a protein family are generated using methods such as PSI-BLAST search against nonredundant (nr) database of protein sequences. The PSSM profiles are reliable and quantitative measures of residue conservation at a given location and are being used as features by machine learning methods for predicting various properties and functional annotation of proteins.

There are a number of methods available in which evolutionary profiles have been utilized for detecting subcellular locations of proteins. These include prediction of mitochondrial proteins in malarial parasite (Verma *et al.*, 2010), prediction of subcellular localization of mycobacterial proteins (Rashid *et al.*, 2007) and prediction of protein subnuclear localization (Mundra *et al.*, 2007). Web servers such as LOCSVMPSI (Xie *et al.*, 2005; URL: http://Bioinformatics.ustc.edu.cn/LOCSVMPSI/LOCSVMPSI. php) and TSSub (Guo & Lin, 2006; URL: http://166.111.24.5/webtools/TSSub/index.html) are available that implement SVM-based methods for prediction of subcellular localization of eukaryotic proteins.

An ANN-based algorithm reports efficient prediction of DNA-binding sites using PSSM profiles (Ahmad & Sarai, 2005). The results observed are claimed to be far better in comparison with the methods based on sequence information alone. Similarly, in an SVM-based approach for predicting RNA-binding sites, greater accuracy is achieved when PSSM profiles are used than that of single sequence-based methods (Kumar *et al.*, 2008; Cheng *et al.*, 2008).

For prediction of fungal adhesins and adhesin-like proteins using SVM, the best classifier performance is obtained when PSI-BLAST derived PSSM matrices are used as features (Ramana & Gupta, 2010). SVM has also been applied to predict proteins secreted by malaria parasite into host erythrocyte (Verma *et al.*, 2008), allergenic proteins (Kumar & Shelokar, 2008) and proline *cis/trans* isomerization in proteins (Song *et al.*, 2006). ANN-based methods that use PSSM profiles have also been developed like PPRODO (Sim *et al.*, 2005a), which predicts domain boundaries of proteins from sequence information while another method predicts beta turn types in proteins (Kaur & Raghava, 2004). A method based on FKNN that uses PSI-BLAST profiles as feature vectors has been developed for prediction of solvent accessibility (Sim *et al,* 2005b).

### 3.4    Sequence Motifs and Patterns

Sequence motifs or patterns are defined as sub-sequences that are conserved across a set of protein sequences, most often belonging to a family of proteins (Bork & Koonin, 1996). Being associated with a characteristic function, presence of motif/pattern in a protein sequence serves as a diagnostic for function prediction. Several machine learning methods have been developed which perform encoding of the protein sequence in terms of features that determine whether a certain motif is present in a sequence. Sequence motifs, thus, can be utilized for feature extraction to predict important functional aspects of proteins.

TargetP (http://www.cbs.dtu.dk/services/TargetP/) is an ANN-based tool that uses only N-terminal sequence information, to predict large-scale subcellular localization of proteins (Emanuelsson *et al.*, 2000). ANN is also used to predict mitochondrial transit peptides in malarial parasite (Bender *et al.*, 2003). An automated motif-finding algorithm combined with ANN has resulted in a prediction server ChloroP (http://www.cbs.dtu.dk/services/ChloroP/) for identifying chloroplast transit peptides and their cleavage sites (Emanuelsson *et al.*, 1999). Based on similar features, SVM has been applied for prediction of protein–protein interactions (Martin *et al.*, 2005), alpha-turn types in proteins (Cai *et al.*, 2003a) and prediction of phosphorylation sites (Kim *et al.*, 2004). An SVM-based prediction server to predict aminoacyl tRNA synthetases using PROSITE domains has also been developed (Panwar & Raghava, 2010). There are many ANN-based methods that are available for prediction of kinase-specific phosphorylation sites (Blom *et al.*, 2004) and to predict mucin type O-glycosylation sites in mammalian proteins (Hansen *et al.*, 1998). Motif-based approach has been used for functional classification of the enzymes by an SVM classifier (Kunik *et al.*, 2005).

### 3.4.1   Analysis of Signal Peptides

The processes through which proteins are routed to their final destination within a cell are referred to as subcellular protein sorting. These are mediated through specialized "sorting signals" in the sequences of proteins. These signals are called as signal peptides and they control entry of almost all proteins to the secretory pathway both in prokaryotes and eukaryotes (von Heijne, 1990; Rapoport, 1992). Computational identification of signal peptides and prediction of their cleavage sites is very important not only for genome analysis and automated annotations (Nielsen, 1999) but also for production of proteins in recombinant systems (Nielsen, 1997).

Machine-learning techniques being well suited for pattern recognition tasks, have been widely applied for prediction of signal peptides. ANNs were utilized extensively for predicting signal peptides in the early 1990s (Ladunga *et al.*, 1991; Schneider and Wrede, 1993). The method SignalP was developed for identification of signal peptides in prokaryotes and eukaryotes and their cleavage sites based on ANN (Nielsen, 1997). An updated version, SignalP 3.0 is based on ANN and HMM algorithms (Bendtsen *et al.*, 2004a). As compared to earlier versions of the method, SignalP 3.0 offers improved accuracy for identification of signal peptides in the proteins from eukaryotes, Gram positive and Gram negative bacteria. SPEPlip is an ANN-based method for prediction of lipoprotein cleavage sites (Fariselli *et al.*, 2003). There are other approaches available too, like, Phobius, which is a combined transmembrane protein topology and signal peptide predictor based on HMMs (Käll *et al.*, 2004). The method Signal-3L predicts signal peptides and their cleavage sites in human, plant, animal, eukaryotic, Gram-positive and Gram-negative bacterial protein sequences based on KNN (Shen & Chou, 2007a). HMM-based method is available for prediction of signal peptides in archaeal proteins (Bagos *et al.*, 2009).

Lipoproteins in bacteria are characterized by the presence of a unique signal sequence at the N-terminal end (Hayashi & Wu, 1990). This signal sequence is referred to as a "lipobox" and is used extensively for computational identification and analysis of bacterial lipoproteins. Machine learning-based approaches for this purpose include HMM-based methods for prediction of lipoprotein signal peptides in gram-negative bacteria (Juncker *et al.*, 2003) and in gram-positive bacteria (Bagos *et al.*, 2008). An HMM-based algorithm has been used for functional assignment of predicted lipoproteins in addition to prediction of signal sequences (Babu *et al.*, 2006). Recently, an SVM-based server LIPOPREDICT has also been developed to predict bacterial lipoproteins (Kumari *et al.*, 2012; URL: http://www.lipopredict.cdac.in).

### 3.4.2   Prediction of MHC-binding Peptides and B-cell Epitopes

The Major Histocompatibility Complex (MHC) constitutes a very important component of the human immune system because of its role in both cell-mediated immune response as well as in the humoral immune response. Antigenic proteins are processed inside a cell so as to present only a specific part of a protein (T-cell epitope) bound to an MHC molecule, to evoke an immune response. Specificity of binding of peptides to various MHC alleles is a well-known characteristic feature that makes precise identification of MHC-binding peptides necessary for the prevention, diagnosis and treatment of different types of diseases. Hence automated prediction of MHC binding peptides is an important part of computational immunology (immunoinformatics).

It has been discovered that peptides binding to specific MHC alleles are of short lengths ranging from 9-12 amino acid residues and share specific conserved positions where amino acids with similar properties are present, making them functionally important (Falk *et al*, 1991; Roetzschke *et al.*, 1991). This led to the conclusion that specific "peptide motifs" are involved in the binding of peptides to both MHC class I and class II molecules. Machine learning algorithms have been used in combination with the peptide motifs extensively for prediction of MHC-binding peptides.

ANN-based classifiers have been used for prediction of peptide binding to both class I (Gulukota *et al.*, 1997; Brusic *et al.*, 1994) and class II alleles (Brusic *et al.*, 1998). In a comparative study it has been shown that  ANN-based method offers high specificity when sufficient experimental data for peptide-MHC binding is available while HMM-based method would be preferred for high sensitivity with increasing peptide data (Yu *et al.*, 2002). Earlier, Mamitsuka developed an HMM-based method to predict peptides binding to MHC (Mamitsuka, 1989). Several groups have utilized SVM for predicting class I and class II binding peptides (Donnes & Elofsson, 2002; Bhasin & Raghava, 2004c; Bozic *et al.*, 2005). SVM has been shown to outperform ANN and DT when smaller training datasets are used for performing predictions (Zhao *et al.*, 2003). Recently, a competition of machine learning methods was held, to assess their accuracies for predicting T-cell epitopes. The results show that machine learning methodologies perform exceptionally well for the prediction task (Zhang *et al.,* 2011a).

Machine learning algorithms have also been widely employed for prediction of linear B-cell epitopes with high efficacies. ABCPred (http://www.imtech.res.in/raghava/abcpred/) is a method that uses recurrent ANNs for predicting linear B-cell epitopes (Saha & Raghava, 2006). BCPred  and FBCPred predict linear B-cell epitopes and flexible length linear B-cell epitopes respectively, using SVM classifiers (El Manzalawy *et al.*, 2008a; El Manzalawy *et al.*, 2008b). COBEpro (http://scratch.proteomics.ics.uci.edu) is based on a two-step procedure involving SVM for predicting linear B-cell epitopes (Sweredoski & Baldi, 2009).

## 3.5   Prediction methods Using Functional Domain Composition

Functional Domain composition is a recent concept introduced by Chou and co-workers (Chou & Cai, 2002) to represent a protein in an effective way to improve the quality of statistical prediction of protein function. In this system, a protein is represented by a specific set of discrete numbers, instead of using 20 amino acid components or pseudo amino acid components. In the studies carried out by Murvai *et al* (2001), native functional domains are used as a vector base to define a protein.

Functional Domain composition combined with SVM is employed for a variety of prediction problems. These include prediction of protein subcellular location (Chou & Cai, 2002) and membrane protein types (Cai *et al.*, 2003b). KNN predictors are routinely applied for different prediction tasks viz.

prediction of subcellular localization (Jia *et al.*, 2007), protein quaternary structures (Yu *et al.*, 2006b), enzyme family class (Cai *et al.*, 2005a) and peptidase identification and classification (Xu *et al.*, 2008). In a study that uses functional domain composition for prediction of functional class of proteins from *Saccharomyces cerevisiae*, KNN algorithm is found to produce better results than SVM (Cai & Doig, 2004). Web-based software Enzyme Classification System (ECS) (http://pcal.biosino.org/) performs efficient identification as well as classification of enzymes, on the basis of functional domain composition (Lu *et al.*, 2007).

## 3.6    Combinations of Different Types of Features

In addition to several methods as described so far, there are methods that combine two or more types of features in an attempt to enhance the accuracy of function prediction. Traditional approaches for sequence analysis mentioned above derive information from the sequences in their raw form, i.e. as a string of amino acids. As discussed above, it is possible to transform this raw sequence information into biologically more meaningful and dependable form. Thus, different sets of features are derived from the sequence, which represent the protein in a more comprehensive manner. These discriminative feature sets can be combined and advantageously utilized for determining functions of uncharacterized protein using standard machine learning methodologies.

### 3.6.1    Combination of Compositional Features and Physico-chemical Properties

Several sequence-derived physico-chemical properties are used in combination with amino acid compositions. These physico-chemical properties are denoted by descriptors that denote numerous features like distribution of hydrophobicity and hydrophilicity, polarity, charge, secondary structures, solvent accessibility, polarizability, surface tension, normalized van der Waals volumes and many others. A database, AAindex, archives various physico-chemical and biochemical properties of amino acids and pairs of amino acids by numerical values (Kawashima *et al.*, 2000). These values can be utilized for the purpose of effectively discriminating proteins into functional classes.

SVM is widely used for different prediction problems like protein structural class (Kurgan *et al.*, 2008), protein subcellular locations (Sarda *et al.*, 2005; Huang *et al.*, 2007), using combination of features. MultiLoc (http://www-bs.informatik.uni-tuebingen.de/Services/MultiLoc/) is a web-based server that uses SVM for predicting subcellular localization by integrating N-terminal targeting sequences, amino acid composition and protein sequence motifs (Hoglund *et al.*, 2006). In a method developed by Wang *et al.*, SVM is combined with conjoint triad features for prediction of enzyme subfamily class (Wang *et al.*, 2010). A highly efficient web server based on SVM, SVM-Prot is developed for functional classification of proteins (Cai *et al.*, 2003c; URL: http://jing.cz3.nus.edu.sg/cgi-bin/svmprot.cgi). SVM has also been used to predict proteins involved in bacterial secretion systems (Pundhir & Kumar, 2011), protein stability changes (Teng *et al.*, 2010), functional class of metal binding proteins (Lin *et al.*, 2006a), lipid binding proteins (Lin *et al.*, 2006b) and allergens (Cui *et al.*, 2007). A recent review provides insights into the potential of SVM-based method in prediction of druggable proteins (Han *et al.*, 2007). Prediction of protein-protein interactions has also been achieved using SVM and combination of sequence derived features (Bock & Gough, 2001; Guo *et al.*, 2008).

KNN algorithm is used for prediction of protein subcellular location using amino acid and dipeptide composition along with physico-chemical properties (Gao *et al.*, 2005). Various RF-based methods have been developed for various tasks using combination of descriptors. These include algorithms for prediction of glycosylation sites (Hamby & Hirst, 2008), DNA-binding residues (Wu *et al.*, 2009), antifreeze proteins (Kandaswamy *et al.*, 2011) and protein fold (Dehzangi *et al.*, 2010). ANNs have been employed to predict protein folding class (Dubchak *et al.*, 1995), antigenic activity in hepatitis C virus protein (Lara *et al.,* 2008), mammalian secretory proteins targeted to the non-classical secretory pathways (Bendtsen *et al.*, 2004b) and membrane spanning amino acid sequences (Lohmann *et al.*, 1994).

### 3.6.2   Combination of Pseudo Amino Acid Composition with Other Features

The pseudo amino acid composition (PseAA) of a protein is combined with PSSM derived protein profiles to create a new type of descriptor, Pseudo Position-Specific Scoring Matrix; PsePSSM (Chou & Shen, 2007). This descriptor has been used to predict transmembrane proteins and their types, using a 2-layered method involving ensemble classifier that is a combination of Optimized Evidence-Theoretic K-Nearest Neighbor (OET-KNN) classifiers. An ensemble classifier method for predicting protein subnuclear location is developed that is based on combination of PseAA and PsePSSM (Shen & Chou, 2007b). PseAA has also been employed in prediction of protein structural class using continuous wavelet transform and principal component analysis (Li *et al.*, 2009). SVM-based methods are found to be effective in predicting protein submitochondrial location using PseAA and physico-chemical features (Du & Li, 2006) as well as combining different descriptors like amino acid and dipeptide composition, gene ontology and evolutionary information into Chou's PseAA (Fan & Li, 2012). SVM is also applied for prediction of DNA-binding proteins, based on combinations of autocross-covariance transform, pseudo-amino acid composition and dipeptide composition (Fang *et al.*, 2008). Cheng and co-workers have developed an algorithm to predict protein folding rates by applying PseAA along with sliding window method (Cheng *et al.*, 2012). RF is used for development of web server iDNA-Prot, by incorporation of PseAA-based grey model (Lin *et al.*, 2011; URL: http://icpr.jci.edu.cn/bioinfo/iDNA-Prot).

### 3.6.3   Combination of PSSM Profiles with Other Features

The position-specific scoring matrices (PSSM) have also found reasonable application when used in combination with other features. SVM is used to develop web servers for different application purposes, which are based on combinations of PSI-BLAST generated PSSM with amino acid composition; dipeptide composition, secondary structure composition etc. These servers include CyclinPred (Kalita *et al.*, 2008; URL: http://bioinfo.icgeb.res.in/cyclinpred/) for predicting cyclin proteins and ATPsite (Chen *et al.*, 2011a; URL: http://biomine.ece.ualberta.ca/ATPsite/) for prediction of ATP-binding residues. ANN and SVM-based models are generated for prediction of GTP interacting residues, dipeptides and tripeptides using similar feature combinations (Chauhan *et al.*, 2010). In the method developed by Mishra & Raghava, PSSM profile information is derived for a fixed window length in a sequence to predict FAD interacting residues via SVM (Mishra & Raghava, 2010). A classifier based on SVM and ANN performs prediction of histidines and cysteines that participate in binding of several transition metals and iron complexes (Passerini *et al.*, 2006). VirulentPred, a freely accessible web server based on bi-layer cascade SVM predicts virulent proteins in bacterial pathogens using PSSM and compositional features (Garg & Gupta, 2008; URL: http://bioinfo.icgeb.res.in/virulent/).

### 3.6.4    Combination of Functional Domain Composition with Other Features

Methods based on this type of combination include a predictor for enzyme subclass (Cai & Chou, 2005b). A web server ProtIdent (http://www.csbio.sjtu.edu.cn/bioinf/Protease) has been developed for identifying proteases and their types by fusing functional domain composition and sequential evolution information (Chou & Shen, 2008) while another algorithm predicts substrate-enzyme-product triads by combining compound similarity and functional domain composition (Chen *et al.*, 2010). There are also some methods that utilize combination of PseAA and functional domain composition, such as ANN classifier for predicting protein subcellular location (Chou & Cai, 2004).

## 4    Machine Learning Approaches Using Structure-Based Features

The 3D structure of a protein determines several of its important functional features. Therefore numerous structure-based machine learning methods have been developed to determine various aspects of protein function. This section describes the approaches that employ structure and shape-based (geometric) features to identify protein function and local active sites in protein structure. Algorithms that are based on combinations of sequence derived and structural features have also been described.

### 4.1    Structure and Shape Based Properties

Local 3D structural patterns, such as the surface cavities of proteins (e.g. the clefts and pockets) represent important functional sites because of their conserved structural features (Liu, 2008). Hence identification of these local patterns (pockets) constitutes a very important aspect of structure-based functional annotation. Relationship of local surface patterns and functions is particularly critical in the context of functions of enzymes as active site of an enzyme consists of several catalytic residues with specific spatial arrangements. Machine-learning methodologies have been applied successfully for determining enzyme active sites and the residues therein.

SVM algorithm is used for prediction of active sites from 3D structure alone to develop methods applicable to any enzyme family, in general, (e.g. Tong *et al.*, 2008) and also for methods applicable for family-specific prediction of active sites. The method developed by Cai and co-workers for example, predicts the catalytic triad of serine hydrolase family (Cai *et al.*, 2004).

SitePredict is an RF-based method for predicting binding sites for specific metal ions or small molecules in protein structures (Bordner, 2008; URL: http://sitepredict.org/). The method SCREEN uses RF algorithm for the accurate characterization of protein surface cavities and prediction of drug-binding cavities (Nayal & Honig, 2006; URL: http://interface.bioc.columbia.edu/screen).

Recently, an SVM classifier is developed for prediction of ligand-binding sites in bacterial lipoproteins, using combinations of structure and shape-based properties (Kadam *et al.*, 2012).

For identification of DNA-binding proteins having helix-turn-helix structural motif, methods based on ANNs, DT models and an SVM-based kernel protocol are available (Ferrer-Costa *et al.*, 2005; McLaughlin & Berman, 2003; Bhardwaj *et al.*, 2005). SVM is employed to predict protein–protein interaction surfaces by using surface patch analysis (Bradford & Westhead, 2004) and local surface properties (Bordner & Abagyan, 2005). Subsequently Bradford and co-workers combined surface patch analysis with a Bayesian network to predict protein–protein binding sites (Bradford *et al.*, 2006).

Methods for prediction of functional sites in proteins using properties such as shape and geometry of the protein surfaces also constitute an important approach for prediction of function. These methods model continuous surface of 3D structure of proteins to represent its shape and geometry with high resolution and provide useful features that help in the identification and analysis of functionally important sites such as voids or pockets on these surfaces. 3D Zernike Descriptors (3DZD) are moment-based descriptors that provide an effective and popular technique to describe molecular surfaces and hence can be used to represent protein surfaces (Novotni & Klein, 2004). The method based on Zernike descriptors has a huge potential in shape-based prediction methods due to its simple representation and high efficiency of protein shape comparison. (Server available at: http://dragon.bio.purdue.edu/3d-surfer/)

Computational identification of conformational epitopes is very critical because it has been shown that majority of B-cell epitopes are conformational epitopes (Walter, 1986). The total numbers of experimentally determined 3D structures of antigen-antibody complexes being limited, structure-based methods for epitope predictions are comparatively few in number (Kulkarni-Kale *et al.*, 2005; Sweredoski *et al.*, 2008). An RF predictor has been employed to identify conformational B-cell epitopes using 3D structures (Zhang *et al.*, 2011b). Liang *et al.* have used support vector regression based on structures for prediction of antigenic epitopes (Liang *et, al.*, 2010).

Metal atoms are often essential for maintenance of protein structure, enzyme catalysis and regulatory roles. Prediction of metal binding sites from structural data therefore, is of immense value for functional annotation of newly solved protein structures. DT and SVM classifiers have been successfully used for detecting metal binding sites in protein structures (Babor *et al.*, 2008; Levy *et al.*, 2009). A machine-learning based method, FEATURE, performs accurate prediction of calcium binding sites (Liu & Altman, 2009). A Bayesian classifier has been employed for prediction of zinc binding sites (Ebert & Altman, 2008).

## 4.2   Combination of Sequence and Structural Features

As has been discussed so far, both sequence information and 3D structures can be utilized very efficiently by machine learning methods for determining various functional aspects of proteins. Both the approaches however, suffer from certain limitations like less reliability of sequence-based methods in conferring common function to remote homologues and availability of limited structural data, respectively. Newer algorithms are being developed that rely on combining both sequence and structure features to overcome the limitations and for more reliable predictions. An example of this approach is the web server ProFunc that facilitates comprehensive prediction of protein function (Laskowski *et al.*, 2005; http://www.ebi.ac.uk/thornton-srv/databases/ProFunc). Different types of features derived from amino acid sequence of a protein can be combined with important structure-based attributes. Feature vectors derived from such combinations provide highly informative clues for specific function of a protein.

A very efficient application based on machine learning has been created that combines computed electrostatics, evolutionary information derived from sequences and pocket geometric features for high-performance prediction of catalytic residues (Somarowthu *et al.*, 2011). SVM is applied to predict catalytic residues in proteins using structure and sequence features (Petrova & Wu, 2006; Pugalenthi *et al.*, 2008). Ota et al developed a KNN predictor for catalytic residues (Ota *et al.*, 2003). ANN classifiers have been successfully employed for prediction of nucleic acid (specifically, DNA-) binding proteins based on the structural and sequence properties of electrostatic patches (Stawiski *et al.*, 2003). An ANN-based method has been developed for prediction of DNA-binding proteins along with prediction of DNA-binding residues using sequence composition and structural information (Ahmad *et al.*, 2004). Method based on RF algorithm is developed for prediction of protein-RNA binding sites (Liu *et al.*, 2010). An online web server RNABindR that uses a Naive Bayes classifier is also available for predicting RNA-binding sites using both sequence and structure features (Terribilini *et al.*, 2007; URL: http://bindr.gdcb.iastate.edu/RNABindR).

Prediction of protein-protein interactions has become an important step in the roadmap to gain insights into systems biology. With increasing repertoire of protein structural data, the need for accurate methods that can use surface features and sequence features to predict potential interacting protein partners is growing. ANNs have been successfully applied in various methods for prediction of protein-protein interacting sites. These include prediction of protein-protein interaction sites in heterocomplexes (Fariselli *et al.*, 2002) and prediction of interface residues in protein-protein complexes (Chen & Zhou, 2005). SVM-based algorithms are available for identification of protein-protein binding (interaction) sites that employ (i) sequence-based properties along with protein interaction sites ratios (Koike & Takagi, 2004) and (ii) information relating to sequence and structural complementarities across protein interfaces (Chung *et al.*, 2007). Sequence profile and accessible surface area information combined with the structure-based conservation score and SVM has also been applied for the same purpose (Chung *et al.*, 2006). An RF predictor is developed to predict protein interaction sites from sequence and structure-derived parameters (Sikic *et al.*, 2009). Using both structure and sequence data, a machine learning based classifier for predicting B-cell epitopes has been developed (Rubinstein *et al.*, 2009a). A web server, Epitopia, provides an approach for prediction of B-cell epitopes (Rubinstein *et al.*, 2009b; URL: http://epitopia.tau.ac.il).

A server for prediction of leucine-rich nuclear export signals in proteins is available online, which is based on ANNs and HMM (La Cour *et al.*, 2004). Sequence and structure information in combination with SVM is utilized in a method to predict specificities within enzyme families (Rottig *et al.*, 2010) as well as in a web server Mupro (http://www.ics.uci.edu/~baldig/mutation.html) to predict protein stability changes in proteins due to single amino acid mutations (Cheng *et al.*, 2006). SVM is used in prediction of phosphorylation sites in eukaryotic proteins (Blom *et al.*, 1999). Both ANNs and SVM have been employed to predict protein backbone torsion angles (Kuang *et al.*, 2004). It has been shown that SVM performs very efficiently in the task of inferring gene functional annotations from a combination of protein sequence and structure data (Lewis *et al.*, 2006). SVM-based approaches have been developed for predicting transmembrane helix packing arrangements (Nugent & Jones, 2010) and also for prediction of membrane-binding proteins (Bhardwaj *et al.*, 2006).

## 4.3   Combination of Evolutionary Profiles and Structural Features

PSSMs / sequence profiles can be advantageously combined with useful structure derived properties. This combination provides reliable clues for the function of a protein and can be utilized for efficient functional annotation.

ANN is used to identify the catalytic residues in enzymes, based on an analysis of the structure and sequence conservation (Gutteridge *et al.*, 2003) while Tang et al integrated ANN with genetic algorithm for prediction of catalytic residues in enzymes using their structures (Tang *et al.* 2008). SVM has proven to be very effective in predicting catalytic residues when structural features along with sequence profiles are used (Youn *et al.*, 2007).

An ANN-based predictor that uses PSI-BLAST derived sequence profiles and solvent accessibilities of each surface residue has been developed to predict DNA-binding sites on protein surfaces (Tjong & Zhou, 2007). An SVM-based algorithm that derives features from composition, evolutionary conservation and structural parameters is applied for characterization and prediction of the binding sites in DNA-binding proteins (Kuznetsov *et al.*, 2006; Dey *et al.*, 2012). SVM classifier is also employed in the method PRINTR, to predict RNA-binding sites in proteins using PSSM profiles and structural information (Wang *et al.*, 2008).

Combination of different types of structure and sequence features along with SVM is used to predict hotspots in protein interfaces (Xia *et al.*, 2010; Chen *et al.*, 2011b). An ensemble method consisting of SVM is employed for predicting protein-protein interaction sites using profiles and other informative features (Deng *et al.*, 2009). Machine learning algorithm based on ANNs is utilized for prediction of protein-protein interaction hotspots (Ofran & Rost, 2007).

An ANN classifier is shown to be very efficient for prediction of mammalian mucin-type O-glycosylation sites using substitution matrix profiles and structural information (Julenius *et al.*, 2005). ANN has also been employed for prediction of protein solvent accessibility, combining PSSM and structural profiles (Bondugula & Xu, 2008) and for prediction of carbohydrate binding sites using structure and profiles (Malik & Ahmad, 2007).

# 5   Conclusions

As has been discussed in the previous sections, machine learning methods have been used extensively in the field of protein function prediction and have significantly contributed in the transformation of huge volume of data into useful knowledge. It has been attempted in this review to provide a glimpse of the vast and ever-expanding realm of machine learning based methods in the area of Bioinformatics. Distinction of machine learning methods lies in the fact that they do not require explicit knowledge of homology and homology-derived parameters to be incorporated for the purpose of function prediction. This distinction therefore makes these classes of methods promising especially for novel targets for which homologs are not available. As the amount of genomic data continues to grow at an exponential rate, the requirement for accurate methods for prediction of protein function remains high. There is also a need to develop meta-servers, which will make the methods developed for a specific purpose/objective such as protein-protein interaction sites available as a portal.  The meta-servers would facilitate developers and users alike, by making the training and testing datasets as well as benchmarking results available in public domain. While there is a need to refine the methods to achieve higher accuracy in each class/group, there is also a growing need to bring various aspects of protein function prediction under the realm of machine learning methods.  To understand and model complex biological functions of proteins, algorithms employing diverse and novel features will be developed and are expected to play critical roles in functional annotations. Hybrid machine learning approaches, which utilize combination of different features along with newer feature selection strategies, will constitute an important part of future protein function prediction methods.

# Acknowledgements

KK is a recipient of Junior Research Fellowship of University Grants Commission (UGC) and gratefully acknowledges funding from UGC, Govt. of India.  SVS and UKK acknowledge financial support under the Center of Excellence programs from the Department of Biotechnology (DBT), Govt. of India as well as the Department of Information Technology (DIT), Ministry of Communications and Information Technology (MCIT), Govt. of India. VKJ acknowledges Council of Scientific and Industrial Research (CSIR), New Delhi, India, for emeritus scientist grant. All the authors acknowledge infrastructural facilities at the Bioinformatics Centre, University of Pune, Pune, India.

# References

Ahmad, S., Gromiha, M.M., Sarai, A. (2004). Analysis and prediction of DNA-binding proteins and their binding residues based on composition, sequence and structural information. *Bioinformatics*, 20, 477–486.

Ahmad, S., Sarai, A. (2005). PSSM-based prediction of DNA binding sites in proteins. *BMC Bioinformatics*, 6, 33.

Al-Shahib, A., Breitling, R., Gilbert, D. R. (2007). Predicting protein function by machine learning on amino acid sequences – a critical evaluation. *BMC Genomics*, 8, 78.

Altschul, S.F., Madden, T.L., Schaffer, A.A., Zhang, J., Zhang, Z., Miller, W., Lipman, D.J. (1997). Gapped BLAST and PSI-BLAST: A new generation of protein database search programs. *Nucleic Acids Res.*, 25, 3389–3402.

Altschul, S.F., et al. (1990). Basic local alignment search tool. *J. Mol. Biol.*, 215, 403–410.

Ashburner, M., Ball, C. A., Blake J. A. et al. (2000). Gene ontology: tool for the unification of biology. The gene ontology consortium. *Nat Genet*, 25, 25-9.

Attwood, T. K., et al. (1994). PRINTS – A database of protein motif fingerprints. *Nucleic Acids Res.*, 22, 3590–3596.

Babor, M., Gerzon, S., Raveh, B., Sobolev, V. and Edelman, M. (2008). Prediction of transition metal-binding sites from apo protein structures. *Proteins*, 70, 208–217.

Babu, M. M., Priya, M.. L., Selvan, A. T., Madera, M., Gough, J., Aravind, L., Sankaran, K. (2006). A database of bacterial lipoproteins (DOLOP) with functional assignments to predicted lipoproteins. *J. Bacteriol.*, 188, 2761–2773.

Bagos, P .G., Tsirigos, K. D., Plessas, S. K., Liakopoulos, T. D., Hamodrakas, S. J (2009). Prediction of signal peptides in archaea. *Protein Eng Des Sel*, 22, 27-35.

Bagos, P. G., Tsirigos, K. D., Liakopoulos, T. D. and Hamodrakas, S. J. (2008). Prediction of Lipoprotein Signal Peptides in Gram-Positive Bacteria with a Hidden Markov Model. *J Proteome Res.*, 7(12), 5082-93.

Bairoch, A. et al. (1995). The PROSITE database, its status in 1995. *Nucleic Acids Res.*, 24, 189–196.

Bender, A., Van Dooren G.G., Ralph, S.A., McFadden, G.I., Schneider, G. (2003). Properties and prediction of mitochondrial transit peptides from Plasmodium falciparum. *Mol Biochem Parasitol*, 132 (2), 59-66.

Bendtsen, J. D., Nielsen, H., Von Heijne, G., Brunak, S. (2004a). Improved prediction of signal peptides: SignalP 3.0. *J Mol Biol*, 340 (4), 783-795.

Bendtsen,, J. D., Jensen, L. J., Blom, N., Von Heijne, G., Brunak, S. (2004b). Feature-based prediction of non-classical and leaderless protein secretion *Protein Eng. Des. Sel.* 17, 349–356.

Benner, S. A., Chamberlin, S. G., Liberles, D. A., Govindarajan, S., Knecht, L (2000). Functional inferences from reconstructed evolutionary biology involving rectified databases – an evolutionarily grounded approach to functional genomics. *Res Microbiol*, 151, 97-106.

Bhardwaj, N., Langlois, R. E., Zhao, G., Lu, H. (2005). Kernel-based machine learning protocol for predicting DNA-binding proteins. *Nucleic Acids Res.*, 33, 6486–6493.

Bhardwaj, N., Stahelin, R.V., Langlois, R.E., Cho, W., Lu, H. (2006). Structural Bioinformatics Prediction of Membrane-binding Proteins. *J Mol Biol*, 359 (2), 486-495.

Bhasin, M. and Raghava, G.P. (2004a). Classification of nuclear receptors based on amino acid composition and dipeptide composition *J. Biol. Chem.*, 279, 23262–23266.

Bhasin, M., Garg A., and Raghava, G. P. S. (2005). PSLpred: prediction of subcellular localization of bacterial proteins. *Bioinformatics*, 21(10), 2522-2524.

Bhasin, M., Raghava, G. P. (2004b). GPCRpred: an SVM-based method for prediction of families and subfamilies of G-protein coupled receptors. *Nucleic Acids Res.*, 32, W383–W389.

Bhasin, M., Raghava, G. P. S. (2004c). SVM based method for predicting HLA-DRB1*0401 binding peptides in an antigen sequence. *Bioinformatics*, 20. 421–3.

Blekas K., Fotiadis, DI., Likas, A. (2005). Motif-based protein sequence classification using neural networks. *J Comput Biol*, 12, 64–82.

Blom, N., Gammeltoft, S. and Brunak, S. (1999). Sequence and structure-based prediction of eukaryotic protein phosphorylation sites. *J. Mol. Biol.*, 294, 1351–1362.

Blom, N., Sicheritz-Pontén, T., Gupta, R., Gammeltoft, S. and Brunak, S. (2004). Prediction of post-translational glycosylation and phosphorylation of proteins from the amino acid sequence. *Proteomics*, 4, 1633–1649.

Bock, J. R. and Gough, D.A. (2001). Predicting protein–protein interactions from primary structure. *Bioinformatics*, 17, 455–462.

Bondugula, R., Xu, D. (2008). Combining sequence and structural profiles for protein solvent accessibility prediction. *Proc LSS Comput Syst Bioinform Conf.*, 7, 195-202.

Bordner, A. J. (2008). Predicting small ligand binding sites in proteins using backbone structure. *Bioinformatics*, 24 (24), 2865-2871.

Bordner, A. J. and Abagyan, R. (2005). Statistical analysis and prediction of protein–protein interfaces. *Proteins*, 60, 353–366.

Bork, P. and Koonin, E. V. (1996). Protein sequence motifs. *Curr Opin Struct Biol.*, 6, 3, 366–376.

Bork, P. and Koonin, E.V. (1998). Predicting functions from protein sequences—where are the bottlenecks? *Nat Genet*, 18, 313–318.

Bozic, I., Zhang, G., Brusic, V. (2005). Predictive vaccinology: optimisation of predictions using support vector machine classifiers. *Lecture Notes in Computer Science*. 3578, 375–81.

Bradford, J. R. and Westhead, D. R. (2004). Improved prediction of protein-protein binding sites using a support vector machines approach, *Bioinformatics*, 21 (8), 1487-1494.

Bradford, J. R., Needham, C. J., Bulpitt, A. J., Westhead D. R. (2006). Insights into Protein-Protein Interfaces using a Bayesian Network Prediction Method. *J Mol Biol*, 362 (2), 365-386.

Breiman, L., (2001). Random Forests. *Mach. Learn.* 45, 5–32.

Breiman, L., Friedman, J., Olshen, R., Stone, C. (1984). *Classification and regression trees*. Chapman & Hall, New York.

Brusic, V., Rudy, G., Harrison, L. C. (1994). Prediction of MHC binding peptides using artificial neural networks. In: *Stonier RJ, Yu XS (eds). Complex Systems: Mechanism of Adaptation. Amsterdam: IOS Press*. 253–60.

Brusic, V., Rudy, G., Honeyman, M. et al. (1998). Prediction of MHC class II-binding peptides using an evolutionary algorithm and artificial neural network. *Bioinformatics*, 14, 121–30.

Cai, Y. D., Chou, K. C. (2005a). Using functional domain composition to predict enzyme family classes. *J Proteome Res*, 4 (1), 109-111.

Cai, Y. D. and Chou, K. C. (2005b). Predicting enzyme subclass by functional domain composition and pseudo amino acid composition, *J Proteome Res*, 4, 967-971.

Cai, Y. D., Hu, J. Liu, X. J., and Chou, K. C. (2002). Prediction of protein structural classes by neural network method. *Internet Electron J Mol Des*, 1, 332-338.

Cai, Y. D., Lin, S. L. (2003). Support vector machines for predicting rRNA-, RNA-, and DNA-binding proteins from amino acid sequence. *Biochimica et Biophysica Acta - Proteins and Proteomics*, 1648 (1-2), 127-133.

Cai, Y. D., Feng, K. Y., Li, Y. X., Chou, K. C. (2003a). Support Vector Machine for predicting α-turn types. *Peptides*, 24 (4), 629-630.

Cai, Y. D., Zhou, G. P., Chou, K. C. (2003b). Support vector machines for predicting membrane protein types by using functional domain composition. *Biophys. J.*, 84 (5), 3257-3263.

Cai, C. Z., Han. L. Y., Ji, Z. L., Chen, X., Chen, Y. Z. (2003c). SVM-Prot: Web-based support vector machine software for functional classification of a protein from its primary sequence. *Nucleic Acids Res*, 31 (13), 3692-3697.

Cai, Y. D., Zhou, G. P., Jen, C. H., Lin, S. L., and Chou, K.C. (2004). Identify catalytic triads of serine hydrolases by support vector machines, *J Theor Biol*, 228, 551-557.

Cai, Y.D. and Doig, A.J. (2004). Prediction of Saccharomyces cerevisiae protein functional class from functional domain composition. *Bioinformatics*, 20, 1292–1300.

Capra, JA., Laskowski, RA., Thornton, JM., Singh, M., Funkhouser, TA. (2009). Predicting Protein Ligand Binding Sites by Combining Evolutionary Sequence Conservation and 3D Structure. *PLoS Comput Biol*, 5(12), e1000585.

Cedano, J., Aloy, P., Perez-Pons, J. A., Querol E. (1997). Relation between amino acid composition and cellular location of proteins. *J Mol Biol*, 266 (3), 594-600.

Chae, M.H., Krull, F., Lorenzen, S., Knapp, E.W. (2010). Predicting protein complex geometries with a neural network. *Proteins*, 78, 1026–1039.

Chandonia, J. M., Karplus, M., (1995). Neural networks for secondary structure and structural class prediction, *Protein Sci.*, 4, 275–285.

Chang, C.-C.; Lin, C.-J. (2011). LIBSVM: A library for support vector machines. *ACM Transactions on Intelligent Systems and Technology*, 2, 27:1–27:27, Software available at http://www.csie.ntu.edu.tw/~cjlin/libsvm.

Chang, DTH., Weng, YZ., Lin, JH. et al. (2006). Protemot: prediction of protein binding sites with automatically extracted geometrical templates. *Nucleic Acids Res*, 34, W303–9.

Chang, DT., Oyang, YJ., Lin, JH. (2005). MEDock: a web server for efficient prediction of ligand binding sites based on a novel optimization algorithm. *Nucleic Acids Res*, 33, W233–W238.

Chang, DT., Syu, YT., Lin, PC. (2010). Predicting the protein-protein interactions using primary structures with predicted protein surface. *BMC Bioinformatics*, 11, Suppl 1S3.

Chauhan, J. S., Mishra, N. K. and Raghava, G. P. S. (2010). Prediction of GTP interacting residues, dipeptides and tripeptides in a protein from its evolutionary information. *BMC Bioinformatics*, 11, 301.

Che, D., Liu, Q., Rasheed, K., Tao, X. (2011). Decision tree and ensemble learning algorithms with their applications in bioinformatics. *Adv Exp Med Biol*, 696, 191-199.

Chen, C., Tian, Y. X., Zou, X. Y., Cai, P. X., Mo J.-Y.. (2006a). Using pseudo-amino acid composition and support vector machine to predict protein structural class. *J Theor Biol*, 243, 444-448.

Chen, C., Zhou, X., Tian, Y., Zou, X., Cai, P. (2006b). Predicting protein structural class with pseudo-amino acid composition and support vector machine fusion network. *Anal Biochem*, 357 (1), 116-121.

Chen, H. and Zhou, H.-X. (2005). Prediction of interface residues in protein–protein complexes by a consensus neural network method: Test against NMR data. *Proteins*, 61, 21–35.

Chen, K., Mizianty, M. J., Kurgan, L. (2011a). ATPsite: sequence-based prediction of ATP-binding residues. *Proteome Sci*, 9(Suppl 1), S4.

Chen R., Chen W., Yang S., Wu D., Wang Y., Tian Y., Shi Y. (2011b). Rigorous assessment and integration of the sequence and structure based features to predict hot spots. *BMC Bioinformatics*, 12, 311.

Chen, L., Feng, K. Y., Cai, Y. D., Chou, K.C., & Li, H.P. (2010). Predicting the network of substrate-enzyme-product triads by combining compound similarity and functional domain composition. *BMC Bioinformatics*, 11, 293.

Chen, Y. L., Li, Q. Z. (2007). Prediction of the subcellular location of apoptosis proteins. *J Theor Biol*, 245 (4), 775-783.

Cheng, C. W., Su, E. C., Hwang, J. K., Sung, T. Y., Hsu, W. L. (2008). Predicting RNA-binding sites of proteins using support vector machines and evolutionary information. *BMC Bioinformatics*, 9, S6.

Cheng, J., Randall, A., Baldi, P. (2006). Prediction of protein stability changes for single-site mutations using support vector machines. *Proteins*, 62, 1125–1132.

Cheng, X., Xiao, X., Wu, ZC., Wang, P., Lin, WZ. (2012). Swfoldrate: Predicting protein folding rates from amino acid sequence with sliding window method. *Proteins*, Aug. 29 (Epub ahead of print).

Chou, K. C. (1999). Using pair-coupled amino acid composition to predict protein secondary structure content. *J. Protein Chem.*, 18, 473–480.

Chou, K. C. (2001). Prediction of protein cellular attributes using pseudo-amino acid composition. *Proteins*, 43, 246–255.

Chou, K. C. and Cai, Y. D. (2004). Predicting subcellular localization of proteins by hybridizing functional domain composition and pseudo-amino acid composition. *J Cell Biochem*, 91, 1197-1203.

Chou, K. C. and Shen, H.B. (2008). ProtIdent: A web server for identifying proteases and their types by fusing functional domain and sequential evolution information. *Biochem Biophys Res Comm*, 376, 321-325.

Chou, K. C. and Zhang, C.T. (1995). Review: Prediction of protein structural classes. *Crit Rev Biochem Mol Biol*, 30, 275-349.

Chou, K. C., Shen, H. B. (2007). MemType-2L: A Web server for predicting membrane proteins and their types by incorporating evolution information through Pse-PSSM. *Biochem Biophys Res Commun*, 360 (2), pp. 339-345.

Chou, K., Cai, Y. (2002). Using functional domain composition and support vector machines for prediction of protein subcellular location. *J. Biol. Chem.* 277, 45765-45769.

Chou, KC. (2011). Some remarks on protein attribute prediction and pseudo amino acid composition (50th Anniversary Year Review). *J Theor Biol*, 273, 236–247.

Chu, W., Huang, Y., Huang, C., Cheng, Y., Huang, C., Oyang, Y. (2009). ProteDNA: a sequence-based predictor of sequence-specific DNA-binding residues in transcription factors. *Nucleic Acids Res.*, 37, W396-W401.

Chung, J. L., Wang, W., Bourne, P. E. (2006). Exploiting sequence and structure homologs to identify protein-protein binding sites. *Proteins*, 62(3), 630-640.

Chung, J. L., Wang, W., Bourne, P. E. (2007). High-Throughput Identification of Interacting Protein-Protein Binding Sites. *BMC Bioinformatics*, 8, 223.

Cui, J., Han, L. Y., Li, H., Ung, C. Y., Tang, Z. Q., Zheng, C. J., Cao, Z. W., Chen, Y. Z. (2007). Computer prediction of allergen proteins from sequence-derived protein structural and physicochemical properties. *Mol Immunol*, 44 (4), 514-520.

De Fonzo V., Aluffi-Pentini, F., Parisi, V. (2007). Hidden Markov models in bioinformatics. *Curr Bioinform*, 2, 49–61.

Dehzangi, A., Amnuaisuk, S. P., Dehzangi, O. (2010). Using Random Forest for Protein Fold Prediction Problem: An Empirical Study. *J. Inf. Sci. Eng.*, 26(6), 1941-1956.

Deng, L., Guan, J., Dong, Q., Zhou, S. (2009). Prediction of protein-protein interaction sites using an ensemble method. *BMC Bioinformatics*, 10, 426.

Dey, S., Pal, A., Guharoy, M., Sonavane, S., and Chakrabarti, P. (2012). Characterization and prediction of the binding site in DNA-binding proteins: improvement of accuracy by combining residue composition, evolutionary conservation and structural parameters. *Nucleic Acids Res.*, May 27.

Ding, Y. S., Zhang, T. L. & Chou, K.C. (2007). Prediction of protein structure classes with pseudo amino acid composition and fuzzy support vector machine network. *Protein Pept Lett*, 14, 811-815.

Dodson, GG.,Lane, DP.,Verma, CS. (2008). Molecular simulations of protein dynamics: new windows on mechanisms in biology. *EMBO Rep*, 9, 144–150.

Donnes, P., Elofsson, A. (2002). Prediction of MHC class I binding peptides, using SVMHC. *BMC Bioinformatics*, 3, 25.

Doytchinova, I.A., Flower, D.R. (2007). Identifying candidate subunit vaccines using an alignment-independent method based on principal amino acid properties. *Vaccine*, 25 (5), 856-866.

Drăghici, S. and Potter, R. B. (2003). Predicting HIV drug resistance with neural networks. *Bioinformatics*, 19(1), 98-107.

Du, P., Li, Y. (2006). Prediction of protein submitochondria locations by hybridizing pseudo-amino acid composition with various physicochemical features of segmented sequence. *BMC Bioinformatics*, 7, 518.

Dubchak, I., Muchnik, I., Holbrook, S., Kim, S. (1995). Prediction of protein folding class using global description of amino acid sequence. *Proc Natl Acad Sci USA*, 92, 8700–8704.

EL-Manzalawy, Y., Dobbs, D., Honavar, V. (2008a). Predicting linear B-cell epitopes using string kernels. *J. Mol. Recognit.*, 21, 243-255.

EL-Manzalawy, Y., Dobbs, D., Honavar, V. (2008b). Predicting flexible length linear Bcell epitopes. *7th International Conference on Computational Systems Bioinformatics*, 121-131.

Ebert, J., Altman, R. (2008). Robust recognition of zinc binding sites in proteins. *Prot Sci*, 17, 54–65.

Eisenberg, D., Marcotte, E. M., Xenarios. I. & Yeates, T. (2000). Protein function in the post-genomic era. *Nature*, 405, 823-826.

Emanuelsson, O., Nielsen, H., Brunak, S., Von Heijne G. (2000). Predicting subcellular localization of proteins based on their N-terminal amino acid sequence. *J Mol Biol*, 300 (4), 1005-1016.

Emanuelsson, O., Nielsen, H., Von Heijne G. Chloro, P. (1999). a neural network-based method for predicting chloroplast transit peptides and their cleavage sites. *Protein Sci.*, 8, 978–984.

Falk, K., Ro¨tzschke O, Stevanovic, S. et al. (1991). Allele-specific motifs revealed by sequencing of self-peptides eluted from MHC molecules. *Nature*, 351, 290–6.

Fan, GL. and Li, QZ. (2012). Predicting protein submitochondria locations by combining different descriptors into the general form of Chou's pseudo amino acid composition. *Amino Acids*, 43, 2, 545-55.

Fang, Y., Guo, Y., Feng, Y., Li, M. (2008). Predicting DNA-binding proteins: approached from Chou's pseudo amino acid composition and other specific sequence features. *Amino Acids*, 34, 103–109.

Fariselli, P., Finocchiaro, G., Casadio, R. (2003). SPEPlip: the detection of signal peptide and lipoprotein cleavage sites. *Bioinformatics*, 19, 2498–2499.

Fariselli, P., Pazos, F., Valencia, A. and Casadio, R. (2002). Prediction of protein–protein interaction sites in heterocomplexes with neural networks. *Eur J Biochem*, 269, 1356–1361.

Favia, A. D. and Nobeli, I. (2011). Using Chemical Structure to Infer Biological Function, In: *Computational Approaches in Cheminformatics and Bioinformatics (eds R. Guha and A. Bender), John Wiley & Sons, Inc.*, Hoboken, NJ, USA.

Ferrer-Costa, C., Shanahan, H. P.,, Jones, S., Thornton, J. M. (2005). HTHquery: A method for detecting DNA-binding proteins with a helix-turn-helix structural motif. *Bioinformatics*, 21 (18), 3679-3680.

Finn, R., Clements, J., Eddy, S. (2011). HMMER Web Server: Interactive Sequence Similarity Searching. *Nucleic Acids Res*, 39, W29-37.

Friedberg, I. (2006). Automated protein function prediction--the genomic challenge. *Brief Bioinform*, 7, 225-242.

Galperin, MY., Walker, DR., Koonin, EV. (1998). Analogous enzymes: independent inventions in enzyme evolution. *Genome Res*, 8, 779-90.

Gao, Q. B., Wang, Z. Z., Yan, C., Du, Y. H. (2005). Prediction of protein subcellular location using a combined feature of sequence. *FEBS Letters*, 579 (16), 3444-3448.

Garg, A., Bhasin M., Raghava G. P. (2005). SVM-based method for subcellular localization of human proteins using amino acid compositions, their order and similarity search. *J. Biol. Chem.* 280, 14427–14432.

Garg, A., Gupta, D. (2008). VirulentPred: a SVM based prediction method for virulent proteins in bacterial pathogens. *BMC Bioinformatics*, 62.

Garg, A., Raghava, G. P.S. (2008). A Machine Learning Based Method for the Prediction of Secretory Proteins Using Amino Acid Composition, Their Order and Similarity-Search. *In Silico Biol*, 8, 129-140.

Glazer, DS., Radmer, RJ., Altman, RB. (2009). Improving structure-based function prediction using molecular dynamics. *Structure*, 17, 919–929.

Gold, ND., Jackson, RM. (2006). Fold independent structural comparisons of protein-ligand binding sites for exploring functional relationships. *J Mol Biol.*, 3, 355(5), 1112-24.

Grill, C. P. & Rush, V. N. (2000). Analysing spectral data: comparison and application of two techniques. *Biol J Linn Soc*, 69, 121–138.

Gulukota, K., Sidney, J., Sette, A., DeLisi, C. (1997). Two complementary methods for predicting peptides binding major histocompatibility complex molecules. *J Mol Biol.* 267, 1258–67.

Guo, J., Lin, Y. (2006). TSSub: eukaryotic protein subcellular localization by extracting features from profiles. *Bioinformatics*, 22, 1784-5.

Guo, Y., Yu, L., Wen, Z., Li, M. (2008). Using support vector machine combined with auto covariance to predict protein-protein interactions from protein sequences. *Nucleic Acids Res.*, 36, 3025–3030.

Gutteridge, A., Bartlett, G.J., and Thornton, J.M. (2003). Using a neural network and spatial clustering to predict the location of active sites in enzymes. *J. Mol. Biol.*, 330, 719–734.

Guyon, I., Weston, J., Barnhill, S., Vapnik, V. (2002). Gene selection for cancer classification using support vector machines. *Mach. Learn.*, 46, 389-422.

Hall, M., Frank, E., Holmes, G., Pfahringer, B., Reutemann, P., Witten, I. H. (2009). The WEKA data mining software: an update. *SIGKDD Explor. Newsl.*, 11, 10–18.

Hamby, S. E., Hirst, J. D. (2008). Prediction of glycosylation sites using random forests. *BMC Bioinformatics*, 9, 500.

Han, L. Y.,, Zheng, C. J., Xie, B., Jia, J., Ma, X. H., Zhu, F., Lin, H. H., Chen, Y. Z. (2007). Support vector machines approach for predicting druggable proteins: recent progress in its exploration and investigation of its usefulness. *Drug Discov Today*, 12 (7-8), 304-313.

Han, L., Cui, J., Lin, H., Ji, Z., Cao, Z., Li, Y., Chen, Y. (2006). Recent progresses in the application of machine learning approach for predicting protein functional class independent of sequence similarity. *Proteomics*, 6, 4023-4037.

Hansen, J. E., Lund, O., Tolstrup, N., Gooley, A. A., et al. (1998). NetOglyc: Prediction of mucin type O-glycosylation sites based on sequence context and surface accessibility. *Glycoconj J*, 15, 115-130.

Harrison A., Pearl F., Sillitoe I., Slidel T., Mott R., Thornton J. M., Orengo C. (2003). Recognising the fold of a protein structure. *Bioinformatics*, 19, 1748-1759.

Hayashi, S. and Wu, H.C. (1990). Lipoproteins in bacteria. *J. Bioenerg. Biomembr.* 22, 451–471.

Henikoff, S. (1996). Scores for sequence searches and alignments. *Curr Opin Struct Biol*, 6 (3), 353-360.

Henikoff, S. and Henikoff, J. G. (1994). Protein family classification based on searching a database of blocks. *Genomics*, 19, 97–107.

Hirose, S., Yokota, K., Kuroda, Y., Wako, H., Endo, S., Kanai, S., Noguchi, T. (2010). Prediction of protein motions from amino acid sequence and its application to protein-protein interaction. *BMC Struct. Biol.*, 10, 20.

Hoglund, A., Donnes, P., Blum, T., Adolph, H. W., Kohlbacher, O. (2006). MultiLoc: Prediction of protein subcellular localization using N-terminal targeting sequences, sequence motifs and amino acid composition. *Bioinformatics*, 22 (10), 1158-1165.

Holm L., Sander C. (1993). Protein structure comparison by alignment of distance matrices. *J Mol Biol*, 233, 123-138.

Hua, S. and Sun, Z. (2001).    Support vector machine approach for protein subcellular localization prediction. *Bioinformatics*, 17(8), 721-728.

Huang, N., Chen, H., and Sun, Z. (2005). CTKPred: an SVM-based method for the prediction and classification of the cytokine superfamily. *Protein Eng Des Sel*, 18(8), 365-368.

Huang, W. L., Tung, C. W., Huang, H. L., Hwang, S. F. Ho, S. Y. (2007). ProLoc: Prediction of protein subnuclear localization using SVM with automatic selection from physicochemical composition features. *BioSystems*, 90 (2), 573-581.

Huang, Y. and Yanda, Li. (2004).   Prediction of protein subcellular locations using fuzzy k-NN method. *Bioinformatics*, 20(1), 21-28.

Hwang, S., Gou, Z. and Igor, B. (2007). DP-Bind: a web server for sequence-based prediction of DNA-binding residues in DNA-binding proteins. *Bioinformatics*, 23, 634-636.

Ishida, T., Kinoshita, K. (2007). PrDOS: prediction of disordered protein regions from amino acid sequence. *Nucleic Acids Res.*, 35, W460–464.

Jain, AK., Duin, RPW., Mao, J. (2000). Statistical Pattern Recognition: A Review. *IEEE Trans Pattern Anal Mach Intell*, 22, 4–37.

Jensen, L. J., Skovgaard, M., Brunak, S. (2002). Prediction of novel archaeal enzymes from sequence-derived features. *Protein Sci.*, 3, 2894–2898.

Jia, P., Qian, Z., Zeng, Z., Cai, Y., Li Y. (2007). Prediction of subcellular protein localization based on functional domain composition. *Biochem Biophys Res Commun*, 357 (2), 366-370.

Johnson, R. and Wichern, D. (1982). *Applied Multivariate Statistical Analysis*. Prentice-Hall, Inc.: Englewood Cliffs, NJ.

Julenius, K., Molgaard, A., Gupta, R., Brunak, S. (2005). Prediction, conservation analysis, and structural characterization of mammalian mucin-type O-glycosylation sites. *Glycobiology*, 15,153-164.

Juncker, A.S., Willenbrock, H., Von Heijne, G, Brunak, S., Nielsen, H., et al. (2003). Prediction of lipoprotein signal peptides in Gram-negative bacteria. *Protein Sci.* 12, 1652–1662.

Juncker, AS., Jensen, LJ., Pierleoni, A., Bernsel, A., Tress, ML., Bork, P., Heijne, Gv., Valencia, A., Ouzounis, CA., Casadio, R., Brunak, S. (2009). Sequence-based feature prediction and annotation of proteins. *Genome Biol.*, 10, 206.

Kadam, K., Prabhakar, P., and Jayaraman, V.K. (2012). SVM prediction of ligand-binding sites in bacterial lipoproteins employing shape and physio-chemical descriptors. *Protein Pept Lett*, 19, 1155-1162.

Kalita, M. K., Nandal, U. K., Pattnaik, A., Sivalingam, A., Ramasamy, G., Kumar, M., Raghava, G. P. S. and Gupta, D. (2008). CyclinPred: a SVM-based method for predicting cyclin protein sequences. *PLoS ONE,* 3(7), e2605.

Kandaswamy, K. K., Chou, K. C., Martinetz, T., Moller, S., Suganthan, P. N., Sridharan, S., Pugalenthi, G. (2011). AFP-Pred: A random forest approach for predicting antifreeze proteins from sequence-derived properties. *J Theor Biol*, 270 (1), 56-62.

Kaur, H. and Raghava, G. P. S. (2004). A neural network method for prediction of β-turn types in proteins using evolutionary information. *Bioinformatics*, 20(16), 2751-2758.

Kawashima, S., Ogata, H., Kanehisa, M. (2000). AAindex: amino acid index database. *Nucleic Acids Res*, 28, 374.

Kim, J. H., Lee, J., Oh, B., Kimm, K., Koh, I. (2004). Prediction of phosphorylaton sites using SVMs. *Bioinformatics*, 20, 3179–3184.

Kingsford, C., Salzberg, SL. (2008). What are decision trees? *Nat Biotechnol.*, 26, 1011-1013.

Kinoshita, K., Kono, H. and Yura, K. (2008). Prediction of Molecular Interactions from 3D-Structures: From Small Ligands to Large Protein Complexes, In: *Prediction of Protein Structures, Functions, and Interactions (ed J. M. Bujnicki), John Wiley & Sons, Ltd*, Chichester, UK.

Koike, A. and Takagi, T. (2004). Prediction of protein–protein interaction sites using support vector machines. *Protein Eng Des Sel*, 17, 165–173.

Kuang, R., Lesliei, CS., Yang, A.-S. (2004). Protein backbone angle prediction with machine learning approaches. *Bioinformatics*, 20, 1612–1621.

Kulkarni-Kale, U., Waman, V., Raskar, S., Mehta S., Saxena, S. (2012). Genome To Vaccinome: Role of Bioinformatics, Immunoinformatics & Comparative Genomics. *Curr Bioinform*, 7, 4, 451-463.

Kulkarni-Kale, U., Bhosle, S., and Kolaskar, A.S. (2005). CEP: A conformational epitope prediction server. *Nucleic Acids Res.*, 33, W168–W171.

Kumar, K. K., Shelokar, P. S. (2008). An SVM method using evolutionary information for the identification of allergenic proteins. *Bioinformation*, 2(6), 253–256.

Kumar, M., Gromiha, M. M. and Raghava, G. P. S. (2008). Prediction of RNA binding sites in a protein using SVM and PSSM profile. *Proteins*, 71, 189-194.

Kumari, R. S., Kadam, K., Badwaik, R., Jayaraman. V. K. (2012). Lipopredict: Bacterial lipoprotein prediction server. *Bioinformation*, 8(8): 394-398.

Kunik, V., Solan, Z., Edelman, S. et al. (2005). Motif extraction and protein classification. *Proc IEEE Comput Syst Bioinform Conf.*, 80, 5.

Kurgan, L., Cios, K., Chen, K. (2008). SCPRED: Accurate prediction of protein structural class for sequences of twilight-zone similarity with predicting sequences. *BMC Bioinformatics*, 9, 226.

Kuznetsov, I. B., Gou, Z., Li, R. and Hwang, S. (2006). Using evolutionary and structural information to predict DNA-binding sites on DNA-binding proteins. *Proteins*, 64, 19–27.

Käll, L., Krogh, A., Sonnhammer, E. L. (2004). A combined transmembrane topology and signal peptide prediction method. *J. Mol. Biol.*, 338, 1027–1036.

La Cour, T., L. Kiemer, A. Mølgaard, R. Gupta, K. Skriver, and S. Brunak. (2004). Analysis and prediction of leucine-rich nuclear export signals. *Protein Eng. Des. Sel.*, 17, 527-536.

Ladunga, I., Czakó, F., Csabai, I., Geszti, T. (1991). Improving signal peptide prediction accuracy by simulated neural network. *Comput Appl Biosci.*, 7(4), 485-7.

Lancashire, LJ., Lemetre, C., Ball, GR. (2009). An introduction to artificial neural networks in bioinformatics–application to complex microarray and mass spectrometry datasets in cancer studies. *Brief Bioinform.*, 10, 315–329.

Lara, J., Wohlhueter, R. M., Dimitrova, Z., Khudyakov, Y. E. (2008) Artificial neural network for prediction of antigenic activity for a major conformational epitope in the hepatitis C virus NS3 protein. *Bioinformatics*, 24 (17), 1858-1864.

Larrañaga, P., Calvo, B., Robles, V., et al. (2006). Machine learning in bioinformatics *Brief Bioinform*, 7(1), 86-112.

Laskowski, R. A., Watson, J. D., Thornton, J. M. (2005). ProFunc: a server for predicting protein function from 3D structure. *Nucleic Acids Res*, 33, W89-93.

Levy, R., Edelman, M. and Sobolev, V. (2009). Prediction of 3D metal binding sites from translated gene sequences based on remote-homology templates. *Proteins*, 76, 365–374.

Lewis, DP., Jebara, T., Noble, WS. (2006). Support vector machine learning from heterogeneous data: an empirical analysis using protein sequence and structure. *Bioinformatics*, 22, 2753-60.

Li, F. M., Li, Q. Z. (2008). Predicting Protein Subcellular Location Using Chou's Pseudo Amino Acid Composition and Improved Hybrid Approach. *Protein Pept Lett*, 15, 612-616.

Li, L., Umbach, DM., Terry, P., Taylor, JA. (2004). Application of the GA/KNN method to SELDI proteomics data. *Bioinformatics*, 20, 1638-1640.

Li, ZC., Zhou, XB., Dai, Z., Zou, XY. (2009). Prediction of protein structural classes by Chou's pseudo amino acid composition: approached using continuous wavelet transform and principal component analysis. *Amino acids*, 37, 2, 415-25.

Li, GZ., Bu, HL., Yang, MQ., Zeng, XQ., Yang, JY. (2008). Selecting subsets of newly extracted features from PCA and PLS in microarray data analysis. *BMC Genomics*, 9, S24.

Liang, S., Zheng, D., Standley, D. M., Yao, B., Zacharias, M., et al. (2010). EPSVR and EPMeta: prediction of antigenic epitopes using support vector regression and multiple server results. *BMC Bioinformatics*, 11, 381.

Liaw, A., M. Wiener. (2002). Classification and regression by randomForest, *R News*, 2, 18–22.

Lin, H. H., Han, L. Y., Zhang, H. L., Zheng, C. J., Xie, B., et al. (2006a). Prediction of the functional class of metal-binding proteins from sequence derived physicochemical properties by support vector machine approach. *BMC Bioinformatics*, 7, S13.

Lin, H. H., Han, L. Y., Zhang, H. L., Zheng, C. J., Xie, B., et al. (2006b) Prediction of the functional class of lipid binding proteins from sequence-derived properties irrespective of sequence similarity. *J Lipid Res*, 47, 824–831.

Lin, W. Z., Fang, J. A., Xiao, X., Chou. K. C. (2011). iDNA-Prot: Identification of DNA Binding Proteins Using Random Forest with Grey Model. *PLoS ONE*, 6(9), e24756.

Liu, T., Altman, R. B. (2009). Prediction of calcium-binding sites by combining loop-modeling with machine learning. *BMC Struct Biol*, 9, 72.

Liu, Z. P., Wu, L. Y., Wang, Y., Zhang, X. S., Chen, L. N. (2010). Prediction of protein-RNA binding sites by a random forest method with combined features. *Bioinformatics*, 26, 1616–1622.

Liu, Z. P., et al. (2008). Bridging protein local structures and protein functions. *Amino Acids*, 35, 627-650.

Lohmann, R., Schneider, G., Behrens, D., Wrede, P. (1994). A neural network model for the prediction of membrane-spanning amino acid sequences. *Protein Sci*, 1597–1601.

Lu, L., Qian, Z., Cai, Y. D., Li, Y. (2007). ECS: An automatic enzyme classifier based on functional domain composition. *Comput Biol Chem*, 31 (3), 226-232.

Lukashin, A.V., Borodovsky, M. (1998). GeneMark.hmm: new solutions for gene finding, *Nucleic Acids* Res, 26, 1107-1115.

Ma, J., Gu, H. (2010). A novel method for predicting protein subcellular localization based on pseudo amino acid composition. *BMB Rep.*, 43(10), 670-6.

Madej, T., Gibrat, JF., Bryant, SH. (1995). Threading a database of protein cores. *Proteins*, 23, 356–69.

Majoros, WH., Pertea, M., Salzberg, SL. (2005). Efficient implementation of a generalized pair hidden Markov model for comparative gene finding. *Bioinformatics*, 21, 1782-8.

Malik, A., Ahmad, S. (2007). Sequence and structural features of carbohydrate binding in proteins and assessment of predictability using a neural network. *BMC Struct Biol*, 7, 1.

Mamitsuka, H. (1989). Predicting peptides that bind to MHC molecules using supervised learning of hidden Markov models. *Proteins*. 33, 460–74.

Martin, S., Roe, D., Faulon, J. L. (2005). Predicting protein–protein interactions using signature products. *Bioinformatics*, 21, 218–226.

McLaughlin, W. A., Berman, H. M. (2003). Statistical models for discerning protein structures containing the DNA-binding helix-turn-helix motif. *J Mol Biol*, 330 (1), 43-55.

Mishra, N.K. and Raghava, G. P. S. (2010). Prediction of FAD interacting residues in a protein from its primary sequence using evolutionary information. *BMC Bioinformatics*, 11, S48.

Mundra, P., Kumar, M., Kumar, K. K., Jayaraman, V. K., Kulkarni, B. D. (2007). Using pseudo amino acid composition to predict protein subnuclear localization: Approached with PSSM. *Pattern Recognit Lett*, 28 (13), 1610-1615.

Murvai, J., Vlahovicek, K., Barta, E., Pongor, S. (2001). The SBASE protein domain library, release 8.0: a collection of annotated protein sequence segments. *Nucleic Acids Res*. 29, 58–60.

Najmanovich, R., Kurbatova, N., Thornton, J. (2008). Detection of 3D atomic similarities and their use in the discrimination of small molecule protein-binding sites. *Bioinformatics*, 24(16), 105-11.

Nakai, K., Horton, P. (1999). PSORT: A program for detecting sorting signals in proteins and predicting their subcellular localization. *Trends Biochem Sci.*, 24 (1), 34-35.

Nayal, M., Honig, B. (2006). On the nature of cavities on protein surfaces: application to the identification of drug-binding sites. *Proteins*, 63, 892–906.

Needleman, SB., Wunsch, CD. (1970). A general method applicable to the search for similarities in the amino acid sequences of two proteins. *J. Mol. Biol.*, 48, 443-453.

Nielsen, H., Brunak, S., Von Heijne, G. (1999). Machine learning approaches for the prediction of signal peptides and other protein sorting signals. *Protein Eng.*, 12, 3–9.

Nielsen, H., Engelbrecht, J., Brunak, S., Von Heijne, G. (1997). Identification of prokaryotic and eukaryotic signal peptides and prediction of their cleavage sites. *Protein Eng.*, 10, 1–6.

Nielsen, H., Engelbrecht, J., von Heijne, G. and Brunak, S. (1996). Defining a similarity threshold for a functional protein sequence pattern: The signal peptide cleavage site. *Proteins*, 24, 165–177.

Novotni, M., Klein, R. (2004). Shape retrieval using 3D Zernike descriptors. *Comput Aided Des*, 36, 1047-1062.

Nugent, T., Jones, DT. (2010). Predicting Transmembrane Helix Packing Arrangements using Residue Contacts and a Force-Directed Algorithm. *PLoS Comput Biol*, 6(3), e1000714.

Ofran, Y., Mysore,V. and Rost, B. (2007). Prediction of DNA-binding residues from sequence. *Bioinformatics*, 23(13), i347-i353.

Ofran, Y., Rost, B. (2007). Protein–Protein Interaction Hotspots Carved into Sequences. *PLoS Comput Biol*, 3(7), e119.

Orengo, CA., Taylor, WR. (1996). SSAP: sequential structure alignment program for protein structure comparison. *Methods Enzymol*, 266, 617-635.

Ota, M., Kinoshita, K., Nishikawa, K. (2003). Prediction of catalytic residues in enzymes based on known tertiary structure, stability profile, and sequence conservation. *J Mol Biol*, 327 (5), 1053-1064.

Panwar, B., Raghava, G. P. (2010). Prediction and classification of aminoacyl tRNA synthetases using PROSITE domains. *BMC Genomics*, 11, 507.

Park, K. J. and Kanehisa, M. (2003). Prediction of protein subcellular locations by support vector machines using compositions of amino acids and amino acid pairs. *Bioinformatics*, 19(13), 1656-1663.

Passerini, A., Punta, M., Ceroni, A., Rost, B. and Frasconi, P. (2006). Identifying cysteines and histidines in transition-metal-binding sites using support vector machines and neural networks. *Proteins*, 65, 305–316.

Pearson, W. R. (1996). Effective protein sequence comparison. *Methods Enzymol.*, 266, 227–258.

Pearson, W. R., Lipman, D. J. (1988). Improved tools for biological sequence comparison. *Proc Natl Acad Sci USA*, 85, 2444-2448.

Petrova, N. V., Wu, C. H. (2006). Prediction of catalytic residues using Support Vector Machine with selected protein sequence and structural properties. *BMC Bioinformatics*, 7, 312.

Pierri, C.L., Parisi, G., Porcelli, V. (2010). Computational approaches for protein function prediction: A combined strategy from multiple sequence alignment to molecular docking-based virtual screening. *Biochimica et Biophysica Acta - Proteins and Proteomics*, 1804 (9), 1695-1712.

Pugalenthi, G., Kumar, K. K., Suganthan, P. N., Gangal, R. (2008). Identification of catalytic residues from protein structure using support vector machine with sequence and structural features. *Biochem Biophys Res Commun*, 367 (3), 630-634.

Pundhir, S. & Kumar, A. (2011). SSPred: A prediction server based on SVM for the identification and classification of proteins involved in bacterial secretion systems. *Bioinformation*, 6(10): 380-382.

Qi, Yanjun. (2012). Random Forest for Bioinformatics. In: *Ensemble Machine Learning: Methods and Applications. Eds. Zhang, C. and Ma, Y. Springer-Verlag* New York Inc, 307.

Qiu, J. D., Huang, J. H., Shi, S. P., Liang, R. P. (2010). Using the Concept of Chou's Pseudo Amino Acid Composition to Predict Enzyme Family Classes: An Approach with Support Vector Machine Based on Discrete Wavelet Transform. *Protein Pept Lett.*, 17(6), 715-22.

Quinlan, J. (1993). *C4.5: programs for machine learning*, Morgan Kaufmann, San Mateo.

Ramana, J., Gupta, D. (2010). FaaPred: a SVM-based prediction method for fungal adhesins and adhesin-like proteins. *PLoS One.*, 5, e9695.

Rapoport, T. A. (1992). Transport of proteins across the endoplasmic reticulum membrane. *Science*, 258, 931–936.

Rappuoli, R. (2001). Reverse vaccinology, a genome-based approach to vaccine development. *Vaccine*, 19, 2688–2691.

Rashid, M., Saha, S., Raghava, G. P. S. (2007). Support Vector Machine-based method for predicting subcellular localization of mycobacterial proteins using evolutionary information and motifs. *BMC Bioinformatics*, 8(1), 337.

Roetzschke, O., Falk, K., Stefanovic, S. et al. (1991). Exact prediction of a natural T cell epitope. *EurJ Immunol*, 21, 2891–4.

Rost, B., Sander, C. (1994). Combining evolutionary information and neural networks to predict protein secondary structure, *Proteins*, 19, 55–72.

Rost, B. (2002). Enzyme function less conserved than anticipated. *J Mol Biol*, 318, 595-608.

Rubinstein, N. D., Mayrose, I., Pupko, T. (2009a). A machine-learning approach for predicting B-cell epitopes. *Mol Immunol*, 46 (5), 840-847.

Rubinstein, N. D., Mayrose, I., Martz, E., Pupko, T. (2009b). Epitopia: a web-server for predicting B-cell epitopes. *BMC Bioinformatics*. 10, 287.

Röttig, M., Rausch, C., Kohlbacher, O. (2010). Combining Structure and Sequence Information Allows Automated Prediction of Substrate Specificities within Enzyme Families. *PLoS Comput Biol*, 6(1), e1000636.

Saeys, Y., Inza, I., Larranaga, P. (2007). A review of feature selection techniques in bioinformatics. *Bioinformatics*, 23 (19), 2507-2517.

Saghatelian, A. & Cravatt, B. F. (2005). Assignment of the protein function in the post genomic era. *Nat Chem Biol*, 1, 130-143.

Saha, S., Raghava, G. (2006). Prediction of continuous B-cell epitopes in an antigen using recurrent neural network. *Proteins*, 65, 40-48.

Sarda, D., Chua, G. H., Li, K. B., Krishnan, A. (2005). pSLIP: SVM based protein subcellular localization prediction using multiple physicochemical properties. *BMC Bioinformatics*, 6, 152.

Schneider, G., Wrede, P. (1993). Development of artificial neural filters for pattern recognition in protein sequences. *J Mol Evol.*, 36(6), 586-95.

Shen, J., Zhang, J., Luo, X., Zhu, W., Yu, K., Chen, K., Li, Y., Jiang, H. (2007). Predicting protein-protein interactions based only on sequences information. *Proc. Natl Acad. Sci. USA.*, 104, 4337-4341.

Shen, H. B., Chou, K. C. (2007a). Signal-3L: A 3-layer approach for predicting signal peptides. *Biochem Biophys Res Commun*, 363 (2), 297-303.

Shen, H. B. & Chou, K.C. (2007b). Nuc-PLoc: A new web-server for predicting protein subnuclear localization by fusing PseAA composition and PsePSSM. *Protein Eng Des Sel*, 20, 561-567.

Shen, H. B., Yang, J., Chou, K. C. (2006). Fuzzy KNN for predicting membrane protein types from pseudo-amino acid composition. *J Theor Biol*, 240 (1), 9-13.

Shi, J. Y., Zhang S. W., Pan Q., Cheng Y. M. and Xie, J. (2007). Prediction of protein subcellular localization by support vector machines using multi-scale energy and pseudo amino acid composition. *Amino Acids*, 33, 69-74.

Šikić, M., Tomić, S., Vlahoviček, K. (2009). Prediction of Protein–Protein Interaction Sites in Sequences and 3D Structures by Random Forests. *PLoS Comput Biol*, 5(1), e1000278.

Sim, J., Kim, S.-Y. and Lee, J. (2005a). PPRODO: Prediction of protein domain boundaries using neural networks. *Proteins*, 59, 627–632.

Sim, J., Kim, S. Y., Lee, J. (2005b). Prediction of protein solvent accessibility using fuzzy k-nearest neighbor method. *Bioinformatics*, 21 (12), 2844-2849.

Sleator, RD. (2012). Prediction of protein functions. *Methods Mol Biol*, 815, 15-24.

Smith, TF., Waterman, MS. (1981). Identification of common molecular subsequences. *J. Mol. Biol.*, 147, 195-197.

Somarowthu, S., Yang, H., Hildebrand, D. G.C. and Ondrechen, M. J. (2011). High-performance prediction of functional residues in proteins with machine learning and computed input features. *Biopolymers*, 95, 390–400.

Song, J., Burrage, K., Yuan, Z., Huber, T. (2006). Prediction of cis/trans isomerization in proteins using PSI-BLAST profiles and secondary structure information. *BMC Bioinformatics*, 7, 124.

Stawiski, E. W., Gregoret, L. M., Mandel-Gutfreund, Y. (2003). Annotating nucleic acid-binding function based on protein structure. *J Mol Biol*, 326 (4), 1065-1079.

Sturrock, S. S. and Collins, J. F. (1993). *MPsrch version 1.3*. Biocomputing Research Unit, University of Edinburgh, Edinburgh, UK.

Sweredoski, MJ., Baldi, P. (2008). PEPITO: improved discontinuous B-cell epitope prediction using multiple distance + thresholds and half sphere exposure. *Bioinformatics*, 24, 1459-1460.

Sweredoski, M., Baldi, P. (2009). COBEpro: a novel system for predicting continuous B-cell epitopes. *Protein Eng Des Sel.*, 22(3), 113-120.

Tamura, T., Akutsu, T. (2007). Subcellular location prediction of proteins using support vector machines with alignment of block sequences utilizing amino acid composition. *BMC Bioinformatics*, 8, 466.

Tan, P.N., Steinbach, M., Kumar, V. (2005). *Introduction to Data Mining*. Addison-Wesley.

Tang, YR., Sheng, ZY., Chen, YZ., Zhang, Z. (2008). An improved prediction of catalytic residues in enzyme structures. *Protein Eng Des Sel*, 21, 295–302.

Tarca, A. L., Carey, V. J., Chen, X-w, Romero R., Drăghici S. (2007). Machine Learning and Its Applications to Biology. *PLoS Comput Biol*, 3(6), e116.

Teng, S., Srivastava, A. K., Wang, L. (2010). Sequence feature-based prediction of protein stability changes upon amino acid substitutions. *BMC Genomics*, (Suppl 2), S5.

Terribilini, M., Lee, J. H., Yan, C., Jernigan, R. L., Honavar, V., Dobbs, D. (2006). Prediction of RNA binding sites in proteins from amino acid sequence. *RNA*, 12, 1450-1462.

Terribilini, M., Sander, J. D., Lee, J. H., Zaback, P., Jernigan, R. L., et al. (2007). RNABindR: a server for analyzing and predicting RNA-binding sites in proteins. *Nucleic Acids Res*, 35, W578–W584.

Terwilliger, TC., Stuart, D., Yokoyama, S. (2009). Lessons from structural genomics. *Annu Rev Biophys.*, 38, 371–383.

Tjong, H., Zhou, H-X., (2007). DISPLAR: an accurate method for predicting DNA-binding sites on protein surfaces. *Nucleic Acids Res*, 35, 1465-1477.

Tong, W., Williams, R. J., Wei, Y., Murga, L. F., Ko, J., Ondrechen, M. J. (2008). Enhanced performance in prediction of protein active sites with THEMATICS and support vector machines. *Protein Sci.* 17, 333–341.

Torrance, J.W., Bartlett, G.J., Porter, C.T., Thornton, J.M. (2005). Using a library of structural templates to recognise catalytic sites and explore their evolution in homologous families. *J Mol Biol*, 347, 565-581.

Vapnik, V. (1995). *The Nature of Statistical Learning Theory*, Springer, New York.

Verma, R., Tiwari, A., Kaur, S., Varshney, G. C., Raghava, G. P. S. (2008). Identification of Proteins Secreted by Malaria Parasite into Erythrocyte using SVM and PSSM profiles. *BMC Bioinformatics*, 9, 201.

Verma, R., Varshney, G., Raghava, G. (2010). Prediction of mitochondrial proteins of malaria parasite using split amino acid composition and PSSM profile. *Amino Acids*, 39, 101-110.

von Heijne, G. (1990). The signal peptide. *J. Membrane Biol.*, 115, 195–201.

Walter, G. (1986). Production and use of antibodies against synthetic peptides. *J. Immunol. Methods*, 88, 149-61.

Wang, D. and Larder, B. (2003). Enhanced Prediction of Lopinavir Resistance from Genotype by Use of Artificial Neural Networks. *J. Infect. Dis.*, 188, 5, 653-660.

Wang, J., Sung, W. K., Krishnan, A., Li, K. B. (2005). Protein subcellular localization prediction for Gram-negative bacteria using amino acid subalphabets and a combination of multiple support vector machines. *BMC Bioinformatics*, 6, 174.

Wang, L., Brown, S. J. (2006a). Prediction Of DNA-Binding Residues from Sequence Features. *J Bioinform Comput Biol*, 4, 6, 1141-1158.

Wang, L. J., Brown, S. J. (2006b). BindN: a web-based tool for efficient prediction of DNA and RNA binding sites in amino acid sequences. *Nucleic Acids Res.*, 34, W243–W248.

Wang, M., Yang, J., Liu, G. P., Xu, Z. J., Chou, K. C. (2004). Weighted-support vector machines for predicting membrane protein types based on pseudo-amino acid composition. *Protein Eng Des Sel*, 17 (6), pp. 509-516.

Wang, T., Yang J. (2010). Predicting subcellular localization of gram-negative bacterial proteins by linear dimensionality reduction method. *Protein Pept Lett.*, 17(1), 32-7.

Wang, Y. C., Wang, X. B., Yang, Z. X., Deng, N. Y. (2010). Prediction of enzyme subfamily class via pseudo amino acid composition by incorporating the conjoint triad feature. *Protein Pept. Lett.*, 17, pp. 1441–1449.

Wang, Y., Xue, Z., Shen, G., and Xu, J. (2008). PRINTR: Prediction of RNA binding sites in proteins using SVM and profiles. *Amino Acids*, 35, 2, 295-302.

Wass, MN., Kelley, LA., Sternberg, MJE. (2010). 3DLigandSite: predicting ligand-binding sites using similar structures. *Nucleic Acids Res*, 38, W469–W473.

Whisstock, JC., Lesk, AM. (2003). Prediction of protein function from protein sequence and structure. *Q Rev Biophys*, 36, 307-40.

Wong, S. L., Zhang, L. V., Tong, A. H., Li, Z., et al. (2004). Combining biological networks to predict genetic interactions. *Proc Natl Acad Sci USA*, 101, 15682-15687.

Wu, J., Liu, H., Duan, X., Ding, Y., Wu, H., Bai, Y. and Sun, X. (2009). Prediction of DNA-binding residues in proteins from amino acid sequences using a random forest model with a hybrid feature. *Bioinformatics*, 25, 1, 30-35.

Xia, JF., Zhao, XM., Song, J., Huang, DS. (2010). APIS: accurate prediction of hot spots in protein interfaces by combining protrusion index with solvent accessibility. *BMC Bioinformatics*, 11, 174–174.

Xie, D., Li, A., Wang, M., Fan, Z., Feng, H. (2005). LOCSVMPSI: a web server for subcellular localization of eukaryotic proteins using SVM and profile of PSI-BLAST. *Nucleic Acids Res*, 33, W105-W110.

Xu, Y., Uberbacher, E. (1997). Computational Gene Identification Using Neural Networks and Similarity Search. Machine Learning and Sequence Pattern Analysis, In: *Computational Biology, Eds. Steven Salzberg, David Searls, Simon Kasifi, Elsevier Publishing Company.*

Xu, X., Yu, D., Fang, W., Cheng, Y., Qian, Z., Lu, W., Cai, Y., Feng, K. (2008). Prediction of peptidase category based on functional domain composition. *J Proteome Res*, 7(10), 4521-4524.

Yang, Z.R. Biological applications of support vector machines. (2004). *Brief. Bioinform.*, 5 (4), 328–338.

Yang, P., Hwa Yang, Y., Zhou, B., Zomaya, Y. (2010). A review of ensemble methods in bioinformatics. *Curr Bioinform*, 5, 296–308.

Yoon, BJ. (2009). Hidden Markov Models and their Applications in Biological Sequence Analysis. *Curr Genomics*, 10, 402–415.

Youn, E., Peters, B., Radivojac, P., Mooney, S. (2007). Evaluation of features for catalytic residue prediction in novel folds. *Prot Sci*, 16, 216–226.

Yu, C. S., Chen, Y. C., Lu, C. H. and Hwang, J. K. (2006a), Prediction of protein subcellular localization. *Proteins*, 64: 643–651.

Yu, X., Wang, C., Li, Y. (2006b). Classification of protein quaternary structure by functional domain composition. *BMC Bioinformatics*, 7, 187.

Yu, C. S., Lin, C. J., Hwang, J. K. (2004). Predicting subcellular localization of proteins for gram-negative bacteria by support vector machines based on n-peptide compositions. *Protein Sci.*, 13, 1402–1406.

Yu, C. Y., Chou, L. C., Chang, D. T. (2010). Predicting protein-protein interactions in unbalanced data using the primary structure of proteins. *BMC Bioinformatics*, 11, 167.

Yu, K., Petrovsky, N., Schonbach, C., et al. (2002). Methods for prediction of peptide binding to MHC molecules: a comparative study. *Mol Med*, 8, 137-48.

Zhang, T. L., Ding, Y. S., Chou, K. C. (2008). Prediction protein structural classes with pseudo-amino acid composition: Approximate entropy and hydrophobicity pattern. *J Theor Biol*, 250 (1), 186-193.

Zhang, G. L., Ansari, H.R., Bradley, P., Cawley, G.C., Hertz ,T., Hu, X., Jojic, N., Brusic, V. (2011a). Machine learning competition in immunology - Prediction of HLA class I binding peptides. *J Immunol Methods*, 374 (1-2), 1-4.

Zhang, W., Xiong, Y., Zhao, M., Zou, H., Ye, X., et al. (2011b). Prediction of conformational B-cell epitopes from 3D structures by random forests with a distance-based feature. *BMC Bioinformatics*, 12, 341.

Zhao, Y., Pinilla, C., Valmori, D., et al. (2003). Application of support vector machines for T-cell epitopes prediction. *Bioinformatics*, 19, 1978–84.

Zhao, XM., Chen, L., Aihara K. (2008). Protein function prediction with high-throughput data. *Amino Acids*, 35 (3), 517–530.

Zhou, X. B., Chen, C., Li, Z. C., Zou, X. Y. (2007). Using Chou's amphiphilic pseudo-amino acid composition and support vector machine for prediction of enzyme subfamily classes. *J Theor Biol*, 248 (3), 546-551.

# Analysis and Characterization of Alu Insertion Sites: A Statistical Method and a Data Mining Solution

Kun Zhang
*Department of Computer Science*
*Xavier University of Louisiana, USA*

Wei Fan
*Huawei Noah Ark's Lab, China*

Andrea Edwards, Augustine Orgah
*Department of Computer Science*
*Xavier University of Louisiana, USA*

Prescott Deininger
*Tulane Cancer Center, School of Public Health and Tropical Medicine*
*Tulane University, USA*

# 1   Introduction

Retrotransposable elements are mobile DNA sequences that can cause diseases and shape genomes by integrating genetic information into chromosomes. These elements can be employed for functional genomics, gene transfer and human gene therapy. However, their insertion site preferences, which are critically important for these potential uses, are still far from being understood. Alus are the primate-specific short interspersed non-autonomous retrotransposable elements whose active retrotransposition depends on reverse transcriptase encoded by autonomous long interspersed element-1 (L1). Full-length Alus are approximately 300 bps in length and are commonly found in introns and intergenic genomic regions. Throughout the evolutionary history of primates, Alu elements have amplified to more than one million copies, comprising roughly 11% of the human genome. Several distinct Alu subfamilies of different genetic ages have been identified. Compared to older subfamilies, the younger class Alu-Y is characterized by an increasing number of disease-causing insertion mutations, and higher proportions that exist in a polymorphic state. Because of their continued amplification and fairly random, non-specific insertional mutagenesis, Alu elements have a major impact on the human genome. A significant proportion of human genetic diseases have been ascribed to the disruptive Alu insertions and mutations (Deininger and Batzer, 1999; Belancio et al., 2008).

Analyzing and characterizing the preferences of Alu insertion sites has been a vital step to further understand the Alu insertion mechanism. The primary work concerning this issue is (Jurka, 1997). By locally aligning 400 sequences near the insertion site, Jurka identified the preferred primary insertion site is the 5' TT-AAAA consensus sequence around the 5' ends of flanking repeats of Alu. This consensus is a potential target for enzymatic nicking by the endonuclease domain provided by the L1 ORF2 product, and some variations in this consensus could also be used as targets. The above results are further validated through a larger scale sequence analyses using the Smith-Waterman local alignment algorithm (Gentles et al., 2005). Using sequences from different Alu subfamilies, Toda (Toda et al., 1998) analyzed merely 5' flanking regions of Alu elements by the information content calculation. Their results suggest: (1) the region between -20 and 5' end of Alu elements is highly adenine-rich and shows significantly higher information content values compared to the rest of the region. (2) younger subfamilies of Alu elements have higher information content values than older subfamilies. Another earlier study also analyzed the patterns of Alu-insertion and restriction-site polymorphisms in ancestral human diversity (Watkins et al., 2001). Although those studies hint at the involvement of sequence-specific enzyme specificity for Alu insertion, there is substantial computational cost in constructing these models. Yet, little is known how the distribution of the 5'-TTAAAA motif influences the Alu density on the genome-wide scale and whether any broader-scale patterns could exist that may also impact the insertion of Alus.

In this chapter, we present a statistical method and a data mining solution to fill this gap. Using a two-step regression analysis, we explore the genome wide gene-level effect of 5'-TTAAAA motif density on Alu density. On the other hand, a divide-conquer and aggregate based approach, from the data mining aspect, provides an integrated algorithmic framework addressing the key computational challenges associated with this problem. Below are our main contributions of this work.

1.  By considering that a single linear model is not sufficient for the observed data where a substantial proportion (e. g. approximately 30% in human genome) of genes contains no Alus, we developed a two-step regression model to analyze the gene-level effect of 5'-TTAAAA motif on the integration of Alu elements. Our results show that the gene-level effect of the motif density on Alu density varied across chromosomes substantially in terms of statistical significance level.

2. We introduce a divide-conquer and aggregate based framework to efficiently predict and characterize the primary Alu insertion site in a unified process. In this framework, the core is an improved frequent pattern classification algorithm coupled with two task-oriented modules for position reserved sequence mapping and target pattern aggregation. Algorithmically, this is the first probabilistic generative model developed for this issue. The concept of two-mode dynamic support, scalability and time complexity analyses are also provided for the proposed approach.

3. Compared to the benchmark biological study, our results provide a further refined analysis of the characteristic patterns involved in the mechanism of Alu insertion. Most importantly in biology, we acquire a 200nt predictive profile around the Alu insertion which not only contains the widely accepted signal consensus, but also suggests a longer pattern $(T)_7AA[G|A]AATAA$. This pattern provides more insight into the favored sequence variations allowed for preferred binding and cleavage by the L1 ORF2 endonuclease that is involved in initiating the insertion process.

4. For bioinformatics and data mining research, we have analytically and empirically shown that, (1) as the data is not in the pre-defined feature vectors, discriminative patterns are good candidates not only for prediction but general pattern approximation. (2) when compact yet predictive pattern discovery suffers from the intractable computation barrier, the proposed method can provide a general solution to similar sequential or structural pattern discovery problems.

The rest of the article is organized as follows. Section 2 presents a two-step regression analysis of the genome-wide gene-level effect of 5'-TTAAAA motif density on Alu density. Section 3 describes a divide-conquer and aggregate based data mining approach exploring the existence of broader-scale patterns that may also impact the insertion of Alus. We conclude this chapter and discuss the future directions in Section 4.

## 2   Two-Step Regression Analysis of the Gene-Level Effect of 5'-TTAAAA Motif Density on Alu Density

It has been widely recognized that the integration of Alu elements is initiated with its endonuclease-dependent cleavage at the 5'-TTAAAA hexanucleotide, and the variants derived by a single base substitution, particularly from A to G and T to C (Jurka, 1997). A recent publication further reported that such motif(s) contributed to $6.1\% - 26.7\%$ of the variation in Alu density of genome sequences of fixed length, depending on the subtypes and the genome regions related to the evolution divergence of human, chimpanzee and orangutan (Kvikstad *et al.*, 2010). The authors divided the entire human genome into around 2400 bins with each of 1M bases long, and measured motif and Alu densities on these sequences of fixed length. In our study, the densities were determined using genes as the units, thus our data structure and representation was quite different from that in (Kvikstad *et al.*, 2010). Considering the scarcity of the retained Alu elements in the exon regions, we focused on the analysis of the motif in introns relative to Alu densities. The substantial level of genes without any Alus makes the method employed in (Kvikstad *et al.*, 2010) not applicable to the statistical analysis conducted here.

A two-step regression model was developed to analyze the gene-level effect of 5'-TTAAAA motif on the integration of Alu elements. The motivation is that a single linear model is not sufficient to analyze the observed data where a substantial proportion (e. g. approximately 30% in human genome) of genes contains no Alu elements and, as a result, we cannot conduct the logarithm transformation of Alu densities to resemble a normal distribution. The proposed method consists of a logistic regression model and a simple linear model. Below are the mathematical expressions of these two models.

Model-1 :

$$\log\left(\frac{P(z_i = 1)}{1 - P(z_i = 1)}\right) = \mu + \alpha l_i + \beta x_i$$

Model-2 :

$$\log(y_j) = \mu^* + \alpha^* l_j + \beta^* x_j + e_j \ , \ y > 0$$

In Model-1, $z_i \in \{1, 0\}$ indicates if gene $i$ has at least one Alu in the intron region(s). $x_i$ is the intron motif density, and $l_i$ is the log10 transformed adjusted sequence length (with Alu sequences excluded from the calculation). In Model-2, for a specific gene, $j$, $x_j$, $y_j$, $l_j$ and $e_j$ are the motif density, Alu density, log10 adjusted sequence length of this gene, and random noise, respectively. $(\mu, \alpha, \beta)$ and $(\mu^*, \alpha^*, \beta^*)$ are the parameter sets of the two models. Model-1 evaluates the effect of the motif density on the presence or absence of Alus in the intron regions for all multi-exon genes; while Model-2 tests the effect of the motif density on the intron Alu density for the genes with at least one Alu element in the intron region(s). We conducted the logistic regression analysis using the procedure *lrm* included in the R package "Design". The pseudo contribution rate of the intron motif to the total variability was measured as the increase of Nagelkerke R2 index (Nagelkerke, 1991) due to adding the density $(x)$ to the reduced model which contained 1 as the only explainable variable. The simple regression analysis was conducted with the procedure lm in the R package "stats" and the contribution rate of intron motif to the total variability was measured as the increase of statistic R2 due to adding the density $(x)$ to the reduced model. The multi-testing across chromosomes was addressed by BH method (Benjamini *et al.*, 1995). It is worth noting that in both models, gene size was included as an independent variable. This is because our preliminary study showed that gene size had a significant effect on the presence or absence of Alu in intron region(s) for most chromosomes.

    Figure 1 shows the results obtained from the proposed two-step regression method. The data points are labeled with chromosome IDs. The X- and Y- coordinates are the negatives of the log10 transformed FDR-adjusted p-values (Benjamini *et al.*,1995) from the two models, respectively. The dashed red lines correspond to 0.05 in the scale of adjusted p-values. As shown in Figure 1, the influence of motif density on the intron Alu density is chromosome-specific. For chromosome-7, the effect is not significant as demonstrated by both models. For chromosomes -4, -6, -13, -X, and -Y, the effect is significant only in Model-1. For chromosomes -18 and -21, the effect is significant only in Model-2. The rest of the chromosomes have the adjusted *p*-values less than 0.05 as reflected by both models. The most significant cases are detected in chromosome-1 where the adjusted p-values are less than $1 \times 10^{-8}$ and $1 \times 10^{-10}$ in the two models, respectively. For chromosome-19 which has the highest genome-wide Alu density, the effect is marginally significant as measured by Model-1. The chromosome-wide gene-level positive association between Alus and the motif are suggested by the facts that all the regression coefficients $\beta$ are positive in the Model-1 and the coefficients $\beta^*$ are positive in model-2 except for chromosomes -7 and X.

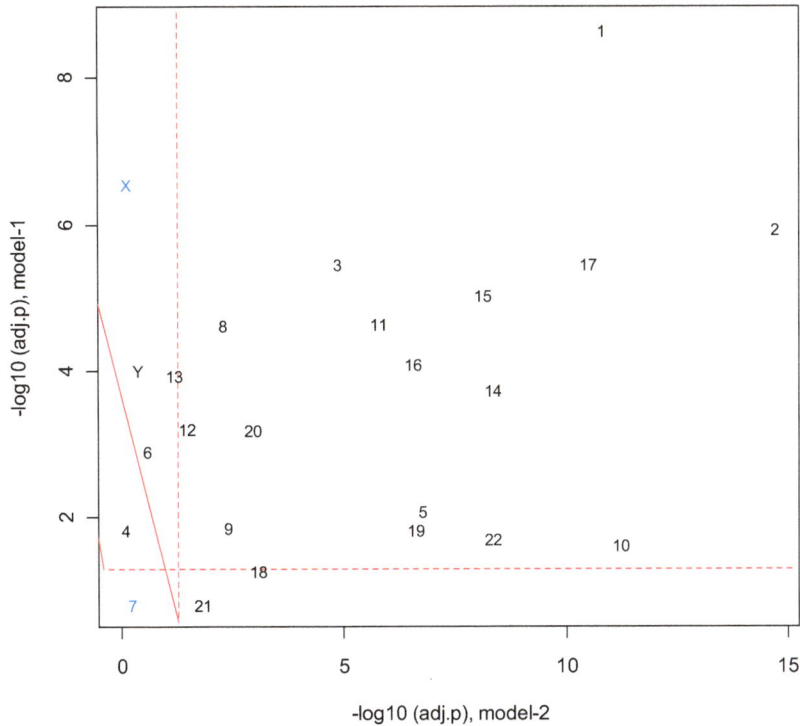

**Figure 1**: The visualization of the gene-level effects of 5'-TTAAAA intron motif density on intron Alu density obtained from the proposed two step regression method. The data points are labeled with chromosome IDs. The X- and Y- coordinates are the negatives of the log10 transformed p-values (adjusted with BH method) from the two models, respectively. The dashed red lines correspond to 0.05 in the scale of adjusted p-values. Model-1 evaluates the effect of the motif density on the presence or absence of Alus in the introns of the genes. Model-2 evaluates the effect of the motif density on the intron Alu density of the genes with at least one Alu repeat in their intron regions. All the regression coefficients β are positive in the model-1 and the coefficients β* are positive in model-1 except for chromosomes 7 and X (marked with blue).

# 3  A Divide-Conquer and Aggregate Based Approach for Alu Insertion Site Characterization

Besides the potential effect of the 5'-TTAAAA motif on the genome-wide Alu density, another question of interest to biologist is whether any broader-scale patterns could exist that may also influence the insertion of Alus. However, several biological specifications present in this application make the problem interesting and challenging. First, due to the costly and time-consuming laboratory studies it takes to enhance the recognition of the Alu insertion mechanism, biologists want to fairly ensure the certainty of a sequence being a target of Alu insertion when it is fed to the model. That is, the predictive precision needs to be maximized while the corresponding recall is maintained at a reasonable level. Unfortunately, the raw data is in the format of DNA sequences, and no pre-defined feature vectors can be directly presented to data mining algorithms to construct predictive models. Second, besides those significant discriminative patterns indicating the possible Alu insertions, biologists are very interested in identifying any potential proximal patterns in a relatively large scale of bases that may also affect the nicking. Nevertheless, without any prior knowledge of the existence of such patterns, it is nontrivial to design methods to catch them. The safest way to address this issue is to acquire a position reserved global predictive profile of the target sequences by aggregating the class exclusive discriminative patterns together, and then present it to biologists for further analysis.

One promising approach to mine biological sequence data is discovering frequent patterns, i.e., patterns which occur in at least as many sequences as specified by a threshold. This approach is motivated by two fundamental biological observations: (1) similar sequences or structures are more likely to have the same or similar function, and (2) large portions of DNA or protein sequences are rather noisy. Thus, if a pattern occurs frequently, it ought to be important or meaningful in some way. The effectiveness of frequent pattern discovery has been demonstrated by much work using both sequential and structured data (Han *et al.*, 2007, Leung *et al.*, 2010). On the other hand, a major obstacle faced by the frequent pattern mining research is how to efficiently discover those essential and discriminative frequent patterns. State-of-the-art frequent pattern mining algorithms (Cheng *et al.*, 2007; Deshpande *et al.,* 2005) usually employ a batch process, which first enumerates patterns above the given support and then performs pattern selection on this initial pool, as shown in Figure 2. Nevertheless, with these methods, there is still limited success in eventually finding those compact yet discriminative patterns. This is due to the four inherent problems of this process. (1) The number of candidate patterns can still be prohibitively large for effective pattern selection. One of the deteriorating factors is the routine of "ordered" enumeration, that is, we cannot enumerate patterns of "min_sup = 10%" without first enumerating all patterns of "min_sup > 10%". Another similar example exists in frequent sequence pattern mining. For example, to discover frequent patterns of length $l$ from a set of DNA sequences, all possible pattern candidates of length $l$ would be enumerated, resulting in $4^l (4^{10} \approx 10^6)$ strings in total. However, before $4^l$ patterns are obtained, up to $\sum_{i=1}^{l} 4^i$ sequences of length $\leq l$ could be first generated, which obviously poses an intractable computational burden on this process. (2) If the frequency of discriminative patterns is below the support value chosen to enumerate the candidates; those patterns won't even be considered even if they have high discriminative information. (3) The discriminative power of each pattern is directly evaluated against the complete dataset, but not on some subsets of data that the other chosen patterns do not predict well. (4) The correlation among multiple patterns is not directly evaluated on their joint predictability. In addition, a common problematic issue in the bioinformatics practice is that frequent patterns are only mined on the bio-data in question. It cannot guarantee that the discovered patterns are solely proprietary to the target data since they may also occur in other category of data of no interest.

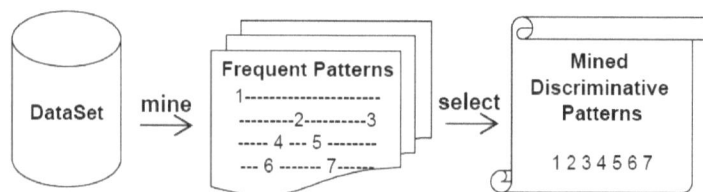

**Figure 2:** Traditional two-step method

In response to these considerations, we develop a systematic divide-conquer and aggregate based framework to tackle the above challenges as a whole. The proposed framework is a significant extension and generalization of our prior work (Fan *et al.*, 2008).

## 3.1   Methods

In this section, we first define the notions of frequent sequence pattern mining, and then present the design and analysis of the proposed method.

### 3.1.1   Notation

In the context of biological sequence mining, a sequence pattern is an ordered list of items defined on a specific alphabet. For example, the DNA alphabet consists of four nucleotides or bases, i.e. $\Sigma=\{A,C,G,T\}$, and each can be viewed as an item. A subset of $\Sigma$ is called an itemset. If not all positions in a pattern are precisely known, a wildcard symbol $n$ can be included in $\Sigma$ accordingly. The number of instances of items in a pattern is called the length of the pattern, and a pattern of length $l$ is denoted as an *l-mer* pattern. A pattern $t = \{t_1 \ t_2 \ ... \ t_m\}$ is a subpattern of $p = \{p_1 \ p_1 \ ... \ p_w\}$ if and only if $\exists \ j_1, j_2,...,j_m$ such that $1 \leq j_1 < j_2 < \cdots < j_m \leq w$ and $t_1 \subseteq p_{j1}$, $t_1 \subseteq p_{j2}$,..., $t_m \subseteq p_{jm}$.

We also call $p$ a superpattern of $t$. Given a sequence database $D$, a pattern $p$ is frequent if at least a fraction of sequences within $D$ contain $p$, i.e., $Support_D(p) \geq min\_sup$, where $min\_sup$ is the pre-defined support value. In general, frequent sequence pattern mining can be viewed as a special case of frequent itemset mining with the sequential constraint reserved among items. As shown in Figure 3, the proposed method contains the following three steps: position reserved sequence mapping, pattern discovery via model based search tree (MBT) and target pattern aggregation.

### 3.1.2   Position Reserved Sequence Mapping

To identify the bases most-likely to receive Alu insertions, we implemented a positional mapping procedure for each nucleotide in a sequence. Without loss of generality, at a specific position $i$ ($1 \leq i \leq L$), the probability of occurrence of each symbol in the alphabet is $1/|\Sigma|$. Therefore, $|\Sigma|$ mapping formulas are needed at position $i$ to uniquely represent a particular character. Figure 3(a) presents an example of this mapping schema if every position is known. According to this mapping, we can obtain the position-reserved numerical representations of the sequences in the dataset for MBT training.

### 3.1.3   Pattern Discovery via MBT

MBT or "model-based" search tree was initially proposed in our previous work (Fan *et al.*, 2008). As shown in Figure 3(b1), the basic flow proceeds by constructing a depth-first search tree on the data from two classes. As each node in the tree is expanded, a frequent pattern mining algorithm is invoked only on the examples within that node to generate a pool of pattern candidates. Then based on some fitness criteria, such as gain ratio or Gini index, one pattern of the highest score among all candidates is chosen as the most discriminative feature and maintained in this node. Finally, depending on whether the examples contain the selected pattern (or whether the pattern is present in the examples), the data at the given node are divided into two disjoint subsets with each corresponding to a child node. The model tree grows by exploring each child separately and recursively. The search and tree construction terminates when (1) either every example in the given node belongs to the same class, or (2) the number of total examples at the node is smaller than a predefined threshold. After the algorithm completes, $K$ discriminative frequent patterns are discovered and the corresponding model-based search tree is constructed. Algorithm 1 presents the detailed implementation.

**(a)**
Position
Reserved
Sequence
Mapping

**Original Binary Sequences**

Seq 1: ATGTAGGTAA +
Seq 2: AGGAATATTT −
: :
Seq n: CTGATAAATC +

| Nucleotides at Position i | Mapping |
|---|---|
| A | 1+4*(i-1) |
| C | 2+4*(i-1) |
| G | 3+4*(i-1) |
| T | 4+4*(i-1) |

**Mapped Training Sequences**

Seq 1: 1 8 11 16 17 23 27 32 33 37 +
Seq 2: 1 7 11 13 17 24 25 32 36 40 −
: :
Seq n: 2 8 11 13 20 21 25 29 36 38 +

**(b)**
Pattern
Discovery
via MBT

mine & select — Data — P1
mine & select — P2, P5
mine & select — P3, P4, P6, P7

+ , Few Data , ........ , − , +

P1
P2
P3
P4
P5
P6
P7

represent

| P1 P2... P7 |
| Data1  1 1 ... 0 |
| Data2  1 0 ... 1 |
| Data3  1 1 ... 0 |

ANN

DT
SVM

LR

Petal.Length< 2.45
setosa  Petal.Width< 1.75
versicolor  virginica

$logit(p) = \ln\left(\frac{p}{1-p}\right) = \alpha + \beta_1 x_{1,} + \cdots + \beta_k x_{k,}$

Any classifiers you can name

*b1: Divide-and-Conquer Based Frequent Pattern Mining*   *b2: Mined Discriminative Patterns*   *b3: Classification via other classifiers*

**(c)**
Target
Pattern
Aggregation
& Reversed
Mapping

**Mined  Positional Patterns of Target Class**

P1: 11 16 23 27 32 37 (8/10)
P3: 11 15 18 23 32 38 (3/5)
P7: 12 15 17 24 31    (1/3)

| Reversed Mapping | Nucleotides at Position i |
|---|---|
| (i-1) % 4 = 0 | A |
| (i-2) % 4 = 0 | C |
| (i-3) % 4 = 0 | G |
| (i-4) % 4 = 0 | T |

PWM

| i | A | C | G | T | Predicted Pattern |
|---|---|---|---|---|---|
| 1 | 0 | 0 | 0 | 0 | n |
| 2 | 0 | 0 | 0 | 0 | n |
| 3 | 0 | 0 | 0.81 | 0.19 | G |
| 4 | 0 | 0 | 0.54 | 0.46 | G |
| 5 | 0.36 | 0.64 | 0 | 0 | C |
| 6 | 0 | 0 | 0.81 | 0.19 | G |
| 7 | 0 | 0 | 1 | 0 | G |
| 8 | 0 | 0 | 0.19 | 0.81 | T |
| 9 | 0 | 0 | 0 | 0 | n |
| 10 | 0.57 | 0.43 | 0 | 0 | A |

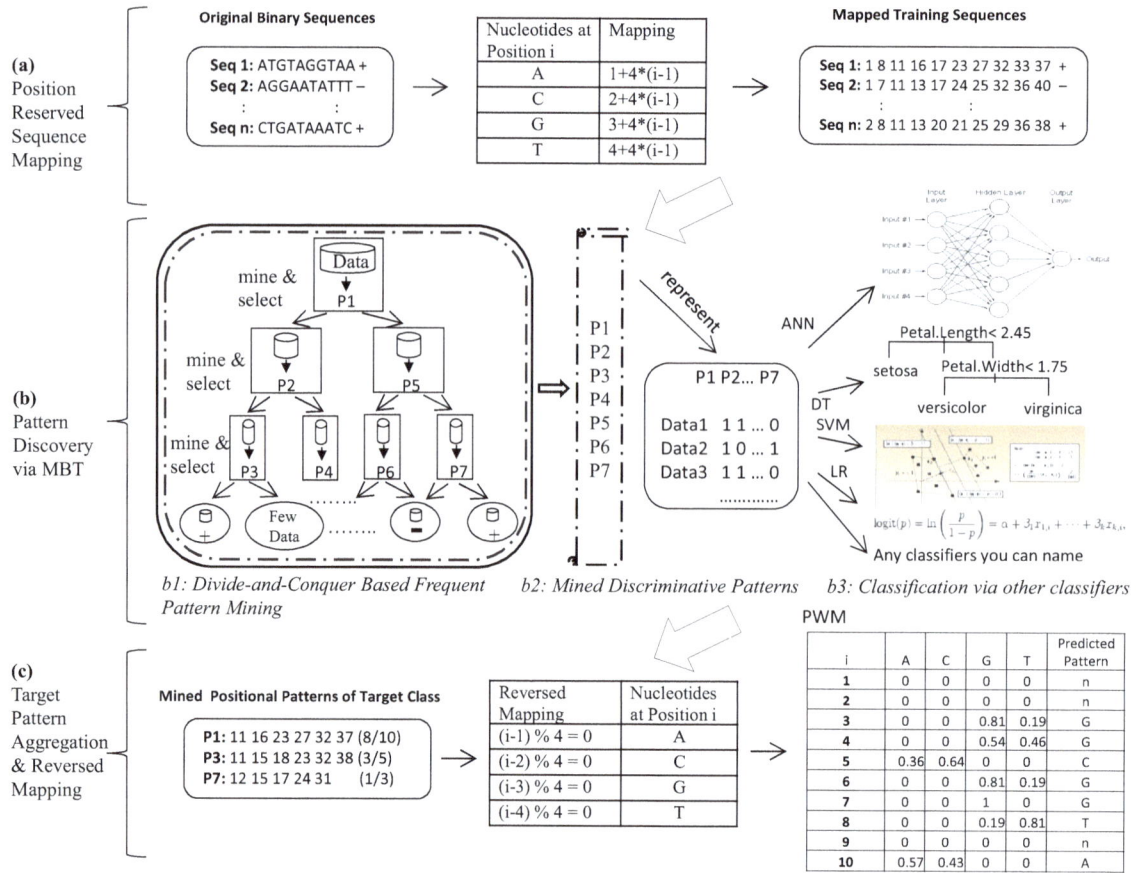

**Figure 3:** Overall flow of proposed method (artificial data for illustration purpose)

---

### Algorithm 1: Build Model-based Search Tree

---

**Input:**   1: A set of examples **D** from which patterns are to be mined
2: A support threshold **p** normalized between 0 and 1
3: A pattern discover algorithm, such as a frequent pattern mining algorithm **fp(. . .)**
4: **m**: minimum node size.

**Output:**  1: A selected set of patterns, **Fs**
2: A model-based search tree **T**.

1: Call the frequent pattern algorithm, which returns a set of frequent patterns **FP = fp(D, p)**
2: Evaluate the fitness of each pattern **α ∈ FP**;
3: Choose pattern **$\alpha_m$** as the most discriminative feature;
4: **Fs = Fs ∪ {$\alpha_m$}**;
5: Maintain pattern **$\alpha_m$** as the testing feature in current node of the tree **T**;
6: **$D_L$** = subset of examples in **D** containing **$\alpha_m$**, and **$D_R = D - D_L$**;
7: for **$\ell \in \{L,R\}$**
8:     if **$|D_\ell| \leq m$** or examples in **$D_\ell$** have the same class label,  make **$T_\ell$** a leaf node;
9:     else recursively construct **$T_\ell$** with **$D_\ell$** and **p**;
10: return **Fs** and **T**

Moreover, as illustrated in Figure 3(b2), once those $K$ discriminative patterns are obtained, the original examples can be transformed into a $K$ dimensional feature space through a binary representation. In this way, we successfully acquire the transformed "feature vectors" that can be given to any data mining s to build predictive models, which is shown in Figure 3(b3). Additionally, based on the divide-and-conquer tree structure, the MBT itself can also serve as an independent classification or probability estimation tree. Its performance has been demonstrated to be comparable to other popular data mining approaches, such as SVM (Fan *et al.*, 2008).

It has been theoretically proven that the number of frequent patterns ever enumerated by MBT can be upper-bounded by $O(N^{N(1-s)})$ during the tree construction process, where $N$ is the number of examples in the dataset ($> 3$) and $s$ is the support in percentage. This enumeration scale can be also applied to the traditional frequent pattern algorithms (Fan *et al.*, 2008). However, It is worth noting that in MBT, the support $s$ is the unified local support at each node, i.e., the same support percentage $s$ is used at each node to generate patterns. On the other hand, in terms of the entire dataset, a pattern with support $s$ at a specific node also has a global support $s'$, which is much smaller than $s$. For example, assume that a node size is 10 and $s = 20\%$, for a problem of size 10000, the global support is $10 \times 20\% / 10000 = 0.02\%$. To discover such patterns, the traditional pattern mining algorithms will return an explosive number of candidates or fail due to resource constraints, since it will generate $O(N^{N(1-s')})$ patterns. As $s'$ approaches 0, traditional frequent pattern mining algorithms could obtain up to $N^N$ patterns. However, the recursive algorithm can identify such patterns without considering every candidate, thus it will not generate an explosive number of patterns. In particular, compared with traditional pattern mining approaches, the "scale down" ratio of the patterns obtained by MBT will be approximately up to $\approx N^{N(1-s)} / N^N = 1/N^{Ns}$. This demonstrates that the proposed recursive algorithm could conquer the barrier of explosive growth of frequent patterns and successfully identify discriminative patterns with very small support.

### 3.1.4  Target Pattern Aggregation

As shown in Figure 3(b), MBT is not only a frequent pattern based predictive model, but also a discriminative feature miner. The discovered features can be either further used to train other classifiers or be aggregated to provide a global solution to the target class. The rationale behind this aggregation is as follows. Enfolding the batch process of frequent pattern generation and selection at each decision node, the proposed algorithm is still a typical application of divide-and-conquer strategy. Once $K$ discriminative frequent patterns are obtained via the tree construction process, each merely occurring in the target class and locally reflecting partial specific of this target class can be aggregated to acquire a large-scale pattern which captures the crucial "signatures" distinguishing the target class from the class of no interest. This aggregation essentially corresponds to the generic "combine" step of divide-and-conquer diagram, and is achieved by the accumulation and normalization of the predicted nucleotide probability at a specific position.

To retrieve the patterns solely of the target class, for each selected pattern at a decision node in the tree, we also track how frequently this pattern occurs in the sequences of different classes within the region defined by this node. As shown in Figure 3(c), the patterns only contained in the target class are collected for aggregation. More specifically, let $P_t$ be a discovered target sequential pattern consisting of a string of numerical positions. Associated with $P_t$ is a frequency value which indicates the number of sequences in the target class at a specific node containing $P_t$.

In general, this frequency value can be distributed to each numerical position within $P_t$ to represent the frequency that we may have a specific nucleotide at this position via the reversed positional mapping. By accumulating and normalizing the frequency value of a specific nucleotide at a particular position using all of the discovered target patterns, we can obtain an aggregated sequential pattern along with an $L \times 4$ position weight matrix (PWM) $M$, where $L$ is the maximal sequence length. The $i^{th}$ row in $M$ contains four probabilities, each indicating the probability we may have a specific nucleotide at the position $i$ in the aggregated sequence. The nucleotide of the highest probability will be chosen as the predicted base at position $i$. It is this aggregation mechanism that allows us to acquire a global predicted probabilistic view of the target sequences, whereby making it possible to characterize the Alu insertion site on a relatively large-scale bases.

### 3.1.5    Time Complexity of the Proposed Method

Given a set of $N$ sequences, in the worst case, the computational complexity of the proposed method can be upper bounded by $O(LN + \log N (FP + dN \log N))$, where $L$ is the maximal sequence length, $d$ is the number of frequent patterns generated at a node, $O(FP)$ denotes the computational cost of the frequent pattern mining algorithm, and $O(LN)$ represents the required computations by position reserved sequence mapping as well as target pattern aggregation and reversed mapping. It is evident that the major computational cost is primarily determined by the frequent pattern mining algorithm employed at each internal node of MBT, and it is $\leq O(\log N (FP + dN \log N))$. Because there are many efficient frequent pattern mining algorithms available (Cheng *et al.*, 2007 and 2008; Grahne and Zhu, 2003; Pei *et al.*, 2001; Yan *et al.*, 2008), the overall computational cost of MBT is acceptable compared to the primitive local alignment algorithm. Typically, the time complexity of applying the Smith-Waterman alignment algorithm to the same set of $N$ sequences is $C_2^N O(L^2)$. As more sequences are involved into the study, simply aligning them using the Smith-Waterman algorithm is obviously impractical because its complexity can be factorial.

### 3.2    Experimental Results

This section discusses the datasets used in the study, and three sets of experiments conducted to evaluate the efficacy of the proposed method. We term our method "MBT" in the following descriptions and Figures. To the best of our knowledge, there is no existing data mining algorithms proposed for Alu or other retrotransposable element insertion site prediction, therefore, we first summarize the MBT's classification results on accuracy, precision, recall and the number of mined patterns, and then we present the characterized Alu insertion site contained in a 200nt predicted profile. Finally, to study the scalability and quality of the patterns discovered by MBT, we compare its results to those of two benchmark approaches, one is the "Pattern Growth" algorithm (Ye *et al.*, 2007), and the other is what has been widely accepted in biology (Jurka, 1997).

### 3.2.1    Datasets

Two sets of Pre-Alu Insertion (PAI) sequences are generated from the human and chimpanzee genomes. For each sequence, we first identified five components as shown in Figure 4(a). Then each sequence is formed by the specifics illustrated in Figure 4(b). Typically, each sequence consists of 100 bases preceding the 3' end of the 5' flanking region, one copy of the target site duplication (TSD, i.e., *flanking repeat*) and some bases from the 5' end of the 3' flanking region. The total length of TSD and the sequence from 3' flanking region is set to be 100, making each sequence 200 bases long. It is worth noting that, for both sets of PAI sequences, we only consider those from Alu Y family and of the perfect TSDs, that is, the 5' TSD exactly matches the 3' TSD. TSDs are indentified by applying TSDFinder (Szak *et al.*, 2002) to the annotated human and chimpanzee genomes available at UCSC Genome Browser (http://genome.ucsc.edu/). In total,

5258 human and 3142 chimpanzee PAI sequences are involved in the study as the positive or target class. To train MBT, we also acquired four sets of 200nt Non-Pre-Alu insertion (NPAI) sequences by random sequence generation (Rouchka and Hardin, 2007) as well as random selection from three species which are known to not have Alu insertions. These species are *S.pombe*, chicken and mouse. We set the number of negative sequences to be 2000 since MBT is rather robust to the varied class distributions (Fan *et al.*, 2008). As a result, eight datasets are generated by respectively combining one of the four sets of NPAI sequences with the human or chimpanzee PAI sequences. Table 1 summarizes the statistics of each dataset.

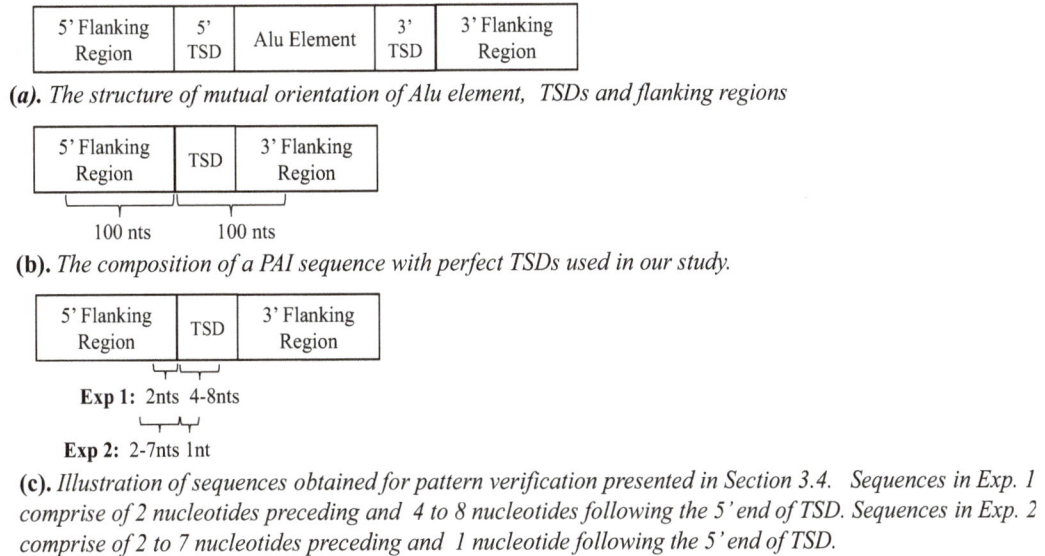

| 5' Flanking Region | 5' TSD | Alu Element | 3' TSD | 3' Flanking Region |
|---|---|---|---|---|

**(a)**. *The structure of mutual orientation of Alu element, TSDs and flanking regions*

| 5' Flanking Region | TSD | 3' Flanking Region |
|---|---|---|

100 nts          100 nts

**(b)**. *The composition of a PAI sequence with perfect TSDs used in our study.*

| 5' Flanking Region | TSD | 3' Flanking Region |
|---|---|---|

**Exp 1:** 2nts  4-8nts

**Exp 2:** 2-7nts 1nt

**(c)**. *Illustration of sequences obtained for pattern verification presented in Section 3.4. Sequences in Exp. 1 comprise of 2 nucleotides preceding and 4 to 8 nucleotides following the 5' end of TSD. Sequences in Exp. 2 comprise of 2 to 7 nucleotides preceding and 1 nucleotide following the 5' end of TSD.*

**Figure 4:** Structures of Alu sequences and PAI sequences used in experiments

| Datasets | | PAI vs NonPAI |
|---|---|---|
| **Human (H)** | *Chicken (C)* | 5258:2000 |
| | *Mouses(M)* | 5258:2000 |
| | *Random* | 5258:2000 |
| | *S. pombe (Sp)* | 5258:2000 |
| **Chimpanzee(C)** | *Chicken (C)* | 3142:2000 |
| | *Mouses(M)* | 3142:2000 |
| | *Random* | 3142:2000 |
| | *S. pombe (Sp)* | 3142:2000 |

**Table 1:** Dataset description

### 3.2.2  Classification Results

Standard 3-fold cross validation (CV) is employed to conduct classification study as well as the parameter selection for *min_sup*. Figure 5 summarizes the average results over 3 runs for the human and chimpanzee when *min_sup* is respectively set to be 5%, 10% and 20%. In general, along with at least a 90.5% recall

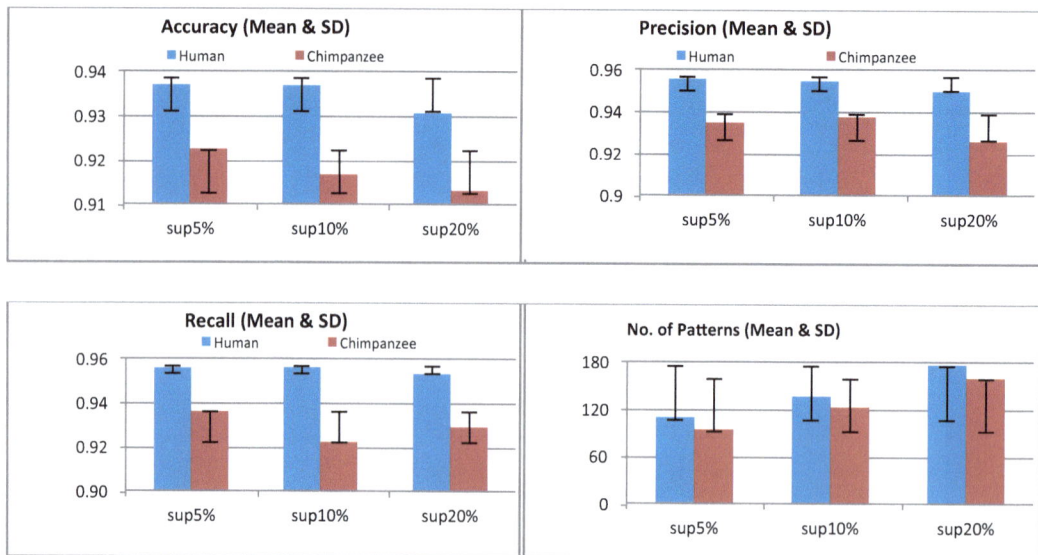

| Min_sup 5% | No. of Mined Patterns | Accuracy (%) | Precision (%) | Recall(%) |
|---|---|---|---|---|
| H-C / C-C | 121 / 99.3 | 92.2 / 90.9 | 94.7 / 92.2 | 94.6 / 93 |
| H-M / C-M | 112 / 93 | 93.2 / 92.4 | 95.5 / 93.6 | 95.1 / 94 |
| H-Random / C-Random | 98 / 87.3 | 93.8 / 92 | 96.5 / 94.2 | 94.9 / 92.7 |
| H-Sp / C-Sp | 106 / 94.3 | 93.6 / 91.7 | 95.4 / 93.8 | 95.7 / 92.6 |
| Min_sup 10% | No. of Mined Patterns | Accuracy (%) | Precision (%) | Recall(%) |
| H-C / C-C | 149 / 130 | 92.6 / 90.1 | 94.9 / 93.1 | 94.9 / 90.5 |
| H-M / C-M | 135.7 / 121.7 | 93 / 90.8 | 95 / 93 | 95.3 / 91.9 |
| H-Random / C-Random | 122.7 / 116.3 | 94.1 / 92.1 | 96.5 / 95.1 | 95.2 / 91.8 |
| H-Sp / C-Sp | 136.3 / 119.7 | 93.1 / 91.6 | 95.4 / 93.6 | 95 / 92.6 |
| Min_sup 20% | No. of Mined Patterns | Accuracy (%) | Precision (%) | Recall(%) |
| H-C / C-C | 191 / 172 | 91.5 / 90.1 | 94.5 / 91.9 | 93.8 / 91.8 |
| H-M / C-M | 186.3 / 159 | 92 / 91.2 | 94.3 / 93 | 94.8 / 92.7 |
| H-Random / C-Random | 152.3 / 149.3 | 94.1 / 91.7 | 96.3 / 93.7 | 95.6 / 92.7 |
| H-Sp / C-Sp | 175.3 / 155.7 | 92.5 / 90.2 | 94.7 / 91.6 | 95 / 92.4 |

**Figure 5:** MBT performance on Human (numbers before "/") and Chimpanzee (numbers after "/").

score, MBT achieves quite good performance on precision, i.e. over 94.3% for the human and 91.6% for the chimpanzee. This suggests that the frequent patterns discovered by MBT not only are very specific to PAI sequences, but also capture the characteristics of a large portion of PAI sequences and only reject a small number of other members in this class. In addition, MBT consistently performs better on the datasets containing the PAI sequences obtained from the human. This observation could be ascribed to the larger number of sequences acquired from the human, which enables MBT to discover more discriminative frequent patterns for the classification purpose.

As a further effort to study the sensitivity of MBT, we also respectively computed the means and standard deviations of the accuracy, precision and recall over the four datasets using the same category of PAI sequences as the positive class. The rather small range of the standard deviation for each evaluation metric ([0.6%, 1.1%] for accuracy, [0.7%, 0.99%] for precision, [0.2%, 0.86%] for recall) indicates that the performance of MBT is fairly stable with respect to different sequences as the negative class. Moreover, for both species, MBT achieves the overall highest accuracy, precision and recall, as well as the most compact set of discovered frequent patterns when it is trained at *min_sup* being 5%. As the value of *min_sup* increases from 5% to 20%, the performance of MBT tends to slightly decline with more frequent patterns obtained. This is because, compared to bigger *min_sup* thresholds, smaller ones can generate a larger pool of candidates from which MBT has a better chance of selecting optimal patterns with higher fitness scores. We also conducted the paired t-test on the accuracies, precisions and recalls achived on the eight datasets (human and chimpanzee) when *min_sup* is respectively 5%, 10% and 20%. P-values of these pairwise tests are presented in Table 2. It is evident that, at 0.05 level of significance, there is no difference between the accuracies, precisions and recalls obtained when *min_sup* is respectively 5% and 10%.

|  | Min_sup: 5% VS 10% | Min_sup: 5% VS 20% | Min_sup: 10% VS 20% |
|---|---|---|---|
| **Accuracy** | 0.239 | 0.006 | 0.054 |
| **Precision** | 0.676 | 0.018 | 0.010 |
| **Recall** | 0.127 | 0.082 | 0.502 |

**Table 2:** P-values of the paired t-test on the accuracies, precisions and recalls achieved on the eight datasets (human and chimpanzee) when min_sup is respectively 5%, 10% and 20%.

### 3.2.3  Characterization of Alu Insertion Site through Frequent Pattern Aggregation

Besides the classification study of the proposed algorithm, we carried out another set of experiments to directly mine the patterns proprietary to the PAI sequences. In particular, MBT is trained on all of the binary sequences in a dataset without conducting 3-fold CV, and only the patterns which occur in the PAI class are aggregated to characterize the potential Alu insertion site. We set min_sup to be 5% due to the overall better performance achieved in the above cross valiation study.

To graphically reveal the global predicted specifics around the Alu insertion site, for each species, we concatenated four aggregated predicted profiles together. Each profile is obtained by solely aggregating the target patterns mined from a data set of different negative (i.e. NAPI) but the same positive (i.e. PAI) sequences. By concatenating the multiple predicted profiles discovered from the varied pools of patterns, we can acquire a more complete and convincing forecast of the conserved subsequences. The logos (Crooks *et al.*, 2004) over four different sequence datasets for the human and chimpanzee are presented in Figure 6. At each specific position, the logo letters are ordered from most to least frequent, and the height of each letter is in proportional to the predicted likelihood that this nucleotide could occur. Instead of no prediction at all, the letter vacancy at a position indicates the possibility of more than three bases. It is evident that the most remarkable signals are detected around the insertion site occurring between positions -1 and 0. To determine the maximum length of the statistically significant patterns contained in the predicted profile, we employ the information content criterion (Schneider et al., 1986) as defined below, where $f_{c,i}$ is the observed frequency of base $c$ at position $i$, and $B_c$ the background or expected frequency of base $c$.

$$IC_i = \sum_{c \in \{A,C,G,T\}} f_{c,i} \log_2 \frac{f_{c,i}}{B_c}$$

For both species, the information content curves suggest that statistically significant patterns do exist in the peak regions surrounding the primary insertion sites, and the safest cutoff for the longest sequence pattern is from positions –7 to +7. It should be noted that, information content is computed on 100 bases from the 5' flanking region and the TSD sequences of varied lengths because we are mainly interested in the primary insertion site in this study.

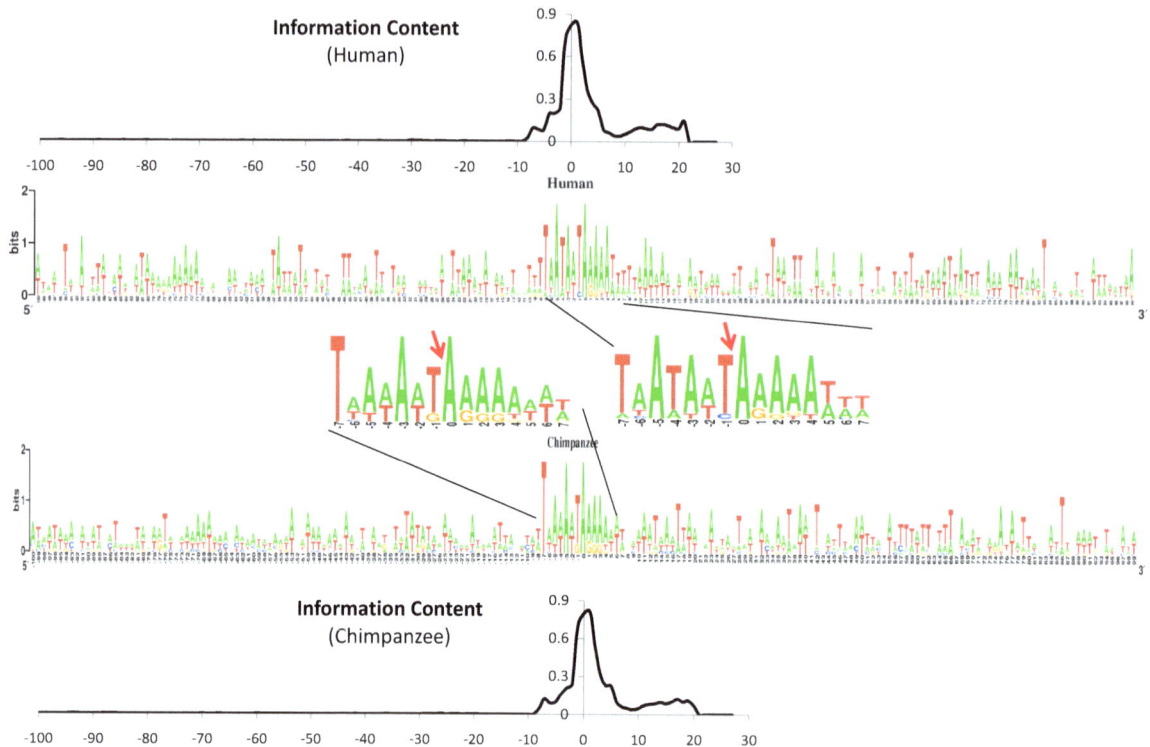

**Figure 6:** Human and Chimpanzee: 200nt predicted profiles and statistically significant patterns identified via information content (arrows indicate primary Alu insertion site).

As highlighted in Figure 6, the two discovered consecutive sequences are highly similar, and the super pattern of both can be generalized as 5' [T|A][A|T|C][A|T][T|A][A|T][A|T][T|G|C][A|A|G][A|G] [A|G|T][A|T|G][T|A|G][T|A|C][T|A|G] with the nucleotides at each position listed from most to least frequent. We underline the sequence in the 3' end to distinguish it from the 5' side. It is evident that the likelihood of the third base prediction at a particular position is essentially quite trivial, whereby dropping it won't damage the mined knowledge much. Thus we have a simplified pattern shown as follows: [T|A][A|T] [A|T][T|A][A|T][A|T][T|G][A][A|G][A|G][A|G][A|T][T|A][T|A][T|A]. Compared to the original search space, we already cut it more than half. The above sequence obviously comprises the reported primary candidates for the nick site (Jurka, 1997), e.g. 5' TTAAAA, which is between –2 and +3. At the same time, more than one nucleotide prediction at most positions also suggests that alternative patterns very likely exist around the insertion site. Moreover, guanine is rather frequent between positions –1 and +3, and its frequency gradually decreases as the pattern extends towards 3' end. Cytosine is seldom observed in the studied region, and most scattered low occurrence is often beyond positions –5 and +5. In addition, the nucleotide profiles of the predicted sequences are obviously A+T-rich, which demonstrate that Alu has a strong bias for insertion into A+T-rich endonuclease target sites. This is consistent with the observations for genomic Alu insertions (Jurka, 1997; Boissinot *et al.*, 2000).

### 3.2.4  Pattern Verification via Algorithm Comparison

"Pattern Growth" (Ye *et al.,* 2007) is one of the state-of-the-art algorithms developed for protein databases without sequence alignment. It essentially employs the principles of pattern growth as PrefixSpan (Pei *et al.*, 2001). To verify that the subsets of the simplified super-pattern identified by MBT are also ranked highly by "Pattern Growth" in terms of relative frequency, we implement the DNA version of this algorithm "DNAPG" by revising the original code. Two experiments are conducted in this study, each focusing on the frequent pattern verification with the majority of bases obtained preceding or following the insertion site. Figure 4(c) illustrates the experimental procedures of sequence acquisition. Due to space limitations, we only report the detailed results of Exp. 1. For each set of sequences of the specific length $l$ ($6 \leq l \leq 10$), DNAPG is trained to discover the consecutive patterns containing the same number of bases. By doing this, we in fact considerably reduce the search space of DNAPG at least by $4^{190}$, and we denote this DNAPG as "Shrunk DNAPG (SDNAPG)". To mine all of such position-specific patterns without any prior knowledge, we have to set the absolute *min_sup* of SDNAPG to be 1. That is, an *l-mer* ($6 \leq l \leq 10$) pattern will be enumerated by SDNAPG as long as it occurs in at least one sequence of length $l$. On the other hand, *l-mer* patterns discovered by MBT are obtained via direct regular expression matching using the superpattern of length $l$. Typically, for MBT, the super pattern used in Exp. 1 guiding the search is 5' [A|T][T|G][A] [A|G][A|G][A|G][A|T][T|A][T|A][T|A].

Figure 7(a) summarizes the number of patterns of varied lengths discovered by SDNAPG and MBT on each species and common to both. On average, the number of patterns identified by MBT is 37.5% of the patterns enumerated by SDNAPG regardless of the pattern composition. Compared to SDNAPG, MBT significantly reduces the cognitive domain from which insightful knowledge could be derived and interpreted by the biologists.

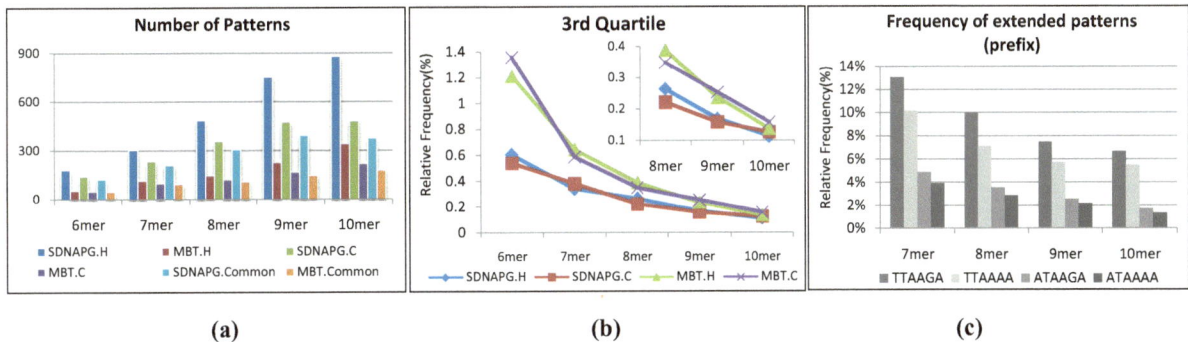

(a)                                          (b)                                          (c)

**Figure 7:** (a). MBT vs SDNAPG: comparison of number of discovered patterns (b). MBT vs SDNAPG: comparison of pattern rankings. (c). Prefix study: frequency of extended patterns

Using the patterns common to both species, we also studied the quality of mined patterns by looking into the distribution of the patterns' relative frequency. The box plots of the relative frequency of the different patterns mined by two algorithms are presented in Figure 8. For each set of the specific composition, the

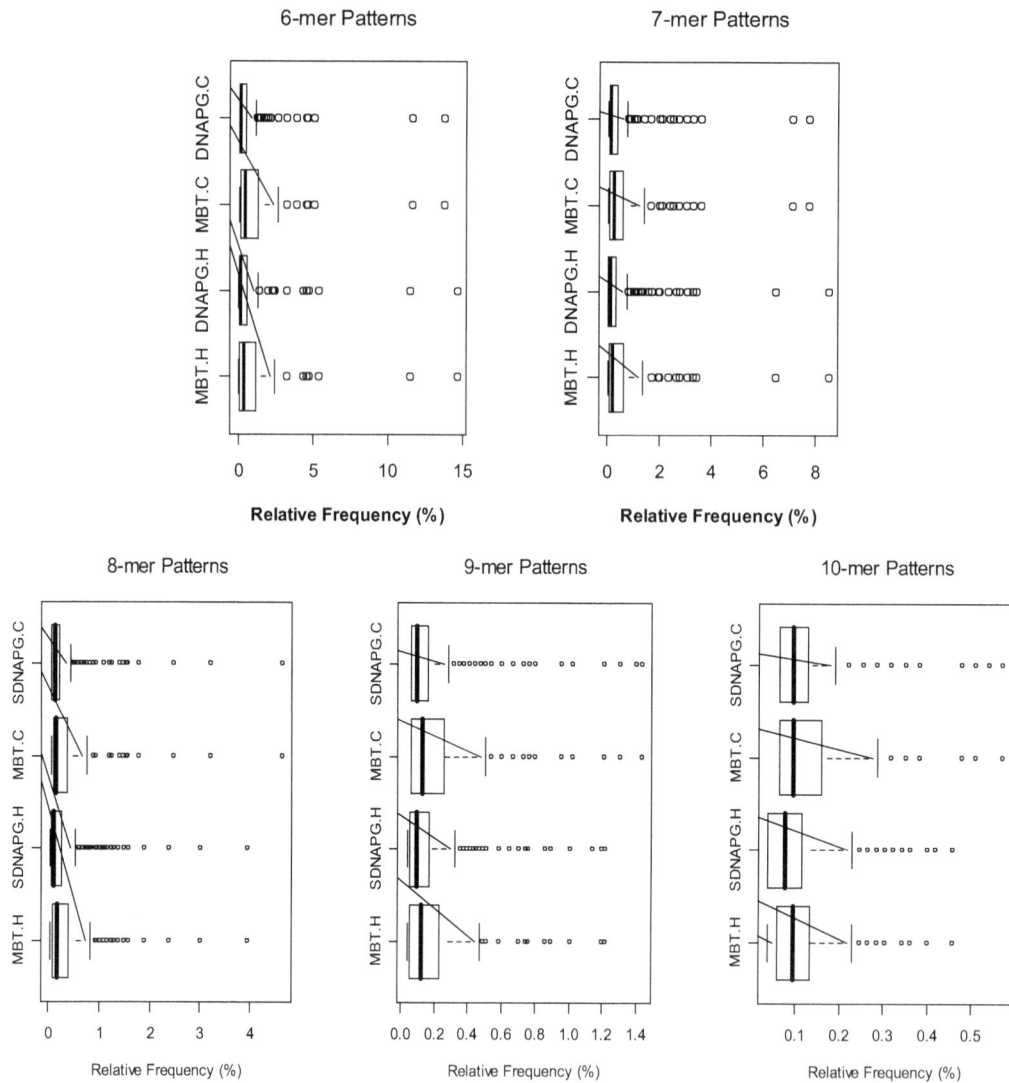

**Figure 8:** MBT vs SDNAPG: distributions of mined patterns' relative frequencies

patterns discovered by MBT consistently demonstrate much higher relative frequency compared to those enumerated by SDNAPG. At the same time, the patterns of the highest relative frequencies, as shown as the "extreme" outliers in each plot, are always captured by MBT for both species. Because the distributions of the relative frequency are all rather skewed, the median and the 3rd quartile are essentially more reasonable statistical summaries than the mean. In particular, the non-parametric Wilcoxon rank test showed that the difference between the medians of the relative frequency distributions of patterns obtained from two algorithms on the same species is constantly statistically significant at 95% confidence level. In addition, as presented in Figure 7(b), on average over two species, the 3rd quartile of the relative frequencies of patterns selected by MBT is respectively 130%, 72%, 52%, 49% and 23% higher than that of SDNAPD as the patterns vary from 6mer to 10mer. A quartile study further reveals that, regardless of the pattern composition, the 75% quartile of the relative frequency of patterns selected by MBT corresponds to at least 83% quartile of the relative frequency of patterns generated by SDNAPG.

As another way to study the quality of mined patterns, we also compared the relative frequencies of 6mer patterns discovered by MBT to those 6mer patterns reported by Jurka (1997) around primary insertion sites associated with 400 sequences. It is worth noting that, 6mer patterns of MBT are mined from the same sequence region that Jurka used for consensus discovery, thus these two results are comparable. Figure 9(a) plots the relative frequencies of all of the 144 patterns reported by Jurka as well as those shared by MBT on the human and chimpanzee. Patterns in the plot are ranked by the relative frequencies of Jurka's patterns in the descending order. In general, the pattern size of MBT is around 33% of that of Jurka's, while the relative frequencies of patterns mined by MBT tend to be higher than those reported by Jurka, which can be observed from the box plot of Figure 9(b). A closer examination presented in the bar chart of Figure 9(b) further reveals that, most of the abundant patterns reported by Jurka are also ranked on the top by MBT, such as the signal consensus pattern TT<u>AAAA</u> and its variants TT<u>AAGA</u>, TT<u>AGAA</u>, TT<u>AAAG</u>, etc. They differ by only one base and share the same prefix character T.

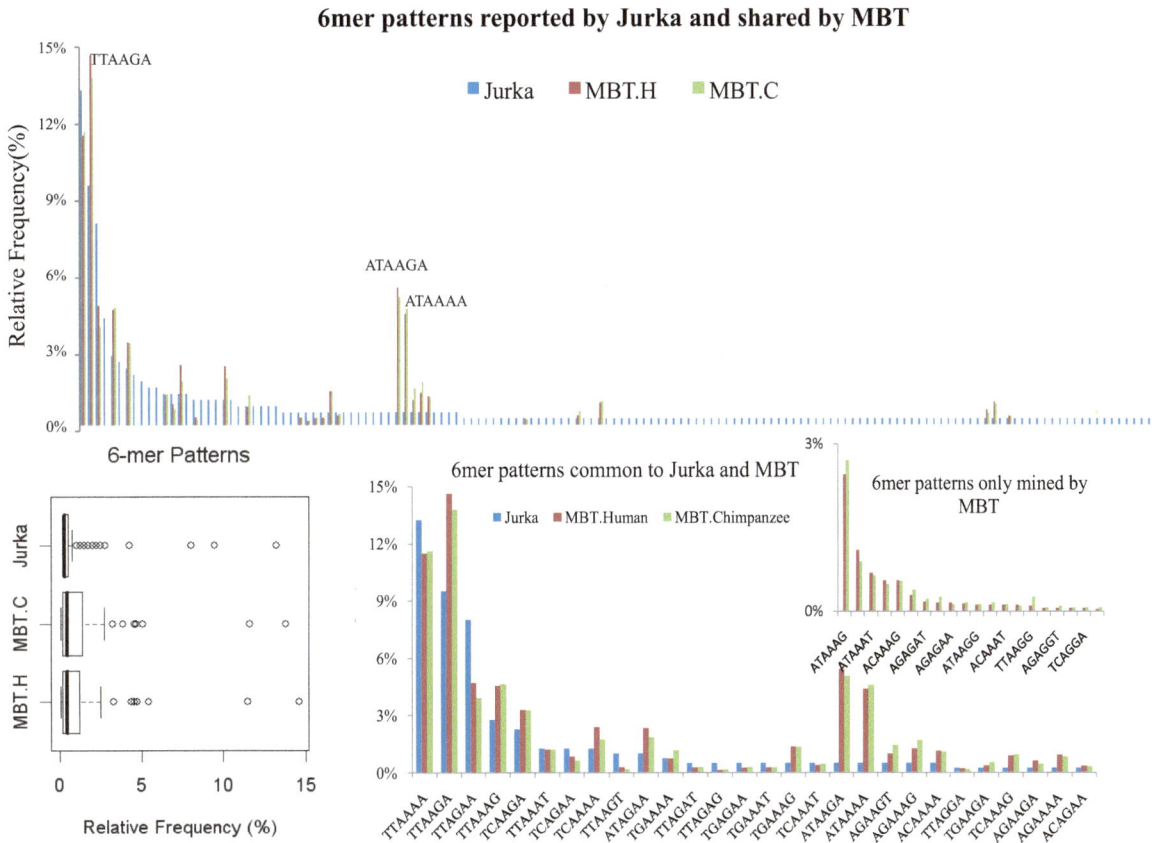

**Figure 9:** 6mer pattern comparison - MBT vs widely accepted in biology (Jurka's study)

In a total of 8400 human and chimpanzee sequences, they represent around 39.1% of the 6mer patterns discovered in the sequence region of 2 nts preceding and 4 nts following the insertion site. However, inconsistency in the patterns' ranking does exist between these two sets of results, and there are two most remarkable observations. First, the pattern of the highest frequency identified by MBT is TTAAGA, instead of TTAAAA, the most frequent pattern reported by Jurka. Among 8400 sequences, 14.3% contain TTAA-GA while TTAAAA is associated with 11.5% of sequences. Typically, the relative frequency of TTAAGA reported by Jurka is about 4.8% lower than ours, while the relative frequency of TTAAAA reported by Jurka is 1.7% higher. If TTAAGA could be another signal pattern, together with its variants of the common prefix T and one base mutation, they exist in 30.1% sequences used in our study. Second, ATAAGA and ATAAAA occur much more often in our sequences compared to Jurka's. If each of them is also treated as a signal sequence, along with its variants of the common prefix A and differing by one nucleotide, they respectively represent 17.1% and 11.6% of 6mer consensus patterns surrounding the insertion site, which are summarized in Table 3. Therefore, [T|A]TAA[G|A]A and its variants could be a more general consensus which accounts for about 62.4% of 6mer patterns in this region.

| Signal Patterns | Variants with the same prefix character (T or A) and one base mutation | Total Frequency |
|---|---|---|
| TTAAAA(11.5%) | TTAAGA, TTAGAA, TTAAAG, TCAAAA, TTAAAT, TGAAAA | 39.1% |
| TTAAGA(14.3%) | TTAAAA,TCAAGA, TGAAGA, TTAAGT, TTAGGA, TTAAGG, | 30.1% |
| ATAAAA(4.5%) | ATAAGA, ATAAAG, ATAGAA, ACAAAA, AGAAAA, ATAAAA | 17.1% |
| ATAAGA(5.3%) | ATAAGA, ATAAAA, ACAAGA, AGAAGA, ATAAGT, ATAAGG, | 11.6% |

**Table 3:** Refined consensus analysis – MBT vs widely-accepted in biology

Using each of the four 6mer patterns as the prefix, we also calculated the total frequency of the corresponding extended patterns. As presented in Figure 7(c), for each pattern category, the patterns with TTAA[G|A]A as the prefix constantly dominate patterns with other 6mer patterns as prefixes. In particular, the most frequent extended pattern would be TTAAGAATAA. The same experimental procedure is used in Exp. 2 to compare MBT with SDNAPG, and we obtain the similar results. A further suffix study shows that the most abundant extended patterns can be captured by $[T|A]T_3[T|A][T|A][T|G]A$ with $T_7A$ ranked highest. Therefore, if we can assemble both groups of patterns together, the longer pattern of the highest frequency would be $T_7AA[G|A]AATAA$, which largely reflects the site-preference shown by the L1 ORF2-encoded endonuclease that initiates the insertion process in the genome.

# 4   Conclusions

In this chapter, we respectively present a statistical method and a data mining solution to the analysis and characterization of Alu insertion sites in primate genomes, a problem of primary interest for the overall recognition of Alu biology and genetic basis of human diseases. By simply aligning 400 sequences around Alu insertion sites, biologists identified the preferred, immediate consensus at the position of Alu insertion. It is well known that these methods are computationally costly, and are not portable from one retrotransposable element to another if biological properties pertaining to a specific element are utilized in the solution. At the same time, little is known how the distribution of the 5'-TTAAAA motif influences the Alu density on the genome-wide scale, and whether any broader-scale patterns could exist that may also influence the insertion of Alu. Furthermore, there is no existing method that can issue the probabilistic certainty of a sequence being a target of Alu insertion.

Using a two-step regression analysis, we study the genome wide gene-level effect of 5'-TTAAAA motif density on Alu density. Our results show that the gene-level effect of the motif density on Alu density varied across chromosomes substantially in terms of statistical significance level. However, except for chromosome-7, all other chromosomes have the adjusted p-values less than 0.05 at least in one of the two proposed statistical models that evaluated the motif effects from different aspects. The (pseudo) contribution rates to the total variability are lower than 11%, in general. One exception occurred in chromosome-Y where the Alu distribution holds special importance in studying the evolution of genome. For this chromosome, the pseudo contribution rate is as high as 33% in Model-1 where the binary dependent variable indicates if a gene contains at least one Alu in its intron region(s). A possible explanation for this exception is that the redistribution of Alus on this sex chromosome was relatively delayed due to the lack of recombination between chromosome pairs (Medstrand *et al.*, 2002); therefore, the initial association between the motif and Alus has been largely retained. Here, one may be puzzled that the adjusted p-value calculated from Model-2 (indicating the gene-level effect of 5'-TTAAAA motif on intron Alu density) for chromosome Y is larger than 0.05. While the reason is still not clear, we tend to attribute the inconsistence to the fact that, in our dataset, chromosome-Y has only 29 genes containing Alus and thus the Model-2 lacks power to detect the Alu-motif association for this chromosome.

On the other hand, from the data mining perspective, we introduce a divide-conquer and aggregate based framework to efficiently characterize the broader-scale patterns of Alu insertion site in a unified process. In this framework, the core is an improved frequent pattern classification algorithm coupled with two task-oriented modules for position reserved sequence mapping and target pattern aggregation. Algorithmically, this is the first probabilistic generative model developed for this issue. The concept of two-mode dynamic support, scalability and time complexity analyses are also provided for the proposed approach. Using 8400 PAI sequences collected from the primate genomes, rather exhaustive classification study, large-scale insertion site characterization as well as pattern verification via algorithm comparison, we have demonstrated that: (1) Inductive learning can be a method of choice for insertions site prediction of retrotransposable elements. In particular, (2) Both the predictive precision and recall on the target PAI sequences are over 90.5%; (3) Compared to the two benchmark approaches, "Pattern Growth" algorithm (Ye *et al.*, 2007) and the study has been widely accepted in biology (Jurka, 1997), the proposed method is able to discover much more compact yet highly ranked patterns; (4) Most importantly, the obtained 200nt predictive profile around the Alu insertion not only contains the widely accepted signal consensus, but also suggests a longer pattern $(T)_7AA[G|A]AATAA$ which indicates a broader surface of preferred binding sites of the L1 ORF2-encoded endonuclease. This is significant and important for biology studies.

For data mining research, we have shown that in general, (1) Discriminative patterns are good candidates not only for classification but general pattern approximation as the data is not in the pre-defined feature vectors. (2) When compact yet predictive pattern discovery suffers from the intractable computation barrier, the proposed divide-conquer and aggregate based MBT can provide a common framework for similar sequential or structural pattern discovery problems, such as other biological sequence pattern mining, intrusion detection and system management. More sophisticated sequence or structure mapping and reversed mapping techniques could be employed to achieve better performance. Studies of the second nick site of Alu on the other strand, as well as applying the proposed method to other retrotransposable elements are also on our agenda.

## Acknowledgments

This study was supported by National Institutes of Health grants (NIMHD-RCMI 8G12MD007595-04, NIGMS P20GM103424), an US Department of Army grant (W911NF-12-1-0066), an NSF grant (EPS-1006891), a Louisiana BOR award (LEQSF(2008-11)-RD-A-32), and the funding from the Louisiana Cancer Research Consortium.

## References

Belancio, V., Hedges, D. and Deininger, P. (2008) 'Mammalian non-LTR retrotransposons: For better or worse, in sickness and in health', Genome Research. Vol. 18, pp. 343-358.

Benjamini Y, Hochberg, Y. (1995) ' Controlling the false discover rate – A practical and powerful approach to multiple testing'. J ROY STAT SOC B MET 1995, 75:289-300.

Boissinot, S., Chevret, P. and Furano, A. (2000) 'L1 (LINE-1) retrotransposon evolution and amplification in recent human history'. Mol Biol Evol, Vol. 17, pp. 915–928.

Cheng, H., Yan X., Han, J. and Yu, P. (2008) 'Direct discriminative pattern mining for effective classification'. Proceedings of the 2008 IEEE 24th International Conference on Data Engineering, pp. 169-178.

Cheng, H., Yan, X., Han, J. and Hsu, C. (2007) 'Discriminative frequent pattern analysis for effective classification'. Proceedings of the 2007 IEEE 23rd International Conference on Data Engineering, pp. 716-725.

Crooks, GE., Hon, G., Chandonia, JM. and Brenner, SE.(2004) 'WebLogo: A sequence logo generator', Genome Research, Vol.14, pp. 1188-1190.

Deininger P. and Batzer M.(1999), 'Alu repeats and human disease'. Mol. Genet. Metab. Vol. 67, pp.183–193.

Deshpande, M., Kuramochi, M., Wale, N. and Karypis G. (2005) 'Frequent substructure-based approaches for classifying chemical compounds'. IEEE Trans. Knowledge & Data Eng.,Vol. 17, No. 8, pp. 1036–1050.

Fan, W., Zhang, K., Cheng, H., Gao, J., Yan, X., Han, J., Yu, P.S. and Verscheure, O. (2008), 'Direct Mining of Discriminative and Essential Graphical and Itemset Features via Model based Search Tree', Proceedings of the 14th ACM SIGKDD International Conference on Knowledge Discovery and Data Mining, pp. 230-238.

Gentles, A., Kohany, O. and Jurka, J.(2005), 'Evolutionary diversity and potential recombinogenic role of integration targets of Non-LTR retrotransposons'. Mol Biol Evol. Vol. 22, No.10, pp.1983-1991.

Grahne, G and Zhu, J.(2003), 'Efficiently using prefix-trees in mining frequent itemsets', ICDM workshop on Frequent Itemset Mining Implementation.

Han, J., Cheng, H., Xin D. and Yan, X., (2007), 'Frequent pattern mining: current status and future directions', Data Mining and Knowledge Discovery, Vol. 15, No. 1, pp.55-86.

Jurka, J.(1997), Sequence patterns indicate an enzymatic involvement in integration of mammalian retroposons, Acad. Sci. USA. Vol. 94, pp. 1872–1877.

Kvikstad EM, Makova KD (2010) ' The (r)evolution of SINE versus LINE distributions in primate genomes: sex chromosomes are important'. Genome Research, 20(5):600-613.

Leung KS, Wong KC, Chan TM, Wong MH, Lee KH, Lau CK, Tsui SK (2010). 'Discovering protein-DNA binding sequence patterns using association rule mining'. Nucleic Acids Res., 38, 19:6324-37.

Medstrand P, van de Lagemaat LN, Mager DL(2002) 'Retroelement distributions in the human genome: variations associated with age and proximity to genes'. Genome Research, 12(10):1483-1495.

Nagelkerke NJD(1991) 'A note on a general definition of the coefficient of determination'. Biometrika (78):691-692.

Pei, J., Han, J., Mortazavi-Asl, B., Pinto, H., Chen, Q., Dayal, U. and Hsu, M.-C.(2001), 'PrefixSpan: Mining sequential patterns efficiently by prefix-projected pattern growth'. Proceedings of the 2001 IEEE International Conference on Data Engineering.

Rouchka, EC. and Hardin, CT.(2007), 'rMotifGen: random motif generator for DNA and protein sequences'. BMC Bioinformatics Vol. 8, pp. 292.

Schneider, TD., Stormo, GD., Gold, L. and Ehrenfeucht, A. (1986), 'Information content of binding sites on nucleotide sequences.', J. Mol. Biol. Vol.188, pp. 415-431.

Szak, S., Pickeral, O., Makalowski, W., Boguski, M., Landsman, D. and Boeke, J.(2002), 'Molecular archeology of L1 insertions in the human genome', Genome Biology, Vol. 3, No. 10.

Toda,Y., Saito, R. and Tomita, M.(1998), 'Comprehensive Sequence Analyses of 5' Flanking Regions of Primate Alu Elements', Genome Inform Ser Workshop Genome Inform. Vol. 9, pp. 41-48.

Watkins WS, Ricker CE, Bamshad MJ, Carroll ML, Nguyen SV, Batzer MA, Harpending HC, Rogers AR, Jorde LB (2001). 'Patterns of ancestral human diversity: an analysis of Alu-insertion and restriction-site polymorphisms'. Am. J. Hum. Genet., 68, 3:738-52.

Yan, X., Cheng, H., Han J. and Yu P. (2008), 'Mining significant graph patterns by leap search'. Proceedings of the 2008 ACM SIGMOD International Conference on Management of Data, pp. 433-444.

Ye, K., Kosters, W. and Ijzerman, A.(2007), 'An efficient, versatile and scalable pattern growth approach to mine frequent patterns in unaligned protein sequences', Bioinformatics, Vol. 23, No. 6, pp. 687-693.

# Identification of Coevolving Amino Acids using Mutual Information

Elin Teppa

*Bioinformatics Unit. Fundación Instituto Leloir*
*Buenos Aires, Argentina*

Diego Javier Zea

*Structural Bioinformatics Unit. Universidad Nacional de Quilmes*
*Buenos Aires, Argentina*

Cristina Marino Buslje

*Bioinformatics Unit. Fundación Instituto Leloir*
*Buenos Aires, Argentina*

# 1   Introduction

The information on important residues in proteins is a topic of concern and many experimental and computational approaches have been applied to tackle this problem.

Changes due to the mutations of amino acids at various points within a protein can be passed on to the next generation. These changes do not occur randomly, functionality and structure impose different constraints on different positions. Important amino acid positions are often conserved; however, mutational studies have shown that many non-conserved positions may also be functionally important. In particular, there may be compensatory mutations. Such is the case of a mutation in a certain point which then induces a coordinated mutation in other position(s) elsewhere within the protein. These coevolving mutations are of key interest since they identify residues that interact within the protein to carry out a particular function such as: catalytic reaction, structure stabilization, protein-protein and substrate interaction and allosteric regulation.

Multiple sequence alignments (MSAs) of homologous proteins carry at least two levels of such evolutionary information. The first level is given by the amino acid conservation at each position within the protein sequence and a second level of information is coded by the inter-relationship between two or more positions. While the first type of information is relatively straightforward to calculate and interpret, the second type is more complex. Mutations of essential residues in a protein sequence may occur, only if a compensatory mutation takes place elsewhere within the protein to preserve or restore activity (Martin *et al.*, 2005). The extent of the mutual coevolutionary relationship between two positions in a protein family can be estimated using mutual information (MI) from information theory (Cover & Thomas, 1991; Dunn *et al.*, 2005; Martin *et al.*, 2005; Tillier & Lui, 2003). As stated by DePristo *et al.*(DePristo *et al.*, 2005) (and other references therein), compensatory mutations are highly frequent and involve not only functional but also biophysical properties such as stability and tendency to aggregation. Figure 1 represents the different types of patterns in an MSA: conserved, variable and coevolved positions. Evolutionary variations in the sequences are constrained by a number of requirements, including the maintenance of favourable interactions in direct residue-residue contacts. This information contained in MSAs allows us to predict residue pairs which are likely to be close to each other in the three-dimensional structure.

The principal goal of this work is to summarise state of the art methods of studying coevolution between residues and their application in functionally important sites prediction.

In the last fifteen years a large number of methods have been developed to infer residue coevolution in proteins. In general, they start from a MSA of homologous protein wherein a coevolution score is calculated for each pair of positions. A review of existing scoring functions can be found in (Halperin *et al.*, 2006).

Some examples of these methods are the Statistical Coupling Analysis (SCA) which uses evolutionary data to measure coupling between positions on a MSA. In this approach, statistical coupling of two sites, $i$ and $j$, is defined as the degree to which amino acid frequencies at site $i$ change in response to a perturbation of frequencies at another site $j$ (Lockless & Ranganathan, 1999).

Another example is the CAPS method (Coevolution Analysis Using Protein Sequences) which compares the correlated variance of the evolutionary rate at two sites corrected by the time since the divergence of the protein sequences. The evolutionary variation at two sites is measured using time-corrected Blosum values for the transition between two amino acids at a particular site when comparing two particular sequences (Fares & McNally, 2006).

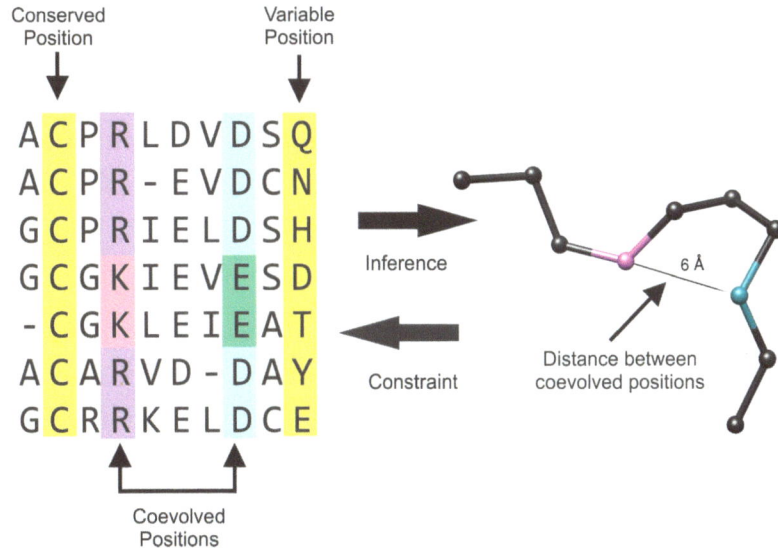

**Figure 1:** Representation of a multiple sequence alignment of homologous proteins (left) and the α-carbon structure of one protein of the alignment (right). Conserved and variable positions are highlighted in yellow. The positions that coevolved are highlighted in purple and light blue. The residues within these positions where change occurred are shown in pink and green. The arrows (middle) represent the interrelation of coevolution and structural information. This Figure is an adaptation of Figure 1 of (Marks *et al.*, 2011).

Also there are several methods based on Pearson's correlation coefficient (r) see equation 1 (Gobel *et al.*, 1994; Pazos *et al.*, 1997)

$$r_{ij} = \frac{1}{N^2} \sum_{k,l=1}^{N} \frac{(S_{i(k,l)} - \bar{S}_i)(S_{j(k,l)} - \bar{S}_j)}{\sigma_i \sigma_j} \; , \tag{1}$$

where N is the total number of sequences in the MSA, $S_{i(k,l)}$ is a weight for a substitution in the position $i$ between the sequences $k$ and $l$, $\bar{S}_i$ is the mean weight for substitution at position $i$ and $\sigma_i$ is the standard deviation of $S_{i(k,l)}$. The weight for residues substitution can be taken for the McLachlan similarity matrix in which substitution values are assigned on the basis of physicochemical properties of residues (McLachlan, 1971). For a discussion about the choice of the similarity matrix see (Di Lena *et al.*, 2011).

Other methods explicitly take into account the protein family's phylogenetic tree information to predict coevolving sites, as the continuous-time Markov process coevolutionary algorithm (Yeang & Haussler, 2007), LnLCorr (Pollock *et al.*, 1999) and CoMap (Dutheil *et al.*, 2005).

Caporaso and co-workers in a comparative study have shown that tree-ignorant like MI and Statistical Coupling Analysis methods detect coevolution with equivalent or better power than tree-aware methods (Caporaso *et al.*, 2008).In this article, we will only discuss the concepts and applications of MI.

## 1.1 Formal Definition of Mutual Information

Mutual Information is a measurement of uncertainty reduction for a MSA of homologous proteins. The MI between two positions (two columns in the MSA) reflects the extent to which knowing the amino acid at one position allows us to predict the amino acid identity at the other position. Intuitively, MI measures the information shared between two columns of the MSA ($x$ and $y$). For example, if $x$ and $y$ are independent, then information on $x$ does not give any information about $y$ and vice versa, so their MI is zero. On the other hand, the MI between two positions (or any two variables) attains it maximum value when they are fully correlated.

MI is a nonlinear statistic that measures the information between two random and discrete variables. Given that any two positions in a MSA can be considered random such as variables $x$ and $y$, the MI between them is given by the relationship shown in equation 2:

$$\mathrm{MI}_{x,y} = \sum_{a,b} P\left(a_x, b_y\right) \cdot \log\left(\frac{P\left(a_x, b_y\right)}{P\left(a_x\right) \cdot P\left(b_y\right)}\right) ,\qquad(2)$$

where $P(a_x, b_y)$ is the frequency of amino acid $a$ occurring at position $x$ and amino acid $b$ occurring at position $y$ in the same sequence, $P(a_x)$ is the frequency of amino acid $a$ at position $x$ and $P(b_y)$ is the frequency of amino acid $b$ at position $y$. The amino acid pair frequency $P(a, b)$ is calculated from $N(a_x, b_y)/N$. Where $N(a_x, b_y)$ is the number of times that an amino acid pair $(a, b)$ is observed at positions $x$ and $y$ and $N$ is the number of sequences in the MSA.

MI is thus a natural measure which makes it possible to identify sites of correlated and compensatory mutations in homologous proteins. Even though in principle the calculation of MI is simple, its interpretation has demonstrated to be very complex. Different approaches have been tested to overcome that difficulty and benefit from that information (Buslje *et al.*, 2009; Dunn, *et al.*,2008; Dutheil, 2012; Gloor *et al.*, 2005; Gouveia-Oliveira & Pedersen, 2007).

The application of MI to MSAs was first introduced by Korber *et al.* (1993) in order to identify covarying sites in viral peptides (Korber *et al.*, 1993). The approach was extended to measure coevolution by Giraud *et al* (1998) (Giraud *et al.*, 1998). However without the introduction of some correction factors, the MI yielded limited success (see below). Distinguishing phylogenetic correlations from functional correlations was a challenge in the methodology of coevolution detection and several methods have been suggested to correct such source of noise inherent to the MI calculation (Buslje *et al.*, 2009; Dunn *et al.*, 2008; Dutheil, 2011; Gouveia-Oliveira & Pedersen, 2007).

One of the problems faced when correlating MI values to the extent of coevolution lies in the fact that protein sequences are not independent, but have an inherent signal due to their evolutionary relationship. This has been clearly demonstrated in the work by Gouveia-Oliveira and Pedersen (2007) (Gouveia-Oliveira & Pedersen, 2007) where they show how sequences that are related through a tree-formed history can result in a covariance signal that resembles coevolution. In Figure 2, two independent events result in a set of sequences with mutual information between sites 1 and 2.

Most sites indeed segregate according to phylogeny, and are therefore hard to separate from true coevolving sites. One possible solution is to use highly divergent sequences in the alignment, in which case the phylogenetic signal is weak. However, it is best to construct methods that effectively counter this obstacle. Likewise, research shows that the degree of sequence conservation of each position strongly correlates to their estimated MI (Fodor & Aldrich, 2004; Martin *et al.*, 2005).

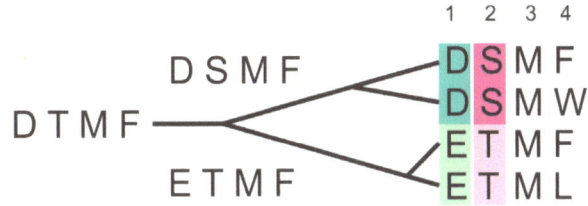

**Figure 2:** The phylogenetic signal mimics coevolution. Two independent mutation events can result in a set of sequences with mutual information. Sites 1 and 2 of this alignment show mutual information, although they did not coevolve. This Figure is based in Figure 1 from (Gouveia-Oliveira & Pedersen, 2007).

A number of different approaches have been proposed to lower the high background signal imposed by phylogeny and noise, thus enabling a more accurate identification of coevolving positions in protein sequences. A simple way to account for shared ancestry is to measure the extent of correlation that would be expected solely due to phylogeny and stochasticity. This is achieved by randomization (also known as bootstrap) procedures, which remove any functional correlation and therefore allow the user to get an empirical null distribution estimation of the correlation statistics. Methods vary according to the type of bootstrap procedure used. Dutheil (2011) gives a list of several existing methods, categorized according to their handling of various correlation sources.

Two examples of corrections to overcome the problems due to common phylogenetic origin and the inherent entropy of each column are the row column weighting (*RCW*) (Gouveia-Oliveira & Pedersen, 2007) and the average product correction (*APC*) (Dunn *et al.*, 2008). The *RCW* method divides all MI values by the average MI value of the two residues, as shown in equation 3.

$$RCW = \frac{MI_{xy}}{(MI_{x\bullet} \cdot MI_{\bullet y}) \div 2} \, , \tag{3}$$

where $MI_{xy}$ is the MI between residues $x$ and $y$, $MI_{x\bullet}$ is the average of the MI value of residue $x$ to all other residues in the MSA and similarly $MI_{\bullet y}$ is the average of the MI value of residue $y$ to all other residues in the MSA.

The APC method defines a term (APC) and subtracts this value from MI giving a corrected MI ($MI_{apc}$) (equation 4 and 5):

$$MI_{apc} = MI_{xy} - APC_{x,y} \, , \tag{4}$$

$$APC_{x,y} = \frac{MI_{x\bullet} \cdot MI_{\bullet y}}{\overline{\overline{MI_{\bullet\bullet}}}} \, , \tag{5}$$

where $MI_{x\bullet}$ is the average MI value of residue $x$ to all other residues in the *MSA* (similarly $MI_{\bullet y}$), and $\overline{\overline{MI_{\bullet\bullet}}}$ is the average MI value over all pairs of residues in the MSA.

Similarly, when dealing with biological data, MSAs will often suffer from a high degree of unnatural sequence bias and redundancy, as a result of multiple-strain sequencing and biased selection of sequenced species. It was therefore expected that the sequence clustering would improve the accuracy of the MI calculation. In (Buslje *et al.*, 2009) is shown the use of a Hobohm 1 algorithm (Hobohm *et al.*, 1992) to define sequence clusters, and assign each sequence within a given cluster a weight corresponding to one divided by the number of sequences in the cluster. In this work clusters were defined at a sequence identity threshold of 62%.

It is also clear that for MSAs of limited size, a large fraction of the $P(a_x, b_y)$ values will be estimated from a very low number of observations, and their contribution to MI could be highly noisy. To deal with such low counts, we introduce a parameter $\lambda$. The initial value for the variable $N(a_x, b_y) = \lambda$ is set for all amino acid pairs. We tested a range of $\lambda$ values $0 - 0.2$ in steps of $0.01$. The maximal performance was achieved for a value of $\lambda$ equal to $0.05$, but similar results were obtained in the range $0.025 - 0.075$. That means that all possible amino acids pairs will be observed at least $0.05$ times ($\lambda$). Only for MSAs with a small number of sequences, where a large fraction of amino acid pairs remain unobserved, $\lambda$ will influence of the amino acids occupancy calculation. For large MSAs, most amino acid pairs will be observed at least once, and the influence of $\lambda$ will be minor. The optimization values for the identity threshold for clustering, as well as $\lambda$ and the comparative performance of different methods including those parameters are described in (Buslje *et al.*, 2009). At last, to make the MI value comparable between families, we applied a $Z$-score transformation. The $Z$-score is then calculated as the number of standard deviations that the observed MI value falls above the mean value obtained from the randomized MSAs.

Hereinafter, whenever MI is cited we are referring to the $Z$-score MI corrected by APC, clustering and low count.

An additional obstacle in coevolution detection is the lack of a benchmark based on real data to test these methods, as we never have had access to the real coevolutionary history of biological data sets. True coevolving pairs are never known, and one has to rely on alternative information sources to label a given pair as truly coevolving or not. As an approximation, it is assumed that all residue pairs in contact (i.e. with a C$\beta$ distance $<8$ Å) are coevolving (Buslje *et al.*, 2009; Choi *et al.*, 2005; Gouveia-Oliveira & Pedersen, 2007; Korber *et al.*, 1993). This is obviously a flawed assumption since many sites that are in contact are non-coevolving and many sites that are coevolving are not necessarily in contact in the final folded structure of the protein. However, the vast majority of coevolving pairs are assumed to be in contact (Choi *et al.*, 2005), therefore this approach seems reasonable when carrying out a comparable study on the performance of different prediction methods. It should be noted that the actual predictive performance of the different methods would most likely be underestimated in such a benchmark.

To really test the performance in detecting coevolving residues (not contact residues) Gouveia-Oliveira and Pedersen (2007) have created a benchmark of *in-silico* generated data. In such a benchmark, they simulated alignments of protein sequences including coevolving pairs of sites. This dataset included MSAs with differing rates of evolution, different rates of pair coevolution, various numbers of taxa and different methods to simulate coevolution (Gouveia-Oliveira & Pedersen, 2007). The benchmark was carefully created to simulate variations that occur in biological data sets. Despite that, method testing with such an artificial data set is only a theoretical exercise, since it depends on a range of assumptions and an evolutionary model that may differ from the natural evolution of biological sequences.

## 1.2    Representations of the MI

The three most common ways of representing the MI between protein residues (Figure 3) are: i) as a contingency table (Figure 3 panel B), and graphically: ii) as a matrix (Figure 3 panel C), or iii) as a network where nodes are the residues and edges are the MI relationships (Figure 3 panel D). It can be observed that although the MI is calculated between a pair of residues, groups of residues that coevolve form a network. Figure 4 illustrates the coevolution network of Pfam (Finn *et al.*, 2008) family PF00890.

A) MSA

```
        1 2 3 4
Seq1    Q A P G
Seq2    C A P G
Seq3    D A P G
Seq4    E A P G
Seq5    F A P G
Seq6    G A P G
Seq7    H A L I
Seq8    I A L I
Seq9    K A L I
Seq10   L A L I
Seq11   M A Y S
Seq12   N A Y S
Seq13   P A Y S
Seq14   Q A Y S
Seq15   R A Y S
Seq16   S A Y S
```

B) Table

| Residues pair | MI score |
|:---:|:---:|
| [1][2] | 0.00 |
| [1][3] | 0.13 |
| [1][4] | 0.13 |
| [2][3] | 0.22 |
| [2][4] | 0.22 |
| [3][4] | 0.34 |

C) MI matrix

|   | 2 | 3 | 4 |
|---|---|---|---|
| 1 |   |   |   |
| 2 |   |   |   |
| 3 |   |   |   |
| 4 |   |   |   |

D) MI network

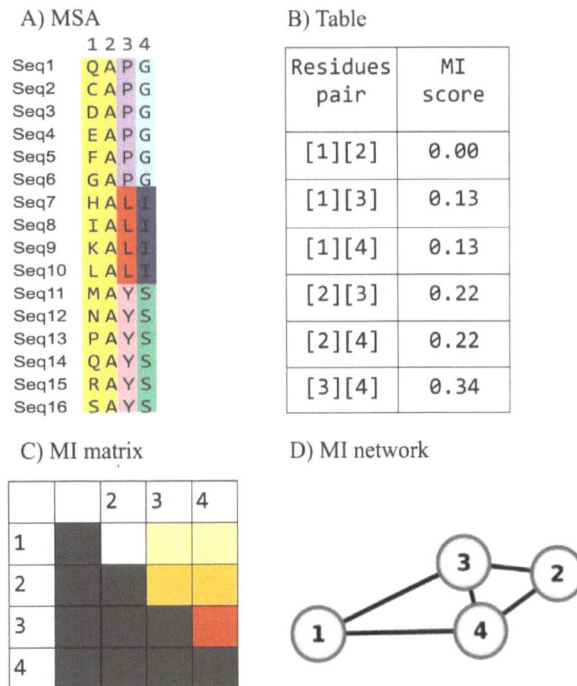

**Figure 3:** MI representations A) MSA representation, B) contingency table; C) MI matrix coloured according to the MI′s strength from white to red (lower to higher) and D) MI network nodes represent the alignment position. Edges are weighted upon MI value (shorter distance means larger MI value).

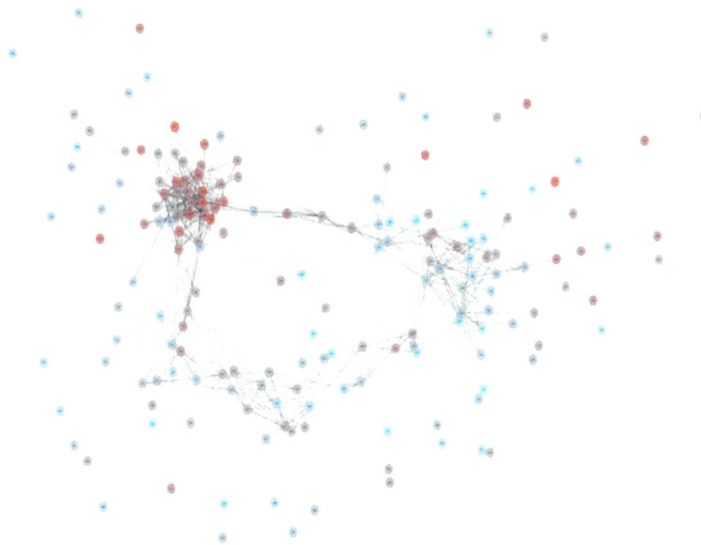

**Figure 4:** MI network of protein family PF00890. Amino acids are represented as coloured circles from light blue to red upon conservation (from lower to higher). Edges are represented as lines binding nodes. Edge length is inversely proportional to the MI value (the closer they are to nodes, the higher their MI value will be)

In that representation, the nodes (positions in the MSA) are coloured according to the conservation of that position in the MSA.

## 2    Assessing the Performance of Prediction Models

The Receiver Operator Characteristic (ROC) curve is widely used to measure the predictive performance of methods in which the outcome is a dichotomous variable. The ROC curve is a representation of the sensitivity (True Positive Rate) as a function of 1- specificity (False Positive Rate) at different threshold settings. As shown on Figure 5, a perfect method should yield a ROC curve with a false positive rate (FPR) equal to 0 and a true positive rate (TPR) equal to 1 as one of its points, indicating the maximum sensitivity and specificity. In this kind of representation, a random predictor will follow a diagonal line. As real methods fall between these two curves, they can be compared using the area under the ROC curve (AUC). The closer the curve is to the (0,1) point, the higher the AUC will be and therefore the better the method. An AUC of 1 indicates a perfect method while an AUC of 0.5 indicates random outcomes. In natural sciences, it is usually more relevant to compute a partial AUC by restricting the comparison to the lower 10% false positive rates, giving rise to the AUC0.1 score. The final value is standardized to fall in the range between 0 and 1. Both the full AUC value and the value integrated for specificities from 1 to 0.9 (AUC0.1) are useful measures to capture the high specificity performance of different methods.

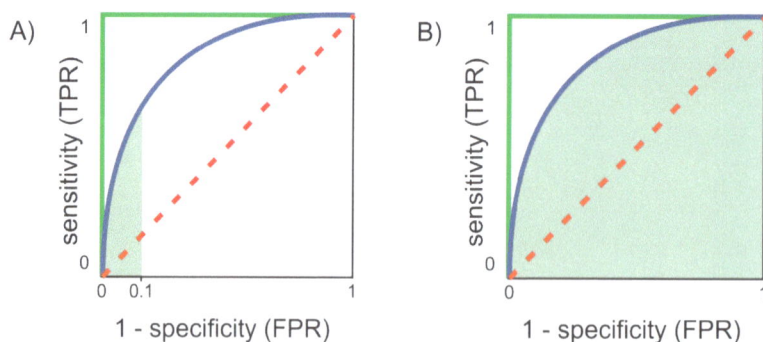

**Figure 5:** Receiver operating characteristic (ROC) curves. Red dashed line represents the ROC curve for a random guess. Green curve represents a perfect prediction method, were values for sensitivity and specificity are maximal. The blue curve represents an example of a real method of classification. The grey area under the curve represents the AUC. A) AUC0.1: Area under the ROC curve integrated up to a false positive rate of 0.1 (10% of FPR). B) The complete AUC.

## 3    MI improves the Prediction of Catalytic Residues

Identification of catalytic residues (CR) is essential for the characterization of enzyme function. Catalytic residues are in general conserved and located in the functional site of a protein in order to attain their function. However, many non-catalytic residues are highly conserved and not all CRs are conserved throughout a given protein family, making true CR identification a challenging task. The structural environment of an active site must be highly conserved in order to maintain its function during the course of evolution. This places strict limitations on the amino acid diversity in the proximity of an active site. Therefore, it seems plausible to hypothesise that catalytic residues would carry a particular signature defined by a network of close proximity residues with high mutual information and this signature can be applied to distinguish functional from other non-functional conserved residues.

A simple strategy to predict CR is based on homology, where annotated protein information is used to infer the CR of homologous protein, based on sequence and/or structure comparison. This approach is limited since it requires an annotated homolog of the target protein and more importantly, proteins with similar three-dimensional structures can carry out different functions and thus differ in the residues responsible for catalysis (Nagano *et al.*, 2002; Todd *et al.*, 2001).

Other approaches combine sequence, structure and evolutionary information to predict CR (Xin *et al.*, 2010). Also, Ota and co-workers (2003) incorporate a stability profile to the conservation and structural information (Ota *et al.*, 2003).

However, the most common way to identify functionally important sites is conservation. CRs are highly conserved and therefore, a natural measure for detection is their conservation score in a MSA. Capra and Singh (2007) (Capra & Singh, 2007) make a comparative analysis of several conservation methods and their performances in predicting CRs. They found that the best in performance is the Jensen-Shannon divergence score (JSD) (out of the 7 methods tested in that work). They also show that incorporating the conservation of neighboring positions into the score for a column (3 residues on either side of each column) improves the performance of all the tested method.

We also inspected how several conservation measurements could be used for the identification of catalytic residues (for details see (Marino Buslje *et al.*, 2010)) on a benchmark dataset based on the Catalytic Site Atlas (CSA) database (version 2.2.11, released August 2009) (Porter *et al.*, 2004). CSA provides catalytic site annotation for enzymes in the PDB. Catalytic residues are defined as those residues thought to be directly involved in some aspect of the reaction catalyzed by an enzyme. Our dataset is comprised of 434 protein families (each one containing at least one PDB entry), covering 8 SCOP classes, 199 folds, 249 super families and 389 families, which in turn included a total of 1212 CSA annotated catalytic residues. In our hands, the conservation method with the highest predictive performance in terms of AUC was the raw Kullback Leibler (KL) (Cover & Thomas, 1991) score with an average AUC value of 0.892 and an AUC0.1 value of 0.485.

We then sought to investigate if mutual information could contribute beyond sequence conservation to the identification of catalytic residues. Thus, a similar analysis was performed by using different measurements of mutual information, and finally the analysis was carried out using a combined measurement of conservation and mutual information.

We analysed the environment of a catalytic residue by means of the mutual information carried in the surrounding residues. MI gives a value for each pair of residues in a MSA. We searched for a mutual information score per residue that characterizes the extent of mutual information in its physical neighbourhood. First, we calculated a cumulative mutual information score (cMI) for each residue. The cMI is the sum of MI values above a certain threshold (fixed at 6 see (Buslje *et al.*, 2009)) for every amino acid pair where the particular residue appears as shown in equation 6. This value defines to what extent a given amino acid takes part in a mutual information network and is only sequence based (no structural information is needed) (see Figure 6 A).

$$cMI_x = \sum_{y, MI(x,y)>t} MI_{(x,y)} \tag{6}$$

Next, we defined a proximity score for each residue as the average of cMI of all the residues within a certain physical distance to the given amino acid (optimized at 7.5 Å, see (Marino Buslje et al., 2010)), as shown in equation 7.

$$pMI_x = \frac{1}{N} \cdot \sum_{y, dxy<t} cMI_{(x,y)} \tag{7}$$

where $N$ is total number of residues in the protein. Finally, we normalized the proximity average values for a given MSA so that they would fall within the range [0 – 1] to obtain the proximity MI (pMI) score (Figure 6 B). The distance between each pair of residues in the structure was calculated as the shortest distance between any two heavy atoms belonging to each of the two residues.

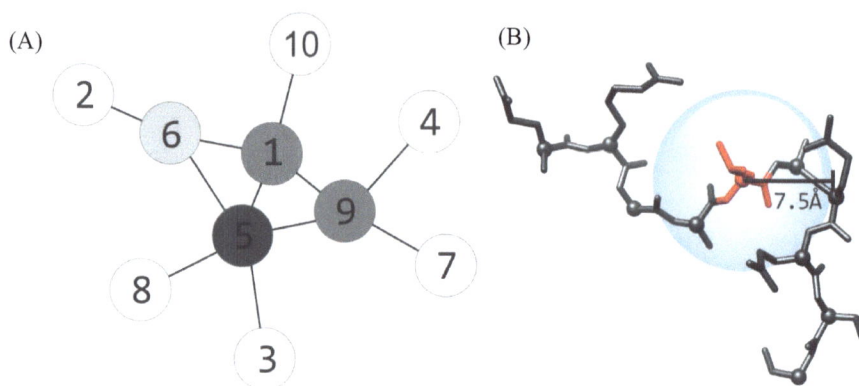

**Figure 6**: Representation of the cMI (A) and pMI (B). (A) Each node represents a residue coloured upon cMI value (calculated as the sum of MI above a 6.0) from dark gray (higher) to white (lower). Edges between nodes indicate that they have a MI value above the threshold. (B) pMI is the average of the cMI of residues closer than 7.5Å.

We noticed that residues in close proximity with CR tend to have high cMI scores. Furthermore, when measuring the pMI, which tells us about the networks of mutual information in the proximity of a residue (within a certain distance threshold) the catalytic residues were observed to have higher pMI than other conserved residues. We exploited this observation in the dataset of 434 protein families described above.

Using a 7.5 Å cut-off distance to define the structural proximity, and a MI threshold of 6.0 to define reliable mutual information interactions (see (Marino Buslje et al., 2010)), the average predictive performance of the pMI measurement in terms of the average AUC and AUC0.1 values on the 434 Pfam entries was 0.843 and 0.342 respectively. In both cases is significantly different from random ($p <$ 0.0001, binomial test excluding ties). As the number of proximity interactions is used to normalize the pMI measurement, this predictive performance does not stem from any implicit bias in the data imposed by catalytic residues in a particular state of solvent exposure.

Similarly, as the active site in most cases is defined in terms of multiple catalytic residues in close proximity, it is natural to suggest that a proximity score based on sequence conservation would also be a strong catalytic residue predictor. Using the same distance cut-off as for the mutual information proximity score, we found that the proximity conservation score, pC, achieved an average predictive performance of 0.854 and 0.379 in terms of AUC and AUC0.1. These values are greater than what was obtained using the pMI score, but not statistically significant (p > 0.05, binomial test excluding ties).

We thus applied a combined catalytic likeliness score (Cls) to identify catalytic residues. The Cls is calculated as a weighted sum of the KL conservation, the pMI and the pC scores (equation 8).

$$\text{Cls} = \left(1 - w_{MI} - w_C\right) \cdot Kl + w_{MI} \cdot \text{pMI} + w_C \cdot p_C \tag{8}$$

Here, pC is the average conservation score of residues within a given proximity distance, while $w_C$, and $w_{MI}$ are adjustable relative weights.

The calculation of the combined catalytic likeliness score depends on three parameters: $Z_{thr}$ (MI Z-score threshold for including an amino acid pair in the cMI score), $D_{MI}$ (distance threshold to include an amino acid in the pMI average score), $D_C$ (distance threshold to include an amino acid in the pC average score), and the relative weights, $w_{MI}$ and $w_C$, on pMI and pC, respectively. These parameters were estimated using five-fold cross validation. The optimal values were obtained using brute force grid-sampling on 4/5 of the data set to optimize the average AUC value and the remaining 1/5 of the data was evaluated next using this set of optimal parameters. This procedure was repeated five times leading to five sets of optimal parameters and evaluation performance values for each MSA in the data set.

The performance of the Cls score to detect catalytic residues was 0.927 and 0.594 (AUC and AUC0.1, respectively) with the optimal set of parameters: $Z_{thr} = 5.5 \pm 0.2$, $D_{MI} = 8.0 \pm 0.1$, $D_C = 5.6 \pm 0.5$, $w_{MI} = 0.6 \pm 0.0$, and $w_C = 0.2 \pm 0.0$. The low standard deviation value on each parameter-estimate indicates that the parameter optimization is robust across the different cross-validation data sets. This performance is significantly higher than the KL conservation, as well as the pMI and the pC individual scoring functions ($p > 0.001$ in all cases using binomial test excluding ties).

In Figure 7 we display the results of the four prediction measurements, KL, pMI, pC and Cls for the identification of the catalytic residues in the Pfam family PF00890 represented on the fumarate reductase of *Shewanella putrefaciens* MR-1 (PDB entry 1D4C). The function of fumarate reductase is carried out by the active site residues His364, Arg401, His503 and Arg544. It can be seen that the KL conservation score of the catalytic residues is relatively low (Figure 7A) while both the pC, and pMI scores are high in the catalytic residue proximity (Figure 7B and 7C). Comparing the Figures 7 B and C, it is evident that the two proximity measurements contribute different information to the combined (Cls) prediction score. Finally, the combined Cls is depicted in Figure 7D. The AUC values for the four prediction measurements shown in Figure 7 are 0.92, 0.94, 0.98 and 0.99 (KL, pC, pMI and Cls respectively). These values translate into a number of false positive predictions at 100% sensitivity (corresponding to the number of non-catalytic residues with a prediction score higher than the lowest score obtained by a CR) yield 47 (Figure 7A), 39 (Figure 7B), 15 (Figure 7C) and 4 (Figure 7D). These results highlight the strong predictive power of the Cls measurements in identifying catalytic residues and eliminating false positive predictions.

The gain in predictive performance for detecting catalytic residues is consistent for all families, independently on the catalytic residue's conservation level. However, the most dramatic gain in performance when including pMI is observed for families where the conservation of the catalytic residues is poor.

The catalytic environment of an active site needs to be conserved for a protein family to maintain its function, and one might speculate that when the conservation of a catalytic residue is weak, the catalytic environment is maintained by coevolution.

In conclusion, through these results we have demonstrated that networks of residues with high MI provide a distinct signature on CR. We propose that such a signature should be present in other classes of functional residues where the requirement to maintain a particular function places limitations on diversification of the structural environment throughout the course of evolution.

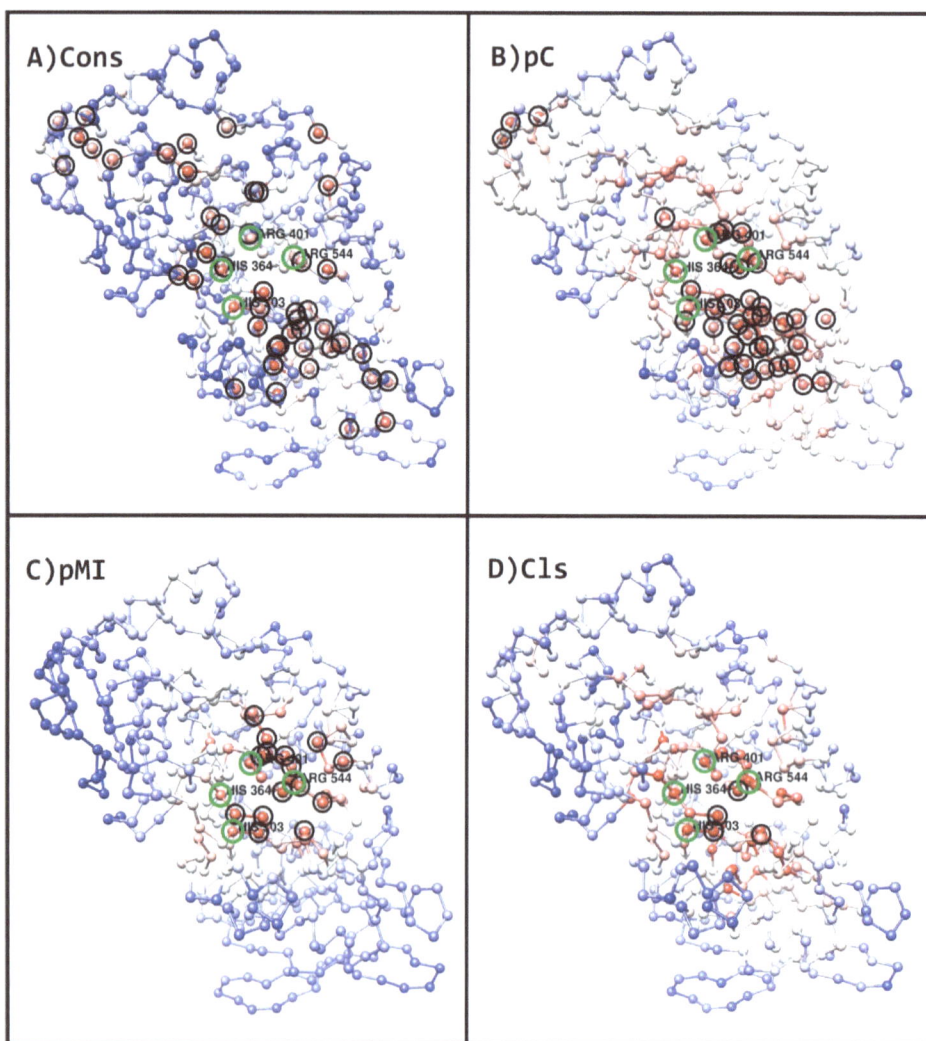

**Figure 7:** Identification of CR using four different prediction scores. Cα representation of the PDB entry 1D4C representing the Pfam PF00890 family. Catalytic residues are encircled in green. The four different prediction scores are shown A) KL Conservation, B) Proximity conservation (pC), C) proximity MI (pMI) and D) Catalytic likeliness score (Cls). The black circles are the predicted false positive residues: 47, 39, 15 and 4 respectively. The prediction scores are represented in blue and red (blue: lowest; red: highest). Molecular graphics images were produced with UCSF Chimera package. (University of California, San Francisco). Figure from (Marino Buslje *et al.*, 2010).

# 4   Mutual Information Network Properties

As it has been stated above, protein functions are maintained by concerted changes of a group of residues forced to coevolve. Studies have shown that protein folds have evolved under constraints imposed by function, so their structure is robust against random mutational events, yet extremely sensitive to perturbations at key positions (del Sol *et al.*, 2006). Likewise, functionally important residues undergo sequence variations as they evolve and form spatial clusters in the protein structure. Such clusters may be part of binding sites, catalytic sites or allosteric pathways (Venner *et al.*, 2010). Using sequence based analysis Halabi *et al.* (Halabi *et al.*, 2009), introduced the concept of groups of correlated amino acids that evolve quasi-independently, called *sectors*. Strikingly, those sectors were observed to be physically in contact in the 3D structure. In addition, the information within a protein must be transmitted, at least partly, between residues in physical contact, some of which are important in maintaining a short path in the distance network (Amitai *et al.*, 2004; del Sol *et al.*, 2006). Thus, it is reasonable to consider a protein as an undirected network of contacting residues. The process of decomposing protein structures into modules of densely-interconnected residues using this kind of network representations has been useful in explaining allosteric communication (del Sol *et al.*, 2007).

In this section we will show the results of analysing the mutual information networks between residues in a set of 172 families of enzymes and describe the relationship between coevolution and the 3D structure of the protein (Aguilar *et al.*, 2012). We selected those families (from the set of 434 enzymes families described above) because they contained more than 400 unique sequences/clusters (sequences with less than 62% identity). This condition was necessary to provide a reliable estimation of MI as shown in (Buslje *et al.*, 2009), so that we could be sure of the reliability of the observations taken from the MI network analysis.

## 4.1   Topological Properties of Mutual Information Networks and Distance Networks

Graph theory can be used to study proteins with vertices or *nodes* and a collection of *edges* that connect pairs of vertices. Some basic definitions applied here are: i) degree: the degree of a node in a network is the number of connections it has to other nodes and the degree distribution is the probability distribution of these degrees over the whole network, ii) clustering coefficient: it quantifies how well connected the neighbours of a vertex are in a graph, iii) modularity: it was designed to measure the strength of division of a network into modules (also called groups, clusters or communities). Networks with high modularity have dense connections between the nodes within modules but sparse connections between nodes in different modules (see Figure 8).

MI networks (MIN) were defined for each Pfam family as graphs G(N,E), where nodes (set N) were defined as positions in the MSA of a family (i.e. the columns of the MSA) and edges (set E) were defined between any pair of nodes with MI > 6 (Buslje *et al.*, 2009) (see Figure 4). Distance networks (DN) were defined for the reference protein of every Pfam family from the dataset as graphs G'(N',E'), where nodes (set N') are the residues (i.e. rcsiduc numbering) of the reference protein, and edges (set E') were defined between pairs of residues at a distance shorter than 5 Å. Figure 9 illustrates the distance network of the representative protein of Pfam family PF00890 (which MI network is depicted in Figure 4).

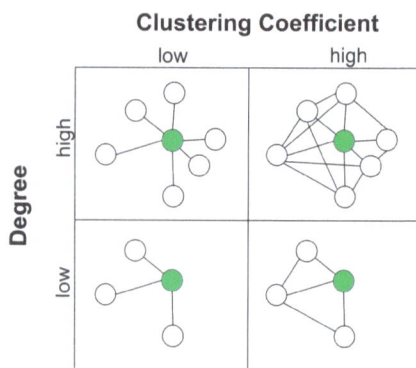

**Figure 8**: Representation of the clustering coefficient and degree. Networks have nodes with different values of degree and clustering coefficient.

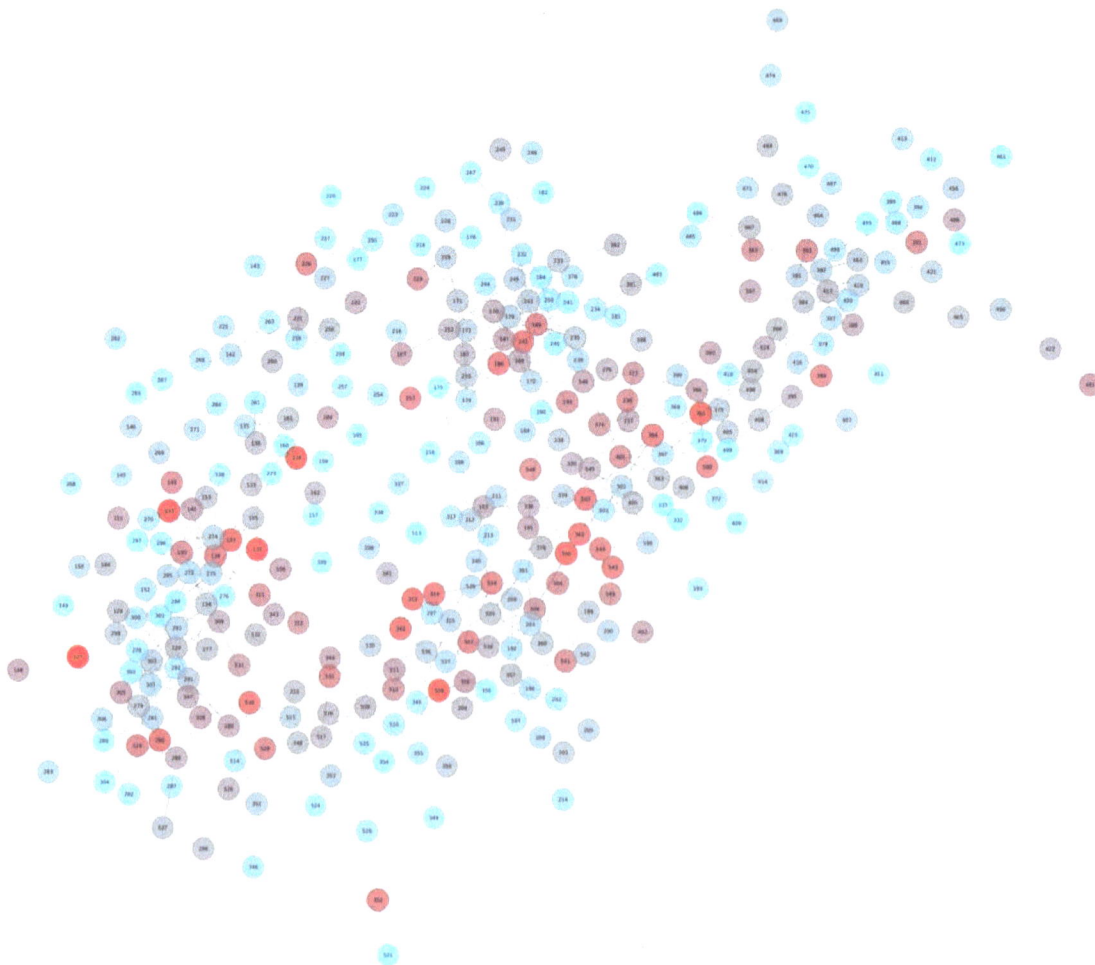

**Figure 9:** Distance network of protein PDB code 1D4C representing the Pfam family PF00890. As in Figure 4, amino acids are represented as circles coloured from light blue to red upon conservation (from lower to higher). Edges are represented as lines binding nodes closer than 5 Å.

We observed that the topological properties of MINs and DNs cannot be inferred from one another. The degree distribution of the DN of any protein structure follows a bell-like Poisson distribution as would be expected for a statistically homogeneous random model (Figure 10). This has been observed by other authors as well, and has been attributed to a restriction in the number of residues occupying a volume within the protein space (Amaral *et al.*, 2000; Atilgan *et al.*, 2004; Greene & Higman, 2003). On the other hand the distribution degree of the MINs displays a mixture of distributions ranging from fast-decaying power-law to Poissonian (Figure 10). Since coevolution demands some degree of physical proximity (Dunn *et al.*, 2008; Shackelford & Karplus, 2007), deviations from a purely scale-free architecture may be due to a limit in the possible number of neighbours that a node can have. Also, there are a number of biological factors influencing the ability of two residues to coevolve (e.g. their functional roles, their biochemical nature, their structural surroundings, etc.) which could possibly hinder the existence of a large number of simultaneously coevolving residues. This would prevent the existence of nodes with distinctly large numbers of neighbours in the MINs, thus truncating the characteristic long tails in power-law degree distributions.

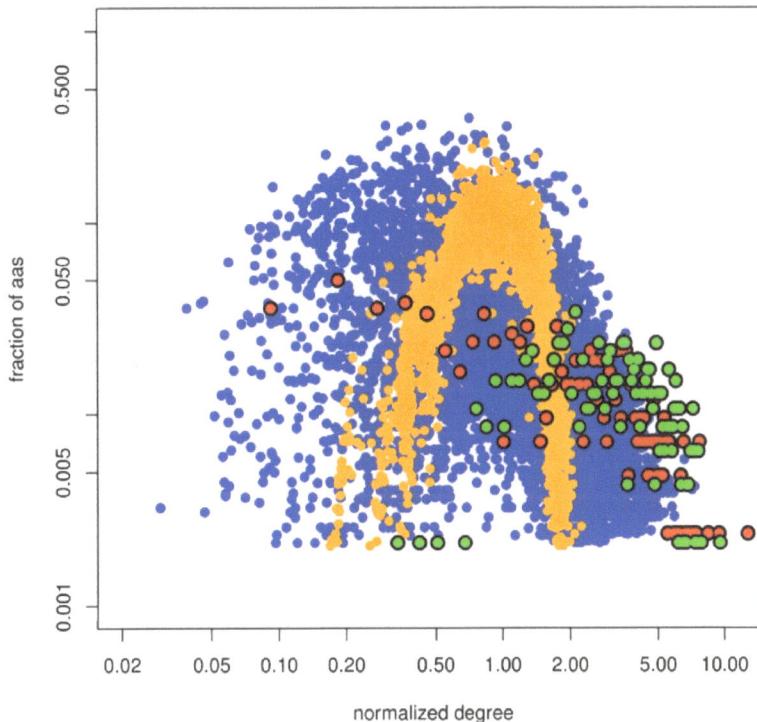

**Figure 10:** Degree distribution of the MIN and DN. Fraction of amino acids versus the normalized degree in MINs (blue dots) and DNs (orange dots). Degrees were normalized with respect to the average degree. All DNs followed a Poisson distribution ($\alpha = 0.01$, KS test). 43.8% of MINs followed a power-law distribution and 29.9% followed a Poisson distribution ($\alpha = 0.01$). Red dots: normalized degree distribution in the MIN for Pfam family PF01432, showing a truncated power-law distribution. Green dots: normalized degree distribution in the MIN for Pfam family PF00118. Logarithmic scale.

The clustering coefficient distribution of the MINs and DNs also shows differences. The mean values for the distributions are 0.365 for MINs, and 0.514 for DNs. This implies networks with very dense regions, which is in line with the observations of some other biological networks (Wagner & Fell, 2001). However, the dispersion of the clustering coefficient in MINs is significantly larger than in DNs ($p$-value $< 2.2 \times 10^{-16}$, KS test). This large dispersion is characteristic in modular architectures (Jeong et al., 2000). The modularity of MINs versus the homogeneity of DNs can be observed by comparing the MIN and DN of the same protein in Figures 4 and 9. This means that residues in MINs tend to form small clusters where all residues evolution influence one another, while there is very little evolutionary dependence between clusters. Finally, analysis of clustering coefficient and characteristic path length shows that MINs and DNs display a small-world structure (See: Aguilar *et al.* (2012) for a detailed description of these results).

## 4.2    Groups of Coevolving Residues (MI clusters) Mapped onto the 3D Structure

The above mentioned modularity of MINs allows us to partition them into clusters based on connectivity parameters. We used the MCL algorithm (Van Dongen, 2000) (which has been extensively used for biological network clustering) to identify clusters of co-evolving residues in MINs, hereinafter called *MI clusters*. These MI clusters contain groups of co-evolving residues, regardless of their distance in the 3D structure of the protein.

We investigated the spatial arrangement of MI clusters by mapping them onto the DN (i.e. onto the 3D structure of the reference protein). In other words, edges between two residues were defined if they had MI and if they were also connected in the DN (less than 5 Å apart). The resulting sub networks are hereinafter defined as *MI3D clusters*. Therefore, MI3D clusters contain groups of co-evolving residues which are close ($< 5$ Å) in the 3D structure of the protein.

About 80% of the MI clusters generate MI3D clusters once mapped onto the DN (clusters with less than four residues were not considered in our analysis). The number of MI3D clusters per Pfam family and their size distribution are shown in Figure 11. We determined that the number of MI and MI3D clusters per Pfam is around 12 (mean 11.97) and 10 (mean 10.47) respectively. These similar numbers show that MI clusters tend to stay as a unit when mapped onto the 3D structure.

Furthermore, about 75% of MI clusters are preserved as a single cluster and about 6% of the MI clusters split into two or more isolated MI3D clusters when mapped onto the structure of the protein. These results confirm that groups of co-evolving amino acids tend to be spatially close (Socolich *et al.*, 2005; Yeang & Haussler, 2007). Although previous studies have shown that co-evolution also occurs between non-contacting residues (Knaggs *et al.*, 2007; Kowarsch *et al.*, 2010), our results confirm that there is a link between co-evolution and physical contact. However, the fact that about 6% of MI clusters are broken into several isolated MI3D clusters can explain that a pair of residues can actually co-evolve even though they are not in physical contact. A common selective pressure in two separated areas of the protein could explain this observation (e.g. two interaction patches, allosterism, etc.).

We next identified the MI3D clusters which either contained a catalytic residue or were close to one (distance $< 5$ Å). We called those clusters *catalytic MI3D clusters*. We found that, on average, non-catalytic MI3D clusters are more than twice as frequent as catalytic MI3D clusters. This can be explained given the singularity of the catalytic site. Another noticeable feature is that, within a Pfam domain, catalytic MI3D clusters are, on average, 4-fold larger than non-catalytic ones (Aguilar *et al.*, 2012).

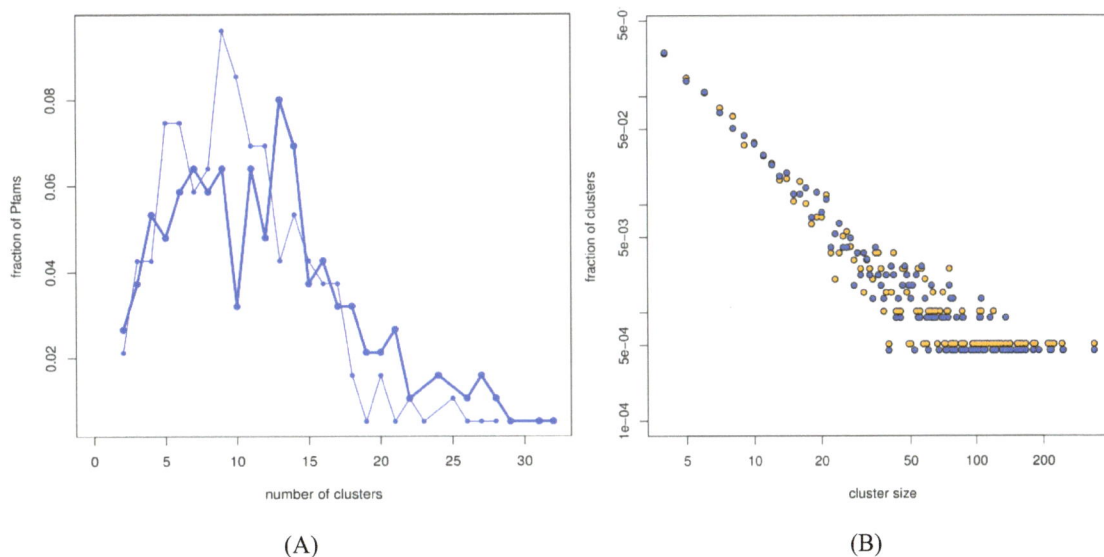

**Figure 11:** Number and size distribution of MI and MI3D clusters per Pfam family. **(A)** Distribution of the number of MI clusters and MI3D clusters: Thick line: distribution of the number of MI clusters (mean=11.97). Thin line: distribution of the number of MI3D clusters (mean=10.47). **(B)** Size distribution of MI and MI3D clusters. Blue dots: size distribution of MI clusters (mean=13.53; median=6). Orange dots: size distribution of MI3D clusters (mean=13.25; median=6).

Although the majority of MI clusters (72.9%) do not produce catalytic MI3D clusters (but produce non-catalytic MI3D clusters), it is worth noting that, when they do, they mostly produce only one (Figure 12). As expected, considering that they originate from different MI clusters, catalytic MI3D clusters within the same Pfam are less likely to co-evolve than at random.

Taking into account that there are, on average, more than 3 catalytic MI3D clusters per Pfam, this implies that catalytic MI3D clusters usually evolve independently despite their physical proximity. This suggests either an integrative process (which "connects" different parts of the protein to the catalytic site) or a fail-safe mechanism where mutual information connects functional residues, for instance, in the event of losing a catalytic MI3D cluster (e.g. due to a mutation).

Furthermore, we observed that a catalytic and a non-catalytic MI3D cluster can actually co-evolve, as 23% of the Pfam families with catalytic and non-catalytic MI3D clusters, at least one catalytic and one non-catalytic MI3D cluster were derived from the same MI cluster. This suggests the presence of catalytic subsites, i.e. positions that determine specificity or other necessary residues for the accomplishment of the catalysis (e.g., allosteric sites).

### 4.3    A protein can be Represented as a Network of MI3D Clusters

For each Pfam family, a network of MI3D clusters was defined as follows: each MI3D cluster is a node, and edges between pairs of nodes exist only if at least two residues (each from a different node) are closer than 5 Å. This network was named *MI3D cluster Network* (3DCN). A graphical representation of the 3DCN and structural mapping for Pfam domain PF00890 is shown in Figure 13.

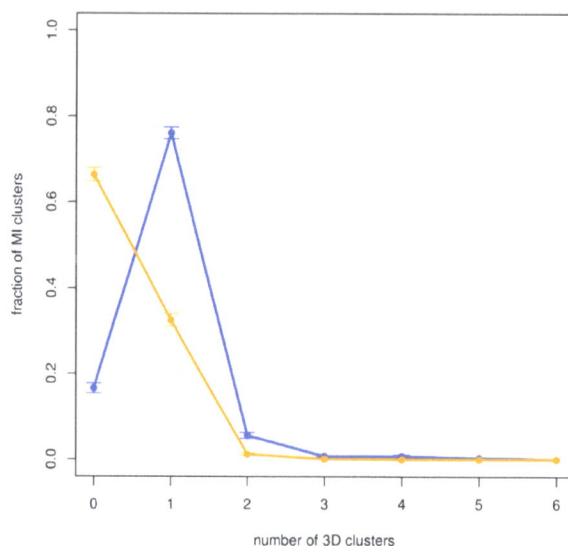

**Figure 12:** Distribution of the number of 3D clusters generated by mapping the MI cluster onto the 3D structure. Blue line: all MI3D clusters. Orange line: only catalytic MI3D clusters. 74.1% of MI clusters are preserved as a single MI3D cluster after mapping. 25.9% of MI clusters produce one catalytic MI3D cluster after mapping.

We then sought distinctive topological characteristics of the 3DCNs´nodes which could be used to identify catalytic clusters in the protein. Catalytic MI3D clusters have significantly higher degrees than non-catalytic ones. Furthermore, catalytic MI3D clusters have, on average, significantly higher values of betweenness centrality in the 3DCN than non-catalytic MI3D clusters (Figure 13). Those values are largely independent from the size of the 3DCN. This suggests a central role of catalytic MI3D clusters in the distribution of information from the catalytic site to the rest of the MI3D clusters.

With these results, we demonstrated that the size (see point 4.2), betweenness centrality and degree of MI3D clusters in the 3DCN could be used to predict catalytic MI3D clusters (Aguilar, *et al.*, 2012).

### 4.4    Prediction of Functional Sites Using MI

It is reasonable to expect important residues to be subject to co-evolutionary pressures. In agreement with the idea of using communities of correlated amino acids to uncover sets of residues defining functional characteristics in a protein family (Bleicher *et al.*, 2011), we investigated whether MI clusters were enriched in residues relevant to enzymatic activity, such as metal-binding residues and residues forming active sites. Our results indicate that the UniProt features ACT_SITE, BINDING, MUTAGEN and METAL are significantly over-represented in MI clusters (Aguilar *et al.*, 2012).

### 4.5    Prediction of Functional Sites Using MI and 3D Information

We then investigated whether MI3D clusters are also enriched in residues important for enzymatic activity. MI3D clusters were significantly enriched in residues with UniProt features ACT_SITE, BINDING, METAL and MUTAGEN as compared to MI clusters. For instance, the enrichment in metal-binding residues increases more than 2-fold in comparison to random expectation. This shows the advantage of combining mutual information with structural information.

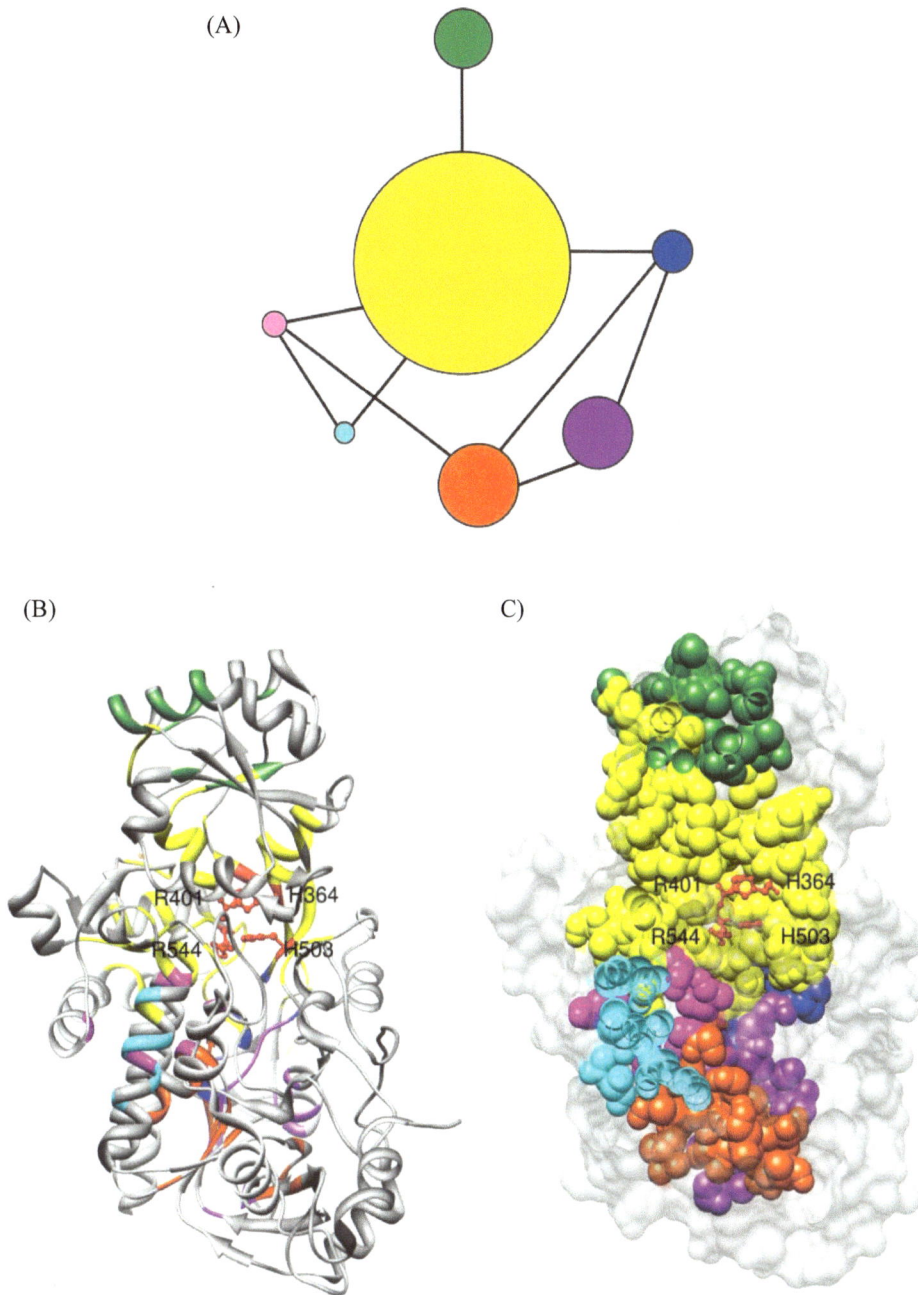

**Figure 13**: A network of MI3D clusters mapped onto the protein structure. 3DCN of the fumarate reductase (pdb code: 1D4C chain A, PF00890). Catalytic MI3D clusters: yellow. Non-catalytic MI3D clusters: magenta, blue, cyan, purple and orange. **(A)** The size of a node in the 3DCN is proportional to the number of residues in the MI3D cluster. **(B)** Ribbon representation of 1D4C. Colours are as in panel A. Catalytic residues are named and represented as red balls and sticks. **(C)** Surface representation of the view in panel B has been cut to show the interior clusters with residues represented as spheres.

Next, we focused on the functional enrichment in catalytic MI3D clusters, finding that UniProt features ACT_SITE, BINDING, METAL and MUTAGEN are significantly enhanced in such clusters. This result is expected for the ACT_SITE feature, but it might be potentially predictive for the other features. Also, the ACT_SITE feature is significantly under-represented in non-catalytic MI3D clusters (on average ten times less likely to occur than random chance) (Aguilar *et al.*, 2012).

In conclusion, in section 4 we have presented a study on the topology of mutual information networks and how that knowledge can be exploited to predict the location of different functional residues of enzymatic protein families. We observed that the combination of co-evolutionary and spatial information unveils a dense network of physically close co-evolving residues within the protein structure, which can be identified by clustering methods. The topological properties of these clustered structures suggest a role in increasing the tolerance to functional disruption and enhancing the adaptativeness of the protein. Also, network properties can be used to functionally characterize the clusters and exploit this information as a prediction tool by reducing the search space when looking for functional sites.

# 5    Online Resources for Coevolution Prediction and Visualization

We've collected a summarized list of servers to help predict and visualize coevolving residues. All of them are available online and free to use for academic purposes.

*Coevolution Analysis of Protein Residues* (Yip *et al.*, 2008). (http://coevolution.gersteinlab.org/coevolution/). It offers a comprehensive set of coevolution score functions including: correlation-based methods (Gobel *et al.*, 1994), statistical coupling analysis (Lockless & Ranganathan, 1999); explicit Likelihood of subset co-variation (Dekker *et al.*, 2004) and mutual information (as described in (Clarke, 1995)). It also provides MSA preprocessing options for improving signal detection, including sequence weighting, site pair filtering by sequence separation and correction for phylogenetic influence as suggested in (Martin *et al.*, 2005), as well as tools to analyze the results. If a 3D structure is available, it can be used to evaluate the effectiveness of the score function for inter-residue distance prediction and to create a scatterplot for coevolutionary scores against inter-residue distances.

*MatrixPlot 1.2* (Gorodkin *et al.*,1999) (http://www.cbs.dtu.dk/services/MatrixPlot/mutualProt/index.php) gives a mutual information matrix. It can be used either with nucleotides or protein alignments. The plot can combine the mutual information between all positions with other sequence information plotted along the edges of the matrix, e.g. contact between residues.

*InterMap3D* (Gouveia-Oliveira *et al.*, 2009) (http://www.cbs.dtu.dk/services/InterMap3D) predicts interacting residues by identifying coevolving pairs. The prediction can be done using one of three different methods: RCW MI, MI/Entropy, DEPENDENCY or by the intersection of the results of any of these.

*MI2Logo* (manuscript in preparation) (http://www.leloir.org.ar/MI2Logo) is a server that allows users to calculate and visualize the MI between residues in a MSA as described in (Buslje *et al.*, 2009). The output is displayed as an interactive MI network (with a cytoscape plug-in (Lopes *et al.*, 2010)) where each node corresponds to a column in the MSA and edges between nodes represent significant MI values. Several parameters can be set in order to calculate and present the data. For example if the structure of the protein is known, structural data can be displayed by adding the PDB numbering scheme to the nodes and distance information for edges. Also, node coloring can be set to match different attributes, such as conservation value, secondary structure, etc. Additionally, by clicking each node the relative frequency of different amino acids for this position is shown. Also, raw data can be downloaded for further user manipulation.

*CAPS* (Coevolution Analysis using Protein Sequences) (Fares & McNally, 2006) (http://bioinf. gen.tcd.ie/caps/) is a software that identifies intra or inter molecular coevolution. The software implements a method to detect intra-molecular coevolution as published in (Fares & Travers, 2006). For inter-molecular coevolution, the program requires two alignment files (one per protein), both containing the same number of sequences from the same taxa and in the same order as in the input files.

# References

Aguilar, D., Oliva, B., & Marino Buslje, C. (2012). Mapping the Mutual Information Network of Enzymatic Families in the Protein Structure to Unveil Functional Features. [doi:10.1371/journal.pone.0041430]. PLoS ONE, 7(7), e41430.

Amaral, L. A. N., Scala, A., Barthélémy, M., & Stanley, H. E. (2000). Classes of small-world networks. Proceedings of the National Academy of Sciences, 97(21), 11149-11152.

Amitai, G., Shemesh, A., Sitbon, E., Shklar, M., Netanely, D., Venger, I., et al. (2004). Network Analysis of Protein Structures Identifies Functional Residues. Journal of Molecular Biology, 344(4), 1135-1146.

Atilgan, A. R., Akan, P., & Baysal, C. (2004). Small-World Communication of Residues and Significance for Protein Dynamics. Biophysical Journal, 86(1), 85-91.

Bleicher, L., Lemke, N., & Garratt, R. C. (2011). Using Amino Acid Correlation and Community Detection Algorithms to Identify Functional Determinants in Protein Families. [doi:10.1371/journal.pone.0027786]. PLoS ONE, 6(12), e27786.

Buslje, C. M., Santos, J., Delfino, J. M., & Nielsen, M. (2009). Correction for phylogeny, small number of observations and data redundancy improves the identification of coevolving amino acid pairs using mutual information. Bioinformatics, 25(9), 1125-1131.

Caporaso, J. G., Smit, S., Easton, B., Hunter, L., Huttley, G., & Knight, R. (2008). Detecting coevolution without phylogenetic trees? Tree-ignorant metrics of coevolution perform as well as tree-aware metrics. BMC Evolutionary Biology, 8(1), 327.

Capra, J., & Singh, M. (2007). - Predicting functionally important residues from sequence conservation. Bioinformatics, 23(15), 1875-1882.

Choi, S., Weimin, L., & Bruce, T. (2005). - Robust signals of coevolution of interacting residues in mammalian proteomes identified by phylogeny-aided structural analysis. Nat Genet, 37(12), 1367-1371.

Clarke, N. D. (1995). Covariation of residues in the homeodomain sequence family. Protein Science, 4(11), 2269-2278.

Cover, T. M., & Thomas, J. A. (1991). Elements of information theory.

Dekker, J. P., Fodor, A., Aldrich, R. W., & Yellen, G. (2004). A perturbation-based method for calculating explicit likelihood of evolutionary co-variance in multiple sequence alignments. Bioinformatics, 20(10), 1565 - 1572.

del Sol, A., Arauzo-Bravo, M., Amoros, D., & Nussinov, R. (2007). Modular architecture of protein structures and allosteric communications: potential implications for signaling proteins and regulatory linkages. Genome Biology, 8(5), R92.

del Sol, A., Fujihashi, H., Amoros, D., & Nussinov, R. (2006). Residues crucial for maintaining short paths in network communication mediate signaling in proteins. Mol Syst Biol, 2.

DePristo, M. A., Weinreich, D. M., & Hartl, D. L. (2005). Missense meanderings in sequence space: a biophysical view of protein evolution. Nat Rev Genet, 6(9), 678-687.

Di Lena, P., Fariselli, P., Margara, L., Vassura, M., & Casadio, R. (2011). - Is there an optimal substitution matrix for contact prediction with correlated mutations? IEEE/ACM Trans Comput Biol Bioinform, 8(4), 1017-1028.

Dunn, R., Dudbridge, F., & Sanderson, C. (2005). The use of edge-betweenness clustering to investigate biological function in protein interaction networks. BMC Bioinformatics, 6, 39.

Dunn, S. D., Wahl, L. M., & Gloor, G. B. (2008). Mutual information without the influence of phylogeny or entropy dramatically improves residue contact prediction. Bioinformatics, 24(3), 333-340.

Dutheil, J. (2012). Detecting coevolving positions in a molecule: why and how to account for phylogeny. Brief Bioinform, 13(2), 228-243.

Dutheil, J., Pupko, T., Jean-Marie, A., & Galtier, N. (2005). A Model-Based Approach for Detecting Coevolving Positions in a Molecule. Molecular Biology and Evolution, 22(9), 1919-1928.

Dutheil, J. Y. (2011). Detecting coevolving positions in a molecule: why and how to account for phylogeny. Briefings in Bioinformatics.

Fares, M., & McNally, D. (2006). - CAPS: coevolution analysis using protein sequences. Bioinformatics, 22(22), 2821-2822.

Fares, M. A., & McNally, D. (2006). - CAPS: coevolution analysis using protein sequences. Bioinformatics, 22(22), 2821-2822.

Fares, M. A., & Travers, S. A. A. (2006). A Novel Method for Detecting Intramolecular Coevolution: Adding a Further Dimension to Selective Constraints Analyses. Genetics, 173(1), 9-23.

Finn, R. D., Tate, J., Mistry, J., Coggill, P. C., Sammut, S. J., Hotz, H.-R., et al. (2008). The Pfam protein families database. Nucl. Acids Res., 36(suppl_1), D281-288.

Fodor, A. A., & Aldrich, R. W. (2004). Influence of conservation on calculations of amino acid covariance in multiple sequence alignments. Proteins, 56(2), 211 - 221.

Giraud, B. G., Lapedes, A., & Liu, L. C. (1998). Analysis of correlations between sites in models of protein sequences. Physical Review E, 58(5), 6312-6322.

Gloor, G. B., Martin, L. C., Wahl, L. M., & Dunn, S. D. (2005). Mutual information in protein multiple sequence alignments reveals two classes of coevolving positions. Biochemistry, 44(19), 7156 - 7165.

Gobel, U., Sander, C., Schneider, R., & Valencia, A. (1994). Correlated mutations and residue contacts in proteins. Proteins, 18(4), 309 - 317.

Gorodkin, J., Staerfeldt, H. H., Lund, O., & Brunak, S. (1999). MatrixPlot: visualizing sequence constraints. Bioinformatics, 15(9), 769 - 770.

Gouveia-Oliveira, R., & Pedersen, A. (2007). Finding coevolving amino acid residues using row and column weighting of mutual information and multi-dimensional amino acid representation. Algorithms for Molecular Biology, 2(1), 12.

Gouveia-Oliveira, R., Roque, F., Wernersson, R., Sicheritz-Ponten, T., Sackett, P. W., Molgaard, A., et al. (2009). - InterMap3D: predicting and visualizing co-evolving protein residues. Bioinformatics, 25(15), 1963-1965.

Greene, L. H., & Higman, V. A. (2003). Uncovering Network Systems Within Protein Structures. Journal of Molecular Biology, 334(4), 781-791.

Halabi, N., Rivoire, O., Leibler, S., & Ranganathan, R. (2009). Protein Sectors: Evolutionary Units of Three-Dimensional Structure. Cell, 138(4), 774-786.

Halperin, I., Wolfson, H., & Nussinov, R. (2006). - Correlated mutations: advances and limitations. A study on fusion proteins and on the Cohesin-Dockerin families. Proteins, 63(4), 832-845.

Hobohm, U., Scharf, M., Schneider, R., & Sander, C. (1992). Selection of representative protein data sets. Protein Sci, 1(3), 409-417.

Jeong, H., Tombor, B., Albert, R., Oltvai, Z. N., & Barabasi, A. L. (2000). The large-scale organization of metabolic networks. [10.1038/35036627]. Nature, 407(6804), 651-654.

Knaggs, M. H., Salsbury Jr, F. R., Edgell, M. H., & Fetrow, J. S. (2007). Insights into Correlated Motions and Long-Range Interactions in CheY Derived from Molecular Dynamics Simulations. [doi: 10.1529/biophysj.106.081950]. Biophysical Journal, 92(6), 2062-2079.

Korber, B. T., Farber, R. M., Wolpert, D. H., & Lapedes, A. S. (1993). Covariation of mutations in the V3 loop of human immunodeficiency virus type 1 envelope protein: an information theoretic analysis. Proceedings of the National Academy of Sciences of the United States of America, 90(15), 7176-7180.

Kowarsch, A., Fuchs, A., Frishman, D., & Pagel, P. (2010). Correlated Mutations: A Hallmark of Phenotypic Amino Acid Substitutions. PLoS Comput Biol, 6(9), e1000923.

Lockless, S. W., & Ranganathan, R. (1999). Evolutionarily Conserved Pathways of Energetic Connectivity in Protein Families. Science, 286(5438), 295-299.

Lopes, C., Franz, M., Kazi, F., Donaldson, S. L., Morris, Q., & Bader, G. D. (2010). - Cytoscape Web: an interactive web-based network browser. Bioinformatics, 26(18), 2347-2348.

Marino Buslje, C., Teppa, E., Di Doménico, T., Delfino, J. M., & Nielsen, M. (2010). Networks of High Mutual Information Define the Structural Proximity of Catalytic Sites: Implications for Catalytic Residue Identification. PLoS Comput Biol, 6(11), e1000978.

Marks, D. S., Colwell, L. J., Sheridan, R., Hopf, T. A., Pagnani, A., Zecchina, R., et al. (2011). Protein 3D Structure Computed from Evolutionary Sequence Variation. [doi:10.1371/journal.pone.0028766]. PLoS ONE, 6(12), e28766.

Martin, L. C., Gloor, G. B., Dunn, S. D., & Wahl, L. M. (2005). Using information theory to search for co-evolving residues in proteins. Bioinformatics, 21(22), 4116-4124.

McLachlan, A. D. (1971). Tests for comparing related amino-acid sequences. Cytochrome c and cytochrome c 551. J Mol Biol, 61(2), 409 - 424.

Nagano, N., Orengo, C., & Thornton, J. (2002). - One fold with many functions: the evolutionary relationships between TIM barrel families based on their sequences, structures and functions. J Mol Biol, 321(5), 741-765.

Ota, M., Kinoshita, K., & Nishikawa, K. (2003). - Prediction of catalytic residues in enzymes based on known tertiary structure, stability profile, and sequence conservation. J Mol Biol, 327(5), 1053-1064.

Pazos, F., Helmer-Citterich, M., Ausiello, G., & Valencia, A. (1997). Correlated mutations contain information about protein-protein interaction. J Mol Biol, 271(4), 511 - 523.

Pollock, D. D., Taylor, W. R., & Goldman, N. (1999). Coevolving protein residues: maximum likelihood identification and relationship to structure. J Mol Biol, 287(1), 187 - 198.

Porter, C. T., Bartlett, G. J., & Thornton, J. M. (2004). The Catalytic Site Atlas: a resource of catalytic sites and residues identified in enzymes using structural data. Nucleic Acids Research, 32(suppl 1), D129-D133.

Shackelford, G., & Karplus, K. (2007). Contact prediction using mutual information and neural nets. Proteins: Structure, Function, and Bioinformatics, 69(S8), 159-164.

Socolich, M., Lockless, S. W., Russ, W. P., Lee, H., Gardner, K. H., & Ranganathan, R. (2005). Evolutionary information for specifying a protein fold. Nature, 437(7058), 512 - 518.

Tillier, E. R., & Lui, T. W. (2003). Using multiple interdependency to separate functional from phylogenetic correlations in protein alignments. Bioinformatics, 19(6), 750 - 755.

Todd, A., Orengo, C. A., & Thornton, J. M. (2001). - Evolution of function in protein superfamilies, from a structural perspective. J Mol Biol, 307(4), 1113-1143.

Van Dongen, S. (2000). Graph clustering by flow simulation. PhD thesis.

Venner, E., Lisewski, A. M., Erdin, S., Ward, R. M., Amin, S. R., & Lichtarge, O. (2010). Accurate Protein Structure Annotation through Competitive Diffusion of Enzymatic Functions over a Network of Local Evolutionary Similarities. PLoS ONE, 5(12), e14286.

Wagner, A., & Fell, D. A. (2001). The small world inside large metabolic networks. Proceedings of the Royal Society of London. Series B: Biological Sciences, 268(1478), 1803-1810.

Xin, F., Myers, S., Li, Y., Cooper, D., Mooney, S., & Radivojac, P. (2010). - Structure-based kernels for the prediction of catalytic residues and their involvement in human inherited disease. Bioinformatics, 26(16), 1975-1982.

Yeang, C.-H., & Haussler, D. (2007). Detecting Coevolution in and among Protein Domains. [doi:10.1371/journal.pcbi.0030211]. PLoS Comput Biol, 3(11), e211.

Yip, K., Patel, P., Kim, P. M., Engelman, D. M., McDermott, D., & Gerstein, M. (2008). - An integrated system for studying residue coevolution in proteins. Bioinformatics, 24(2), 290-292.

# Evaluation of Multiple-locus Variable-number Tandem-repeat Analysis for Typing Polyclonal Hospital- and Community-acquired Methicillin-resistant Staphylococcus Aureus Populations

Belinda Rivero-Pérez, Julia Alcoba-Florez and Sebastian Méndez-Alvarez

*Research Unit*
*Hospital Universitario Ntra. Sra. de Candelaria, Santa Cruz de Tenerife, Spain*

# 1   Introduction

The first methicillin-resistant *Staphylococcus aureus* (MRSA) isolate was detected in 1961 (Eriksen *et al.*, 1963). Since then, MRSA has become one of the most worrisome pathogens worldwide. Many efforts to design an ideal method to type these bacteria and to control their dissemination have been employed (Criso´stomo *et al.*, 2001). Up to now, the gold standard for short-term epidemiological surveillance of *S. aureus* has been pulsed-field gel electrophoresis (PFGE) (Crossley *et al.*, 1979; El Helali *et al.*, 2005; Enright *et al.*, 2002). However, this method is demanding and time-consuming and needs expensive reagents. Multilocus sequence typing (MLST) is the ideal method for long-term epidemiological studies, but its routine application is very unfeasible in clinical laboratories (Enright *et al.*, 2000). In 2003, a new method for typing *S. aureus* strains, multiple-locus variable-number tandem-repeat analysis (MLVA), was applied (Sabat *et al.*, 2003). This technique consists of simultaneous amplification of variable-number tandem repeats of different genes. Several works have tried to determine if MLVA provides enough information to be performed routinely instead of PFGE or MLST in clinical microbiology laboratories (Tenover *et al.*, 2007).

Our first aim was to determine if MLVA could predict MRSA clones present in the Hospital Universitario Nuestra Señora de Candelaria (HUNSC), Tenerife, Spain, that were previously characterized by PFGE, MLST, and staphylococcal cassette chromosome *mec* (SCC*mec*) typing (reported here as PFGE/MLST-SCC*mec* type) (Pérez-Roth *et al.*, 2004) and to establish possible criteria of clustering MLVA patterns, looking for high concordance levels. This study expected to validate MLVA to introduce it as a routine typing method in the HUNSC (Rivero-Pérez *et al.*, 2010). On the other hand, other goal of this study was also to find out the situation of community-acquired methicillin-resistant *Staphylococcus aureus* (CA-MRSA) isolates in Tenerife Island. With this objective, one hundred CA-MRSA isolates were collected and their molecular features investigated, applying PFGE, MLST, SCC*mec* and *spa* typing methods as in the case of HA-MRSA was previosly done (Rivero-Pérez *et al.*, 2012).

# 2   Typing Parameters and Quantification Indexes

During last years, different methods employed in the typing of MRSA isolates have been compared with the aim of finding the best one to analyse staphylococcal populations. When methods are evaluated two important traits have to be taken into account: method efficiency and efficacy (Trindade *et al.*, 2003). Efficiency is valued by its quickness, easiness to be executed and understood, and prize; whilst, efficacy is measured by:

1. Typing capacity: Percentage of bacterial strains that can be assigned to a marker by the method.

2. Reproducibility: Percentage of strains that yield the same result each time that the method is repeated.

3. Discriminatory power: method ability to distinguish between non related isolates. It is determined by the number of types identified and the relative frequencies of these types.

These two traits cannot be defined by a unique value, what make them inappropriate to compare methods. For this reason, the Simpson's Diversity Index (*D*) is applied (Hunter *et al.*, 1988). This index measures the probability that two related strains were allocated in two different typing groups (Simpson, 1949). Simpson's Index is calculated by applying the following formula:

$$D = \frac{1}{N(N-1)} \sum_{j=1}^{s} n_j(n_j - 1) \qquad \text{(Ec. 1)}$$

where $N$ is the total number of isolates, $S$ is the total number of described types and $n_j$ is the number of isolates belonging to type $j$. An acceptable discrimination level depends on the method but a process with a discrimination power over 0.9 is advised. Distinct discriminatory indexes can be applied to different techniques and depending on the discrimination level they yield the best index to use is decided. $D$ is neutral estimation of the real diversity of a population on the base of a sample of individuals ($n$) (Abramson & Sexton, 1999). $D$ values will vary depending on the collected samples. Moreover, the variavility of our analyses will be based on the real variability, which is calculated by using the variance ($\delta^2$) (Gould, 2006):

$$\delta^2 = \frac{4}{n} \left[ \sum_j \pi_j^3 - (\sum \pi_j^2)^2 \right] \qquad \text{(Ec. 2)}$$

where $n$ is the total number of isolates, $\pi_j$ is the number of isolates belonging to type $j$, and $\pi$ is the frequency resulting when $n_j$ is divided by $n$. Typical deviation is suggested to behave as a measure of the divergence existing between $D$ over 1. Then, two times at each side of $D$ value would include the 95% of all expected distribution, and subsequently it is an approximated measure of the confidence when estimating more than one diversity indexes. This value is called confidence interval (IC):

$$IC = \left[ D - 2\sqrt{\delta^2}, D - 2\sqrt{\delta^2} \right] \qquad \text{(Ec. 3)}$$

In conclusion, using the $IC$ when $D$ is being used increases the truthfulness of the comparison between the genetic diversity calculated under different conditions. Accordingly, considering the $IC$ also augment the reliability of the discriminatory power of different typing systems (Grundmann et al., 2001).

Furthermore, the method to employ should be chosen taking into account also the time scale and the environment the study is going to considerer. Thus, e.g., PFGE is the most used method for local comparisons in short time periods since it presents difficulties in the reproducibility and in the reliability among different laboratories. Currently, multi centre studies using this technique are achievable by the standardization of the electrophoresis conditions and the software normalization. However, MLST has the advantage of sequences being unambiguous, conducting to an easier comparison between laboratories. MLST is moreover complemented with the determination of the SCC*mec* type, applying the Enright *et al.* nomenclature, which was accepted in Tokyo in 2002 by the International Union of Microbiologic Societies. Under this nomenclature, the ST is combined with the general phenotype and the SCC*mec* type; e.g., ST22 – MRSA - IV (Enright *et al.*, 2000; Feil *et al.*, 2003).

At the moment, tools to evaluate each technique independently are available but recently a method for quantitatively calculating the accordance between different systems has been proposed (Carriço *et al.*, 2006; Hubert *et al.*, 1985). It is based on two coefficients that compare two kinds of groups resulting from the same group of isolates (Grundmann *et al.*, 2001). These two coefficients are:

1.  **Adjusted Rand (AR) index:** It is a correction of Rand (Rand, 1971) coefficient, which is commonly used to quantify the congruence between two typing methods (Pinto *et al.*, 2007). The

Rand Index represents the proportion of presence and absence of common bands in the two compared methods:

$$R = \frac{a+d}{a+b+c+d}$$ (Ec. 4)

where, $a$ constitutes the isolates that belong to the same group by both methods; $b$ those isolates that belong to the same group by method 1 but does not by method 2; $c$ are that isolates belonging to the same group by method 2 but not by method 1; $d$ is the number of isolates belonging to different groups by both methods. A limitation of this method is that when we compare to divisions randomly, the index never reaches a null value, indicating that congruence between methods does not exist. This limitation is solved in the adjusted Rand method, which introduces a correction factor ($n_c$; that corresponds with $a$ and $d$ if both typing methods were totally independent) permitting a better quantitative evaluation of the global congruence between two divisions.

$$AR = \frac{a+d-n_c}{a+b+c+d-n_c}$$ (Ec. 5)

$$n_c = \frac{n(n^2+1)-(n+1)\sum n_i^2 -(n+1)\sum n_j^2 +2\sum\sum \frac{n_i^2 n_j^2}{n}}{2(n-1)}$$ (Ec. 6)

2. **Wallace Index:** This index improves the comparison between two methods because it yields an unique value that indicates the probability of classifying two strains as the same type by those two methods. The index gives up a value from 0 to 1, indicating that the results shown by one of the two methods are more predictable by the other method as much as the value of the index is nearer to 1 (Wallace, 1983). Then, that is an asymmetric index, since one method could show definite capacity to predict the results obtained by other, but this capacity was not the same in the reciprocal order.

$$W_1(1,2) = \frac{a}{a+b} \qquad W_2(1,2) = \frac{a}{a+c}$$ (Ec. 7)

Moreover, since the grade of congruence between two methods depends on the particular population in which the study is developed, some variability exists respecting the real population. By this reason, the Wallace value should be accompanied by a confidence interval (Pinto et al., 2008).

$$IC = W_{A\to B} \pm 2\sqrt{\delta^2(W_{A\to B})}$$ (Ec. 8)

where $W_{A\to B}$ is defined as the ratio between the number of pairs of individuals equally classified by methods $A$ and $B$ and the number of pairs of individuals equally classified by $A$. In conclusion, this combination of methods (Adjusted Rand Index and Wallace Index) improves the information that can be obtained, if two methods present a high global relation and, moreover, if one of the methods can predict the other and vice versa.

# 3    Typing of hospital acquired MRSA by Multiple-Locus Variable number tandem repeat Analysis (MLVA)

A relatively new method for typing *S. aureus* strains is the multiple-locus variable-number tandem-repeat analysis (MLVA) (Trindade *et al.*, 2003). This technique consists of simultaneous amplification of variable-number tandem repeats of different genes. Several works have tried to determine if MLVA provides enough information to be performed routinely instead of PFGE or MLST, which are more laborious, in the clinical setting. In our laboratory, MLVA was performed as previously described (Sabat *et al.*, 2003) but slightly modified to obtain optimal results and to accelerate the process (Rivero-Pérez *et al.*, 2010) concluding that the utilization of MLVA allows distinguishing among different MRSA reservoirs and other circulating MRSA strains.

The 292 HA-MRSA isolates included in the study belonged to the clones included in Table 2. MLVA was performed as previously described (Moser *et al.*, 2009; Sabat *et al.*, 2003) but slightly modified to obtain optimal results and to accelerate the process. The PCR mixture was prepared with 1x reaction buffer, 1.5 mM $MgCl_2$, 0.2 mM deoxynucleoside triphosphates (dNTPs), 1.2 mM each of ClfA-F, ClfA-R, ClfB-F, ClfB-R, SdrCDE-F, and SdrCDE-R primers, 0.5 mM each of Spa-F and Spa-R primers, 1 mM each of Sspa-F and Sspa-R primers, and 0.05 U of *Taq* DNA polymerase (Bioline). Cycling conditions (MyCycler; Bio-Rad) were 94°C for 5 min, 20 cycles of 94°C for 30 s, 58.2°C for 45 s, and 72°C for 1.5 min, and finally 72°C for 5 min (Figure 1). To assess reproducibility, 10 randomly chosen isolates of different MLVA types were used for three independent MLVA experiments. The dendrogram obtained by Dice's coefficient with a 1% tolerance value was analyzed using three different cut-offs (Table 1). Simpson's index of diversity, *D* (Feil *et al.*, 2003), was employed to measure the discriminatory powers of MLVA and PFGE/MLST-SCC*mec* typing (Clinical and Laboratory Standards Institute, 2007; David *et al.*, 2008). Moreover, concordance levels between these methods were quantified using two coefficients, adjusted Rand (AR) (Rand, 1971) and Wallace (W) (Pinto *et al.*, 2007, 2008; Wallace, 1983), as Carrico et al. suggested (Carriço *et al.*, 2006).

| | MLVA (one band) | | MLVA (80%) | | MLVA (70%) | |
|---|---|---|---|---|---|---|
| | AR | W (%) | AR | W (%) | AR | W (%) |
| Tipo PFGE-ST-SCC*mec* | 0.794 | 98.71 (97.93-99.45) | 0.976 | 98.29 (97.11-99.33) | 0.967 | 96.08 (93.35-98.08) |
| Subtipo PFGE-ST-SCC*mec* | 0.644 | 69.21 (61.01-77.38) | 0.696 | 65.86 (58.51-73.12) | 0.688 | 64.62 (57.15-71.59) |
| Tipo PFGE-ST-SCC*mec*-CC | 0.794 | 98.71 (97.93-99.45) | 0.976 | 98.29 (97.11-99.33) | 0.967 | 96.08 (93.35-98.08) |
| Subtipo PFGE-ST-SCC*mec*-CC | 0.644 | 69.21 (61.01-77.38) | 0.696 | 65.86 (58.51-73.12) | 0.688 | 64.62 (57.15-71.59) |
| CC | 0.765 | 100 | 0.957 | 100 | 0.986 | 100 |

Table 1: MLVA correlation, analysed under three different cut off points: PFGE-MLST-SCC*mec*, adjusted Rand index and Wallace index. Red squares indicate the best results obtained. Abbreviations: MLVA: Multiple-Locus Variable number tandem repeat Analysis; AR: Adjusted Rand index; W: Wallace index; Tipo: Type; Subtipo: Subtype; PFGE: Pulsed Field Gel Electrophoresis; ST: Sequence Type; SCC*mec*: Staphylococcal Chromosome Cassette *mec*; CC: Clonal Complex.

| CC | PFGE/MLST-SCCmec type, no. (%) of isolates | No. (name(s)) of PFGE subtypes at >80% cut off | >80% cutoff | | | >70% cutoff | | |
|---|---|---|---|---|---|---|---|---|
| | | | Total no. of MLVA types in CC | MLVA type | No. (name(s)) of MLVA subtypes | Total no. of MLVA types in CC | MLVA type | No. (name(s)) of MLVA subtypes |
| 8 | PFGE-A/ST247-IA, 58 (15.59) | 12 (A1 to A12) | 4 | b | 7 (b1 to b7) | 4 | c | 7 (c1 to c7) |
| | PFGE-L/ST8-IVA, 1 (0.34) | 1 (L1) | | fi | 1 (d1) | | i | 1 (i1) |
| | PFGE-V/ST8-IV, 1 (0.34) | 1 (V1) | | o | 1 (o1) | | j | 1 (j1) |
| | PFGE-O/ST239-III, 1 (0.34) | 1 (O1) | | g | 1 (g1) | | g | 1 (g1) |
| 30 | PFGE-B/ST36-II, 164 (55.41) | 9 (B1 to B9) | 2 | a | 8 (a1 to a8) | 1 | a | 9 (a1 to a9) |
| | PFGE-F/ST30-IV, 1 (0.34) | 1 (F1) | | h | 1 (h1) | | | |
| 5 | PFGE-C/ST125-IVA, 50 (16.89) | 3 (C1 to C3) | 6 | c, d, n | 4 (c1 to c4), 1 (d1), 1 (n1) | 2 | b | 6 (b1 to b3, b5, b6, b8) |
| | PFGE-D/ST146-IVA, 8 (2.70) | 1 (D1) | | c, d, k, m | 1 (c1), 1 (d1), 1 (k1), 1 (m1) | | b, e | 3 (b1, b4, b7), 1 (e2) |
| | PFGE-D/ST471-IV, 1 (0.34) | 1 (N1) | | l | 1 (l1) | | e | 1 (e3) |
| 22 | PFGE-E/ST22-IV, 5 (1.69) | 2 (E1, E2) | 1 | e | 1 (e1) | 1 | d | 1 (d1) |
| Unknown | PFGE-M/ST80-IV, 1 (0.34) | 1 (M1) | 1 | f | 1 (f1) | 1 | f | 1 (f1) |
| | PFGE-U/ST88-IV, 1 (0.34) | 1 (U1) | 1 | i | 1 (i1) | 1 | h | 1 (h1) |
| Total | 12[a] | 34 | 16 | | 31 | 10 | | 32 |

**Table 2:** Classification of different MRSA clones by applying the 80% and 70% cut-offs criteria. MLVA types and subtypes are indicated. [a] Total number of different PFGE/MLST-SCCmec types.

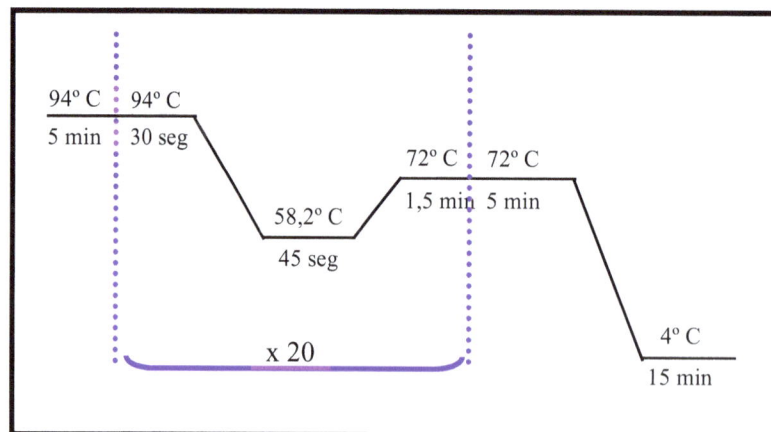

**Figure 1:** Optimized PCR program for MLVA amplification.

# 4   Results of Typing HA-MRSA by MLVA

All 292 HA-MRSA were type-able by MLVA. Interestingly, it was possible to optimize the results by running the five pairs of primers in the same reaction, described as a difficult technique (Figure 2) (Tenover *et al.*, 2007). Also, the PCRs were performed successfully from cellular suspensions without DNA extraction. The intralaboratory reproducibility of MLVA was very high (100%), as previously noted by other authors (Sabat *et al.*, 2003; Tenover *et al.*, 2007).

By application of the previously established criterion in which two isolates with any different band were classified as two distinct MLVA types (Sabat *et al.*, 2003), MLVA produced 35 distinct patterns, showing a *D* value of 71.33% (range, 66.14 to 76.52%). Although PFGE showed a lower value, *D* of 68.47% (64.07 to 72.88%), the difference was not significant. The isolates were divided into 14 clusters (*a* to *n*), and 21 organisms had unique MLVA pattern (ñ to ah). The PFGE-A/ST247-IA, PFGE-

B/ST36-II, PFGE-C/ST125-IVA, and PFGE-D/ST146- IVA clones were divided into different MLVA types. All of the PFGE-E/ST22-IV isolates were clustered together, and each sporadic MRSA clone corresponded with one MLVA type. Therefore, we are able to rule out relationships but not to establish them. The quantitative analyses showed low congruence values and even lower values when the PFGE subtypes were considered (Table 1). Tenover *et al.* obtained similar results with a visual analysis determining if MLVA could predict USA strain PFGE types. Then, they applied the ≥ 80% and ≥ 75% relatedness cutoff criteria (Tenover *et al.*, 1995, 2007;). We tested other criteria and the ≥ 80% and ≥ 70% relatedness cutoffs, as previously proposed (Malachowa *et al.*, 2005; Tenover *et al.*, 2007).

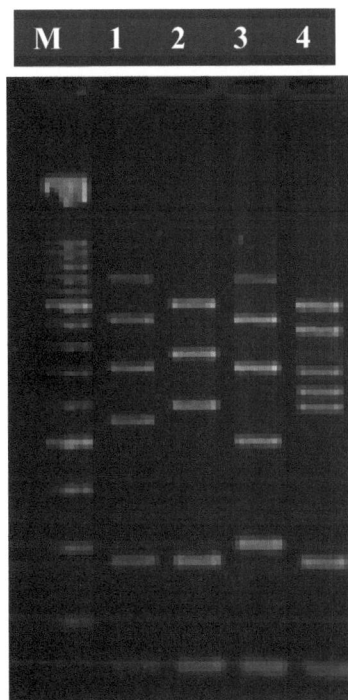

**Figure 2:** Electrophoresis gel where different band patterns can be observed. Lane M shows Marker XIV (Roche Diagnostics); Lanes 1 and 3 show patterns with 6 bands; Lane 2 shows only 5 bands and, finally, lane 4 shows a complete pattern with the 7 MLVA bands.

By using the > 80% relatedness cutoff, the number of MLVA types was reduced from 35 to 17, reducing the *D* value to 61.82% (57.00 to 66.04%). The 17 MLVA types included 5 clusters of > 1 organism and 12 unique MLVA patterns (Rivero-Pérez *et al.*, 2010). The PFGE-A/ST247-IA, PFGE-B/ST36-II and PFGE-E/ ST22-IV clones corresponded with the MLVA types *b*, *a* and *e*, respectively. Therefore, we were successful in grouping MRSA isolates to the same clone, although the distributions of the MLVA subtypes and the PFGE subtypes did not correspond. Subtype A1, the so-called Iberian clone, showed the same MLVA pattern as the other A subtypes (A2 to A13) (Figure 3), and the same happened with subtypes B1 (Figure 3) and E1, the so-called EMRSA-16 and EMRSA-15 clones, respectively. Therefore, MLVA could predict the PFGE/MLST-SCC*mec* types, but it could not distinguish the possible outbreaks of particular PFGE subtypes, being important above all in epidemic clones, such as the Iberian, EMRSA-16, and EMRSA-15 clones, present in our hospital. The quantitative analysis with and without PFGE subtype data demonstrated this observation (Table 1). On the other hand, the PFGE-C/ ST125-IVA and PFGE-D/ST146-IVA clones were difficult to distinguish by MLVA, since both clones showed mixed MLVA types c and d. These clustering differences of MLVA were observed by Tenover *et al.*, applying the 80% and 75% cutoff criteria, with USA strain PFGE types (Rivero-Pérez *et al.*, 2010; Tenover *et al.*, 1995, 2007). For example, USA100 isolates were clustered together in the same MLVA type, whereas USA800 isolates were separated into six different MLVA types. They suggested that the variability of the MLVA patterns may be strain dependent (Tenover *et al.*, 2007). Even so, congruence levels in our study upon application of this criterion were very high (Table 1). Therefore, MLVA typing could be a useful tool to localize and to follow the movement of these MRSA strains inside the hospital and, thus, to reduce the number of nosocomial infections, just as was described previously (Chaberny *et al*, 2008; Huang *et al.*, 2006).

Use of the > 70% relatedness cutoff reduced the number of MLVA types from 17 to 11, showing a *D* of 60.48% (55.92 to 65.04%). The 11 MLVA types included 5 clusters of > 1 organism and 6 unique MLVA patterns (Rivero-Pérez *et al.*, 2010). As with the > 80% cutoff, the PFGE-A/ST247-IA, PFGE-B/ST36-II, and PFGE-E/ST22-IV isolates each belonged to a different MLVA type (Figure 1). However, by use of this less stringent criterion, the single isolate PFGE-F/ST30-IV was clustered together with the PFGE-B/ST36-II isolates, both belonging to clonal complex 30 (CC30). The PFGE-C/ST125-IVA and PFGE-D/ ST146-IVA clones were mixed again, except one PFGE-D/ ST146-IVA isolate that was clustered together with the PFGEN/ ST471-IV clone, both belonging to CC5 (Table 2). Therefore, the MLVA types represented MRSA isolates with different PFGE/MLST-SCC*mec* types, what was proved with the quantitative analysis (Table 1). Malachowa *et al.* determined a good correlation between MLVA and PFGE by applying a 70% cutoff for MLVA but a 75% cutoff for PFGE (Malachowa *et al.*, 2005). Nevertheless, we do not agree with the change from an 80% cutoff for PFGE, since it is a justified and internationally accepted criterion (Tenover *et al.*, 2007). In that study, Malachowa *et al.* found that MLVA (70% cutoff) grouped isolates with the same CC, although with some exceptions. The exception in our study was CC8, where the different strains were not grouped together (Rivero-Pérez *et al.*, 2010). At a quantitative level, the values obtained in the analysis including the corresponding CCs together with PFGE/ MLST-SCC*mec* types did not vary, while in the analysis comparing MLVA *vs* CCs only, the AR and W values increased to 0.98 and 100%, respectively (Table 1).

Developing an efficient strategy to prevent the dissemination of MRSA clones and to provide optimal treatment for patients is of paramount importance. However, in many hospitals, the resources are not available for PFGE or MLST, techniques par excellence chosen in epidemiological studies. As a result, our aim has been to validate a method described as cheap, fast, and easy to use for analysis of hospital-acquired MRSA. Our efforts validate MLVA as a routine typing technique, reaching an agreement between the efficacy and the efficiency, as Trindade *et al.* (2003) suggested. Since the concordance levels between typing methods can vary depending on the collection of isolates, different studies of the correlation of MLVA and other techniques have led to various conclusions (Moser *et al.*, 2009; Sabat *et al.*, 2003; Tenover *et al.*, 2007). In our analysis, MLVA could predict MRSA clones previously identified by PFGE/MLST-SCC*mec* typing (Ruimy *et al.*, 2008), with the highest congruence between both methods achieved when we applied the 80% cutoff criterion. Also, the 70% cutoff criterion could be used to cluster isolates that belong to the same CC. Once the method was validated for the collection of HUNSC-MRSA isolates, MLVA typing was also applied in the characterization of the 95 CA-MRSA isolates, which were also typed by PCR, PFGE, SCC*mec*, MLST, and *spa*-typing. Furthermore, MLVA has been

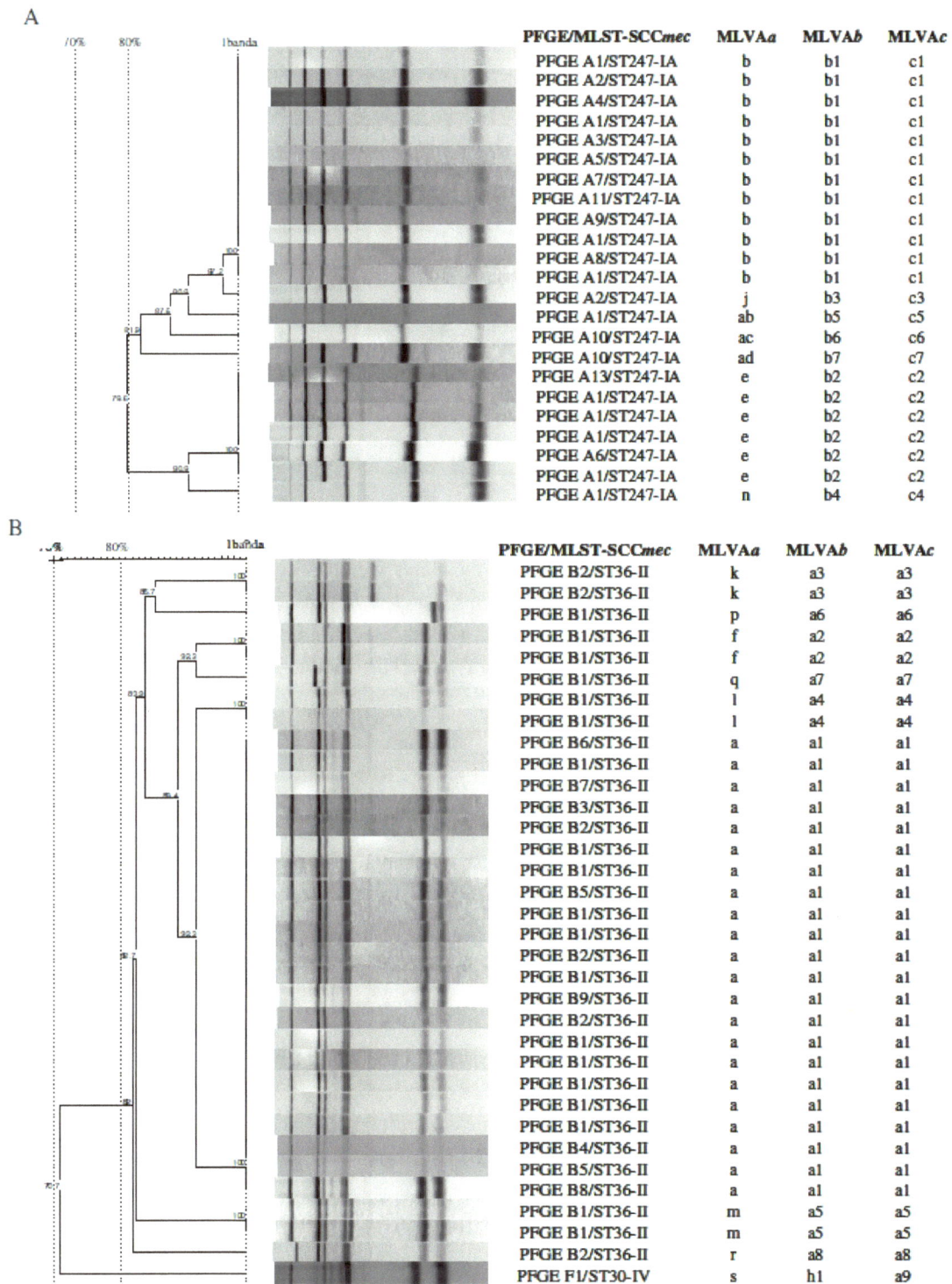

**Figure 3:** A. Iberic clone classification, PFGE A1/ST247-IA. And B. epidemic clone EMRSA16, PFGE A1/ST36-II; Classifications obtained by MLVA analysed under the three cut offs employed in this study (a=1 band, b=80% and c=70%), as well as other subtypes from the same group.

described to provide a solid basis for the assignment of different genetic variants, which is useful information for epidemiological tracking (Melles *et al.*, 2009).

In conclusion, this study demonstrates the ability of MLVA to distinguish among different MRSA reservoirs and other circulating MRSA strains in the HUNSC. The proven simplicity, low cost, and speed of MLVA enable the performance of routine checkups in patients, mainly via admission screening on surgical wards and in intensive care units, hampering the spread of these strains and therefore reducing the morbidity, mortality, and costs (Abramson & Sexton, 1999; Centres for Disease Control and Prevention (CDC), January 2010; Faria *et al*, 2005).

# 5     Typing of community acquired MRSA (CA-MRSA) by Multiple-Locus Variable number tandem repeat Analysis (MLVA)

With the recent detection of MRSA infections in patients lacking health care-related risk factors the term community-acquired methicillin-resistant *Staphylococcus aureus* (CA-MRSA) has been become known (Manzur *et al.*, 2008; Ribeiro *et al.*, 2005). Many cases of CA-MRSA spreading to the community have been described worldwide. The aim of this study was to find out the situation of CA-MRSA isolates in Tenerife Island. In this respect, one hundred MRSA isolates were collected from eight different health regions and their molecular features investigated. This study revealed a wide variety of MRSA clones, including the description of an emergent ST: ST1434 (CC8), and two new *spa* types: t7575 (ST125) and t7678 (ST22). The PVL genes were found only in five isolates belonging to unrelated lineages: ST8, ST30 and ST22, which could indicate at least three independent introductions of PVL+ strains in Tenerife. Moreover, we detected that hospital MRSA clones, like EMRSA-15 and EMRSA-16, had spread to the community and are now circulating in both environments (Table 1). Therefore, in our study, the CDC's rules were not enough to distinguish CA-MRSA from HA-MRSA (Centres for Disease Control and Prevention (CDC), January 2010; Clinical and Laboratory Standards Institute, 2007; David *et al.*, 2008). Thus, we think that the epidemiological information is not enough to discriminate between both MRSAs and it is indispensable that prevention guidelines include the routine determination of at least the genetic background for each MRSA isolate, the antimicrobial susceptibility profile, and the PVL genes content (Broseta *et al.*, 2006; Cercenado *et al.*, 2008; Cercenado & Ruiz de Gopegui, 2008).

## 5.1    Clinical Settings, Patients, Bacterial Isolates and Surveillance Period

This study was performed in the Hospital Universitario Nuestra Señora de Candelaria (HUNSC), which is a tertiary medical center in Tenerife, Spain. Tenerife is organized into 31 Health Regions (HRs), which are different areas of the Island with a regional healthcare center each. Everybody is attached to a healthcare center depending on where they live. Eight HRs participated in this study: Puerto de la Cruz, Tacoronte, La Laguna, Candelaria, Güímar, Granadilla, Abona, and Santa Cruz de Tenerife, where the HUNSC is located. The healthcare centers of these HRs routinely refer possible infectious samples to the Clinical Microbiology Laboratory in the HUNSC, which then pass onto the Research Unit those MRSA samples which match the CA-MRSA according to the CDC's criteria, herein expounded. The following clinical and epidemiological data were registered for each CA-MRSA infection case: sex, age, date, specimen, HR, hospitalization or residency in a long-term facility and history of MRSA. The surveillance period was from July, 2004 to May, 2007, a period of 34 months.

From all isolates recovered, those fitting the criteria suggested by the CDC (Centres for Disease Control and Prevention (CDC), January 2010; Clinical and Laboratory Standards Institute, 2007) were selected as CA-MRSAs. According to the CDC, a bacterial infection is caused by a CA-MRSA if:

1. The isolate was recovered from an external patient or from an internal patient of the hospital if the isolate was recovered within the first 48 hours after patient admission.

2. The patient has not clinical anamnesis including MRSA infection or colonization.

3. The patient has not suffered during last year hospital admission, surgery, dialysis neither has lived in an elder residence.

4. The patient has not permanent catheter or any medical indwelling feature.

## 5.2    Strain Characterization

For each CA-MRSA isolate the susceptibility testing was performed with the automatic Vitek2 system (AST-P559 card) (BioMérieux, Francia) according to the manufacturer's instructions for a panel of 10 antibiotics: penicillin, clindamycin, erythromycin, gentamicin, oxacillin, ciprofloxacin, trimethoprim-sulfamethoxazole, mupirocin, teicoplanin and vancomycin. The antimicrobial susceptibility profiles were interpreted according to the Clinical and Laboratory Standards Institute (CLSI, 2007) (Clinical and Laboratory Standards Institute, 2007). Antibiotypes were considered different if at least one difference was observed in the antibiotic resistance profile. Antimicrobial multiresistance was defined as resistance to ≥ 3 different classes of non-beta-lactam antimicrobials. Moreover, the resistance to oxacillin and mupirocin were estimated by Etest, and the inducible resistance to clindamycin was determined by Dtest. The species identification and the methicillin and mupirocin resistance were confirmed by multiplex PCR (Pérez-Roth et al., 2001), and also the presence of the PVL genes (lukF-PV and lukS-PV) (Daskalaki et al., 2010; Ribeiro et al., 2005).

SCCmec type I-IV was detected firstly by the Oliveira and de Lencastre strategy (Oliveira & de Lencastre, 2002) and then the discrimination between SCCmec IV and V was performed as previously described (Milheiriço et al., 2007). All MRSA isolates were typed by MLVA and PFGE and analyzed by InfoQuest (version 4.5; Bio-rad) using Dice coefficient and the unweighted-pair group method with arithmetic means. A similarity coefficient of ≥ 80% was applied to both methods (Rivero-Pérez et al., 2010, 2012; Tenover et al., 1995). Spa typing was performed for on each MRSA isolate and analyzed using the Ridom StaphType software (Ridom GmbH, Germany) (Harmsen et al., 2003).

MLST was performed for representative isolates distributed among the 29 PFGE types (Enright et al., 2000). In each PFGE type, the chosen isolates were the predominant subtypes and those with the greatest number of band differences from the predominant subtypes. Based on previous studies, we assumed that all MRSA isolates with the same PFGE type belong to the same MLST. Sequence types (STs) and clonal clusters (CCs) were assigned using the S. aureus MLST database (www.mlst.net) hosted by The Imperial College in London, UK.

## 5.3    Spa Typing

Spa typing was performed on each MRSA isolate and analysed using the Ridom StaphType soft-ware (Ridom GmbH, Germany) (Harmsen et al., 2003). MLST was performed on 29 representative isolates distributed among the PFGE types (Enright et al., 2000). In each PFGE type, the chosen isolates were the predominant subtypes and those with the greatest number of band differences compared with the predominant subtypes. Based on previous studies, we assumed that all MRSA isolates with the same PFGE type belong to the same MLST. Sequence types (STs) and clonal clusters (CCs) were assigned using the S. aureus MLST database (www.mlst.net) hosted by The Imperial College in London, UK.

### 5.4    Results of CA-MRSA Typing.

One hundred MRSA isolates, catalogued as CA according to CDC's rules, were collected during the surveillance period. Later, 95 isolates were confirmed as MRSA, but 5 isolates resulted methicillin-sensible *S. aureus* (MSSA) owing to the absence of the *mecA* gene, so they were excluded from the study. The female-to-male ratio was 1.2 and the median age of the patients was 60.09 years old, with an age range between 4 – 92 years (standard deviation [SD], ± 18.6 years). Clustering the patients into 10 groups in periods of 10 years, a peak was observed in patients whose age covered from 71 – 80 years, and also, another peak was noted in between the ages of 31 – 40 years.

The 95 MRSA isolates were distributed among the 8 HRs, and we observed the highest number of isolates came from the Santa Cruz and Puerto de la Cruz HRs. In general, considering the number of people living in each HR (http://www2.gobiernodecanarias.org/istac/estadisticas/php/) which coincides with the number of people referring to each healthcare centre, the prevalence of sampled infectious caused by CAMRSA was < 0.1% across each region (Figure 4).

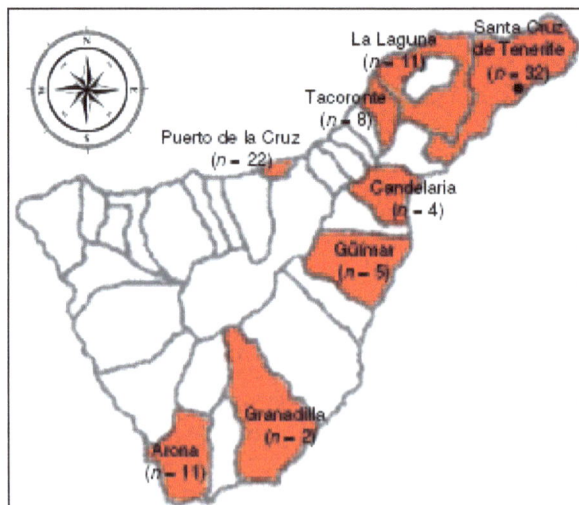

**Figure 4:** Tenerife Island simplified map. Areas from which samples included in the study were recovered are coloured in red. (*n*) indicates the number of MRSA isolates recovered in each of them. ● indicates the HUNSC location.

Of the 95 MRSA isolates, the majority were associated with SSTIs (82.1%; *n* = 79), distributed among ulcers (*n* = 49), skin lesions (*n* = 29), and abscesses (*n* = 1) (Daskalaki *et al.*, 2010; Moran *et al.*, 2005). The remaining isolates were from otic exudates (6.3%; *n* = 6), nasal exudates (4.2%; *n* = 4), pharynx exudates (3.2%; *n* = 3), sputum (1.1%; *n* = 1), seroma (1.1%; *n* = 1), and urine (1.1%; *n* = 1) (Pérez-Roth *et al.*, 2010).

## 5.5  Antimicrobial Susceptibility

Heterogeneous antimicrobial susceptibility phenotypes were determined for CA-MRSA isolates, detecting thirteen different profiles (Rivero-Pérez *et al.*, 2012). All MRSA isolates were resistant to beta-lactams and susceptible to trimetropim-sulfametoxazol, teicoplanin and vancomycin. Only one isolate showed inducible resistance to clindamycin. Remarkably, 60% of isolates were multiresistant, whereas 3.2% were susceptible to all non-betalactam antimicrobials.

## 5.6  PVL Genes

The presence of PVL was investigated in every MRSA isolate, and *pvl* genes were detected in only 5 MRSA isolates distributed among the CC groups: CC8 (*n* = 3), CC30 (*n* = 1), and CC22 (*n* = 1) (Dufour *et al.*, 2002; López-Aguilar *et al.*, 2007). Oddly enough, all PVL+ CA-MRSA isolates were obtained from Arona and Granadilla de Abona, HRs located in the south of the island, where a higher number of tourists arrive each year (Holmes *et al.*, 2005).

## 5.7  Typing

All isolates showed an identifiable SCC*mec* pattern by the used methods. SCC*mec* type II was found in 24.2% of the isolates, all of them being multiresistant CC30 (ST36). SCC*mec* type IV was detected in 26.3% of the isolates distributed between CC22 (ST22), CC8 (ST8), CC97 (ST97), and one CC30 (ST30) isolate. Finally, SCC*mec* variant IVA was found in 49.5% of the isolates distributed between CC5 (ST125 and ST146) and one CC8 isolate (ST1434). SCC*mec* type V was not detected. All SCC*mec*II MRSA isolates were multiresistant, although 11/25 SCC*mec*IV isolates and 15/47 SCC*mec*IVA isolates were also multiresistant. The MLST clustered the MRSA into 5 CC groups, including 9 MLST types, 15 PFGE types, 12 MLVA types, and 17 *spa* types. The molecular typing data are summarized in the Table 2. Group CC5, with 47 isolates, was the most numerous and diverse having profiles which included PFGE, MLVA profiles, and *spa* types, followed by groups CC30 and CC22. The remaining MRSA isolates corresponded to only 5.3% of the total. Three of the 4 MRSA isolates belonging to cluster CC8 were ST8 related to the PVL+ USA300 (t008) strain and the remaining one was of the new ST1434, a PVL-variant (t148). The MRSA ST1434 (t148) isolated was obtained from a pharyngeal exudate sample, showed resistant to β-lactams, clindamycin, erythromycin, and induced resistance to ciprofloxacin, and is a single-locus variant, triple nucleotide variant of ST72 (CC8) in the gene encoding acetyle coenzyme A acetyltransferase (*yqiL*), turning out to be the unknown intermediate genetic state between the ST72 and the ST990.

Besides, in the community of Santa Cruz de Tenerife (Figure 4) we found a case of familial furunculosis associated with community-acquired leukocidin-positive methicillin-susceptible *Staphylococcus aureus* (PVL_CA-MSSA) ST152 (Pérez-Roth *et al.*, 2010).

# 6  Discussion

The emergence of infections caused by CA-MRSA clones is causing global concern at present. However, due to the different definitions to CA-MRSA, an open debate exists about whether CA-MRSA must be considered as an epidemiologically independent group from HA-MRSA or not (Naimi *et al.*, 2003). In this study, we wanted to research the CA-MRSA strains present in several communities of Tenerife, starting from the minimum requirable characteristics: the CDC's rules. Although several CA-MRSA epidemiological studies have been previously performed in Spain, the special characteristics derived from the insularity, make it necessary to undertake a specific study here (Broseta *et al.*, 2006; Cercenado *et al.*, 2008; Manzur *et al.*, 2008; O'Brien *et al.*, 2009).

The CA-MRSA prevalence found was low, but the real frequency in Tenerife cannot be estimated from this study because the clinical samples sent to the laboratory was from only 8 of the 31 HRs (25.8%). A global study in Tenerife, including all the HRs, is necessary due to the wide variety of nationalities located here. Even so, the current data seems to indicate that HA-MRSA strains continue being a bigger problem than CAMRSA strains here in Tenerife. Although, considering other countries as a reference, an increase in this prevalence is predictable (Moran *et al.*, 2005). Among the antimicrobial susceptibility phenotypes, a high percentage of isolates showed multiresistance, which is not expected of community isolates (Cercenado *et al.*, 2008; Kaplan *et al.*, 2005; Manzur *et al.*, 2008; Naimi *et al.*, 2003). However, recently it has been proposed that this condition is progressively changing and CA-MRSA strains are acquiring new resistances (David *et al.*, 2008; Ribeiro *et al.*, 2005).

Controversy exists about the relationship between CA-MRSA strains and PVL. In our study, PVL was found to be in low frequency, suggesting that is not required for the spread of MRSA in this community, as has just been previously proposed (Rossney *et al.*, 2007). On the other hand, the presence of the PVL in unrelated genetic backgrounds had been described previously (Cercenado *et al.*, 2008; Huang *et al.*, 2006; Vandenesch *et al.*, 2003), and in our case, we think that at least 3 different introductions of PVL carrying strains have occurred (CC30, CC22, CC8) in the south of the island. This hypothesis is in accordance with Vandenesch *et al* (2003), who proposed multiple independent clonal origins for the PVL+ strains and is supported by the location of these PVL+ strains in the HRs strongly exposed to MRSA carriers from worldwide. Oddly enough, we found the PVL+ ST8-IV strain, which is predominant in the USA and probably introduced into Spain due to the presence of an elevated number of immigrants from South America (Cercenado *et al.*, 2008; Manzur *et al.*, 2008; Vandenesch *et al.*, 2003), but we did not find the so-called European clone, the PVL+ ST80-IV (Holmes *et al.*, 2005). In some European countries such as Denmark or Ireland there has been a serious increment in PVL+ CA-MRSA. In the study developed by Faria *et al.* (2005), PVL+ genes were detected in 100% of all the cases of ST80-IV isolates. In Ireland, the emergence of a multidrug-resistant PVL+ ST8-MRSA-IVa/USA300 is alarming and requires ongoing surveillance (Shore *et al.*, 2010). Interestingly, we detected also family transmission and spread of community-acquired leukocidin-positive methicillin-susceptible *S. aureus* ST152 isolates associated with severe clinical symptoms. Remarkably, ST152 isolates recovered in Tenerife were MSSA although ST152 globally distributed is known as an epidemic MRSA clone. Since the Canary Islands are very near the west coast of Africa (15 km), our finding of PVL-positive ST152 MSSA fits with the speculation of Ruimy *et al.* supposing a migration from Africa to Europe, where PVL-positive ST152 MSSA acquired methicillin resistance (Ruimy *et al.*, 2008; Pérez-Roth *et al.*, 2010).

Two *spa* types described only in Germany until now, t1560 (CC5) and t2781 (CC22), were detected among our isolates, and here in Tenerife, the highest percentage of tourism comes from Germany, so these isolates could have been introduced directly from that country. This hypothesis is supported by other studies, where the rise of CA-MRSA diversity due to the presence of people coming from other countries was described (Manzur *et al.*, 2008; Ruimy *et al.*, 2008; Rossney *et al.*, 2007; Salgado *et al.*, 2003).

A 24.2% of our isolates corresponded with the ST36-II clone (EMRSA-16), clone previously detected at the HUNSC (Pérez-Roth *et al.*, 2003, 2004), so we think that these isolates should not be considered CA-MRSA, but CO-MRSA (community-onset), as Salgado *et al.* (2003) proposed. The flow of

MRSA between hospital and community has been already described (David *et al.*, 2008; Dufour *et al.*, 2002; Salgado *et al.*, 2003), and in this case, could explain the presence of the hospital clone ST36-II, the high percentage of multiresistance and the peak of MRSA infections in people from 71-90 years (Naimi *et al.*, 2003; Ruimy *et al.*, 2008; Pérez-Roth *et al.*, 2003). The ST22-IV clone (EMRSA-15) had been also detected into the HUNSC (Pérez-Roth *et al.*, 2004), but in this case we cannot discern its origin because it has been related with community infections too.

Clearly, the identification in our community of the CA-MRSA isolates only based on the CDC's criteria overestimated the number of isolates collected, because included also CO-MRSA isolates. Therefore, we think that the epidemiological information is not enough to discriminate between CA-MRSA and HA-MRSA, corroborating data obtained by other authors (David *et al.*, 2008; Rossney *et al.*, 2007). Definitively, MRSA epidemiology is a cornerstone for human health. That makes necessary to continuously improve our arsenal not only of clinical drugs but also of diagnostic methods that permits rapid and precise frightening plans. In this sense, MLVA has been recently improved by using sixteen VNTR loci amplified in two multiplex PCRs and analyzed by capillary electrophoresis ensuring a high throughput and high discriminatory power (Sobral *et al.*, 2012). This type of high throughput approach has been more recently chip extended (Sabat *et al.*, 2012). It is possible that a prospective study based on our community would reveal not recognized or yet-unknown risks factors here. Moreover, according to David *et al.* (2008) the importance of distinguishing between HA-MRSA and CA-MRSA lies in taking decisions about empirical therapy, because CA-MRSA is more likely to be clindamycin susceptible.

However, among our CA-MRSA isolates the frequency of clindamycin resistance was high, and this empirical treatment should be discarded community (Kaplan *et al.*, 2005; Milheiriço *et al.*, 2007). This fact seems to match with the observed before that the CA- MRSA strains are gradually becoming entrenched as nosocomial pathogens, and that both CA-MRSA and HA-MRSA strains now circulate in both environments (David *et al.*, 2008; Salgado *et al.*, 2003). Also, it has been determined that the MRSA colonization can persist for months or years, so an infection can develop in a different setting from the one in which the organism was initially acquired (Salgado *et al.*, 2003). For all these reasons, in order to apply the appropriate treatment, and to prevent MRSA infections, it is indispensable that prevention guidelines include the routine determination of at least the genetic background for each MRSA isolate, the antimicrobial susceptibility profile and the PVL genes (Kazakova *et al.*, 2005; Ruimy *et al.*, 2008; Pérez-Roth *et al.*, 2006, 2010, 2011; Udo *et al.*, 1993).

# Acknowledgment

We thank Santiago Basaldua Lemarchand for his mathematical support and Joao Carriço for his helpful availability. This work was partially supported by grants FIS06/0002 and FIS10/00125 from the INSTITUTO DE SALUD CARLOSIII (Spanish Health Ministry) to S.M.-A. We thank the MAPFRE Foundation and COFARTE, a pharmaceutical company from Tenerife, for their founding contributions for the development of this study. B.R.-P. was supported partially by the MAPFRE Foundation and by COFARTE.

# References

Abramson, M. A., and D. J. Sexton. 1999. Nosocomial methicillin-resistant and methicillin-susceptible Staphylococcus aureus primary bacteremia: at what costs? Infect. Control Hosp. Epidemiol. 20:408–411.

Broseta, A., Chaves, F., Rojo, P., Otero, J.R. 2006. Emergence of a single clone of community-associated methicillin-resistant Staphylococcus aureus in southern Madrid children. Enferm. Infecc. Microbiol. Clin. 24: 31-35.

Carriço, J.A., C. Silva.Costa, J. Melo-Cristino, F.R. Pinto, H. De Lencastre, J.S. Almeida, M. Ramirez. 2006. Illustration of a common framework for relating multiple typing methods by application to Macrolide-Resistant Streptococcus pyogenes. J. Clin. Microbiol. 44: 2524-2532.

Centres for Disease Control and Prevention (CDC). January 2010, posting date. Community associated MRSA information for clinicians. Infection control topics. http://www.cdc.gov/ncidod/dhqp/ar_mrsa_ca_clinicians.html.

Cercenado, E., Cuevas, O., Marín, M., Bouza, E., Trincado, P., Boquete, T., Padilla, B., Vindel, A. 2008. Community-acquired methicillin-resistant Staphylococcus aureus in Madrid, Spain: transcontinental importation and polyclonal emergence of Panton-Valentine leukocidin-positive isolates. Diagn. Microbiol. Infect. Dis. 61: 143-149.

Cercenado, E., Ruiz de Gopegui, E. 2008. Community-acquired methicillin-resistant Staphylococcus aureus. Enferm. Infecc. Microbiol. Clin. 26: 19-24.

Chaberny, I. F., F. Schwab, S. Ziesing, S. Suerbaum, and P. Gastmeier. 2008. Impact of routine surgical ward and intensive care unit admission surveillance cultures on hospital-wide nosocomial methicillin-resistant Staphylococcus aureus infections in a university hospital: an interrupted time-series analysis. J. Antimicrob. Chemother. 62:1422–1429.

Clinical and Laboratory Standards Institute. 2007. Performance standards for antimicrobial susceptibility testing; 17th informational supplement. Clinical and Laboratory Standards Institute, Wayne, PA. CLSI M100-S17.

Criso´stomo, M. I., H. Westh, A. Tomasz, M. Chung, D. C. Oliveira, and H. de Lencastre. 2001. The evolution of methicillin resistance in Staphylococcus aureus: similarity of genetic backgrounds in historically early methicillinsusceptible and -resistant isolates and contemporary epidemic clones. Proc. Natl. Acad. Sci. U. S. A. 98:9865–9870.

Crossley, K., B. Landsman, and D. Zaske. 1979. An outbreak of infections caused by strains of Staphylococcus aureus resistant to methicillin and aminoglycosides. II. Epidemiologic studies. J. Infect. Dis. 139:280–287.

Daskalaki, M.P., Rojo, P., Marin-Ferrer, M., Barrios, M., Otero, J.R., Chaves, F. 2010. Panton–Valentine leukocidin-positive Staphylococcus aureus skin and soft tissue infections among children in an emergency department in Madrid, Spain. Clin. Microbiol. Infec. 16: 74-77.

David, M.Z., Glikman, D., Crawford, S.E., Peng, J., King, K.J., Hostetler, M.A., Boyle- Vavra, S., Daum, R.S. 2008. What is Community-associated methicillin-resistant Staphylococcus aureus? J. Infect. Dis. 197 : 1235-1243.

Dufour, P., Gillet, Y., Bes, M., Lina, G., Vandenesch, F., Floret, D., Etienne, J., Richet, H. 2002. Community-acquired methicillin-resistant Staphylococcus aureus infections in France: Emergence of a single clone that produces Panton-Valentine Leukocidin. Clin. Infect. Dis. 35: 819-824.

El Helali, N., A. Carbonne, T. Naas, S. Kerneis, O. Fresco, Y. Giovangrandi, N. Fortineau, P. Nordmann, and P. Astagneau. 2005. Nosocomial outbreak of staphylococcal scalded skin syndrome in neonates: epidemiological investigation and control. J. Hosp. Infect. 61:130–138.

Enright, M.C., D.A. Robinson, G. Randle, E.J. Feil, H. Grundmann, B.G. Spratt. 2002. The evolutionary history of methicillin-resistant Staphylococcus aureus (MRSA). Proc. Natl. Acad. Sci. U S A. 99: 7687-7692.

Enright, M.C., Day, N.P., Davies, C.E., Peacock, S.J., Spratt, B.G. 2000. Multilocus sequence typing for characterization of methicillin-resistant and methicillin susceptible clones of Staphylococcus aureus. J. Clin. Microbiol. 38: 1008-1015.

Eriksen, K.R., and I. Erichsen. 1963. Clinical occurrence of methicillinresistant strains of Staphylococcus aureus. Ugeskr. Laeg. 125:1234–1240.

Faria, N.A., Oliveira, D.C., Westh, H., Monnet, D.L., Larsen, A.R., Skov, R., de Lencastre, H. 2005. Epidemiology of emerging methicillin-resistant Staphylococcus aureus (MRSA) in Denmark: a nationwide study in a country with low prevalence of MRSA infection. J. Clin. Microbiol. 43: 1836-1842.

Feil, E.J., J.E. Cooper, H. Grundmann, D.A. Robinson, M.C. Enright, T. Berendt, S.J. Peacock, J.M. Smith, M. Murphy, B.G. Spratt, C.E. Moore, N.P. Day. 2003. How clonal is Staphylococcus aureus? J. Bacteriol. 185: 3307-3316.

Gould, I.M. 2006. Costs of hospital-acquired methicillin-resistant Staphylococcus aureus (MRSA) and its control. Int. J. Antimicrob. Agents. 28: 379-384.

Grundmann, H., S. Hori, G. Tanner. 2001. Determining confidence intervals when measuring genetic diversity and the discriminatory abilities of typing methods for microorganisms. J. Clin. Microbiol. 39: 4190-4192.

Harmsen, D., Claus, H., Witte, W., Rothganger, J., Claus, H., Turnwald, D., Vogel, U. 2003. Typing of methicillin-resistant Staphylococcus aureus in a university hospital setting by using novel software for spa repeat determination and database management. J. Clin. Microbiol. 41: 5442-5448.

Holmes, A., Ganner, M., McGuane, S., Pitt, T.L., Cookson, B.D., Kearns, A.M. 2005. Staphylococcus aureus isolates carrying Panton-Valentine Leucocidin genes in England and Wales: Frequency, characterization, and association with clinical disease. J. Clin. Microbiol. 43: 2384-2390.

Huang, S. S., D. S. Yokoe, V. L. Hinrichsen, L. S. Spurchise, R. Datta, I. Miroshnik, and R. Platt. 2006. Impact of routine intensive care unit surveillance cultures and resultant barrier precautions on hospital-wide methicillinresistant Staphylococcus aureus bacteremia. Clin. Infect. Dis. 43: 971–978.

Hubert, L., and P. Arabie. 1985. Comparing partitions. J. Classification 2: 193–218.

Hunter, P. R., and M. A. Gaston. 1988. Numerical index of the discriminatory ability of typing systems: an application of Simpson's index of diversity. J. Clin. Microbiol. 26: 2465–2466.

Kaplan, S.L. 2005. Treatment of community-associated methicillin-resistant Staphylococcus aureus infections. Pediatr. Infect. Dis. J. 24: 457-458.

Kazakova, S.V., Hageman, J.C., Matava, M., Srinivasan, A., Phelan, L., Garfinkel, B., Boo, T., McAllister, S., Anderson, J., Jensen, B., Dodson, D., Lonsway, D., McDougal, L.K., Arduino, M., Fraser, V.J., Killgore, G., Tenover, F.C., Cody, S., Jernigan, D.B. 2005. A clone of methicillin-resistant Staphylococcus aureus among professional football players. N. Engl. J. Med. 352: 468-475.

López-Aguilar, C., Perez-Roth, E., Moreno A, Duran MC, Casanova C, Aguirre-Jaime A, Mendez-Alvarez, S. 2007. Association between the presence of the Panton-Valentine leukocidin-encoding gene and a lower rate of survival among hospitalized pulmonary patients with staphylococcal disease. J Clin Microbiol. 45: 274-276.

Malachowa, N., A. Sabat, M. Gniadkowski, J. Krzyszton-Russjan, J. Empel, J. Miedzobrodzki, K. Kosowska-Shick, P. C. Appelbaum, and W. Hryniewicz. 2005. Comparison of multiple-locus variable-number tandem repeat analysis with pulsed-field gel electrophoresis, spa typing and multilocus sequence typing for clonal characterization of Staphylococcus aureus isolates. J. Clin. Microbiol. 43: 3095–3100.

Manzur, A., Domínguez, A.M., Pujol, M., González, M.P., Limón, E., Hornero, A., Martín, R., Gudiol, F., Ariza, J. 2008. Community-acquired methicillin-resistant Staphylococcus aureus infections: an emerging threat in Spain. Clin. Microbiol. Infect. 14: 377-380.

Melles, D. C., L. Schouls, P. Franc¸ois, S. Herzig, H. A. Verbrugh, A. van Belkum, and J. Schrenzel. 2009. High-throughput typing of Staphylococcus aureus by amplified fragment length polymorphism (AFLP) or multi-locus variable number of tandem repeat analysis (MLVA) reveals consistent strain relatedness. Eur. J. Clin. Microbiol. Infect. Dis. 28: 39–45.

Milheiriço, C., Oliveira, D.C., de Lencastre, H. 2007. Update to the multiplex PCR strategy for assignment of mec element types in Staphylococcus aureus. Antimicrob. Agents Chemother. 51: 3374-3377.

Moran, G.J., Amii, R.N., Abrahamian, F.M., Talan, D.A. 2005. Methicillin-resistant Staphylococcus aureus in community-acquired skin infections. Emerg. Infect. Dis. 11: 928-930.

Moser, S. A., M. J. Box, M. Patel, M. Amaya, R. Schelonka, and K. B. Waites. 2009. Multiple-locus variable-number tandem-repeat analysis of methicillinresistant Staphylococcus aureus discriminates within U. S. A. pulsed-field gel electrophoresis types. J. Hosp. Infect. 71: 333–339.

Naimi, T.S., LeDell, K.H., Como-Sabetti, K., Borchardt, S.M., Boxrud, D.J., Etienne, J., Johnson, S.K., Vandenesch, F., Fridkin, S., O'Boyle, C., Danila, R.N., Lynfield, R. 2003. Comparison of community- and health care-associated methicillin resistant Staphylococcus aureus infection. JAMA. 290: 2976-2984.

O'Brien, F.G., Coombs, G.W., Pearman, J.W., Gracey, M., Moss, F., Christiansen, K.J., Grubb, W.B. 2009. Population dynamics of methicillin-susceptible and –resistant Staphylococcus aureus in remote communities. J. Antimicrob. Chemother. 64: 684-693.

Oliveira, D.C., de Lencastre, H. 2002. Multiplex PCR strategy for rapid identification of structural types and variantes of the mec element in methicillin-resistant Staphylococcus aureus. Antimicrob. Agents Chemother. 46: 2155-2161.

Pérez-Roth E, Armas-González E, Alcoba-Flórez J, Méndez-Álvarez S. 2011. PCR-based amplification of heterogeneous IS257-ileS2 junctions for molecular monitoring of high-level mupirocin resistance in staphylococci. J Antimicrob Chemother. 66: 471-475.

Pérez-Roth E, Kwong SM, Alcoba-Florez J, Firth N, Méndez-Alvarez S. 2010. Complete nucleotide sequence and comparative analysis of pPR9, a 41.7-kilobase conjugative staphylococcal multiresistance plasmid conferring high-level mupirocin resistance. Antimicrob Agents Chemother. 54:2252-2257.

Pérez-Roth E, López-Aguilar C, Alcoba-Florez J, Méndez-Alvarez S. 2006. High-level mupirocin resistance within methicillin-resistant Staphylococcus aureus pandemic lineages. Antimicrob Agents Chemother. 50: 3207-3211.

Pérez-Roth E, Lorenzo-Díaz F, Méndez-Alvarez S. 2003. Establishment and clonal dissemination of the methicillin-resistant Staphylococcus aureus UK-16 epidemic strain in a Spanish hospital. J. Clin. Microbiol. 41: 5353.

Pérez-Roth, E., Alcoba-Flórez, J., López-Aguilar, C., Rivero-Pérez, B., Gutiérrez- González, I., Méndez-Álvarez, S. 2010. A case of familial furunculosis associated to community-acquired leukocidin-positive methicillin-susceptible Staphylococcus aureus ST152. J. Clin. Microbiol. 48: 329-332.

Pérez-Roth, E., Claverie-Martín, F., Villar, J., Méndez-Alvarez, S. 2001. Multiplex PCR for simultaneous identification of Staphylococcus aureus and detection of methicillin and mupirocin resistance. J. Clin. Microbiol. 39: 4037-4041.

Pérez-Roth, E., Lorenzo-Díaz, F., Batista, N., Moreno, A., Méndez-Álvarez, S. 2004. Tracking methicillin-resistant Staphylococcus aureus clones during a 5-year period (1998 to 2002) in a Spanish hospital. J. Clin. Microbiol. 42: 4649-4656.

Pinto, F.R., J. Melo-Cristino, M. Ramírez. 2008. A confidence interval for the Wallace coefficient of concordance and its application to microbial typing methods. PLoS One. 3: e3696.

Pinto, F.R., J.A. Carriço, M. Ramirez, J.S. Almeida. 2007. Ranked Adjusted Rand: integrating distance and partition information in a measure of clustering agreement. BMC Bioinformatics. 8: 44.

Rand, W.M. 1971. Objective criteria for the evaluation of clustering methods. J. Am. Stat. Assoc. 66: 846-850.

Ribeiro, A., Dias, C., Silva-Carvalho, M.C., Berquó, L., Ferreira, F.A., Santos, R.N., Ferreira-Carvalho, B.T., Figueiredo, A.M. 2005. First Report of Infection with Community-Acquired Methicillin-Resistant Staphylococcus aureus in South America. J. Clin. Microbiol. 43: 1985-1988.

Rivero-Pérez, B., Alcoba-Florez, J., Méndez-Álvarez, S. 2012. Genetic diversity of community-associated methicillin-resistant Staphylococcus aureus isolated from Tenerife Island, Spain. Infect Genet Evol. 12: 586-590.

Rivero-Pérez, B., Pérez-Roth, E., Méndez-Álvarez, S. 2010. Evaluation of multiplelocus variable-number tandem-repeat analysis for typing a polyclonal hospital acquired methicillin-resistant Staphylococcus aureus population in an area where such infections are endemic. J. Clin. Microbiol. 48: 2991-2994.

Rossney, A.S., Shore, A.C., Morgan, P.M., Fitzgibbon, M.M., O'Connell, B., Coleman, D.C. 2007. The emergence and importation of diverse genotypes of methicillinresistant Staphylococcus aureus (MRSA) harboring the Panton-

Valentine Leukocidin gene (pvl) reveal that pvl is a poor marker for community-acquired MRSA strains in Ireland. J. Clin. Microbiol. 45: 2554-2563.

Ruimy, R., A. Maiga, L. Armand-Lefevre, I. Maiga, A. Diallo, A. K. Koumaré, K. Ouattara, S. Soumaré, K. Gaillard, J. C. Lucet, A. Andremont, and E. J. Feil. 2008. The carriage population of Staphylococcus aureus from Mali is composed of a combination of pandemic clones and the divergent Panton-Valentine leukocidin-positive genotype ST152. J. Bacteriol. 190: 3962-3968.

Sabat AJ, Chlebowicz MA, Grundmann H, Arends JP, Kampinga G, Meessen NE, Friedrich AW, van Dijl JM. 2012. Microfluidic-Chip-Based Multiple-Locus Variable-Number Tandem-Repeat Fingerprinting with New Primer Sets for Methicillin-Resistant Staphylococcus aureus. J. Clin Microbiol. 50:2255-2262.

Sabat, A., J. Krzyszton-Russjan, W. Strzalka, R. Filipek, K. Kosowska, W. Hryniewicz, J. Travis, and J. Potempa. 2003. New method for typing Staphylococcus aureus strains: multiple-locus variable-number tandem-repeat analysis of polymorphism and genetic relationships of clinical isolates. J. Clin. Microbiol. 41: 1801–1804.

Salgado, C.D., Farr, B.M., Calfee, D.P. 2003. Community-acquired methicillin-resistant Staphylococcus aureus: a meta-analysis of prevalence and risk factors. Clin. Infect. Dis. 36: 131-139.

Shore, A.C., Brennan, O.M., Ehricht, R., Monecke, S., Schwarz, S., Slickers, P., Coleman, D.C. 2010. Identification and characterization of the multidrug resistance gene cfr in a Panton-Valentine leukocidin-positive sequence type 8 methicillin-resistant Staphylococcus aureus IVa (USA300) isolate. Antimicrob. Agents Chemother. 54: 4978-4984.

Simpson, E. H. 1949. Measurement of species diversity. Nature 163: 688.

Sobral D, Schwarz S, Bergonier D, Brisabois A, Feßler AT, Gilbert FB, Kadlec K, Lebeau B, Loisy-Hamon F, Treilles M, Pourcel C, Vergnaud G. 2012. High throughput multiple locus variable number of tandem repeat analysis (MLVA) of Staphylococcus aureus from human, animal and food sources. PLoS One 7: e33967.

Takizawa, Y., Taneike, I., Nakagawa, S., Oishi, T., Nitahara, Y., Iwakura, N., Ozaki, K., Takano, M., Nakayama, T., Yamamoto, T. 2005. A Panton-Valentine Leucocidin (PVL)-positive community-acquired methicillin-resistant Staphylococcus aureus (MRSA) strain, another such strain carrying a multiple drug resistance plasmid, and other more-typical PVL-negative MRSA strains found in Japan. J. Clin. Microbiol. 43: 3356-3363.

Tenover, F. C., R. R. Vaughn, L. K. McDougal, G. E. Fosheim, and J. E. McGowan, Jr. 2007. Multiple-locus variable-number tandem-repeat assay analysis of methicillin-resistant Staphylococcus aureus strains. J. Clin. Microbiol. 45: 2215–2219.

Tenover, F.C., Arbeit, R.D., Goering, R.V., Mickelsen, P.A., Murray, B.E., Persing, D.H., Swaminathan, B. 1995. Interpreting chromosomal DNA restriction patterns produced by pulsed-field gel electrophoresis: criteria for bacterial strain typing. J. Clin. Microbiol. 33: 2233-2239.

Trindade, P.A., J.A. McCulloch, G.A. Oliveira, E.M. Mamizuka. 2003. Molecular Techniques for MRSA Typing: Current Issues and Perspectives. Braz. J. Infect. Dis. 7: 32-43.

Udo, E.E., Pearman, J.W., Grubb, W.B. 1993. Genetic analysis of community isolates of methicillin-resistant Staphylococcus aureus in Western Australia. J. Hosp. Infect. 25: 97-108.

Vandenesch, F., Naimi, T., Enright, M.C., Lina, G., Nimmo, G.R., Heffernan, H., Liassine, N., Bes, M., Greenland, T., Reverdy, M.E., Etienne, J. 2003. Community-acquired methicillin-resistant Staphylococcus aureus carrying Panton-Valentine leukocidin genes: worldwide emergence. Emerg. Infect. Dis. 9: 978-984.

Wallace, D.L. 1983. A method for comparing two hierarchical clusterings: comment. J. Am. Stat. Assoc. 78: 569-576.

# Sorting Genomes by Rearrangements and Its Application to Phylogeny Reconstruction

Chin Lung Lu
*Department of Computer Science*
*National Tsing Hua University, Taiwan*

Chuan Yi Tang
*Department of Computer Science and Information Engineering*
*Providence University, Taiwan*
*Department of Computer Science*
*National Tsing Hua University, Taiwan*

# 1   Introduction

During evolution, the gene order in a genome is generally not well conserved, because it is subject to be changed by rearrangements, such as reversals (Bafna & Pevzner, 1996; Hannenhalli & Pevzner, 1999; Kaplan et al., 1999; Bader et al., 2001), transpositions (Bafna & Pevzner, 1998; Hartman & Sharan, 2005; Elias & Hartman, 2006), block-interchanges (Christie, 1996; Lin et al., 2005; Huang et al., 2010a), fusions/fissions (Lu et al., 2006) and translocations (Kececioglu & Ravi, 1995; Hannenhalli, 1996; Bergeron et al., 2006a). The studies for analyzing the differences between the gene orders of a set of species genomes have been increasingly recognized as a useful tool in phylogenetic tree reconstruction, because they have helped biologists to gain a better understanding of the evolution of several groups of genomes, such as animal mitochondria (Blanchette et al., 1999; Xu et al., 2006), bacteria (Suyama & Bork, 2001; Belda et al., 2005) and mammals (Bourque & Pevzner, 2002; Zhao & Bourque, 2009). The combinatorial problems considered in these studies, typically called *genome rearrangement problems*, can be formulated as follows. Given the gene (or synteny block) orders of a set of genomes, each represented by a signed permutation, and a set of possible rearrangements, the problem aims to find a shortest series of rearrangements (or a series of rearrangements with minimum weight when rearrangements are weighted according to the probabilities of their occurrences) required to transform (or sort) those genomes into one another (Fertin et al., 2009). The length (or weight) of an optimal series of rearrangements is then called *genome rearrangement distance*. The genome rearrangement distance can serve as a measure of an evolutionary distance between species. In contrast to the sequence-based approaches in which local mutations (i.e., substitutions, insertions and deletions of nucleotides/amino acids) accumulate rather quickly, genome rearrangements are global (or large-scale) and relatively rare mutations and, therefore, their distances are believed to allow for evolutionary reconstructions of more divergent species.

## 1.1   Rearrangement Operations

The genome rearrangements studied in the literature to date can be classified into two categories: (i) *intra-chromosomal* rearrangements, such as reversals (also called *inversions* in biology), transpositions and block-interchanges (here also called *generalized transpositions*), and (ii) *inter-chromosomal* rearrangements, such as fusions, fissions and translocations (see Figure 1 for graphical illustration). *Reversals* reverse a segment on a chromosome and also exchange its strands. *Transpositions* move a segment on a chromosome to another location or, equivalently, exchange two adjacent and non-overlapping segments on the chromosome. *Block-interchanges* are a kind of generalized transpositions that exchange two non-overlapping but not necessarily adjacent segments on a chromosome. *Fusions* join two chromosomes into a bigger one and *fissions* break a chromosome into two smaller ones. *Translocations* exchange an end segment of a chromosome, which contains a telomere of this chromosome, with an end segment of another chromosome. Notice that translocations are equivalent to fusions for circular chromosomes (Alekseyev, 2008; Alekseyev & Pevzner, 2008). However, for linear chromosomes, fusions and fissions are just special cases of translocation that either act on two chromosomes one of which is empty (i.e., fissions), or result in two chromosomes one of which is empty (i.e., fusions).

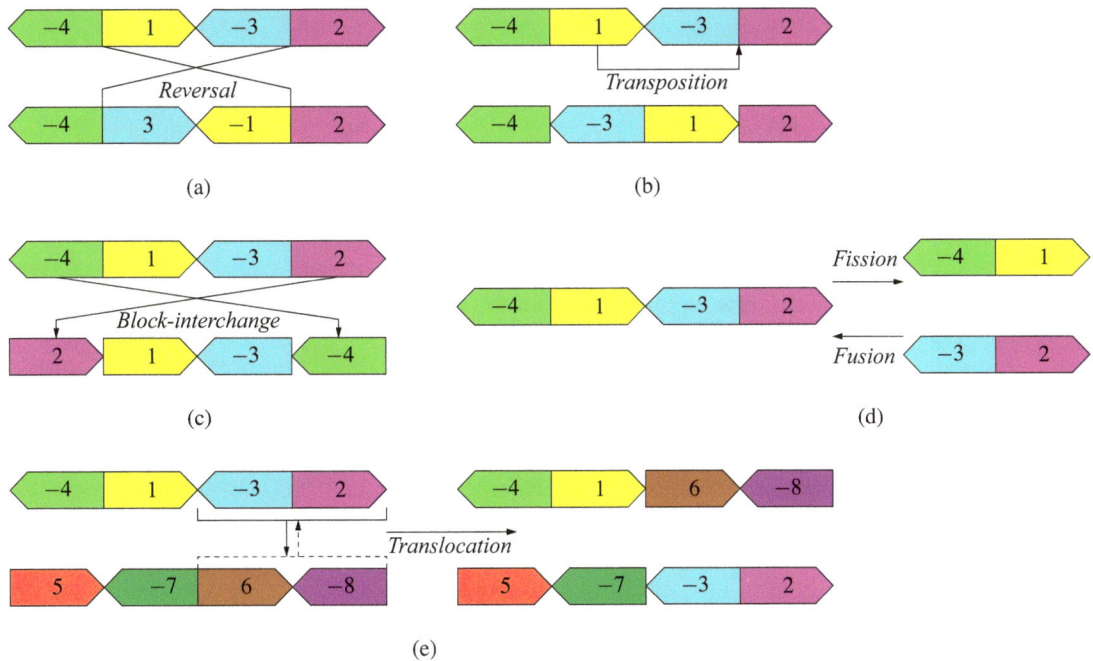

**Figure 1:** Chromosomal rearrangements: (a) reversal, (b) transposition, (c) block-interchange, (d) fission and fusion, and (e) translocation, where a gene (or marker or synteny block) is represented by a signed integer and the associated sign indicates the strandedness of the corresponding gene.

## 1.2    Double Cut and Join Operation

Yancopoulos et al. (Yancopoulos et al., 2005) have introduced and studied the so-called *double cut and join* (DCJ) operation, which cuts the chromosome(s) in two places and rejoins the four cut ends in a new way (see Figure 2), as a basis for modelling all the rearrangement operations described above. In this formulation, both reversals and translocations (including fusions and fissions) can be modelled by a DCJ operation, while block-interchanges (including transpositions) by two consecutive DCJ operations, one for generating a small circular chromosome from a chromosome and the other for re-incorporating this circular chromosome at a new site on the same chromosome. In addition, Yancopoulos et al. (Yancopoulos et al., 2005) designed an $\mathcal{O}(\delta n)$ time algorithm for sorting a genome with linear, multiple chromosomes by reversals, block-interchanges and translocations (including fusions and fissions) with the weight ratio 1:2:1, where $n$ is the number of genes to be considered and $\delta$ is the number of needed DCJ operations. Later on, Bergeron et al. (Bergeron et al., 2006b) reconsidered the DCJ model by allowing the small circular chromosome generated by a DCJ operation not necessarily to be re-incorporated immediately by the following DCJ operation. Since then, this re-formulated DCJ operation has received increased attention, because it can not only provide a unifying model for genome rearrangements, but also result in a relatively simple distance formula that can be calculated by a simpler algorithm (Lin & Moret, 2008; Bergeron et al., 2009).

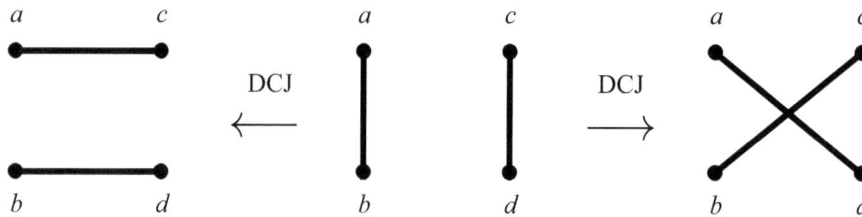

**Figure 2:** Illustration of the DCJ operation, where letters $a, b, c$ and $d$ denote gene ends and black lines denote connections between genes. After cutting two black lines in the middle genome, there are two ways to rejoin the four cut ends.

## 1.3    Multi-break Operation

Recently, Alekseyev and Pevzner (Alekseyev, 2008; Alekseyev & Pevzner, 2008) introduced a more general rearrangement model by defining a new and more powerful operation called *multi-break* operation (or simply *k-break*) acting on a breakpoint graph. Given two genomes, say $P$ (the initial genome) and $Q$ (the target genome), for a genome rearrangement problem, their *breakpoint graph* is an edge-colored graph $G(P,Q)$ defined as follows: (i) Each gene is represented by two vertices in $G(P,Q)$ that denote the two ends of the gene and are labelled as tail and head, respectively, where the direction from tail to head corresponds to the sign (strand) of the gene. (ii) There is a black (respectively, gray) edge to connect two vertices in $G(P,Q)$ if their corresponding gene ends are adjacent in $P$ (respectively, $Q$). Given $k$ black edges, forming a matching on $2k$ vertices, in a breakpoint graph, a *k-break* is defined as replacement of these edges with a set of $k$ black edges that form another matching on the same set of $2k$ vertices (see Figure 3 for an example of 2-break). Notice that an $h$ break is a special case of a $k$ break for $h < k$, in which case only $h$ edges are replaced and the others remain the same. Basically, reversals, translocations, fusions and fissions can be modelled by 2-breaks, while transpositions and block interchanges can be modelled by 3-breaks and 4-breaks, respectively. Although the $k$-break rearrangements may be unlikely to occur for $k > 3$ in chromosomal evolution, they can provide a unifying and simpler model for studying genome rearrangements. In fact, the 2-breaks are equivalent to the DCJ operations described above.

## 1.4    Web Servers of Genome Rearrangements

Currently, as listed in Table 1, there are several web servers that involve one or several of rearrangement operations, such as GRIMM (Tesler, 2002), MGR (Bourque & Pevzner, 2002), ROBIN (Lu et al., 2005), SPRING (Lin et al., 2006), DCJ (Bergeron et al., 2006b) and webMGR (Lin et al., 2010). More recently, we have proposed two novel algorithms (Huang & Lu, 2010) based on permutation groups in algebra to optimally sort a linear and a circular multi-chromosomal genome, respectively, by reversals, generalized transpositions and translocations (including fusions and fissions) in $\mathcal{O}(\delta n)$ time, where here $\delta$ is the minimum number of rearrangement operations that usually is much less than $n$. We have implemented these two algorithms into a novel web server called $\text{SoRT}^2$ (short for "<u>So</u>rting genomes by <u>R</u>eversals, generalized <u>T</u>ranspositions and <u>T</u>ranslocations") that allows the user to perform the analysis of genome rearrangements by calculating the genome rearrangement distance between any pair of input genomes and displaying a corresponding optimal scenario of rearrangement operations (Huang et al., 2010b). For more practical applications, we have also implemented and incorporated the following three related algorithms into the

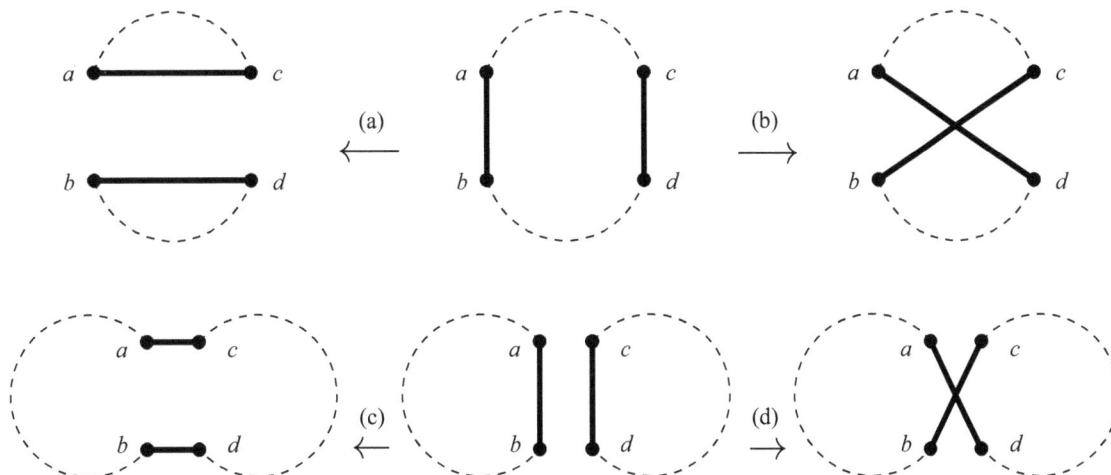

**Figure 3:** A 2-break operating on two edges $(a,b)$ and $(c,d)$ from a circular chromosome models a fission (a) or reversal (b), and a 2-break operating on two edges $(a,b)$ and $(c,d)$ from two different circular chromosomes models a translocation/fusion (c and d).

SoRT$^2$ web server: (i) sorting by reversals only (Kaplan et al., 1999), (ii) sorting by block-interchanges only (Lu et al., 2005), and (iii) sorting by reversals and block-interchanges (Lin et al., 2006; Huang & Lu, 2010). Moreover, we have equipped the SoRT$^2$ web server with the capability of inferring phylogenetic trees of multiple genomes being considered based on their pairwise genome rearrangement distances and the capability of evaluating the statistical reliability of the tree branches using the jackknife resampling approach (Farris et al., 1996). In this chapter, we shall first introduce the SoRT$^2$ web server, including its implementation and basic usage. Then we shall demonstrate the ability of the SoRT$^2$ tool in reconstruction of phylogenetic trees by testing it on some simulated datasets, as well as three biological datasets of gene orderings from mitochondrial, mammalian and bacterial genomes, respectively, and also comparing it to another similar tool GRIMM (Tesler, 2002). For simplicity, when we say "gene" in the rest of this chapter, it also means "marker" or "synteny block" that represents a conserved sequence region shared by all genomes to be considered.

| Web Server | URL | Year | Reference |
|---|---|---|---|
| GRIMM | http://grimm.ucsd.edu/GRIMM/ | 2002 | (Tesler, 2002) |
| MGR | http://grimm.ucsd.edu/MGR/ | 2002 | (Bourque & Pevzner, 2002) |
| ROBIN | http://genome.cs.nthu.edu.tw/ROBIN/ | 2005 | (Lu et al., 2005) |
| SPRING | http://algorithm.cs.nthu.edu.tw/tools/SPRING/ | 2006 | (Lin et al., 2006) |
| DCJ | http://bibiserv.techfak.uni-bielefeld.de/dcj/ | 2006 | (Bergeron et al., 2006b) |
| webMGR | http://webmgr.gis.a-star.edu.sg/ | 2010 | (Lin et al., 2010) |
| SoRT$^2$ | http://genome.cs.nthu.edu.tw/SORT2/ | 2010 | (Huang et al., 2010b) |

**Table 1:** Some currently exiting web servers of genome rearrangements.

## 2    Methods

The program of the SoRT$^2$ web server for sorting a multi-chromosomal genome (that can be linear or circular) into another using reversals, generalized transpositions and translocations (including fusions and fissions) was implemented based on the algorithms that we have recently proposed using permutation groups in algebra (Huang & Lu, 2010), where generalized transpositions are weighted 2 and the others are weighted 1. Usually, transpositions are observed much less frequently than reversals and translocations in many evolutionary scenarios (Yancopoulos et al., 2005; Blanchette et al., 1996). Blanchette et al. (Blanchette et al., 1996) have conducted experiments on real biological data to conclude that the most probable weights are 1 for reversals and 2 for transpositions. In addition, Eriksen (Eriksen, 2002) and his coworkers have used simulations to find that optimal weights for reversals and transpositions are 1 and 2, respectively. On the other hand, if the weight ratio between reversals and transpositions is 1:1, then transpositions are generally favored over reversals, because a reversal (or translocation) removes at most two breakpoints, while a transposition removes at most three breakpoints (and a generalized transposition four breakpoints) (Fertin et al., 2009). According to the above results and discussion, it seems to be biologically meaningful to assign at least twice the weight to generalized transpositions than to the others. However, if generalized transpositions are at least three times the weight of reversals, then there is always an optimal solution for the problem that contains nothing but only reversals and translocations, because a generalized transposition (block-interchange) can be mimicked by three reversals. For example, three consecutive genes $(x, y, z)$ can be transformed into $(z, y, x)$ by a block-interchange or by three reversals with scenario of $(x, -z, -y)$, $(z, -x, -y)$ and $(z, y, x)$. Therefore, it should be reasonable to assign generalized transpositions a weight equal to 2 and the others a weight equal to 1.

### 2.1    Permutation Groups

Permutation groups have been proved to be a useful tool in the study of genome rearrangements (Lin et al., 2005; Lu et al., 2006; Huang et al., 2010a; Huang & Lu, 2010; Huang et al., 2011). Given a set $E = \{1, 2, \ldots, n\}$, a *permutation* is defined to be a one-to-one function from $E$ into itself and usually expressed as a product of cycles. For instance, as illustrated in Figure 4, $\alpha = (1, 3, 2)(4)(5, 6)$ is a product of three cycles to represent a permutation of $E = \{1, 2, \ldots, 6\}$ and means that $\alpha(1) = 3, \alpha(3) = 2, \alpha(2) = 1, \alpha(4) = 4, \alpha(5) = 6$ and $\alpha(6) = 5$. The elements in a cycle can be arranged in any cyclic order and hence the cycle $(5, 6)$ in the permutation $\alpha$ exemplified above can be rewritten as $(6, 5)$. Moreover, if the cycles in a permutation are all disjoint (i.e., no common element in any two cycles), then the product of these cycles is called the *cycle decomposition* of the permutation. Notice that a permutation in the cycle decomposition can be used to model a genome containing several circular chromosomes, with each disjoint cycle representing a circular chromosome (see Figure 4 for an example). A cycle with $k$ elements is further called a $k$-cycle. In convention, the 1-cycles in a permutation are not written explicitly since their elements are *fixed* in the permutation. For instance, the above exemplified permutation $\alpha$ can be written as $\alpha = (1, 3, 2)(5, 6)$. If the cycles in a permutation are all 1-cycles, then this permutation is called an *identity permutation* and denoted by **1**. Suppose that $\alpha$ and $\beta$ are two permutations of $E$. Then their product $\alpha\beta$, also called their *composition*, defines a permutation of $E$ satisfying $\alpha\beta(x) = \alpha(\beta(x))$ for all $x \in E$. If both $\alpha$ and $\beta$ are disjoint, then $\alpha\beta = \beta\alpha$. If $\alpha\beta = \mathbf{1}$, then $\alpha$ is called the *inverse* of $\beta$, denoted by $\beta^{-1}$, and vice versa. Moreover, the *conjugation* of $\beta$ by $\alpha$, denoted by $\alpha \cdot \beta$, is defined to be the permutation $\alpha\beta\alpha^{-1}$. It can be verified that if $y = \beta(x)$, then $\alpha(y) = \alpha \cdot \beta(\alpha(x))$. Hence, $\alpha \cdot \beta$ can be obtained from $\beta$ by just changing its element $x$ with $\alpha(x)$. In other words, if $\beta = (b_1, b_2, \ldots, b_k)$, then $\alpha \cdot \beta = (\alpha(b_1), \alpha(b_2), \ldots, \alpha(b_k))$.

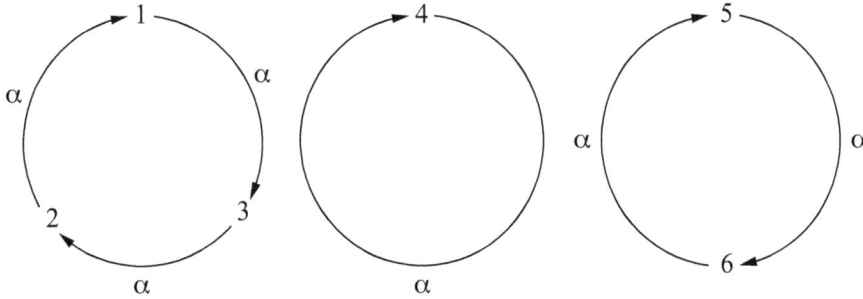

**Figure 4:** A permutation $\alpha = (1,3,2)(4)(5,6)$ in the cycle decomposition, which can be used to represent a genome with three circular chromosomes.

It is a fact that every permutation can be expressed into a product of 2-cycles, in which 1-cycles are still written implicitly. Given a permutation $\alpha$ of $E$, its *norm*, denoted by $\|\alpha\|$, is defined to be the minimum number, say $k$, such that $\alpha$ can be expressed as a product of $k$ 2-cycles. In the cycle decomposition of $\alpha$, let $n_c(\alpha)$ denote the number of its disjoint cycles, notably including the 1-cycles not written explicitly. Given two permutations $\alpha$ and $\beta$ of $E$, $\alpha$ is said to *divide* $\beta$, denoted by $\alpha|\beta$, if and only if $\|\beta\alpha^{-1}\| = \|\beta\| - \|\alpha\|$. In (Huang & Lu, 2010), it has been shown that $\|\alpha\| = |E| - n_c(\alpha)$ and for any $k$ elements in $E$, say $a_1, a_2, \ldots, a_k$, they all appear in a cycle of $\alpha$ in the ordering of $a_1, a_2, \ldots, a_k$ if and only if $(a_1, a_2, \ldots, a_k)|\alpha$. Let $\alpha = (a_1, a_2)$ be a 2-cycle and $\beta$ be an arbitrary permutation of $E$. If $\alpha|\beta$, that is, both $a_1$ and $a_2$ appear in the same cycle of $\beta$, then the composition $\alpha\beta$, as well as $\beta\alpha$, has the effect of fission by breaking this cycle into two smaller cycles. For instance, let $\alpha = (1,3)$ and $\beta = (1,2,3,4)$. Then $\alpha|\beta$, since both 1 and 3 are in the cycle $(1,2,3,4)$, and $\alpha\beta = (1,2)(3,4)$ and $\beta\alpha = (4,1)(2,3)$. On the other hand, if $\alpha \nmid \beta$, that is, $a_1$ and $a_2$ appear in different cycles of $\beta$, then $\alpha\beta$, as well as $\beta\alpha$, has the effect of fusion by joining the two cycles into a bigger cycle. For example, if $\alpha = (1,3)$ and $\beta = (1,2)(3,4)$, then $\alpha \nmid \beta$ and, as a result, $\alpha\beta = (1,2,3,4)$ and $\beta\alpha = (2,1,4,3)$.

## 2.2   A Model for Representing DNA Molecules

To model a double-stranded DNA, we first let $E = \{-1, 1, -2, 2, \ldots, -n, -n\}$ and $\Gamma = (1,-1)(2,-2)\ldots(n,-n)$. We then use an *admissible* cycle $\pi_1$, which is a cycle containing no $i$ and its opposite $-i$ simultaneously for some $i \in E$, to represent a DNA strand, and use $\pi_2 = \Gamma \cdot \pi_1^{-1}$, which is the *reverse complement* of $\pi_1$, to represent the opposite strand of $\pi_1$. As demonstrated in (Huang & Lu, 2010), it is useful to represent a double stranded DNA $\pi$ by the product of its two strands $\pi_1$ and $\pi_2$, that is, $\pi = \pi_1\pi_2 = \pi_2\pi_1$, because we can model elementary rearrangement operations acting on $\pi$ in a simple way as follows. Notice that this representation of a DNA molecule (or chromosome) can certainly be applied to a genome with multiple chromosomes.

- $(v, \pi\Gamma(u))(u, \pi\Gamma(v))$ acts on $\pi$ as a reversal, if $u$ and $v$ are in the same strand of $\pi$, that is, $(u,v)|\pi$.

- $(v,x)(u,w)(\pi\Gamma(x), \pi\Gamma(v))(\pi\Gamma(w), \pi\Gamma(u))$ acts on $\pi$ as a block-interchange, if $u, v, w$ and $x$ are in the same strand of $\pi$ in this order, that is, $(u,v,w,x)|\pi$.

- $(u,v)(\pi\Gamma(v),\pi\Gamma(u))$ acts on $\pi$ as a fission, if $u$ and $v$ are in the same strand of $\pi$, that is, $(u,v)|\pi$.

- $(u,v)(\pi\Gamma(v),\pi\Gamma(u))$ acts on $\pi$ as a fusion, if $u$ and $v$ are in different chromosomes of $\pi$, that is, $(u,v) \dagger \pi$ and $(u,\Gamma(v)) \dagger \pi$.

- $(u,w)(v,x)(\pi\Gamma(w),\pi\Gamma(u))(\pi\Gamma(x),\pi\Gamma(v))$ acts on $\pi$ as a translocation, if $u$ and $v$ are in the same strand of $\pi$ (i.e., $(u,v)|\pi$), $w$ and $x$ are also in the same strand of $\pi$ (i.e., $(w,x)|\pi$), and $u$ and $w$ are at the ends of $\pi$.

## 2.3   Algorithms for Sorting by Weighted Reversals, Block-Interchanges and Translocations

As mentioned early, translocations and fusions are not distinguishable for circular chromosomes and hence the problem of sorting a circular, multi-chromosomal genome $\Pi$ into another circular, multi-chromosomal genome $\Sigma$ by reversals, block-interchanges and translocations (including fusions and fissions) is equivalent to that of sorting by reversals, block-interchanges, fusions and fissions. Suppose that block-interchanges are weighted 2 and the others are all weighted 1. Then according to our previous work in (Lu et al., 2006), it is not hard to show that in this case there is an optimal scenario of events to transform $\Pi$ into $\Sigma$ in the so-called *canonical order*, in which all fusions come before all reversals/block-interchanges, which then come before all fissions. In addition, it can be shown that we can derive a minimum series of 2-cycles from $\Sigma\Pi^{-1}$, acting on $\Pi$ as fusions, to transform $\Pi$ into $\Pi'$, and then derive a minimum series of 2-cycle from $\Pi'\Sigma^{-1}$, acting on $\Sigma$ as fusions, to transform $\Sigma$ into $\Sigma'$ (conversely, these fusions become fissions for transforming $\Sigma'$ into $\Sigma$), and finally derive a minimum weighted series of reversals and block-interchanges from $\Sigma'\Pi'^{-1}$ to transform $\Pi'$ into $\Sigma'$ using the algorithm we proposed in (Huang & Lu, 2010). All of the above procedures actually can be done in $\mathcal{O}(\delta n)$ time, where $\delta$ is the number of fusions, reversals, block-interchanges and fissions needed to transform $\Pi$ into $\Sigma$. In other words, given two circular, multi-chromosomal genomes $\Pi$ and $\Sigma$, the problem of sorting $\Pi$ into $\Sigma$ by using a minimum weighted sequence of reversals, block-interchanges and fusions (or, equivalently, translocations) and fissions can be solved in $\mathcal{O}(\delta n)$ time, where block-interchanges are weighted 2 and the others are weighted 1. On the other hand, for linear chromosomes, fusions and fissions are special cases of translocations. In this case, we still can design an $\mathcal{O}(\delta n)$ time algorithm on the basis of the permutation groups to sort a linear, multi-chromosomal genome $\Pi$ into another $\Sigma$ by reversals, block-interchanges and translocations (including fusions and fissions) with a weight proportion 1:2:1. For details, we refer the reader to our paper (Huang & Lu, 2010).

## 2.4   Tool Implementation and Usage

We have implemented the above algorithms in (Huang & Lu, 2010) into a web server called SoRT[2] (short for "Sorting genomes by Reversals, generalized Transpositions and Translocations") that allows the user to perform the analysis of genome rearrangements by calculating the genome rearrangement distance between any pair of input genomes and displaying a corresponding optimal scenario of rearrangement operations (Huang et al., 2010b). For more practical applications, we have also implemented and incorporated the following three related algorithms into the SoRT[2] web server: (i) the algorithm proposed by Kaplan et al. (Kaplan et al., 1999) for sorting by reversals only, (ii) the algorithm of our ROBIN (Lu et al., 2005) for sorting by block-interchanges only, and (iii) the redesigned algorithm of our SPRING (Lin et al., 2006) for sorting by reversals and block-interchanges based on permutation groups (Huang & Lu, 2010). Furthermore, we have equipped our SoRT[2] with the capability of inferring the phylogenetic tree of multiple genomes being considered based on their pairwise genome rearrangement distances using distance-based approaches of building trees, such as neighbor-joining (NJ) method (Saitou & Nei, 1987), unweighted pair group method with arithmetic mean (UPGMA) method (Sokal & Michener, 1958) and Fitch-Margoliash (FM) method (Fitch & Margolia.E, 1967). Finally, we have also adopted the jackknife resampling approach (Farris et al., 1996), as described as follows, to further calculate statistical reliability of clades (or internal nodes) in the NJ, UPGMA and FM trees. We randomly remove 50% of the input set of genes, while retaining the relative orderings of remaining genes, and calculate the genome rearrangement distance between every pair of genomes. This procedure will be repeated as many times as specified by the user. Suppose that the replicate number specified by the user is 100. We then apply the NEIGHBOR/FITCH program in the PHYLIP package (Felsenstein, 1989) to the 100 matrices of pairwise genome rearrangement distances to obtain 100 jackknife trees. Finally, we apply the CONSENSE program in the PHYLIP package to these 100 jackknife trees to obtain a majority-rule consensus tree with the numbers at each internal node representing the percentage of times that the clade defined by this node appears in the 100 jackknife trees.

The kernel programs of SoRT$^2$ were written in C and its web interface was written in PHP. It is currently installed on IBM PC with 2.8 GHz processor and 3 GB RAM under Linux system and can be freely accessed at http://genome.cs.nthu.edu.tw/SORT2/. The SoRT$^2$ web server provides a user interface (Figure 5a) that is intuitive and easy to operate. It takes as input two or more linear/circular multi-chromosomal gene orders in a kind of FASTA-like format (see the instance depicted in Figure 5a), which follows the syntax used in GRIMM (Tesler, 2002) to represent a genome consisting of $n$ genes that spread over $m$ chromosomes by beginning with a single-line description that starts with a right angle bracket (">"), followed by a signed permutation of $1, 2, \ldots, n$ with $m - 1$ delimiters "$" inserted between the chromosomes (or with a "$" at the end of each chromosome). When the input is two genomes, SoRT$^2$ will calculate their genome rearrangement distance, as well as a corresponding optimal scenario by highlighting the genes involved in each rearrangement operation (e.g., see Figure 5b). In the case of multiple genomes, SoRT$^2$ will output a matrix of pairwise genome rearrangement distances (e.g., see Figure 5c), in which each entry denotes the genome rearrangement distance between its two corresponding genomes and its hyperlink accordingly points to an optimal scenario of used rearrangements. Based on this pairwise rearrangement distance matrix, SoRT$^2$ will further construct a phylogenetic tree of input multiple genomes using the NJ, UPGMA or FM method (e.g., see Figure 5d). In addition, if the function of computing jackknife support values is selected, SoRT$^2$ will also perform the jackknife analysis according to the replicate number specified by the user to evaluate the statistical reliability of clades in the NJ, UPGMA and FM trees. SoRT$^2$ also provides a hyperlink through which the user can further view a consensus tree and more detailed jackknife support values of clades included or not included in the consensus tree. We refer the user to the help page of SoRT$^2$ for the step-by-step guide of its detailed usage.

## 3  Experimental Results

Below, we tested our SoRT$^2$ on some simulated datasets, as well as three biological datasets of gene orderings from mitochondrial, mammalian and bacterial genomes, respectively, to demonstrate its ability in reconstruction of phylogenetic trees, and also compared it to another similar tool GRIMM (Tesler, 2002). Notice that GRIMM utilizes another tool, called MGR (Bourque & Pevzner, 2002), to infer its phylogenetic trees, where MGR constructs the phylogenetic trees by using a heuristic of maximum parsimony approach,

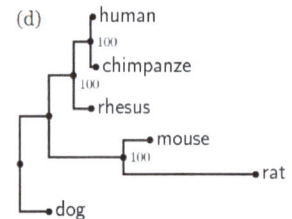

**Figure 5:** (a) User interface of the SoRT² web server. (b) Display of an optimal rearrange-ment scenario in which the genes involved in rearrangements are highlighted. (c) A pairwise rearrangement distance matrix obtained when applying SoRT² to six mammalian genomes with 1,360 synteny blocks. (d) A phylogenetic tree of six mammalian genomes produced by SoRT² with jackknife support values on its clades.

instead of distance-based approach, based on the genome rearrangement distance involving reversals, fu-sions, fissions and translocations (Bourque & Pevzner, 2002). For a fair comparison, we also used the NJ method to reconstruct the phylogenetic trees based on the pairwise rearrangement distances computed by GRIMM and denoted such a kind of GRIMM by GRIMM-NJ for a distinction from the original GRIMM using MGR for its phylogenetic tree reconstruction. All these testing datasets, as well as their experimental results in details, are available on the help page of SoRT².

## 3.1   Performance on Simulated Datasets

First of all, we generated a random rooted binary tree with $m$ multi-chromosomal genomes (or species), where $m$ was varied from 10 to 46 in steps of 4, and assigned a random number $x$ to each edge, where $x$ was an integer between 1 and 5. Then we evolved the randomly generated tree starting from its root with a uni-chromosomal genome of 200 genes by performing $x$ random rearrangement events to each edge until we obtained the gene orders of all the species genomes at the leaves of the tree. Since transpositions generally occur less frequently than reversals and translocations in real biological data, we used three different ratios in our simulations to randomly generate reversals, transpositions and translocations: (i) 1:0:1, (ii) 2:1:2 and

(iii) 1:1:1. Finally, for each choice of species number and rearrangement ratio, we repeated the experiment 100 times and compared SoRT$^2$ with GRIMM-NJ using their average tree similarity. The tree similarity of a tree reconstruction method was calculated as follows based on the property that each branch (edge) divides the set of species at the leaves of a tree into two groups, with one group connected to one end of the branch and the other group connected to the other end. We first used the TREEDIST program in the PHYLIP package (Felsenstein, 1989) to calculate the symmetric difference, say $d$, between the randomly generated tree and the tree produced by the method, where the *symmetric difference* is defined as the number of partitions that are not shared between the two trees (i.e., the number of partitions of the first tree that are not present in the second tree plus the number of partitions of the second tree that are not present in the first tree). Next, we converted this symmetric difference to a tree similarity measure using a simple formula that is $1 - \frac{d}{2m-6}$, where $2m - 6$ is the maximum symmetric difference between two binary trees (Felsenstein, 1989). The average tree similarities calculated in our experiments for SoRT$^2$ and GRIMM-NJ are shown in Figure 6. In the simulated model without transpositions (whose ratio of randomly selected rearrangements is 1:0:1), the average tree similarities achieved by our SoRT$^2$ are almost the same as those by GRIMM-NJ, as shown in Figure 6a, and their overall average tree similarities are both equal to 99.2%. However, in the models with transpositions, our SoRT$^2$ generally performs better than GRIMM-NJ, as illustrated in Figures 6b and 6c, where the overall average tree similarities of SoRT$^2$ and GRIMM-NJ are 99.4% and 99.2%, respectively, for the simulated dataset with ratio of 2:1:2, and 99.4% and 99.1%, respectively, for that with ratio of 1:1:1.

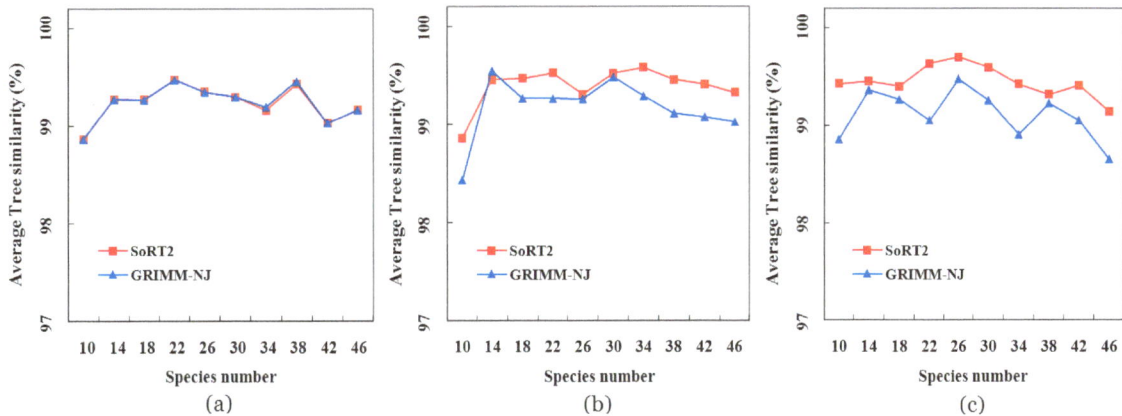

**Figure 6:** Accuracy comparison of SoRT$^2$ and GRIMM-NJ for their phylogenetic tree reconstruction based on three different ratios of reversals, transpositions and translocations: (a) 1:0:1, (b) 2:1:2 and (c) 1:1:1, where vertical axis indicates average tree similarity (%) and horizontal axis indicates species number.

Table 2 shows the average CPU time of SoRT$^2$ and GRIMM for computing the matrix of pairwise genome rearrangement distances, when applying them to simulated datasets that were randomly generated according to the above simulation method using 10 multi-chromosomal species with 100, 200, 500, 1,000, 1,500 and 2,000 genes, respectively. The experiment was repeated 100 times for each choice of gene number. As indicated in Table 2, both GRIMM and SoRT$^2$ can finish their jobs within a second for multi-chromosomal species with no more than 500 genes. For the species with 1,500 to 2,000 genes, GRIMM is clearly faster than our SoRT$^2$, but our SoRT$^2$ still takes only a few seconds to complete its work.

| Gene number | GRIMM | SoRT$^2$ |
|---|---|---|
| 100 | 0.19 s | 0.31 s |
| 200 | 0.19 s | 0.46 s |
| 500 | 0.21 s | 0.90 s |
| 1,000 | 0.24 s | 1.68 s |
| 1,500 | 0.28 s | 2.54 s |
| 2,000 | 0.31 s | 3.46 s |

**Table 2:** Average CPU time for GRIMM and SoRT$^2$ to compute the matrix of pairwise genome rearrangement distances for 10 multi-chromosomal species with gene number varying from 100 to 2,000.

### 3.2    Eleven Metazoan mtDNAs

In this experiment, we applied our SoRT$^2$ to a gene order dataset of 11 metazoan mitochondrial DNAs (mtD-NAs) with 36 genes that was studied by Blanchette et al. (Blanchette et al., 1999), where the 11 metazoan species are human (abbreviated as HU), *Asterina pectinifera* (sea star, abbreviated as SS), *Strongylocentrotus purpuratus* (sea urchin, SU), *Drosophila yakuba* (insect, DR), *Artemia franciscana* (crustacean, AF), *Albinaria coerulea* (snail, AC), *Cepaea nemoralis* (snail, CN), *Katharina tunicata* (chiton, KT), *Lumbricus terrestris* (earthworm, LU), *Ascaris suum* (AS) and *Onchocerca volvulus* (OV). Although many debating trees for metazoan phylogeny have been proposed, the one shown in Figure 7a is most widely accepted (Blanchette et al., 1999) and, therefore, serves as a reference tree for comparing the accuracy of different tools used in this experiment. According to our experimental results, the NJ tree obtained by SoRT$^2$ (Figure 7b) is the same as the one by GRIMM-NJ (Figure 7c) in topology, in which the species in the same group were placed together as sister taxa, except for three Mollusk species KT, AC and CN. Such an inconsistency also occurred in the phylogenetic tree produced by MGR (Figure 7d), but the two Mollusk AC and CN were placed in the branch of deuterostomes (HU, SS and SU).

### 3.3    Six Mammalian Genomes

In (Zhao & Bourque, 2009), Zhao and Bourque created a dataset with 1,360 synteny blocks of six mammalian genomes (human, chimpanzee, rhesus macaque, mouse, rat and dog) to study how to recover their ancestral rearrangement events on a fixed phylogenetic tree as shown in Figure 8a, where the 1,360 synteny blocks in this dataset cover 91.1% of the human genome. In this experiment, we applied our SoRT$^2$, as well as GRIMM-NJ, to this mammalian dataset. As a result, the NJ tree obtained by our SoRT$^2$ (Figure 8b), as well as the GRIMM-NJ tree (Figure 8c), is the same as the one in Figure 8a in topology and has jackknife support values of 100% on almost all its clades. Actually, we had also tested MGR on this mammalian dataset and, unfortunately, MGR was unable to analyze this dataset in a reasonable amount of time so that we did not have its phylogenetic tree in this experiment.

### 3.4    Seven Bacterial Genomes

In this experiment, we tested our SoRT$^2$, as well as GRIMM-NJ and MGR, on a dataset of seven γ-Proteobacterial genomes with 103 genes that came from the study by Belda et al. (Belda et al., 2005). This dataset consists of *Escherichia coli* 0157-H7 (abbreviated as ecs, NC_002695), *Escherichia coli* 0157:H7

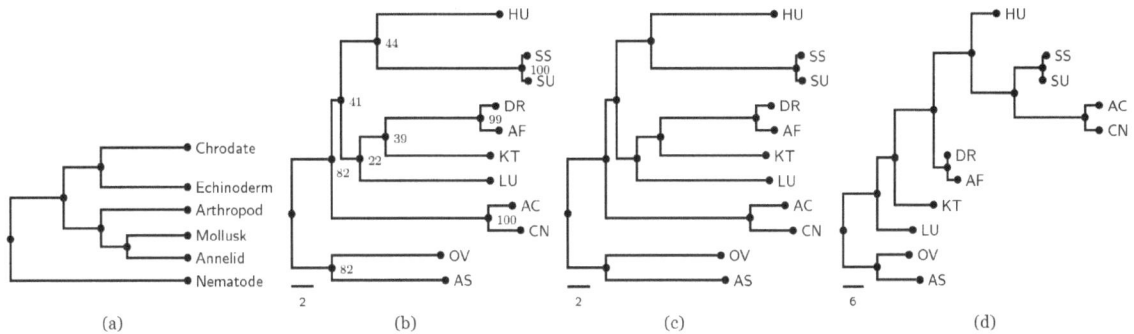

**Figure 7:** (a) The reference tree of 11 metazoan gene orders adopted from (Blanchette et al., 1999), where the 11 metazoan organisms are grouped into six major groupings: Chordate (with HU), Echinoderm (with SS and SU), Arthropod (with DR and AF), Mollusk (with KT, AC and CN), Annelid (with LU) and Nematode (with OV and AS). (b) The NJ tree produced by SoRT$^2$ using a jackknife analysis of 100 replicates, where numbers on internal nodes denote the support values. (c) The NJ tree based on the pairwise rearrangement distances calculated by GRIMM. (d) The phylogenetic tree reconstructed by MGR.

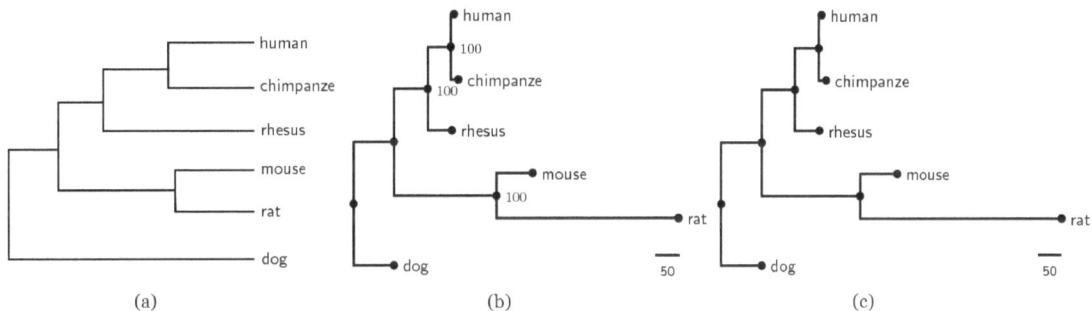

**Figure 8:** (a) The reference tree of six mammalian genomes adopted from (Zhao & Bourque, 2009), where its edges were not drawn to scale. (b) The NJ tree created by SoRT$^2$ using a jackknife analysis of 100 replicates, where numbers on internal nodes are the support values. (c) The NJ tree based on the pairwise rearrangement distances returned by GRIMM.

EDL933 (ece, NC_002655), *Shigella flexneri* 2a str. 301 (sfl, NC_004337), *Shigella flexneri* 2a str. 2457T (sfx, NC_004741), *Salmonella typhimurium* LT2 (stm, NC_003197), *Salmonella enterica* subsp. *enterica* serovar Typhi Ty2 (stt, NC_004631), and *Salmonella enterica* subsp. *enterica* serovar Typhi str. CT18 (sty, NC_003198). Basically, these seven γ-Proteobacteria are closely related enteric bacteria. Figure 9a shows the NJ tree created by our SoRT$^2$, which clearly and correctly divided the seven γ-Proteobacteria into three monophyletic clades. However, both GRIMM-NJ and MGR failed to do that, as shown in Figures 9b and 9c, respectively, because the two *E. coli* strains and the three Salmonella species did not form mutually exclusive monophyletic clades

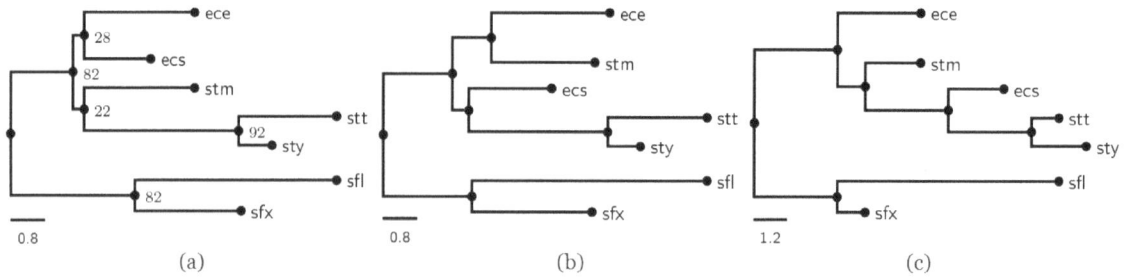

**Figure 9:** (a) The NJ tree constructed by SoRT$^2$ using a jackknife analysis of 100 replicates, where numbers on internal nodes are the support values. (b) The NJ tree based on the pairwise rearrangement distances computed by GRIMM. (c) The phylogenetic tree created by MGR.

# 4  Conclusion

SoRT$^2$ is a web-based tool for the analysis of genome rearrangements involving reversals, generalized transpositions and translocations (including fusions and fissions). It allows the user to quickly calculate pairwise rearrangement distances between input genomes and explore their corresponding optimal scenarios of required rearrangements. In addition, SoRT$^2$ allows the user to quickly infer phylogenetic trees of input multiple genomes based on their pairwise genome rearrangement distances and further evaluate statistical reliability of tree branches. It is worth mentioning that the computation of optimal rearrangement distance involving reversals, generalized transpositions and translocations and the statistical evaluation of trees are not available in other currently existing web servers. Particularly, as was mentioned in (Adam & Sankoff, 2008), a generalized transposition (block-interchange) acting on a chromosome can be viewed as a process of fragment excision, circularization, linearization and re-incorporation, which exactly happens in the configuration of the immune response in higher animals, although the existence and biological significance of generalized transpositions have not yet been discussed in the current biological literature. Therefore, it can be expected that SoRT$^2$ is able to provide interesting insights into the studies of genome rearrangements, particularly involving the generalized transpositions, and phylogenetic reconstruction.

# References

Adam, Z. & Sankoff, D. (2008). The ABCs of MGR with DCJ. Evolutionary Bioinformatics, 4, 69–74.

Alekseyev, M. A. (2008). Multi-break rearrangements and breakpoint re-uses: from circular to linear genomes. Journal of Computational Biology, 15, 1117–1131.

Alekseyev, M. A. & Pevzner, P. A. (2008). Multi-break rearrangements and chromosomal evolution. Theoretical Computer Science, 395, 193–202.

Bader, D. A., Yan, M., & Moret, B. M. W. (2001). A linear-time algorithm for computing inversion distance between signed permutations with an experimental study. Journal of Computational Biology, 8, 483–491.

Bafna, V. & Pevzner, P. A. (1996). Genome rearrangements and sorting by reversals. SIAM Journal on Computing, 25, 272–289.

Bafna, V. & Pevzner, P. A. (1998). Sorting by transpositions. SIAM Journal on Discrete Mathematics, 11, 221–240.

Belda, E., Moya, A., & Silva, F. J. (2005). Genome rearrangement distances and gene order phylogeny in γ-Proteobacteria. Molecular Biology and Evolutionary, 22, 1456–1467.

Bergeron, A., Mixtacki, J., & Stoye, J. (2006a). On sorting by translocations. Journal of Computational Biology, 13, 567–578.

Bergeron, A., Mixtacki, J., & Stoye, J. (2006b). A unifying view of genome rearrangements. Lecture Notes in Computer Science, 4175, 163–173.

Bergeron, A., Mixtacki, J., & Stoye, J. (2009). A new linear time algorithm to compute the genomic distance via the double cut and join distance. Theoretical Computer Science, 410, 5300–5316.

Blanchette, M., Kunisawa, T., & Sankoff, D. (1996). Parametric genome rearrangement. Gene, 172, GC11–GC17.

Blanchette, M., Kunisawa, T., & Sankoff, D. (1999). Gene order breakpoint evidence in animal mitochondrial phylogeny. Journal of Molecular Evolution, 49, 193–203.

Bourque, G. & Pevzner, P. A. (2002). Genome-scale evolution: reconstructing gene orders in the ancestral species. Genome Research, 12, 26–36.

Christie, D. A. (1996). Sorting by block-interchanges. Information Processing Letters, 60, 165–169.

Elias, I. & Hartman, T. (2006). A 1.375-approximation algorithm for sorting by transpositions. IEEE/ACM Transactions on Computational Biology and Bioinformatics, 3, 369–379.

Eriksen, N. (2002). (1+ε)-approximation of sorting by reversals and transpositions. Theoretical Computer Science, 289, 517–529.

Farris, J. S., Albert, V. A., Kallersjo, M., Lipscomb, D., & Kluge, A. G. (1996). Parsimony jackknifing outperforms neighbor-joining. Cladistics, 12, 99–124.

Felsenstein, J. (1989). Phylip: phylogeny inference package (version 3.2). Cladistics, 5, 164–166.

Fertin, G., Labarre, A., Rusu, I., Tannier, E., & Vialette, S. (2009). Combinatorics of Genome Rearrangements. Cambridge: The MIT Press.

Fitch, W. M. & Margolia.E (1967). Construction of phylogenetic trees. Science, 155, 279–284.

Hannenhalli, S. (1996). Polynomial algorithm for computing translocation distance between genomes. Discrete Applied Mathematics, 71, 137–151.

Hannenhalli, S. & Pevzner, P. A. (1999). Transforming cabbage into turnip: polynomial algorithm for sorting signed permutations by reversals. Journal of the ACM, 46, 1–27.

Hartman, T. & Sharan, R. (2005). A 1.5-approximation algorithm for sorting by transpositions and transreversals. Journal of Computer and System Sciences, 70, 300–320.

Huang, K.-H., Chen, K.-T., & Lu, C. L. (2011). Sorting permutations by cut-circularize-linearize-and-paste operations. BMC Genomics, 12, S26.

Huang, Y.-L., Huang, C.-C., Tang, C. Y., & Lu, C. L. (2010a). An improved algorithm for sorting by block-interchanges based on permutation groups. Information Processing Letters, 110, 345–350.

Huang, Y.-L., Huang, C.-C., Tang, C. Y., & Lu, C. L. (2010b). SoRT$^2$: a tool for sorting genomes and reconstructing phylogenetic trees by reversals, generalized transpositions and translocations. Nucleic Acids Research, 38, W221–W227.

Huang, Y.-L. & Lu, C. L. (2010). Sorting by reversals, generalized transpositions and translocations using permutation groups. Journal of Computational Biology, 17, 685–705.

Kaplan, H., Shamir, R., & Tarjan, R. E. (1999). Faster and simpler algorithm for sorting signed permutations by reversals. SIAM Journal on Computing, 29, 880–892.

Kececioglu, J. D. & Ravi, R. (1995). Of mice and men: algorithms for evolutionary distances between genomes with translocation. In Proceedings of the 6th ACM-SIAM Symposium on Discrete Algorithms (SODA1995) (pp. 604–613). San Francisco: Society for Industrial and Applied Mathematics.

Lin, C. H., Zhao, H., Lowcay, S. H., Shahab, A., & Bourque, G. (2010). webMGR: an online tool for the multiple genome rearrangement problem. Bioinformatics, 26, 408–410.

Lin, Y. & Moret, B. M. E. (2008). Estimating true evolutionary distances under the DCJ model. Bioinformatics, 24, i114–i122.

Lin, Y. C., Lu, C. L., Chang, H.-Y., & Tang, C. Y. (2005). An efficient algorithm for sorting by block-interchanges and its application to the evolution of vibrio species. Journal of Computational Biology, 12, 102–112.

Lin, Y. C., Lu, C. L., Liu, Y.-C., & Tang, C. Y. (2006). SPRING: a tool for the analysis of genome rearrangement using reversals and block-interchanges. Nucleic Acids Research, 34, W696–W699.

Lu, C. L., Huang, Y.-L., Wang, T. C., & Chiu, H.-T. (2006). Analysis of circular genome rearrangement by fusions, fissions and block-interchanges. BMC Bioinformatics, 7(295).

Lu, C. L., Wang, T. C., Lin, Y. C., & Tang, C. Y. (2005). ROBIN: a tool for genome rearrangement of block-interchanges. Bioinformatics, 21, 2780–2782.

Saitou, N. & Nei, M. (1987). The neighbor-joining method: a new method for reconstructing phylogenetic trees. Molecular Biology and Evolution, 4, 406–425.

Sokal, R. R. & Michener, C. D. (1958). A statistical method for evaluating systematic relationships. University of Kansas Science Bulletin, 38, 1409–1438.

Suyama, M. & Bork, P. (2001). Evolution of prokaryotic gene order: genome rearrangements in closely related species. Trends in Genetics, 17, 10–13.

Tesler, G. (2002). GRIMM: genome rearrangements web server. Bioinformatics, 18, 492–493.

Xu, W., Jameson, D., Tang, B., & Higgs, P. G. (2006). The relationship between the rate of molecular evolution and the rate of genome rearrangement in animal mitochondrial genomes. Journal of Molecular Evolution, 63, 375–392.

Yancopoulos, S., Attie, O., & Friedberg, R. (2005). Efficient sorting of genomic permutations by translocation, inversion and block interchange. Bioinformatics, 21, 3340–3346.

Zhao, H. & Bourque, G. (2009). Recovering genome rearrangements in the mammalian phylogeny. Genome Research, 19, 934–942.

# Optimization of Sequence Alignment for Microsatellite Regions

Abdulqader Jighly, Khaled El-Shamaa, Aladdin Hamwieh
*International Center for Agricultural Research in the Dry Areas (ICARDA), Syria*

Reem Joukhadar
*University of Aleppo, Syria*

Francis C. Ogbonnaya
*Grains Research and Development Corporation (GRDC), Australia*

# 1   Introduction

Microsatellites, or simple sequence repeats (SSRs), are tandemly repeated DNA sequences with a period of from 1 to 6 base pairs (Tautz, 1989). An SSR which contains one type of repeats, is called a *simple SSR* (e.g. $(CA)_{15}$) and those which have more than one type are called *compound SSRs* (e.g. $(CA)_8(CG)_{12}$) (Peakall *et al.*, 1998). When the tandem repeat interrupted with one nucleotide or more (e.g. $(CA)_8G(CA)_5$) then the SSR called *imperfect SSR*. The repeat units are generally di-, tri- tetra- or penta-nucleotides. They are commonly found in non-coding regions of the genome and less in the coding ones. They are ubiquitously distributed almost in all eukaryotic and prokaryotic genomes (Merkel & Gemmell, 2008).

SSR flanking regions stand very high stability even between different taxa and there is a negative correlation between microsatellite length and substitution rate in nearby flanking sequence (Santibanez-Koref *et al.*, 2001; Sekar *et al.*, 2009). The stability of the SSR flanking regions was investigated in different organisms; three *Phytophthora* species (algaes) (Schena *et al.*, 2008); rice and bamboo (Chen *et al.*, 2010); cotton cotton (Altaf-Khan *et al.*, 2009); *Brassica rapa* and *Arabidopsis thaliana* (Suwabe *et al.*, 2006); cowpea, mung bean and adzuki bean (Vir *et al.*, 2009); 16 different species of *Castanea* spp. (Akkak *et al.*, 2009); different species of the genus *Carya* (Herrera *et al.*, 2011) and wheat (Zhang *et al.*, 2007). Similar studies have also been carried out in different animals such as fish (Zardoya *et al.*, 1996); coral-Acropora (Tang *et al.*, 2010); cattle, sheep, yak, buffalo and goat (Shakyawar *et al.*, 2009); *Probarbus jullienii* (Ghiasi *et al.*, 2009) and gerbils (Du *et al.*, 2010). Further, similar results were obtained from human genome studies when different SSR's flank regions associated with genes expressed in the developing nervous system were compared (Riley and Krieger 2009). Moreover, studying the flanking regions of EST-SSR loci demonstrates a common evolutionary origin of grass fungal endophytes taxa (de Jong *et al.*, 2011).

Despite the high stability of the SSR flanking regions, the abundance and the tandem repeated nature of SSRs make them highly mutable loci (Gow, *et al.*, 2005). In animals, observed SSR mutation rates have been of the order of $10^{-3}$ for autosomal repeat loci (Wiessenbach, *et al.*, 1992; Weber and Wong, 1993). However the average of mutations in SSR loci is $10^{-2}$ in one generation (Ellegren, 2000).

Chistiakov, *et al.*, (2006) suggested that two mechanisms are responsible for the high mutability in SSRs. First, motif repetition makes SSRs prone to mutation by DNA polymerase slippage during replication allowing one strand to hybridize with one of the multi-complimentary tandem sequences on the other strand (Figure1a), and second, unequal crossing over or related processes (Figure1b) (Jakupciak, *et al.*, 2000; Ellegren, 2004; Kelkar, *et al.*, 2008). The slippage rate is correlated to SSR length and this makes longer SSRs more variable than shorter ones (Whittaker, *et al.*, 2003; Sainudiin, *et al.*, 2004). However, there is no threshold length for slippage mutations (Leclercq, *et al.*, 2010). Besides, position in genome (coding or non-coding sequences), presence on leading or lagging strand and the distance from origin of replication also affect SSR mutations. Further, fidelity of replication and repair mechanisms as well as epigenetic factors may influence repeat stability (Choudhary and Trivedi, 2010). The mutations that happen because of the polymerase slippage could be considered as special types of insertion/deletion (indels) mutations that usually occur when adding or erasing sequences without any substitution. Substitution is considered as another kind of mutation called single nucleotide polymorphism (SNPs). In general, SNPs occur much more frequently than indels (Zhang and Gerstein, 2003). But SSR replication slippage generates more genetic change in eukaryotes than do all base substitution per generation (Bell, 1996), so it increases the frequency of indels. In addition, it has been reported that the perfect SSR motifs are significantly more variable compared to imperfect repeated motifs (Kruglyak, *et al.,* 1998; Brandström and El-legren, 2008).

SSRs are increasingly being used as genetic markers. The main features that make SSRs amenable for use as molecular markers are that they are highly mutable loci and their flanking regions are highly conserved, allowing the use of specific PCR primers to amplify the same SSR even across different taxa (Santibanez-Koref, *et al.,* 2001; Sekar, *et al.,* 2009). They have been used for wide range of applications such as evolutionary and diversity studies, marker assisted selection, gene tagging, genome mapping and forensic studies, due to their multi-allelic nature, co-dominant mode of inheritance, their high polymor-phism, abundance in the genome and extensive genome coverage (Powell, *et al.,* 1996; Kantety, *et al.,* 2002; Schlotterer, 2004). The polymorphism of SSR depends on the differences in the numbers of re-peated units among alleles at a single locus.

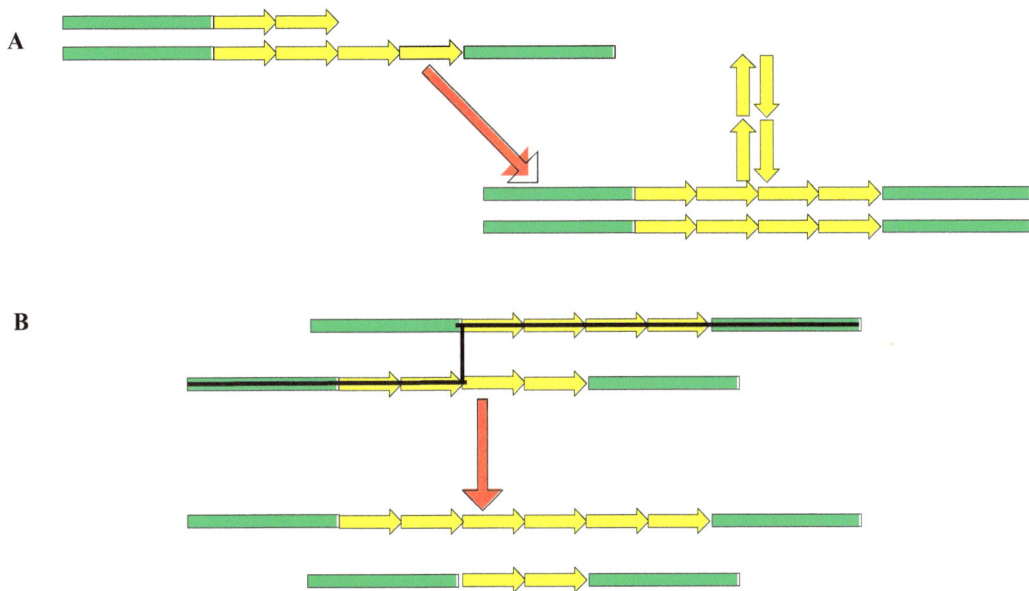

**Figure 1:** Microsatellite mutation mechanisms. **(A)** Polymerase Slippage. **(B)** Unequal crossing-over.

With the ongoing technical improvement within the last three decades, studying differences on se-quence level has become the norm. Integrating such development with the recent advances in bioinfor-matics field opens up opportunities hitherto thought impossible by detecting sequence differences and mutations by different methods such as sequence alignment (Egan *et al.,* 2012). Sequence alignment in-volves the identification of the correct location of different mutations that have occurred since their di-vergence from a common precursor. The accurate sequence alignment should reflect real evolutionary relationships and thus, differences between sequences are weighted based on biological evidences. Be-cause single nucleotide polymorphism mutations (SNPs) are more frequent than insertion/deletion (IN-DELs) mutations (INDELs) (Zhang and Gerstein 2003), all similarity matrixes are being build based on this fact. This would still be applicable for most of the genomic regions but not for microsatellites (Jighly *et al.,* 2011). The increases or decreases on the number of repeated units make the INDEL mutations more frequent than SNP, therefore all alignment methods that use dynamic programming would not be applicable for microsatellites especially for the ones that consist of more than one repeated unit types (compound microsatellites). When aligning such regions, we can clearly notice a lot of overlaps between different repeated units (Jighly *et al.*, 2011). In this chapter, we would discuss the SSR alignment algorithm with artificial and actual genomic SSR sequences and we would present the features of the first SSR aligning tool version as well as the second one (Jighly and El-Shamaa, in preparation).


# 2    The Development of SSR Alignment Tool (SALT)

The first version of the SSR alignment tool (SALT) was generated to test the aligning algorithm but it had so many limitations so it wasn't really applicable especially in cases were many SSRs could be found in the sequence. The users were not able to align their sequences if they have no previous knowledge of the composition of his sequences whether they have SSRs or not. The old version of SALT entails the user to determine the position of the first and the last nucleotide of the SSR in his sequence. Moreover, it also requires the user to indicate the motif sequence and define whether it is simple or compound. Furthermore, the user must align his SSRs one by one after running a global alignment with any other alignment software. Those restrictions combined create a need to update the current version so it could be more relevant and user friendly.

SALT version 2 utilized the same algorithm for aligning SSRs in a full tool for global sequence alignment. This version starts with a *fasta* file which contains raw sequences. The first step is to run ClustalW alignment on the sequences then it would search for SSRs on the consensus sequence. The final step is to align the determined SSRs according to (Jighly *et al.*, 2011).

## 2.1    SALT Algorithm

The SSR alignment tool version 2 algorithm would deal with each SSR according to the following major steps (Jighly and El-Shamaa, in preparation):

1. Call "ClustalW.exe" to align sequences from the input *fasta* file with the IUB weight matrix

2. Detect microsatellite position using regular expression techniques in all aligned sequences or the consensus sequence after determining the following parameters by the user

    a. The minimum repeated unit length

    b. The maximum repeated unit length (e.g. 2 and 6, so we are looking after di-, tri-, tetra-, penta-, and hexa- nucleotide repeats)

    c. Minimum number of repeats to tag it as SSR

    d. The maximum number of stretches may be included in one compound microsatellite

    e. The maximum length of nucleotides between stretches of compound microsatellite

    f. The maximum percentage of accepted non-repeated nucleotides within the microsatellite motifs

3. In the case of microsatellite detection in all sequences, use the position of the sequence the contains the longest microsatellite for the following step

4. Align the detected SSRs by ding the follows for each one (Figure 2)

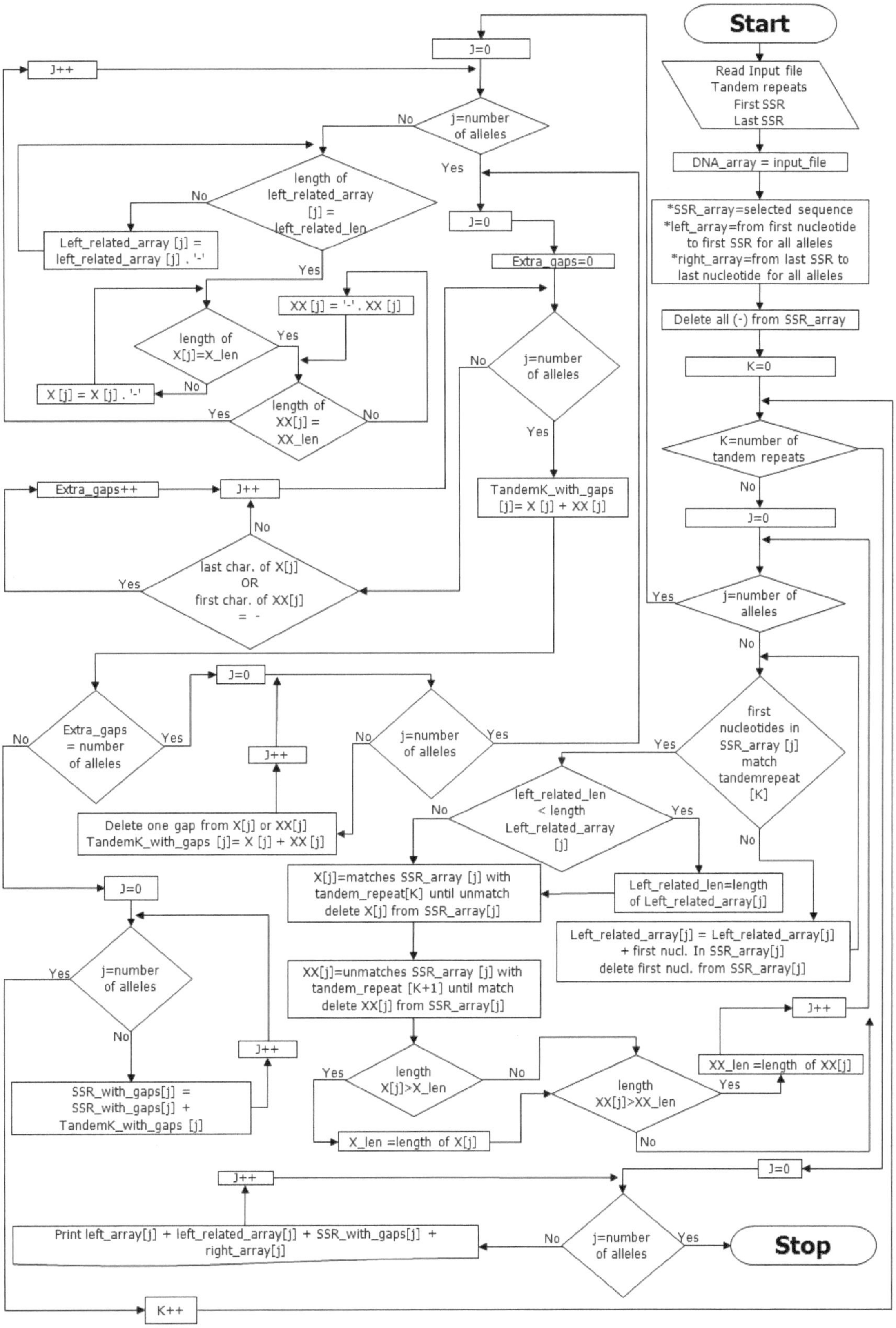

**Figure 2:** The full SSR aligning flow chart (check the algorithm step 4 in the previous page).

a.  Define the first and the last nucleotide position and the repeated unit sequences from the previous step

b.  Extract the aligned SSR from all sequences

c.  Remove all gaps

d.  Identify the sequences that do not match the first repeated unit from the beginning of the selected SSR region

e.  Do the follows for each repeated unit

f.  Put the tandem repeat in a temporary tandem array

g.  Check if the next nucleotides match the next repeated unit

h.  If not, put the unmatched nucleotides from all sequences in another temporary imperfect array and go back to step (f)

i.  If yes, go back to step (f)

j.  Fill all sequences in all arrays with gaps until their length match the longest sequence in the each array

k.  Merge each imperfect array with the previous tandem array

l.  Do the follows for each merged array

m.  Check if there is a sequence without any gap

n.  If not, delete the last gap from all sequences and go back to step (m)

o.  If yes, go back to step (l)

p.  Merge all temporary arrays in one array

5.  Put the final merged array instead of the original aligned SSR

Figure 2 provide the full flow chart of the alignment algorithm (the major step 4 only). The main difficulty that faces the SSR alignment algorithm is to determine the gap position when applying it to an imperfect SSR. According to Kruglyak *et al.,* (1998) and Bandström and Ellegren (2008), the imperfect repeats within the SSR region reduces the occurrences of slippage, resulting in the imperfect SSR changing its tandem nature and fixing the region by prohibiting replication slippage. This is because the bases do not find their complementary bases during replication. However, the best place for the imperfect nucleotides is after the gap and before the next repeated unit (Figure 3).

## 2.2   The Software Development

SALT is a new tool for generating an alignment for SSR loci using the previously described algorithm. It was written using the PERL programming language [URL: http://www.perl.org/]. The Tk package was used to make the user friendly graphical interface [URL: http://www.tcl.tk/]. The main window of the version 2 (In press) is consisted of four textboxes to determine the input and the output files and their directories and another two textboxes to determine the alignment parameters (opening gap and extension gap penalties). The input file should contain raw sequences in *fasta* format. The software uses the ClustalW algorithm to generate the global alignment using the IUB matrix. There is also four buttons, two for browsing the input and the output files, the third for generating the alignment, and the last for closing the program.

TATATATATA**G**TA
TATATATATATATATA

More appropriate

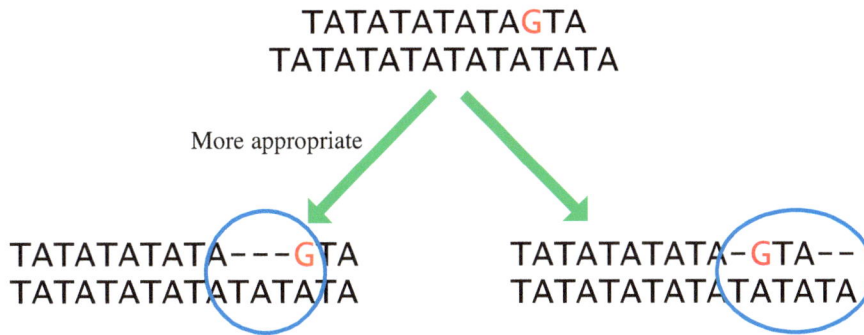

TATATATATA---**G**TA
TATATATATATATA

TATATATATA-**G**TA--
TATATATATATATA

**Figure 3:** The appropriate alignment for the imperfections.

Figure 4 shows the main window of SALT version 1 which was differing from the second one. It was consisted of five textboxes, two of them were for the names or the directories for the input and the output files as same as the second version. Since the first version forced the user to determine the position of his microsatellite and its tandem sequences, it had three extra textboxes for identifying the first and the last nucleotide position of the SSR locus in the whole sequence and another one for the tandem sequences. The user should determine his tandem repeats by separating each repeated from the next one with the space character. There is also four buttons the same as version 2. The accepted input format should be *aligned* sequences in *fasta* format or a ".txt" format as follow:

1.  The first line contains the number of samples, followed by any kind of separator (space or tab…) and, subsequently, the number of nucleotides.

2.  Each of the next lines contains the name of the allele, followed by any kind of separator, then the sequence; thereafter press the Enter button to start the next allele.

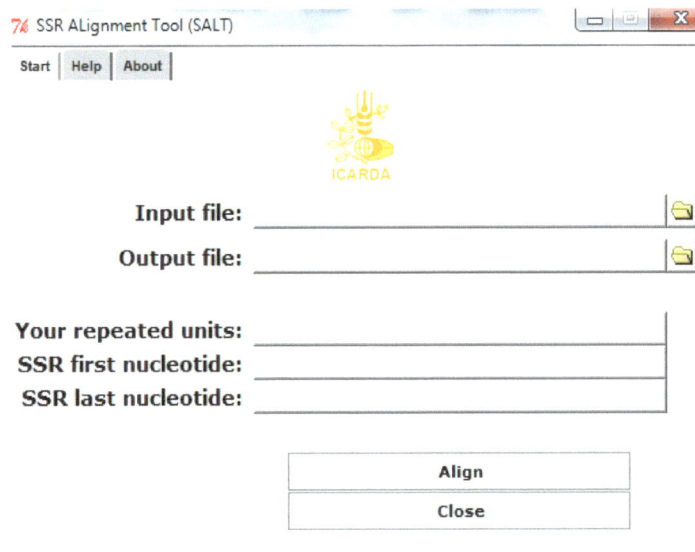

**Figure 4:** The main window of Ssr ALignment Tool (SALT) version 1.

# 3    Testing and Results

## 3.1    Tested Sequences

Five different sequences (Table 1) of SSR motifs the first four (A, B, C and D) are artificial sequences that share the same microsatellite flanking sequences while the last one obtained from a biotechnology laboratory (Genetic Resources Section, ICARDA), were used in the following examples. These sequences were obtained from 26 plants representing 26 alleles. The sequences were aligned using the ClustalW algorithm implemented in SALT version 2 with the following default parameters: gap opening penalty 15, gap extension penalty 6.66, IUB weight matrix, transition weight 0.5, and delay divergent cut-off 30. The phylogenic trees were drawn with the UPGMA method included in MEGA 4 software (Tamura, *et al.,* 2007).

| Case | SSR type | SSR repeat | Seq. length (bp.) | SSR length (bp.) | SSR (%) |
|------|----------|------------|-------------------|------------------|---------|
| A | Simple Perfect | $(TA)_{10}$ | 351 | 54 | 15.4 |
| B | Compound Perfect | $(TA)_{10}(CA)_{16}$ | 397 | 100 | 25.2 |
| C | Compound Perfect | $(TA)_{10}(CA)_{16}(CG)_{14}$ | 457 | 160 | 35 |
| D | Compound Perfect | $(TA)_{10}(CA)_{16}(CG)_{14}(TG)_{18}$ | 479 | 182 | 38 |
| E | Compound Imperfect | $(GAA)_4(GAT)_6(GAGGAT)_3$ | 769 | 72 | 9.4 |

**Table 1:** Five microsatellite motifs vary in their types and lengths, representing most SSR types in the genome sequences.

The first four artificial sequences share the same flanking regions. In this case, all the differences between the phylogenic trees among the four cases would be due to the differences in the SSRs. The following parts of this chapter would discuss the alterations in the aligned sequences and their evolutionary relations (the phylogenic trees).

## 3.2    Results

The sequence case A contained a simple perfect SSR with the tandem TA, which represents about 15.4% of the whole sequence. After applying the alignment in the MEGA 4 alignment and our modifications, one minor difference was shown clearly in the gap sites in some alleles (alleles number 20, 22, 23 and 24) (Figure 5). For the alleles 22 and 24 there were two separate gaps before applying the SSR alignment algorithm (Figure 5a), but after that we got one gap (Figure 5b) which is more reliable.

However, these differences did not reveal any considerable variations in the phylogenic tree before and after applying the SSR alignment algorithm (Figure 6), and the whole aligned sequence length equals 351 bp. in both cases. The Case A could be considered as the simplest case we can ever deal with and there is maybe no need for special considerations to align such case. The following cases are more complicated and they would reflect the need for such algorithm.

The sequence case B contained a compound SSR with two tandem sequences TA and CA, which represents about 25.2% of the whole sequence. The aligned sequence length was increased from 397 bp. to 413 bp. after applying the SSR alignment algorithm which resulted due to the decrement in the overlaps among different sequences and the increment in the gap lengths because of aligning each repeated

```
A   1   TTGTAATATATATATATATATA--------------------------------GATAGAAA
    2   TTGTAATATATATATATATATATATATATATATATATATATATATA--------GATAGAAA
    3   TTGTAATATATATATATATATATATATATATATA--------------------GATAGAAA
    4   TTGTAATATATATATATATATATATATATATATATA------------------GATAGAAT
    5   TTGTAATATATATATATATATA--------------------------------GATAGAAA
    6   TTGTAATATATATATATATATATATATATATATATATATATATA----------GATAGAAA
    7   TTGTAATATATATATATATA----------------------------------GATAGAAA
    8   TTGTAATATATATATATATATATATATA--------------------------GATAGAAA
    9   TTGTAATATATATATATATATA--------------------------------GATAGAAA
   10   TTGTAATATATATATA--------------------------------------GATAGAAA
   11   TTGTAATATATATATATATATATATATATATATATATATATATATATATA----GATAGAAA
   12   TTGTAATATATATATATATATATATATATATATATATATATATA----------GATAGAAT
   13   TTGTAATATATATATATATATA--------------------------------GATAGAAA
   14   TTGTAATATATATATATA------------------------------------GATAGAAA
   15   TTGTAATATATATATATATATATATATATATATATA------------------GATAGAAA
   16   TTGTAATATATATATATATA----------------------------------GATAGAAA
   17   TTGTAATATATATATATATATATATATATATATATATATATATA----------GATAGAAA
   18   TTGTAATATATATATATATATA--------------------------------GATAGAAA
   19   TTGTAATATATATATATATATATATATATATATA--------------------GATAGAAA
   20   TTGTAATATATATATATATATATATATATATATATATATATATA----------TAGATAGAAA
   21   TTGTAATATATATATATATATA--------------------------------GATAGAAA
   22   TTGTAATATATATATAT-----------------ATA-----------------GATAGAAA
   23   TTGTAATATATATATATATATATATATATATATATATATATAT ATATATATATATATATATA--TAGATAGAAT
   24   TTGTAATATATATAT-------------------ATA-----------------GATAGAAA
   25   TTGTAATATATATATATATATATATAT TATATATATATATATATATATATAGATAGAAA
   26   TTGTAATATATATATATATATATATATATA------------------------GATAGAAA

B   1   TTGTAATATATATATATATA----------------------------------GATAGAAA
    2   TTGTAATATATATATATATATATATATATATATATATATATATATA--------GATAGAAA
    3   TTGTAATATATATATATATATATATATATATA----------------------GATAGAAA
    4   TTGTAATATATATATATATATATATATATATA----------------------GATAGAAT
    5   TTGTAATATATATATATATATA--------------------------------GATAGAAA
    6   TTGTAATATATATATATATATATATATATATATATATATATATA----------GATAGAAA
    7   TTGTAATATATATATATATA----------------------------------GATAGAAA
    8   TTGTAATATATATATATATATATATATATA------------------------GATAGAAA
    9   TTGTAATATATATATATATATA--------------------------------GATAGAAA
   10   TTGTAATATATATATA--------------------------------------GATAGAAA
   11   TTGTAATATATATATATATATATATATATATATATATATATATATATA------GATAGAAA
   12   TTGTAATATATATATATATATATATATATATATATATATATATA----------GATAGAAT
   13   TTGTAATATATATATATATATA--------------------------------GATAGAAA
   14   TTGTAATATATATATATA------------------------------------GATAGAAA
   15   TTGTAATATATATATATATATATATATATATATATA------------------GATAGAAA
   16   TTGTAATATATATATATATA----------------------------------GATAGAAA
   17   TTGTAATATATATATATATATATATATATATATATATATATATA----------GATAGAAA
   18   TTGTAATATATATATATATATA--------------------------------GATAGAAA
   19   TTGTAATATATATATATATATATATATATATATA--------------------GATAGAAA
   20   TTGTAATATATATATATATATATATATATATATATATATATATA----------GATAGAAA
   21   TTGTAATATATATATATATATA--------------------------------GATAGAAA
   22   TTGTAATATATATATATATA----------------------------------GATAGAAA
   23   TTGTAATATATATATATATATATATATATATAT ATATATAT TATATATATATA--GATAGAAT
   24   TTGTAATATATATATATA------------------------------------GATAGAAA
   25   TTGTAATATATATATATATATATATAT TATAT ATATATATATATATAGATAGAAA
   26   TTGTAATATATATATATATATATATATATA------------------------GATAGAAA
```

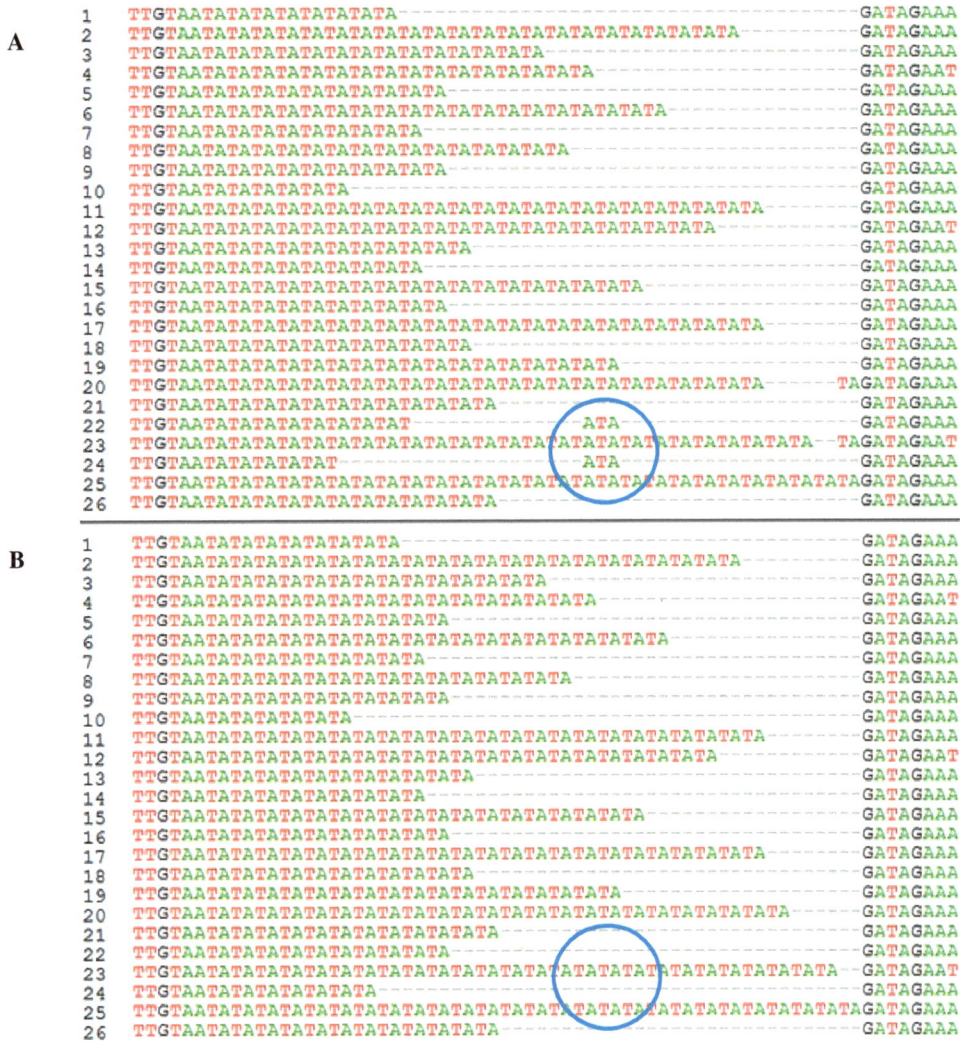

**Figure 5:** Part of the case (A) sequence which contains the SSR region before (A) and after (B) applying the algorithm.

unit separately. However, the phylogenic trees indicated that 50% of the samples –or 13 alleles– showed similar clusters before and after the SSR alignment algorithm being applied (Figure 7). Of those, the alleles 11, 14 and 15 were in the same cluster in both treatments and they were almost the same after applying the algorithm but before that the allele 14 was a little bit distant from the other two alleles. On the other hand, some closely related alleles appear to be closer or almost the same (e.g. the alleles 3 and 7 were very close before applying the algorithm but after that they seem to be exactly the same). Contrariwise, other separate clusters seem to be related and they have been merged in one cluster (e.g. before applying the algorithm there were a cluster contains the alleles 3 and 7, and another separate cluster contains the alleles 1 and 10 but after applying the algorithm both of them have merged in one group). The genetic distance of the most 25 related sequences had been decreased from 0.0085 to 0.0073, while the average distance had been decreased from 0.015 to 0.012.

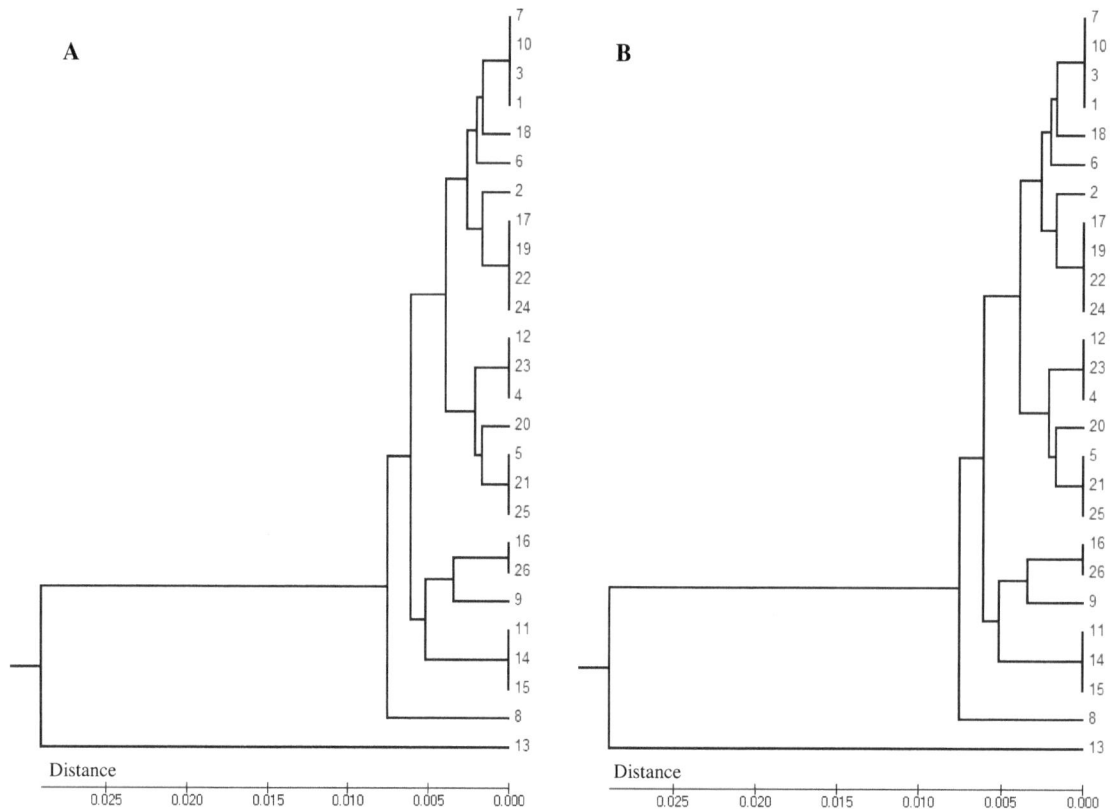

**Figure 6:** Case (A) phylogenic tree before (A) and after (B) applying the algorithm.

The sequence case C contained a compound SSR of TA, CA, and CG tandem repeats representing about 35% of the whole sequence. Applying the SSR alignment algorithm for case C increased the length of the aligned sequence from 457 bp. to 478 bp. The final alignment length differs with 21 nucleotides for this case while it differs with only 16 nucleotides for the case B which reveals higher decrement in the overlapping among the repeated unit and higher increment in the gap lengths among different sequences. However, the comparison of the phylogenic trees before and after applying the SSR alignment algorithm showed that only seven alleles, about 26.9% of the whole sequence, clustered similarly (Figure 8). In case B, the alleles 11, 14 and 15 were in the same cluster in both treatments with some differences with the distances for the allele 14 (Figure 7) but this allele became very distant in case C and distance between the alleles 11 and 15 changed to about 0.007 (Figure 8). After applying the algorithm the alleles 1, 3, 7 and 10 were grouped in the same cluster in case B and C, but before applying it the alleles 1 and 10 were grouped in one cluster while the alleles 3 and 7 grouped in a very distant cluster in the case B. In case C, the alleles 1, 3 and 10 were grouped in the same cluster while the allele 7 was included in another distant cluster. These results reveal the instability of the clustering analysis when dealing with SSRs.

The sequence case D contained compound SSR with the repeated units (TA, CA, CG, and TG). The length of this tandem repeats represents 38% of the whole sequence. The whole aligned sequence length was changed after the SSR alignment algorithm was applied from 479 bp. to 539 bp. The final alignment length differs with 60 nucleotides for this case while it differs with only 16 and 21 nucleotides for the

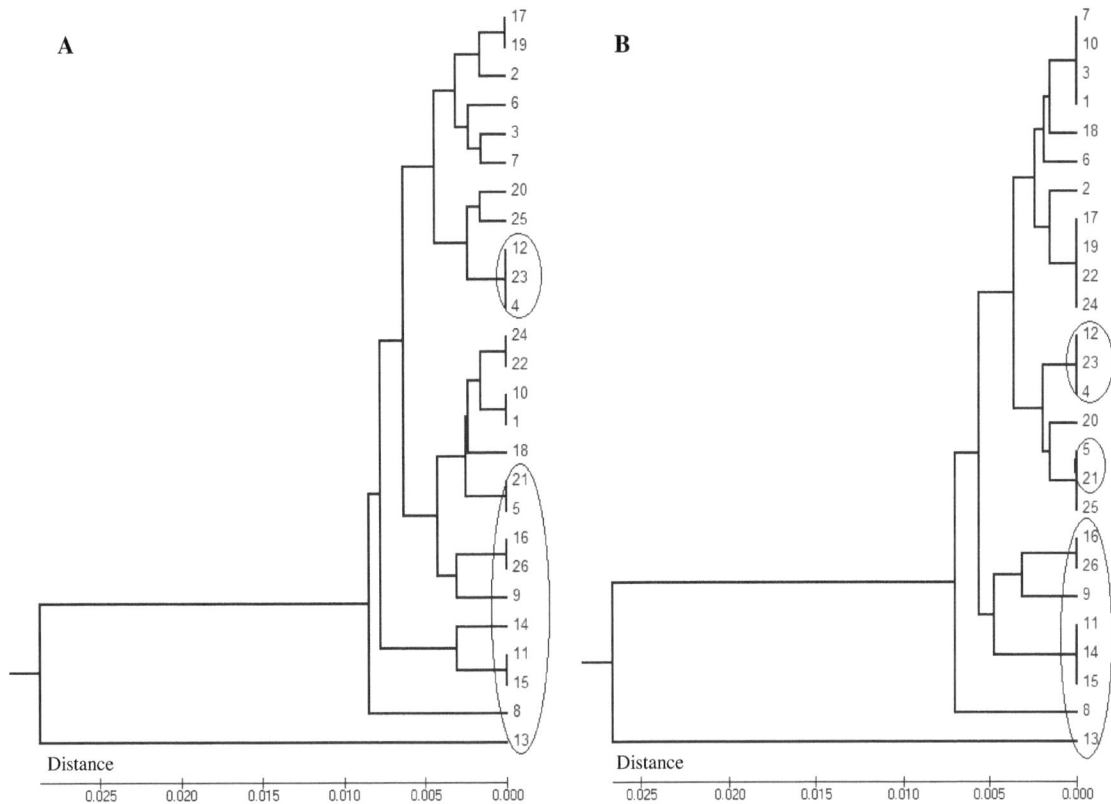

**Figure 7:** Case (B) phylogenic tree before (A) and after (B) applying the algorithm.

cases B and C respectively. These results reveal a particularly high decrement in the overlapping among the repeated unit and increment in the gap lengths among different sequences whenever the SSR became more complex. The cluster analysis resulted in completely different phylogenic trees before and after applying the SSR alignment algorithm (Figure 9). For this case, only three pairs of alleles were similar with the SSR alignment algorithm and still had close relation with the ClustalW alignment without any correction and those alleles are 5 and 21, 3 and 18, 1 and 10. These results reveal the critical need for such correction with the more complex SSRs.

The average pairwise value for cases A, B, C, and D before applying the SSR alignment algorithm indicated that these values were increased whenever the sequence contained more repeated units (Figure 10) and the phylogenic trees showed a huge unreliable differences in the evolutionary relations among different alleles every time we increased the SSR length and complexity. In contrast, after the SSR alignment algorithm was applied to the same sequences the phylogenic trees for all cases were almost the same and there are no considerable differences among those trees. Moreover, the average pairwise values were decreased after applying the SSR alignment algorithm which exposes more stable distances by preventing the creation of various overlaps among different alleles. Those overlaps would make the studied alleles look like as they have many SNPs among them. Furthermore, the average pairwise values have a slight decrease, which may be attributed to the additional aligned repeated unit. The additional units increased the SSR length giving more similarity because it does not contain any overlap or mismatch and

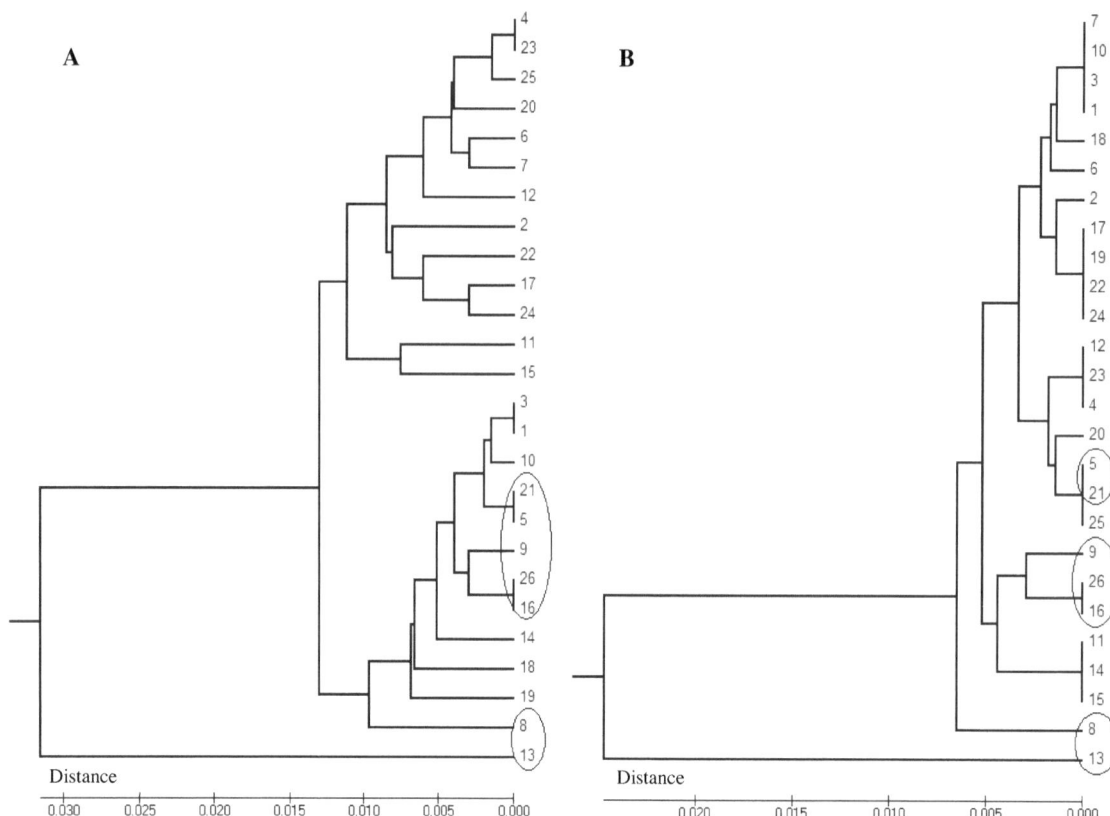

**Figure 8:** Case (C) phylogenic tree before (A) and after (B) applying the algorithm

the only difference among different alleles could be attributed to the opening gap position. The interval values between the two average pairwise values (before and after applying the SSR alignment algorithm) were increased for all cases (A, B, C, and D) indicating that the general alignment methods revealed more genetic distances for the complex SSRs.

The previous cases are based on artificial sequences. The following case (case E) is bases on actual sequences representing 26 alleles of one SSR locus of lentil crop. The Case E showed a compound-imperfect SSR repeat with the tandems GAA, GAT, and GAGGAT respectively. This imperfect SSR represents 9.4% of the sequence tested in case E. The alignment processes showed clear differences before and after the SSR region was treated with the SSR alignment algorithm (Figure 11). Many overlaps could be clearly detected before applying the SSR alignment algorithm (Figure 11a). Those overlaps were corrected after applying the algorithm and figure 11b showed three distinct regions each of them contains one repeated unit.

Applying SSR alignment algorithm for case E increased the length of the aligned sequence from 769 bp. to 784 bp. Despite the small percentage of this SSR in the whole sequence for case E, the phylogenic trees showed that the genetic distance of the most 24 related sequences was decreased from 0.00317 to 0.002 (Figure 12). However, the phylogenic trees indicated that about 26.9% of the samples – or 7 alleles– showed exactly the same clusters before and after the SSR alignment algorithm being applied with one different in the distant with the allele 9 in the cluster that contain the alleles 1, 9 and 16.

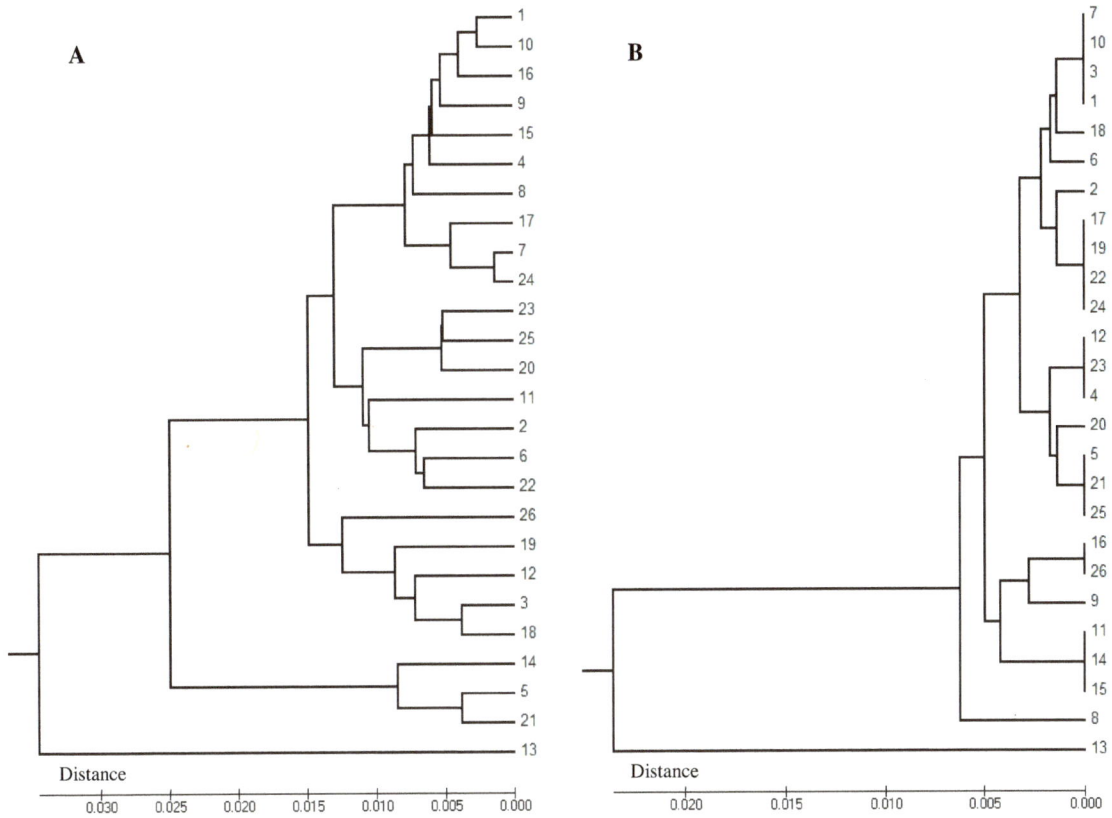

**Figure 9:** Case (D) phylogenic tree before (A) and after (B) applying the algorithm

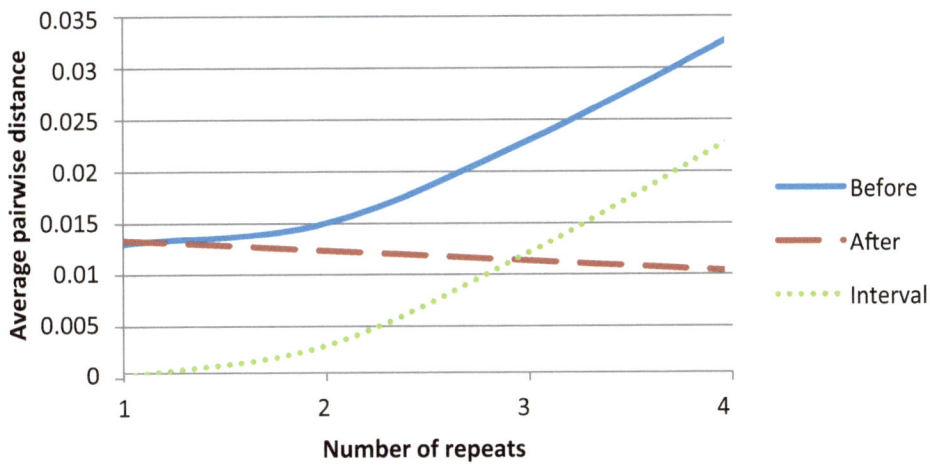

**Figure 10:** The average pairwise distance differences in cases A, B, C and D

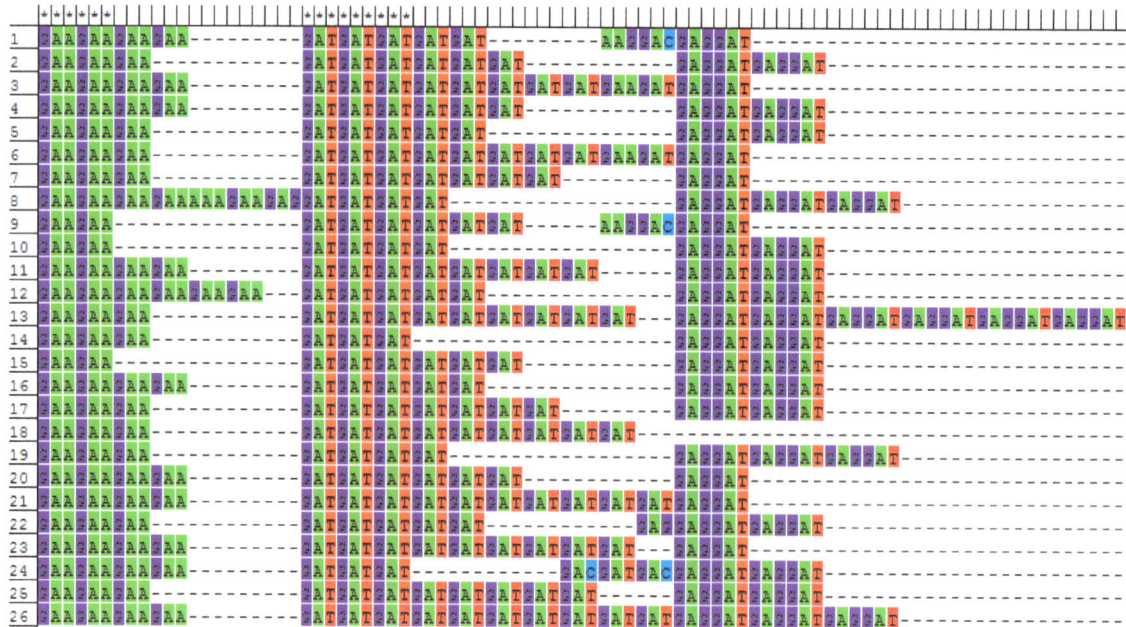

**(A)**

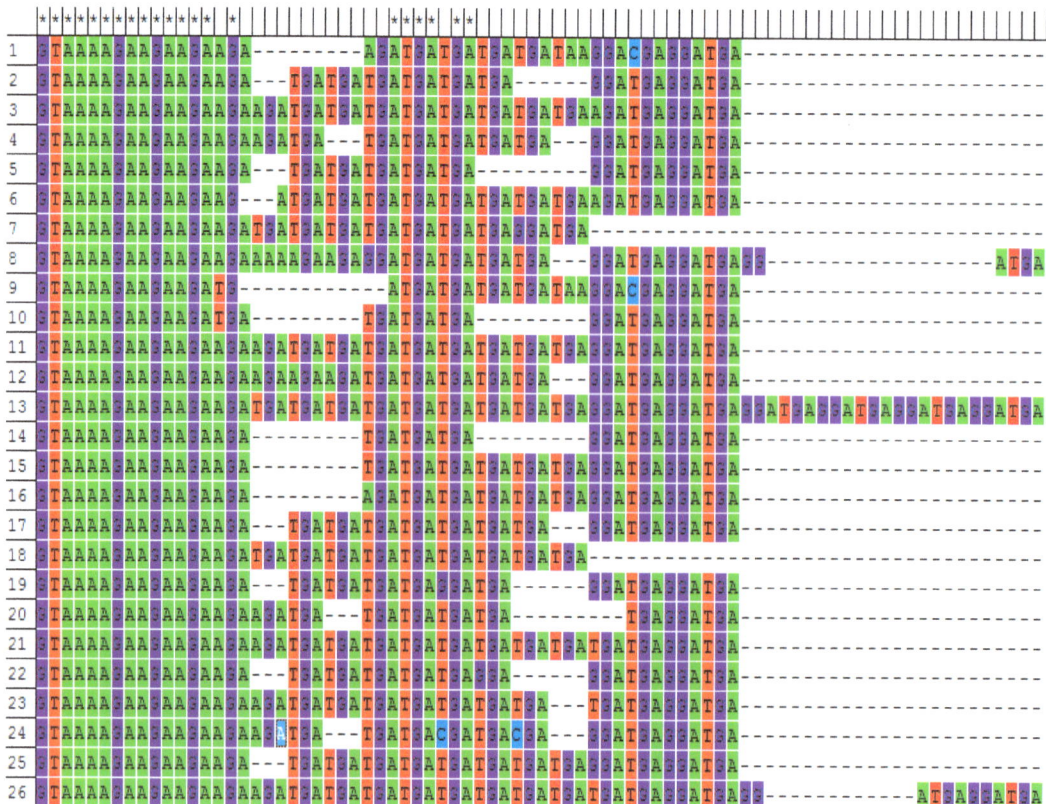

**(B)**

**Figure 11:** A comparison between two alignments of the sequence of case (A) using MEGA4 software (A) and the new software prepared in this paper (B).

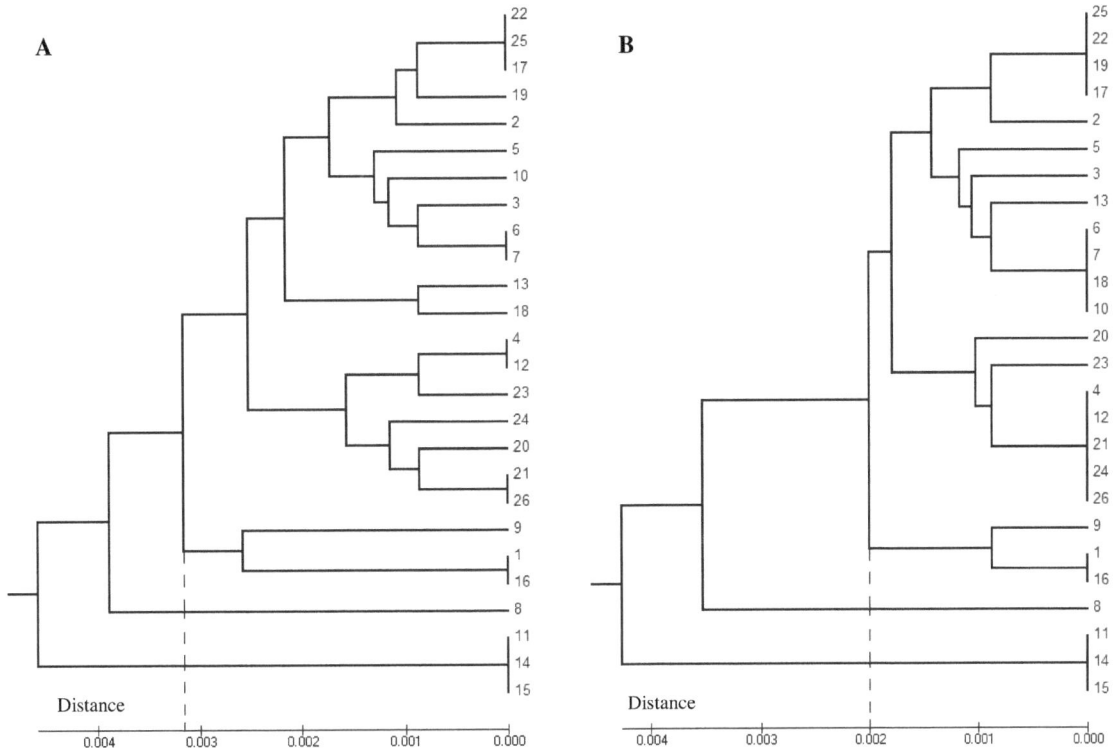

**Figure 12:** Case (E) phylogenic tree before (A) and after (B) applying the algorithm

The alleles 17, 19, 22 and 25 were almost the same after applying the algorithm but before that the allele 19 was a little bit distant from the other three alleles. The alleles 6, 7, 10 and 18 were almost the same after applying the algorithm but before that the allele 10 was distant from the alleles 6 and 7, while the allele 18 was more distant from the other three alleles (Figure 12).

We can deduce from the last examples that (1) the SSR alignment algorithm could be a powerful tool for aligning microsatellites especially for imperfect and compound SSRs, but less so for a simple ones, (2) the SSR alignment algorithm increases the similarity between sequences during alignment by minimizing the overlaps among different repeated units, and (3) it might be necessary to apply it on sequences containing long and complicated SSRs.

## 4    Conclusions

The development and optimization of the last algorithm provides a solution to a fundamental flaw in the current software used for sequence alignment. Scientists usually exclude microsatellites when studying phylogenic trees because of the unrealistic phylogenic relations that results when applying algorithms which are unadjusted to microsatellite regions. They usually settle for counting the number of incidences for each repeated unit or studying the phylogenic relations for the SSR flanking regions. Many overlaps would be generated between different repeated units especially with the imperfect or compound SSRs when applying any previous alignment algorithm whatever we adjust its parameters to fit the SSR case. With the mentioned algorithm, we can include this important source of genetic variation in phylogenic studies without getting untrusted evolutionary relationships. Moreover, with the increasing amount of data which results from the next generation sequencing methods (NGS), searching for microsatellites and realigning them would be as hard as excluding them. The newly developed algorithm and software (SALT version 2) would overcome this limitation and increase the efficiency in mining for SSR for various biological uses.

# 5    Online Resources

1. PERL, v5.8.8 Copyright 1987–2006, Larry Wall. Binary build provided by ActiveState [http://www.ActiveState.com]. The Perl Home Page [http://www.perl.org/].

2. Tk, the extension that makes GUI programming in PERL possible [http://www.tcl.tk/]. Tcl (Tool Command Language) and Tk (ToolKit) was created by Professor John Ousterhout: University of California, Berkeley.

3. SALT version 1 is available as a supplementary material in Jighly et al., 2011.

4. SALT version 2 would be available at ICARDA website [http://www.icarda.org/] soon after acceptance.

# Acknowledgments

The authors gratefully acknowledge Dr. Michael Baum and Dr. Mohammad Imtaiz for their valuable comments to improve the final copy of this chapter.

# References

Akkak, A., Boccacci, P. & Marinoni, D. T. (2010). Cross-Species Amplification of Microsatellite Markers in Castanea spp. And Other Related Species. Acta Hort. (ISHS), 866, 195-201.

Altaf-Khan, M., Qureshi, S. N., Saha, S., Jenkins, J. N., Brubaker, C. L. & Reddy, O. U. (2006). Usefulness of SSR Derived from Tetraploid Gossypium spp. for Analyses of Diploid Gossypium spp. Journal of Crop Improvement, 16, 1-20.

Bell, G. I. (1996). Evolution of simple sequence repeats. Comput.Chem., 20, 41–48.

Brandström, M. & Ellegren, H. (2008). Genome-wide analysis of microsatellite polymorphism in chicken circumventing the ascertainment bias. Genome Res., 18, 881–887.

Chen, S., Lin, Y., Lin, C., Chen, W., Yang, C. H. & Ku, H. (2010). Transferability of rice SSR markers to bamboo. Euphytica, 175, 23–33.

Chistiakov, D. A., Hellemans, B., Haley, C. S., Law, A. S., Tsigenopoulos, C. S., Kotoulas, G., Bertotto, D., Libertini, A. & Volckaert, F. A. (2006). A microsatellite linkage map of the European sea bass Dicentrarchus labrax L. Genetics, 170, 1821–1826.

Choudhary, O. P. & Trivedi, S. (2010). Microsatellite or simple sequence repeat (SSR) instability depends on repeat characteristics during replication and repair. Journal of Cell and Molecular Biology, 8(2), 21-34.

De Jong, E., Guthridge, K. M., Spangenberg, G. C. & Forster, G. W. (2011). Sequence Analysis of SSR-Flanking Regions Identifies Genome Affinities between Pasture Grass Fungal Endophyte Taxa. International Journal of Evolutionary Biology, 10, 1-11.

Du, X., Chen, Z., Li, W., Tan, Y., Lu, J., Zhu, X., Zhao, T., Dong, G. & Zeng, L. (2010). Development of Novel Microsatellite DNA Markers by Cross-Amplification and Analysis of Genetic Variation in Gerbils. Journal of Heredity, 101(6), 710–716.

Egan, A.N., Schlueter, J. & Spooner, D. M. (2012). Applications of next-generation sequencing in plant biology. American Journal of Botany 99(2), 175-185.

Ellegren, H. (2000). Microsatellite mutations in the germline: implications for evolutionary inference. Trends in Genet, 16, 551–558.

Ellegren, H. (2004). Microsatellites: simple sequences with complex evolution. Nat. Rev. Genet, 5, 435–445.

Ghiasi, N., Rashid, Z. A., Hooshmand, S., Yusoff, K., Tan, S. G. & Bhassu, S. (2009). The use of locus specific microsatellite markers for detecting genetic variation in hatchery bred Probarbus jullienii. Biotechnology, 8, 166-170.

Gow, C., Noble, J. L., Rollinson, D. & Jones, C. (2005). A high incidence of clustered microsatellite mutations revealed by parent-offspring analysis in an African freshwater snail, Bulinus forskalii (Gastropoda, Pulmonata). Genetica, 124, 77–83.

Herrera, A. M., Grauke, L. J. & Klein, P. (2011). Validation Of 14 Nuclear SSR Markers Among Different Species Of The Genus Carya. Town & Country Convention Center, P153.

Jakupciak, J. P. & Wells, R. D. (2000). Genetic instabilities of triplet repeat sequences by recombination. IUBMB Life, 50, 355–359.

Jighly, A., Hamwieh, H. & Ogbonnaya, F. C. (2011). Optimization of sequence alignment for SSR (Simple Sequence Repeat) regions. BMC Res. Notes, 4, 239.

Jighly, A. & El-Shamaa, K. (2012). SALT2: A new tool for global sequence alignment considering microsatellite. (**In preparation**).

Kantety, R. V., Rota, M. L., Matthews, D. E. & Sorrells, M. E. (2002). Data mining for simple sequence repeats in expressed sequence rags from barley, maize, rice, sorghum and wheat. Plant Molecular Biol, 48, 501–510.

Kelkar, Y. D., Tyekucheva, S., Chiaromonte, F. & Makova, K. D. L. (2008). The genome-wide determinants of human and chimpanzee microsatellite evolution. Genome Res, 18(1), 30–38.

Kruglyak, S., Durrett, R., Schug, D. & Aquadro, C. (1998). Equilibrium distributions of microsatellite repeat length resulting from a balance between slippage events and point mutations. Proc. Natl. Acad. Sci. USA, 95, 10774–10778.

Leclercq, S., Rivals, E. & Jarne, P. (2010). DNA slippage occurs at microsatellite loci without minimal threshold length in humans: a comparative genomic approach. Genome Biol. Evol., 2, 325–335.

Merkel, A. & Gemmell, N. (2008). Detecting short tandem repeats from genome data: opening the software black box. Briefings in Bioinformatics, 9(5), 355-366.

Peakall, R., Gilmore, S., Keys, W., Morgante, M. & Rafalski, A. (1998). Cross-species amplification of soybean (Glycine max) simple sequence repeats (SSRs) within the genus and other legume genera: implications for the transferability of SSRs in plants. Mol Biol Evol., 15, 1275–1287.

Powell, W., Machray, G. C. & Provan, J. (1996). Polymorphism revealed by simple sequence repeats. Trends Plant Sci., 1, 215–222.

Riley, D. E. & Krieger, J. N. (2009). Embryonic nervous system genes predominate in searches for dinucleotide simple sequence repeats flanked by conserved sequences. Gene., 429:74-79.

Sainudiin, R., Durrett, R. T., Aquadro, C. F. & Nielsen, R. (2004). Microsatellite mutation models: insights from a comparison of humans and chimpanzees. Genetics, 168(1), 383–395.

Santibanez-Koref, M. F., Gangeswaran, R. & Hancock, J. M. (2001). A relationship between lengths of microsatellites and nearby substitution rates in mammalian genomes. Mol Biol Evol, 18(11), 2119–2123.

Schena, L., Cardle, L. & Elcooke, D (2008). Use of genome sequence data in the design and testing of SSR markers for Phytophthora species. BMC Genomics, 9, 620.

Schlotterer, C. (2004). The evolution of molecular markers just a matter of fashion. Nat. Rev. Genet., 5, 63–69.

Sekar, M., Suresh, E., Kumar, N. S., Mayak, S. K. & Balakrishna, C. (2009). Microsatellite DNA markers, a fisheries perspective. Aquaculture Asia Magazine, 27–29.

Shakyawar, S. K., Joshi, B. K. & Kumar, D. (2009). SSR repeat dynamics in mitochondrial genomes of five domestic animal species. Bioinformation, 4(4), 158-163.

Suwabe, K., Tsukazaki, H., Iketani, H., Hatakeyama, K., Kondo, M., Fujimura, M., Nunome, T., Fukuoka, H., Hirai, M. & Matsumoto, S. (2006). Simple Sequence Repeat-Based Comparative Genomics Between Brassica rapa and Arabidopsis thaliana The Genetic Origin of Clubroot Resistance. Genetics, 173, 309–319.

Tamura, K., Dudley, J., Nei, M. & Kumar, S. (2007). MEGA4: molecular evolutionary genetics analysis (MEGA) software version 4.0. Mol Biol Evol, 24, 1596–1599.

Tang, P., Wei, N. V., Chen, C., Wallace, C. C. & Allen, C. (2010). Comparative Study of Genetic Variability of AAT and CTGT Microsatellites in Staghorn Coral, Acropora (Scleractinia Acroporidae). Zoological Studies, 49(5), 657-668.

Tautz, D. (1989). Hypervariability of simple sequences as a general source for polymorphic DNA markers. Nucl Acids Res, 17, 6563–6571.

Vir, R., Bhat, K. V. & Lakhanpaul, S. (2009). Transferability of sequence tagged microsatellite sites (STMS) primers to pulse yielding taxa belonging to Phaseolae. IJIB, 5, 62-66.

Weber, J. & Wong, C. (1993). Mutation of human short tandem repeats. Hum. Mol. Genet., 2, 1123–1128.

Whittaker, J. C., Harbord, R. M., Boxall, N., Mackay, I., Dawson, G. & Sibly, R. M. (2003). Likelihood-based estimation of microsatellite mutation rates. Genetics, 164(2), 781–787.

Wiessenbach, J., Gyapay, G., Dib, C., Vignal, A. & Moresette, J. (1992). A second generation map of the human genome. Nature, 359, 794–801.

Zardoya, R., Vollmer, D. M., Craddock, C., Streelman, J. T., Karl, S. & Meyer, A. (1996). Evolutionary conservation of microsatellite flanking regions and their use in resolving the phylogeny of cichlid fished (Pisces:Perciformes). Proc. R. Soc. Lond. B, 263, 1589-1598.

Zhang, Z. & Gerstein, M. (2003). Patterns of nucleotide substitution, insertion and deletion in the human genome inferred from pseudogenes. Nucleic Acids Res, 31, 5338–5348.

Zhang, L., Sun, G., Yan, Z., Chen, Q., Yuan, Z., Lan, X., Zheng, Y. & Liu, D. (2007). Comparison of Newly Synthetic Hexaploid Wheat with Its Donors on SSR Products. Journal of Genetics and Genomics, 34(10), 939-946.

# Regulation of Endosomal Membrane Trafficking with RUN Domain Proteins

Yasuko Kitagishi
*Department of Environmental Health Science*
*Nara Women's University, Japan*

Mayumi Kobayashi
*Department of Environmental Health Science*
*Nara Women's University, Japan*

Satoru Matsuda
*Department of Environmental Health Science*
*Nara Women's University, Japan*

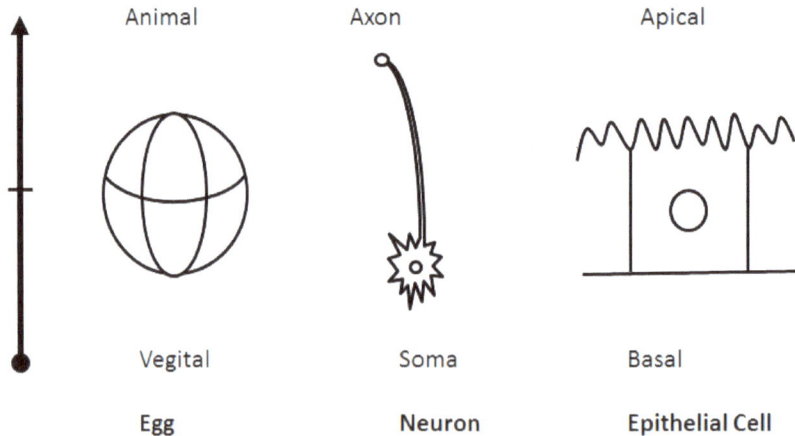

**Figure 1:** Cell polarity is observed in many cases. Left arrow indicates the direction of polarity. Eggs, epithelial, and neuronal cells are asymmetric with discrete regions responsible for different roles that may underlie the generation of specific compartments within cells, which is distinct in biochemical composition, function and structure. The establishment of the cell polarity is not only required for the functioning of the individual cell but is a prerequisite for the development of whole organs.

# 1    Introduction

Cell polarization is required for the cell to function properly (Horton & Ehlers, 2003). The asymmetric organization of cellular components and structures is called the cell polarity (Figure 1). For example, the presence of axon in neuronal cells determines the directional flow of the signal. The formation of distinct membrane in epithelial cells is required for the directional uptake of nutrients from the lumen of the gut to blood vessels (Datta *et al.*, 2011). Establishment of the cell polarity involves many processes including signaling cascades (Happé *et al.*, 2011), membrane trafficking events (Santiago-Tirado & Bretscher, 2011) and cytoskeletal dynamics (Baum & Georgiou, 2011), which is implicated in differentiation, proliferation and morphogenesis of various organisms (Wu *et al.*, 2011) (Figure 1). Dysregulation of cell polarity can cause developmental disorders and cancer (Martin-Belmonte & Perez-Moreno, 2011). Studies have revealed links between cell polarity establishment and cellular membrane traffic (Santiago-Tirado & Bretscher, 2011). So, membrane trafficking is also important in neurodevelopment human diseases (Carrard *et al.*, 2011). The function of endosome-associated proteins has been implicated in the membrane trafficking and cell polarity (Golachowska *et al.*, 2010). Endosomes exchange their contents with each other through membrane fusion processes, which are essential for many cellular functions including protein transport, signaling transduction, and lysosomal degradation (Lin *et al.*, 2012). Based on the membrane function, endosomes can be classified as early endosomes, recycling endosomes, and late endosomes (Figure 2). Upon endocytosis, plasma membrane associated molecules are first delivered to early endosomes, where they are either sorted to recycling endosomes to be trafficked back to the plasma membrane, or are processed through the late endosome and lysosome-pathway for degradation. The initial trafficking of down-regulated proteins is performed by clathrin-mediated internalization and sorting into the lumen of the endosomes (Traub, 2009).

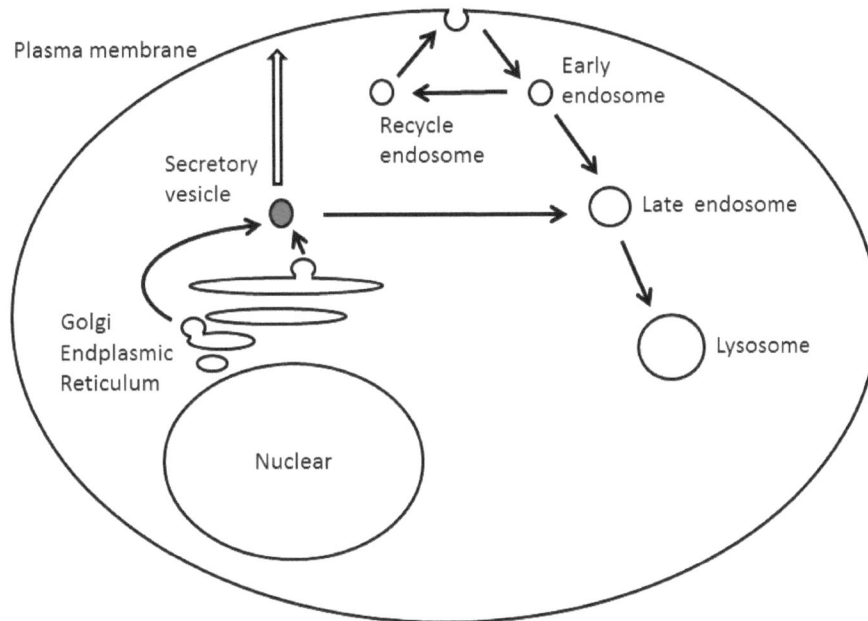

**Figure 2:** Schematic representation of intracellular transport. The model depicts the pathways used by biosynthetic secretory and internalized endocytotic cargoes to reach their final destinations. Note that some critical trafficking routes have been omitted for clarity.

Selective movement of proteins from the plasma or Golgi membrane serves as a comprehensive mechanism to control various cellular processes (Derby & Gleeson, 2007). The movement is mediated by internalization from the cell surface, followed by sorting into intracellular vesicles of endosomes and subsequent delivery to the lysosome. The direction and specificity of endosomal membrane trafficking is definitely regulated by various membrane-bound factors including protein receptors, small GTPases, and phosphoinositides (Mayinger, 2012). While many components of trafficking pathways have been assigned, there may be additional factors that remain unidentified, which precisely controls the direction and specificity of the membrane trafficking. In the present brief review, we summarize the function of RUN domain proteins and the binding partners such as Rab proteins at a viewpoint of endosomal membrane trafficking, covering what is known about the function of RUFY family protein signaling. These findings are initially based on studies of sequence and genome analysis.

## 2   Cell polarity and Membrane trafficking

Cell polarity and vesicle sorting are significant processes that influence normal cell function including cell adhesion and migration, development, pathogen entry, and neurotransmission (Valtorta et al., 2011). Specific molecular targeting has been studied to understand the generation of asymmetric domains inside cells. The pathway is then recognized as a key regulator of endocytic membrane traffic, protein-sorting, and various signaling (Connord et al., 2012). Endosomal membrane trafficking is a spatiotemporally regulated process that confirms suitable delivery of cargo via the pathway (MacGurn, et al., 2012). Endosomes can bud inwardly from the membranes to form vesicles. The endosomal pathway is a complicated system comprising numerous membrane-bound organelles. Endosomes receive cargo from the cell surface via endocytosis, and biosynthetic cargo from the late Golgi complex (Pfeffer, 2009). The trafficking has been shown to be a critical component of many signaling pathways, which is indispensable for a wide range of developmental processes (González-Gaitán, 2003). The lysosomes can fuse with late endosomes to get macromolecules that are sorted for lysosomal degradation (Bright *et al.*, 1997), and to acquire synthesized hydrolytic enzymes from the Golgi complex. In addition, membrane fission also facilitates the recycling of materials acquired from late endosomes or lysosomes (Wenk & De Camilli, 2004). When lysosomal trafficking is interrupted, a variety of lysosomal storage diseases can develop (Vitner, 2010). The endosomal trafficking is regulated by sequential recruitment of a variety of cytosolic and membrane-bound proteins and factors. Studies have also elucidated many of the key components of membrane fusion events that take place during exocytosis. For example, soluble NSF attachment protein receptors (SNAREs) have been identified as the basic components needed for membrane fusion events (Hanson *et al.*, 1997; Gurkan *et al.*, 2007). For the regulation of the priming fusion steps, small GTPases of Rab family, its effectors, Ca2+ levels, and phosphoinositides may be important (Yu *et al*, 2007). Intracellular fusion events in the endosomal pathway are regulated by mechanisms similar to those used in exocytosis. Previous studies have demonstrated that $Ca^{2+}$ influx through voltage-gated $Ca^{2+}$ channels triggers the final step in exocytotic membrane fusion events during neurotransmission (Monck & Fernandez, 1994). Endosomal $Ca^{2+}$ channels may be modulated by lipids enriched in endosomes, similar to various channels of the plasma membrane (Martin *et al.*, 1997).

Evidence suggests that SNAREs can also regulate Rab effectors (Honda *et al.*, 2005; Hammer & Wu, 2002). Similarly, phosphoinositides have been shown to be important not only for the recruitment of Rab family proteins and the binding factors (Zaid *et al.*, 2008), but also for interactions with SNAREs and $Ca^{2+}$ sensors (Vergne *et al*, 2003). Plasma membrane channels are known to be regulated by Rab proteins, SNAREs, and phosphoinositides, which also are molecules that determine the vesicular identity and direction of membrane trafficking. PIP3 is essential for membrane trafficking of early endosome (Cockcroft, 1999). The PIP3 has lots of effector proteins in mammalian cells, all of which contain PIP3 binding motifs such as FYVE or PH domains (Kutateladze, 2007; Saito *et al.*, 2007). Selective recruitment of these effectors by PIP3 may provide a mechanism by which the directionality for incoming vesicles and endosomes is established. The PIP3 is thus critical for the maturation of endosomes, and for fusion events with intracellular organelles (Stenmark & Gillooly, 2001). Consistently, disruption of PIP3 synthesis by wortmannin affects the formation of internal vesicles and the maturation of endosomes (Shisheva, 2008). While phosphoinositides can recruit phosphoinositide-binding proteins to regulate the activity of GTPases, GTPases can in turn control the activity of PIP metabolizing enzymes (Oude Weernink *et al.*, 2007).

## 3    Some small GTPases associate with endosome functions

The Rab proteins are a family of small GTPases that participate in regulating the membrane trafficking pathways. Some Rab proteins recruit effectors to promote membrane fusion and vesicle formation and play a key role in early endocytic pathways (Wang *et al.*, 2011). Rab effectors include sorting adaptors, binding factors, lipid kinases, and lipid phosphatases, which are present on the surface of the acceptor compartment. Binding factors mediate vesicle fusion by interacting with molecules on the acceptor membrane, while lipid kinases produce phosphoinositides to further define vesicular identity and the direction of membrane trafficking (Wang *et al.*, 2011). Rab proteins are classified in specific organelle membrane proteins, establishing the elementary tags to define organelle identity. Briefly, the endosomal Rab proteins such as Rab 4, 5 and 9 are characterized by their localization and function with effector proteins (Mohrmann, & van der Sluijs,, 1999). Rab4 and Rab11 regulate recycling of receptors from early endosomes to the cell surface via distinct pathways (Jones *et al.*, 2006). Rab4 functions at the level of early endosomes, and Rab11 is involved in the trafficking of cargo through recycling endosomes (Nachury et al., 2010). Rab4 has also an important role in Glut4 trafficking in adipocytes, skeletal muscle and cardiocytes (Foster & Klip, 2000). Rab5 functions in clathrin-mediated endocytosis (Cavalli *et al.*, 2001) and in endosome to endosome fusion. EEA1, a Rab5 effector, is recruited selectively onto the early endosomes, whereas Rab5 is symmetrically distributed between the clathrin-coated vesicles and early endosomes (Hayakawa *et al.*, 2007). While Rab5 is localized in the early endosome, Rab7 is localized to late endosome and lysosomes (Wang et al., 2011). Endsomal trafficking is also controlled by Rab6. In addition, Rab8 plays an important role in exocytic membrane trafficking from Golgi complex to plasma membrane (Dugani & Klip, 2005). The Rab8 is associated with myosinVI via optineurin, and the Rab8optineurinmyosin VI complex might be involved in presenting the secretory vesicle to plasma membrane (Chibalina *et al.*, 2008). Rab9 is associated with trafficking to the Golgi network (Chia *et al.*, 2011). Rab11 and Rab11-family interacting protein 3, which plays a role in regulation of actin dynamics, are both required to support the formation of filamentous virions (Bruce *et al.*, 2010). Rab11 is also involved in recycling endosomes back to the plasma membrane. Rab14 has been implicated in phagosome and early endosome fusion. The Rab14 also localizes to the Golgi complex. The Rab27A indirectly recognizes myosin Va on melanosomes via Slac2-a (Kuroda *et al.*, 2005). The Rab27B, a closely related isoform of Rab27A, is also associated with Myosin Va/VIIa via Slac2c/MyRIP (Westbroek *et al.*, 2004). Rab27 and Slac2c/MyRIP are part of a complex mediating the interaction of secretory granules with actin cytoskeleton and participate to the regulation of exocytosis. Rab35 regulates neurite-outgrowth (Chua *et al.*, 2010). Rap-family proteins are small GTPases closely related to Ras. Rap1 is involved in various cellular processes such as regulation of integrin mediated cell adhesion and cadherin-mediated cell junction formation. It has been demonstrated that interaction between Rap proteins and profilin II, an important activator of actin polymerization is mediated via Rgl3, a RalGDS-related protein (Xu *et al.*, 2007). RAPL, a Rap1-associating molecule localizes on microtubules and the activated Rap1 and RAPL control the directional migration of vascular endothelial cells (Kinashi & Katagiri, 2004). Rap2 interacts with the platelet cytoskeleton by direct binding to the actin filament, which is the polymerized but not the monomeric form of actin (Kardassis *et al.*, 2009). In this way, several small GTPases associate with motor proteins and/or filamentous molecules. While small GTPases are essential for membrane trafficking, actin remodeling is also critical. Actin is polymerized at the site of particle attachment and directs membrane extension (Coppolino *et al.*, 2002). Many actin associated proteins are enriched at the phagocytic cup and play important roles in phagocytosis (Fehrenbacher *et al.*, 2003). Importantly, it is the interactions of these small GTPase proteins to the effector molecules that form a functional interaction to regulate the membrane trafficking. Rabs and their effectors can also interact with SNAREs and their accessory proteins to regulate the formation of SNARE complexes, modulating membrane fusion processes (Mller *et al.*, 2003).

# 4   RUN domain proteins involved in the small GTPase-mediated membrane trafficking

The RUN domains, named from RPIP8, UNC-14, and NESCA proteins (MacDonald *et al.*, 2004), might function as effectors of the small GTPase superfamily (Yoshida *et al.*, 2011). Because many RUN domain containing proteins are involved in small GTPase signaling including members of the Rap and Rab families, the RUN domain has been suggested to be involved in the small GTPase-mediated membrane trafficking. The sequence and genome analysis showed the RUN domain containing proteins enclosed hydrophobic amino acids in conserved positions (Wang *et al.*, 2003). The RUN domain is composed of six conserved blocks, which constitute the core of globular structure. The overall crystal structure of the RUN domain adopts a single globular fold consisting of eight alpha-helices (Kukimoto-Niino *et al.*, 2006; Sun *et al.*, 2012). It is a conserved protein motif that consists of approximately 70 amino acids with binding activity to small GTP-binding proteins. However, it is not the all function of a RUN domain to bind a GTPase. The RUN domain binds to some molecules, those are related to motor proteins, and the RUN domain might be responsible for an interaction with a filamentous network (Yoshida *et al.*, 2011).

The RUN domain containing proteins have been shown to promote endosomal fusion and are important for vesicular transport, and the RUN domains appear to be required for localization to detergent-insoluble endosomal microdomains (Mari et al., 2001; Yoshida *et al.*, 2011). The physical interaction between RUN proteins and filamentous materials has been confirmed by several biochemical experiments using wild type and mutant proteins. The association among the small GTPases, RUN proteins, and motor proteins might reflect a new function for these proteins in transport of vesicular cargoes within cells (Yoshida *et al.*, 2011). Small GTPases bound to RUN domain -containing proteins are summarized previously (Yoshida *et al.*, 2011). It has been reported that FYCO1 functions as an adapter linking autophagosomes to microtubule molecular motors, and the Rab7 is implicated in the phagosomal transport and fusion (Pankiv *et al.*, 2010). Nesca, a RUN-domain protein, binds to F-actin, microtubules, and acetylated α-tubulin, which functions as an adapter involved in neuronal vesicular transport (MacDonald *et al*, 2012). We hypothesize that there is a common function underlying the mechanism of association of RUN domain proteins with Rab GTPase for motor proteins.

# 5   Characteristics of RUFY family proteins

The RUFY, designated as the RUN and FYVE domain-containing, protein family contains an amino-terminal RUN domain, and a carboxyl-terminal FYVE domain, which associates with phosphatidylinositol 3-phosphate in membranes of early endosomes (Yang *et al.*, 2002). Actually, RUFY proteins are localized predominantly to endosomes. A RUFY protein is tyrosine-phosphorylated and the mutant lacking the phosphorylation sites fails to go to the endosomes. It has been suggested Rab4, Rab14 and RUFY protein play an important role in the membrane trafficking (Mari *et al.*, 2006; Yamamoto *et al.*, 2012). Sequence and genome analyses have revealed that a RUFY family consists of 4 members of RUFY proteins (Cormont *et al.*, 2001; Yoshida *et al.*, 2010) (Figure 3).

RUFY1, also known as RABIP4 or ZFYVE12, is a 708 amino acid protein that localizes to the cytoplasm and the early endosome membrane (Cormont *et al.*, 2001). RUFY1 has been identified as the downstream effector of Etk protein, which is highly expressed in testis, lung, brain and kidney (Cormont *et al.*,

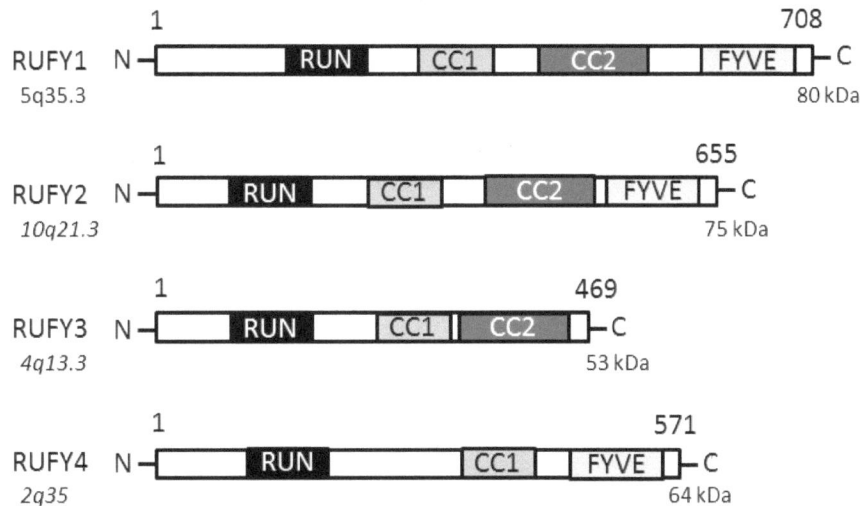

**Figure 3:** Schematic diagram indicating the domain structures of the RUFY1, RUFY2, RUFY3, and RUFY4 proteins. The functionally important sites are shown. Genomic locations of each the genes and approximate molecular mass of each the proteins are also shown. RUN = RPIP8, UNC-14, and NESCA proteins, FYVE = Fab-1, YGL023, Vps27, and EEA1 proteins, CC = Coiled-Coil

2001). RUFY1 functions to bind PIP3-containing phospholipid vesicles and participates in early endosomal trafficking (Cormont *et al.*, 2001). The downstream effects of PI3-kinase signaling are in many cases mediated by proteins containing a PIP3 binding module indicated FYVE finger domain. Lots of FYVE domain containing proteins are localized at endosomes and play an important role in endocytosis. The Etk interacts with RUFY1 through the SH3 and SH2 domains and that tyrosine phosphorylation, Tyr-281 and Tyr-292, of RUFY1 by the Etk is essential for the endosomal localization (Cormont *et al.*, 2001). The Etk plays an important role in the regulation of endocytosis as a downstream effector of PI3-kinase. Two coiled-coil domains also determine endosomal localization of RUFY1 (Cormont *et al.*, 2001). The PI3-kinase inhibitor Wortmannin blocks the endosomal localization of RUFY1. Rab14 engages in a GTP-dependent interaction with RUFY1. The active Rab14 regulates RUFY1 recruitment onto endosomal membranes, and Rab4 allows endosomal fusion (Yamamoto *et al.*, 2010). The Rab14 seems to be primary determinant of RUFY1 recruitment to endosomes and that the FYVE domain may assist RUFY1 targeting to PIP3 enriched early endosomes (Yamamoto *et al.*, 2010). Rab14 and RUFY1 are also involved in Rab4-dependent recycling endosome. Enlargement of early endosomes mediated by RUFY1 needs the interaction with Rab4 Mari *et al.*, 2006). The RUFY1 is present in the sorting endosomes, while Rab4 is present both on sorting and recycling endosomes. This would provide directional trafficking way from the recycling endosomes to the sorting endosomes. RUFY1 can also modify the kinetic parameters of Glut 1 recycling (Cormont *et al.*, 2001).

RUFY2, also known as RABIP4R or ZFYVE13, contains a RUN domain and a carboxyl terminal FYVE zinc finger with two coiled-coil domains in-between (Yang *et al.*, 2002; Barbe *et al.*, 2008). Localizing to nucleus, RUFY2 is expressed in brain, lung and testis (Yang *et al.*, 2002; Barbe *et al.*, 2008).

Believed to be involved with zinc ion binding, RUFY2 as well as RUFY1 interacts with the Etk, a tyrosine kinase involved in regulation of various cellular processes. The carboxyl domain of RUFY2 weakly binds to negative form of Rab33A. RUFY3, also known as RIPX or SINGAR1, is localized in hippocampal neurons and accumulated in the axons (Mori *et al.*, 2007). RUFY3 ensures the robustness of neuronal polarity by suppressing formation of surplus axons. RUFY3 also contains the RUN domain and seems to play important roles in multiple Ras-like GTPase signaling pathways. Rab5 engages in a GTP-dependent interaction with RUFY3. RUFY3 can bind to the active Rab5 and weakly associates to Rap2 (Yoshida *et al.*, 2010). RUFY3 may function as a docking protein for distinct two small GTPases. It has been reported that oxidized LDL -containing immune complexes affect the gene expression of RUFY3 in human U937 monocytic cells (Hammad *et al.*, 2009). RUFY4 is a 571 amino acid protein that contains a RUN domain and a FYVE zinc finger (Kimura *et al.*, 2006). RUFY4 is also believed to be involved with zinc ion binding. As for RUFY2 and for RUFY4, little is known about the precise intracellular functions.

# 6   Perspective

Mis-trafficking is an important pathophysiological feature of motor and sensory neuropathy (Salin-Cantegrel *et al.*, 2011). For example, impaired palmitoyl acyltransferases activity, which is involved in endosomal trafficking, is linked to neurodevelopmental and neuropsychiatric disorders, suggesting critical roles for palmitoylation in neuronal function (Thomas *et al.*, 2012). In addition, a lot of neurodegenerative diseases including Alzheimer's disease exhibit defective endsomal trafficking. The transport would be necessary to ensure neuronal organelle homeostasis. While several storage diseases have been characterized by a progressive accumulation of sphingolipids and mucopolysaccharides in endosomes, the abnormal lipid accumulation may lead to the endosome trafficking deficiency. The functional significance of membrane trafficking in the signaling pathways remains to be more established. Indeed, the RUN domain containing proteins will be an active focus of investigation of this field. The RUFY proteins may be activated in endosomal microdomains enriched in some unidentified cytoskeletal elements. The localization of RUFY proteins during membrane trafficking seems to be dynamic. Although specific kinetic information would be required, RUFY and Rab proteins have an inhibitory function in endocytosis, which is similar to the case of Rab15 in neuronal system (Strick & Elferink, 2005). This inhibitory effect could result from a negative regulation of the recycling. Likewise, RUFY3 may ensure the strength of neuronal cell polarity by suppressing formation of surplus axons. The molecular details of how RUFY3 inhibits the formation of surplus axons remain important issues for future sequence and genome investigation. Deciphering the precise mechanisms involved will provide new insight into the physiological roles of these interesting proteins in regulating vesicle traffic (Figure 4). It is anticipated that future studies would address to get a better knowledge of the potential partners and roles of the RUFY and RUN domain proteins.

## Acknowledgments

This work was supported by grants-in-aid from the Ministry of Education, Culture, Sports, Science and Technology in Japan. In addition, this work was supported in part by the grant from SHIN-EI Pharmaceutical Co., Ltd.

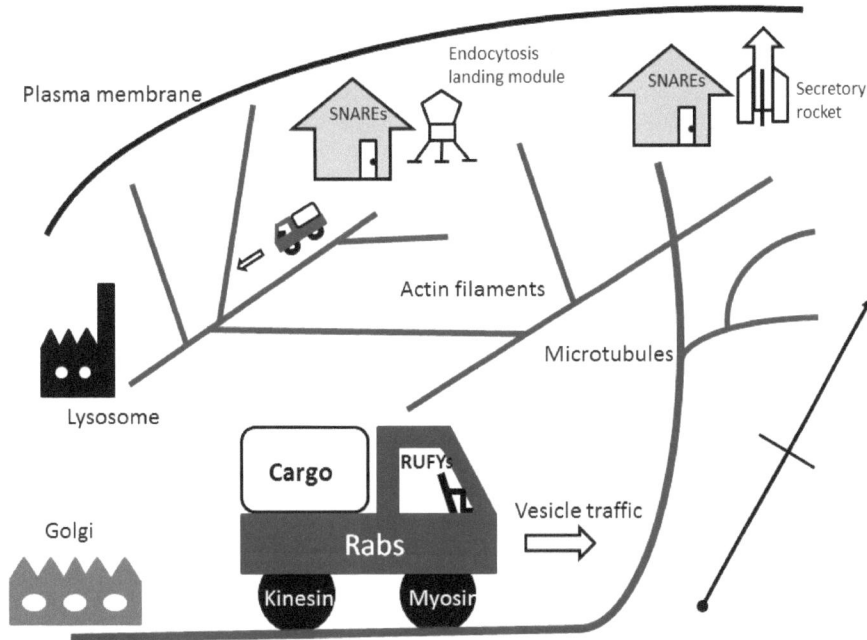

**Figure 4:** Schematic cartoon illustration of membrane-trafficking to the plasma membrane, involving exocytic and endocytic routes, Golgi, lysosome, and endosomal compartments. Examples of the molecule known to act on the regulatory compartments are shown. Cargo leaves the Golgi-network or recycling endosomes in vesicular carriers to the plasma membrane during secretory exocytosis. Intracellular transport may be essential for the proper establishment of cell polarity. Note that several critical molecules have been omitted for clarity. SNAREs = soluble NSF attachment protein receptors, RUFYs = RUN and FYVE domain-containing proteins.

## Competing interests statement

The authors declare that they have no competing financial interests.

## Appendix – Abbreviations

- SNAREs: soluble NSF attachment protein receptors

- RUFY: RUN and FYVE domain-containing proteins.

- RUN: RPIP8, UNC-14, and NESCA proteins,

- FYVE: Fab-1, YGL023, Vps27, and EEA1 proteins,

- CC: Coiled-Coil

- PIP: phosphoinositidephosphate

- PIP3: Phosphatidylinositol (3,4,5)-trisphosphate

# References

Barbe, L., Lundberg, E., Oksvold, P., Stenius, A., Lewin, E., Björling, E., Asplund, A., Pontén, F., Brismar, H., Uhlén, M., & Andersson-Svahn, H. (2008). Toward a confocal subcellular atlas of the human proteome. Mol Cell Proteomics 7, 499-508.

Baum, B., & Georgiou, M. (2011). Dynamics of adherens junctions in epithelial establishment, maintenance, and remodeling. J Cell Biol, 192, 907-917. Bright N. A., Reaves B. J., Mullock B. M., Luzio J. P. (1997). Dense core lysosomes can fuse with late endosomes and are re-formed from the resultant hybrid organelles. J Cell Sci 110 , 2027-2040.

Bruce, E. A., Digard, P., & Stuart, A. D. (2010). The Rab11 pathway is required for influenza A virus budding and filament formation. J Virol, 84, 5848-5859. Carrard, A., Salzmann, A., Perroud, N., Gafner, J., Malafosse, A., & Karege, F. (2011). Genetic association of the Phosphoinositide-3 kinase in schizophrenia and bipolar disorder and interaction with a BDNF gene polymorphism. Brain Behav 1, 119-124.

Cavalli, V., Corti, M., & Gruenberg, J. (2001). Endocytosis and signaling cascades: a close encounter. FEBS Lett, 498, 190-196. Chia, P. Z., Gasnereau, I., Lieu, Z. Z., & Gleeson, P. A. (2011). Rab9-dependent retrograde transport and endosomal sorting of the endopeptidase furin. J Cell Sci 124, 2401-2413.

Chibalina, M. V., Roberts, R. C., Arden, S. D., Kendrick-Jones, J., & Buss, F. (2008). Rab8-optineurin-myosin VI: analysis of interactions and functions in the secretory pathway. Methods Enzymol 438, 11-24.

Chua, C. E., Lim, Y. S., & Tang, B. L. (2010). Rab35–a vesicular traffic-regulating small GTPase with actin modulating roles. FEBS Lett 584, 1-6.

Cockcroft S. (1999). Mammalian phosphatidylinositol transfer proteins: emerging roles in signal transduction and vesicular traffic. Chem Phys Lipids 98, 23-33.

Coppolino M. G., Dierckman R., Loijens J., Collins R. F., Pouladi M., Jongstra-Bilen J., Schreiber A. D., Trimble W. S., Anderson R., Grinstein S. (2002). Inhibition of phosphatidylinositol-4-phosphate 5-kinase Ialpha impairs localized actin remodeling and suppresses phagocytosis. J Biol Chem 277, 43849-43857.

Gonnord P., Blouin C. M., Lamaze C. (2012). Membrane trafficking and signaling: two sides of the same coin. Semin Cell Dev Biol 23, 154-164.

Cormont, M., Mari, M., Galmiche, A., Hofman, P., & Le, Marchand-Brustel, Y. (2001). A FYVE-finger-containing protein, Rabip4, is a Rab4 effector involved in early endosomal traffic. Proc Natl Acad Sci U S A 98, 1637-1642.

Datta A., Bryant D. M., Mostov K. E. (2011). Molecular regulation of lumen morphogenesis. Curr Biol 21, R126-136.

Derby M. C., Gleeson P. A. (2007). New insights into membrane trafficking and protein sorting. Int Rev Cytol 261, 47-116.

Dugani, C. B., & Klip, A. (2005). Glucose transporter 4: cycling, compartments and controversies. EMBO Rep 6, 1137-1142.

Fehrenbacher, K., Huckaba, T., Yang, H. C., Boldogh, I., & Pon, L. (2003). Actin comet tails, endosomes and endosymbionts. J Exp Biol 206, 1977-198 4.

Foster, L. J., & Klip, A. (2000). Mechanism and regulation of GLUT-4 vesicle fusion in muscle and fat cells. Am J Physiol Cell Physiol 279, C877-C890.

Golachowska, M. R., Hoekstra, D., & van IJzendoorn, S. C. (2010). Recycling endosomes in apical plasma membrane domain formation and epithelial cell polarity. Trends Cell Biol 20, 618-626.

Gonzlez-Gaitn, M. (2003). Endocytic trafficking during Drosophila development. Mech Dev 120, 1265-1282.

Gurkan, C., Koulov, A. V., & Balch, W. E. (2007). An evolutionary perspective on eukaryotic membrane trafficking. Adv Exp Med Biol 607, 73-83.

Hammad, S. M., Twal, W. O., Barth, J. L., Smith, K. J., Saad, A. F., Virella, G., Argraves, W. S., & Lopes-Virella, M. F. (2009). Oxidized LDL immune complexes and oxidized LDL differentially affect the expression of genes involved with inflammation and survival in human U937 monocytic cells. Atherosclerosis 202, 394-404.

Hammer, J. A. 3rd, & Wu, X. S. (2002). Rabs grab motors: defining the connections between Rab GTPases and motor proteins. Curr Opin Cell Biol 14, 69-75.

Hanson P. I., Heuser J. E., Jahn R. (1997). Neurotransmitter release - four years of SNARE complexes. Curr Opin Neurobiol 7, 310-315.

Happ, H., de Heer, E., & Peters, D. J. (2011). Polycystic kidney disease: the complexity of planar cell polarity and signaling during tissue regeneration and cyst formation. Biochim Biophys Acta 1812, 1249-1255.

Hayakawa, A., Hayes, S., Leonard, D., Lambright, D., & Corvera, S. (2007). Evolutionarily conserved structural and functional roles of the FYVE domain. Biochem Soc Symp 74, 95-105.

Honda A., Al-Awar O. S., Hay J. C., Donaldson J. G. (2005). Targeting of Arf-1 to the early Golgi by membrin, an ER-Golgi SNARE. J Cell Biol, 168, 1039-1051. Horton A. C., & Ehlers M. D. (2003). Neuronal polarity and trafficking. Neuron 40, 277-295.

Jones, M. C., Caswell, P. T., & Norman, J. C. (2006). Endocytic recycling pathways: emerging regulators of cell migration. Curr Opin Cell Biol 18, 549-557.

Kardassis, D., Murphy, C., Fotsis, T., Moustakas, A., & Stournaras, C. (2009). Control of transforming growth factor beta signal transduction by small GTPases. FEBS J 276, 2947-2965.

Kimura, K., Wakamatsu, A., Suzuki, Y., Ota, T., Nishikawa, T., Yamashita, R., Yamamoto, J., Sekine, M., Tsuritani, K., Wakaguri, H., Ishii, S., Sugiyama, T., Saito, K., Isono, Y., Irie, R., Kushida, N., Yoneyama, T., Otsuka, R., Kanda, K., Yokoi, T., Kondo, H., Wagatsuma, M., Murakawa, K., Ishida, S., Ishibashi, T., Takahashi-Fujii, A., Tanase, T., Nagai, K., Kikuchi, H., Nakai, K., Isogai, T., & Sugano, S. (2006). Diversification of transcriptional modulation: large-scale identification and characterization of putative alternative promoters of human genes. Genome Res 16, 55-65.

Kinashi, T., & Katagiri, K. (2004). Regulation of lymphocyte adhesion and migration by the small GTPase Rap1 and its effector molecule, RAPL. Immunol Lett 93, 1-5.

Kukimoto-Niino M., Takagi T., Akasaka R., Murayama K., Uchikubo-Kamo T., Terada T., Inoue M., Watanabe S., Tanaka A., Hayashizaki Y., Kigawa T., Shirouzu M., Yokoyama S. (2006). Crystal structure of the RUN domain of the RAP2-interacting protein x. J Biol Chem 281, 31843-31853.

Kuroda, T. S., Itoh, T., & Fukuda, M. (2005). Functional analysis of slac2-a/melanophilin as a linker protein between Rab27A and myosin Va in melanosome transport. Methods Enzymol 403, 419-431.

Kutateladze T. G. (2007). Mechanistic similarities in docking of the FYVE and PX domains to phosphatidylinositol 3-phosphate containing membranes. Prog Lipid Res 46, 315-327.

Lin, W. J., Yang, C. Y., Li, L. L., Yi, Y. H., Chen, K. W., Lin, Y. C., Liu, C. C., & Lin, C. H. (2012). Lysosomal targeting of phafin1 mediated by Rab7 induces autophagosome formation. Biochem Biophys Res Commun 417, 35-42.

MacDonald J. I., Dietrich A., Gamble S., Hryciw T., Grant R. I., Meakin S. O. (2012). Nesca, a novel neuronal adapter protein, links the molecular motor kinesin with the pre-synaptic membrane protein, syntaxin-1, in hippocampal neurons. J Neurochem 121, 861-880.

MacDonald, J. I., Kubu, C. J., & Meakin, S. O. (2004). Nesca, a novel adapter, translocates to the nuclear envelope and regulates neurotrophin-induced neurite outgrowth. Cell Biol 164, 851-862.

MacGurn J. A., Hsu P. C., Emr S. D. (2012). Ubiquitin and membrane protein turnover: from cradle to grave. Annu Rev Biochem 81, 231-259.

Mari M., Macia E., Le Marchand-Brustel Y., Cormont M. (2001). Role of the FYVE finger and the RUN domain for the subcellular localization of Rabip4. J Biol Chem 276, 42501-42508.

Mari M., Monzo P., Kaddai V., Keslair F., Gonzalez T., Le Marchand-Brustel Y., Cormont M. (2006). The Rab4 effector Rabip4 plays a role in the endocytotic trafficking of Glut 4 in 3T3-L1 adipocytes. J Cell Sci 119, 1297-1306.

Martin, T. F., Loyet, K. M., Barry, V. A., & Kowalchyk, J. A. (1997). The role of PtdIns(4,5)P2 in exocytotic membrane fusion. Biochem Soc Tran 25, 1137-1141.

Martin-Belmonte, F., & Perez-Moreno, M. (2011). Epithelial cell polarity, stem cells and cancer. Nat Rev Cancer 12, 23-38.

Mayinger P. (2012). Phosphoinositides and vesicular membrane traffic. Biochim Biophys Acta 1821, 1104-1113.

Mohrmann, K., & van der Sluijs, P. (1999). Regulation of membrane transport through the endocytic pathway by rabGTPases. Mol Membr Biol 16, 81-87.

Monck, J. R., & Fernandez, J. M. (1994). The exocytotic fusion pore and neurotransmitter release. Neuron 12, 707-716.

Mori, T., Wada, T., Suzuki, T., Kubota, Y., & Inagaki, N. (2007). Singar1, a novel RUN domain-containing protein, suppresses formation of surplus axons for neuronal polarity. J Biol Chem 282, 19884-19893.

Mller I., Wagner W., Vlker A., Schellmann S., Nacry P., Kttner F., Schwarz-Sommer Z., Mayer U., Jrgens G. (2003). Syntaxin specificity of cytokinesis in Arabidopsis. Nat Cell Biol 5, 531-534.

Nachury, M. V., Seeley, E. S., & Jin, H. (2010). Trafficking to the ciliary membrane: how to get across the periciliary diffusion barrier? Annu Rev Cell Dev Biol 26, 59-87.

Oude Weernink P. A., Han L, Jakobs K. H., Schmidt M. (2007). Dynamic phospholipid signaling by G protein-coupled receptors. Biochim Biophys Acta 1768, 888-900.

Pankiv, S., Alemu, E. A., Brech, A., Bruun, J. A., Lamark, T., Overvatn, A., Bjrky, G., & Johansen ,T. (2010). FYCO1 is a Rab7 effector that binds to LC3 and PI3P to mediate microtubule plus end-directed vesicle transport. J Cell Biol 188, 253-269.

Pfeffer, S. R. (2009). Multiple routes of protein transport from endosomes to the trans Golgi network. FEBS Lett 583, 3811-3816.

Saito, K., Tautz, L., & Mustelin, T. (2007). The lipid-binding SEC14 domain. Biochim Biophys Acta 1771, 719-726.

Salin-Cantegrel A, Rivire JB, Shekarabi M, Rasheed S, Dacal S, Laganire J, Gaudet R, Rochefort D, Lesca G, Gaspar C, Dion PA, Lapointe JY, Rouleau GA. (2011). Transit defect of potassium-chloride Co-transporter 3 is a major pathogenic mechanism in hereditary motor and sensory neuropathy with agenesis of the corpus callosum. J Biol Chem 286, 28456-28465.

Santiago-Tirado, F. H., & Bretscher, A. (2011). Membrane-trafficking sorting hubs: cooperation between PI4P and small GTPases at the trans-Golgi network. Trends Cell Biol 21, 515-525.

Shisheva, A. (2008). Phosphoinositides in insulin action on GLUT4 dynamics: not just PtdIns(3,4,5)P3. Am J Physiol Endocrinol Metab 295, E536-E544.

Stenmark, H., & Gillooly, D. J. (2001). Intracellular trafficking and turnover of phosphatidylinositol 3-phosphate. Semin Cell Dev Biol 12, 193-199.

Strick, D. J., & Elferink, L. A. (2005). Rab15 effector protein: a novel protein for receptor recycling from the endocytic recycling compartment. Mol Biol Cell 16, 5699-5709.

Sun Q., Han C., Liu L., Wang Y., Deng H., Bai L., Jiang T. (2012). Crystal structure and functional implication of the RUN domain of human NESCA. Protein Cell 3, 609-617.

Thomas, G. M., Hayashi, T., Chiu, S. L., Chen, C. M., & Huganir R. L. (2012). Palmitoylation by DHHC5/8 targets GRIP1 to dendritic endosomes to regulate AMPA-R trafficking. Neuron 73, 482-496.

Traub, L. M. (2009). Tickets to ride: selecting cargo for clathrin-regulated internalization. Nat Rev Mol Cell Biol 10, 583-596.

Valtorta F., Pozzi D., Benfenati F., Fornasiero E. F. (2011). The synapsins: multitask modulators of neuronal development. Semin Cell Dev Biol 22, 378-386.

Vergne I., Chua J., Deretic V. (2003). Mycobacterium tuberculosis phagosome maturation arrest: selective targeting of PI3P-dependent membrane trafficking. Traffic 4, 600-606.

Vitner E. B., Platt F. M., Futerman A. H. (2010). Common and uncommon pathogenic cascades in lysosomal storage diseases. J Biol Chem 285, 20423-20427.

Wang S., Zhang Z., Ying K., Chen J. Z., Meng X. F., Yang Q. S., Xie Y., Mao Y. M. (2003). Cloning, expression, and genomic structure of a novel human Rap2 interacting gene (RPIP9). Biochem Genet 41, 13-25.

Wang, T., Ming, Z., Xiaochun, W., & Hong, W. (2011). Rab7: role of its protein interaction cascades in endo-lysosomal traffic. Cell Signal 23, 516-521.

Wenk, M. R., & De Camilli, P. (2004). Protein-lipid interactions and phosphoinositide metabolism in membrane traffic: insights from vesicle recycling in nerve terminals. Proc Natl Acad Sci U S A 101, 8262-8269.

Westbroek, W., Lambert, J., De, Schepper, S., Kleta, R., Van, Den, Bossche, K., Seabra, M. C., Huizing, M., Mommaas, M., & Naeyaert, J. M. (2004). Rab27b is up-regulated in human Griscelli syndrome type II melanocytes and linked to the actin cytoskeleton via exon F-Myosin Va transcripts. Pigment Cell Res 17, 498-505.

Wu, G., Ge, J., Huang, X., Hua, Y., & Mu, D. (2011). Planar cell polarity signaling pathway in congenital heart diseases. J Biomed Biotechnol 2011, 589414.

Xu, J., Shi, S., Matsumoto, N., Noda, M., & Kitayama, H. (2007). Identification of Rgl3 as a potential binding partner for Rap-family small G-proteins and profilin II. Cell Signal 19, 1575-1582.

Yamamoto, H., Koga, H., Katoh, Y., Takahashi, S., Nakayama, K., & Shin, H. W. (2010). Functional cross-talk between Rab14 and Rab4 through a dual effector, RUFY1/Rabip4. Mol Biol Cell 21, 2746-2755.

Yamamoto H., Koga H., Katoh Y., Takahashi S., Nakayama K., Shin H. W. (2012). Functional cross-talk between Rab14 and Rab4 through a dual effector, RUFY1/Rabip4. Mol Biol Cell 21, 2746-2755.

Yang, J., Kim, O., Wu, J., & Qiu, Y. (2002). Interaction between tyrosine kinase Etk and a RUN domain- and FYVE domain-containing protein RUFY1. A possible role of ETK in regulation of vesicle trafficking. J Biol Chem, 277, 30219-30226. Yoshida, H., Kitagishi, Y., Okumura, N., Murakami, M., Nishimura, Y., & Matsuda, S. (2011). How do you RUN on? FEBS Lett 585, 1707-1710.

Yoshida, H., Okumura, N., Kitagishi, Y., Shirafuji, N., & Matsuda, S. (2010). Rab5(Q79L) interacts with the carboxyl terminus of RUFY3. Int J Biol Sci 6, 187-189.

Yu M., Kasai K., Nagashima K., Torii S., Yokota-Hashimoto H., Okamoto K., Takeuchi T., Gomi H., Izumi T. (2007). Exophilin4/Slp2-a targets glucagon granules to the plasma membrane through unique Ca2+-inhibitory phospholipid-binding activity of the C2A domain. Mol Biol Cell 18, 688-696.

Zaid, H., Antonescu, C. N., Randhawa, V. K., & Klip, A. (2008). Insulin action on glucose transporters through molecular switches, tracks and tethers. Biochem J 413, 201-215

# Decoding the Cis-Regulatory Grammar Behind Enhancer Architecture

Jacqueline M. Dresch
*Mathematics Department*
*Harvey Mudd College, USA*

Robert A. Drewell
*Biology Department*
*Harvey Mudd College, USA*

# 1   Introduction

The process of gene regulation and understanding the intricate machinery involved in controlling it poses a very important question in modern biology: what physical properties drive DNA sequences to control complex interactions with proteins leading to the precise expression of genes? All living organisms have genes that are turned on and off to regulate life processes, many of which depend on expression at precise levels, spatial locations and times. Often the molecular factors controlling gene regulation are divided into two groups, cis-acting elements and trans-acting factors. *Cis*-acting elements, also referred to as *cis*-regulatory modules (CRMs) or enhancers, are the regions of DNA containing binding sites for protein factors involved in gene regulation (see Figure 1). *Trans*-factors, on the other hand, are proteins that bind to these *cis*-elements to control expression. These factors are actively transported through the cell, and bind to enhancers to regulate to the spatial and temporal dynamics of gene expression (see Figure 1).

In prokaryotes, enhancers typically have a very small number of binding sites and the protein-DNA and protein-protein interactions involved in gene expression are often well understood. In eukaryotes, however, many of the rules governing gene regulation remain almost entirely unknown due to the complexity of the regulatory systems, involving the concerted occupancy of many trans-factors; including multiple transcription factors ($TF$s), cofactors, and histones on enhancers (Figure 1). A major research goal is therefore to not only understand the basic properties of protein-binding effects involved in gene regulation (i.e., the quantitative change in mRNA levels as one protein blocks or enhances the activity of another), but also gain the ability to model some of the *cis*-acting elements and trans-acting factors which contribute to the complex nature of eukaryotic regulation.

In this chapter we describe research focused on gene expression during the early blastoderm stage of development in the eukaryotic organism *Drosophila melanogaster*. *Drosophila*, more commonly known as the "fruit fly", offers particular advantages for studying gene regulation. As metazoans, their transcriptional machinery closely resembles that of all other animal species, including humans. In addition, flies have very short life spans and large birth rates, making experiments much more feasible in terms of preparation time as well as increasing the amount of data acquired for quantitative analyses. Powerful genetic tools make them a natural choice for studies involving transgenes or genetic crosses. Using the *Drosophila* experimental system in combination with detailed mathematical modeling of CRMs we have learned a great deal about the regulation of gene expression, providing a basis for hypotheses about transcriptional control, development, and evolution in many other eukaryotic species. Large-scale mathematical models of gene regulatory networks have helped further our understanding of general protein network structures, both static and dynamic, including the coregulation of genes, feedback and feedforward loops. On the other hand, smaller-scale models which focus on DNA level information and the fine details of biochemical interactions taking place at the CRM, such as those described later in this chapter, have begun to answer many of the underlying questions regarding enhancer architecture. These models were first derived in the context of prokaryotic systems, but have now been extended and implemented to study both yeast and *Drosophila*. As the amount of available data continues to grow and inform mathematical models, the extension of such approaches to higher organisms is an appealing prospect.

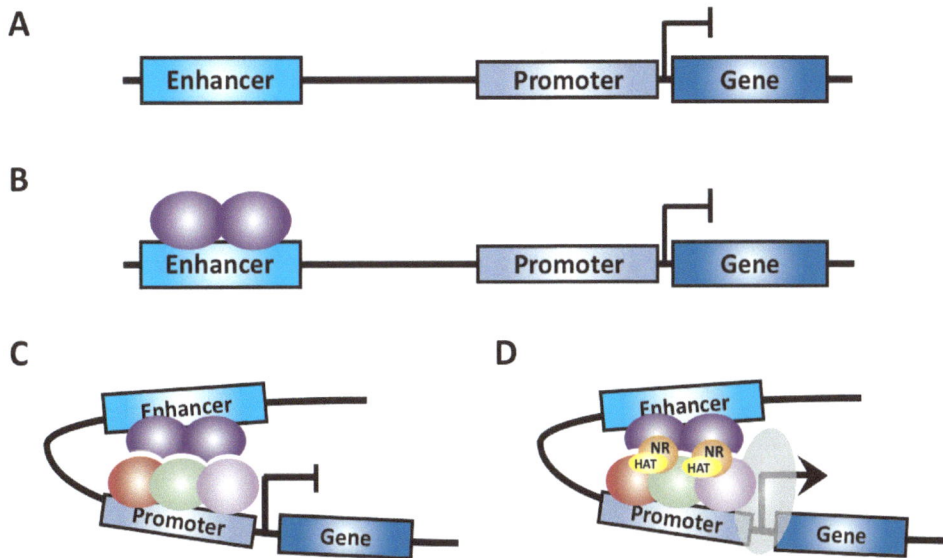

**Figure 1:** Defining a functional enhancer cis-regulatory module: An enhancer is an orientation-independent region of non-protein coding DNA in the genome that is associated with a promoter and target gene (A). Transcription factor (TF) proteins (purple spheres) bind to the enhancer (B) and interact with the transcriptional machinery (red, green and pink spheres) (C) and eventually recruit RNA polymerase II (gray ellipse) at the promoter of target genes to enhance the transcription of the gene (D). The $TF$s bound at an enhancer often also recruit chromatin-modifying enzymes such as histone acetyltransferases (HAT, yellow ellipses) and nucleosome remodeling factors (NR, orange spheres) that facilitate changes to the chromatin environment to allow transcription to proceed. Historically, enhancers were often initially identified in genetic screens, as mutation of the enhancer module disrupts $TF$ binding and results in an associated loss of target gene expression. Later, the use of transposon-mediated mutagenesis in *Drosophila* and plants allowed more sophisticated 'enhancer trap' reporter gene constructs. Enhancers identified in these types of genetic screens include those in the bithorax complex of D. *melanogaster* responsible for regulating the *Abdominal-B* gene (Karch *et al.*, 1985; Celniker *et al.*, 1990) (for a detailed review on enhancer trapping see (Bellen, 1999)). The functional sequences of the enhancer module are often resolved in detailed transgenic reporter gene studies (for early resolution of the eve stripe enhancers see (Goto *et al.*, 1989; Harding *et al.*, 1989)). More recently, global genome-wide approaches to identifying $TF$ binding sites, such as by using Chromatin immunoprecipitation combined with a tiled genomic microarray (ChIP on chip) (Zeitlinger *et al.*, 2007; Visel *et al.*, 2009a) or bioinformatic analysis using comparative genomics to identify genomic regions with potential cis-regulatory function (Nobrega *et al.*, 2003; Peterson *et al.*, 2009), have been successful at identifying an increasing number of enhancers. (Figure obtained from: Borok, *et al.* (2010): http://dev.biologists.org/content/137/1/5)

## 2    Interdisciplinary Approaches to Dissect *Cis*-Regulatory Modules

In *Drosophila* development precise patterns of gene expression regulated by CRMs are required to establish the anterior to posterior axis of the embryo. The best understood CRM is the enhancer (see Figure 1). For many years, researchers have sought to identify these modules and their respective target genes. However, recent interest has shifted towards a more complex analysis of individual enhancers in order to elucidate their molecular activity. Key questions include: which transcription factor binding sites are responsible for functional activity, how these binding sites are organized, and what their affinities for different transcription factors are.

Experimental biologists use diverse techniques to gather information regarding transcriptional regulation by CRMs. Some studies identify the developmental patterns linked to a particular gene's expression, some determine which proteins are physically interacting to control a single gene or group of genes' expression, and others classify the environmental conditions under which gene expression patterns are altered. Although each study only provides us with a subset of information on gene regulation, together they have greatly increased our knowledge of when, where, and how certain genes are expressed. A common and successful methodology involves the discovery of direct physical and functional characteristics of CRMs. Proteins binding to these DNA elements can be assayed by *DNaseI* footprinting. Functional studies to determine the minimal enhancer regions and the effects of *TF*s binding to specific sites involve generating transgenic *Drosophila* with reporter genes linked to small fragments of genomic DNA from CRMs (Pan *et al.*, 1991; Thisse *et al.*, 1991; Jiang and Levine, 1993). Historically these studies have typically only addressed questions about regulation at specific genes.

Other studies, addressing wider questions of gene circuitry begin in the lab and then further test hypotheses using statistical or computational tools. One general approach has involved utilizing synthetic reporter constructs to learn more about protein-protein interactions and enhancer 'grammar' (see Figure 2 for definition) (Szymanski and Levine, 1995; Arnosti *et al.*, 1996a; Kulkarni and Arnosti, 2005; Fakhouri *et al.*, 2010). On a much larger scale, recent studies acquiring protein binding profiles by whole-genome surveys are aimed at discovering the locations of CRMs and groups of genes regulated by the same set of *TF*s. These studies typically use microarray, referred to as chip, chromatin immunoprecipitation (ChIP)-chip or ChIP-sequencing (seq) experiments to search for specific protein binding regions. Recent studies have highlighted the powerful nature of these approaches. Utilizing ChIP-seq to identify specific chromatin signatures, in particular high levels of H3K4me1 and H3K27ac combined with low levels of H3K4me3, has shown success in predicting the genomic location of active enhancers in the examined cell types (Heintzman *et al.*, 2007; Visel *et al.*, 2009b; Bonn *et al.*, 2012; Gorkin *et al.*, 2012). Indeed, there is increasing evidence that the activity of many CRMs is mediated by epigenetic modifications in the genome (Barkess and West, 2012; Buecker and Wysocka, 2012; Ong and Corces, 2012; Spitz and Furlong, 2012). These epigenetic modifications include DNA methylation and post-translational modification of specific amino acid residues on histone tails. In some cases, the specific modifications can be targeted by non-coding RNAs (ncRNAs) (Sinkkonen *et al.*, 2008). However, due to the dynamic nature of chromatin states, linking these histone modifications to the activity of enhancers is still quite challenging and should be analyzed at cell-type specific resolution. In parallel, surveys on groups of genes regulated in the same time period of development or by the same set of *TF*s are aimed at understanding the dynamics of binding events, building gene regulatory networks, and gaining insight on possible protein interactions (Bergman *et al.*, 2005; Sandmann *et al.*, 2007; Zeitlinger *et al.*, 2007; Noyes *et al.*, 2008; MacArthur, 2009; Zinzen *et al.*, 2009; He *et al.*, 2011;

Ozdemir *et al.*, 2011). More recently, some studies have combined these binding profiles with expression measurements to learn more about spatio-temporal expression patterns (Zinzen *et al.*, 2009).

When experiments answer qualitative questions, such as when and where certain genes are expressed, or give a picture of how one node fits into a large gene regulatory network, there arise opportunities for further detailed inquiry. Such inquiries can be readily explored through modeling or statistical analysis. For genome-wide studies, it is often necessary to go through multiple levels of statistical analysis to tease out the important interactions between genes and proteins. For example, ChIP-chip and ChIP-seq studies have compared binding profiles using Pearson Correlation Coefficients to identify possible combinatorial relationships between $TF$s (He *et al.*, 2011). For studies aimed at explicitly describing the physical interactions taking place at CRMs, modelers often take the system of interest and derive deterministic or stochastic models based on the new assumptions that the experimental data has provided. For example, studies involving a cascade of gene expression can begin with a set of genes that have been found to bind the same set of $TF$s or have correlated expression profiles in development and through differential equation modeling, explicitly incorporate parameters representing the level of positive and negative effects one gene has on another (Jaeger *et al.*, 2004). These approaches are aimed at extracting as much information as possible from the experimental data and mathematically analyzing it to provide a direction for future experimentation. The wealth of information emerging from these recent cross-discipline approaches is reviewed in this chapter. These analyses have provided answers to some of the central questions concerning the function of enhancers, but have also brought controversy to the field.

# 3    The Building Blocks of Gene Regulation: the Functional Characteristics of Enhancers

Enhancers were first identified in the SV40 viral genome as regions of non-coding DNA critical for the transcription of adjacent genes (Banerji *et al.*, 1981; Benoist and Chambon, 1981). Functional activity of an enhancer depends upon the binding of specific transcription factor proteins (activators, see Figure 2) within the enhancer DNA sequence, which help to recruit RNA polymerase II and associated protein factors to the promoter of a target gene (detailed in Figure 1) (Wildeman *et al.*, 1984; McEwan *et al.*, 1993). In the years after these initial observations, enhancers were discovered for many genes in a wide range of model organisms (Banerji *et al.*, 1983; Struhl, 1984; Shepherd *et al.*, 1985). In complex eukaryotes, many of the identified enhancers are responsible for directing spatio-temporally restricted patterns of gene expression in the developing embryo (Hiromi *et al.*, 1985; Choi and Engel, 1986). While a number of enhancers are often able to activate transcription at a given eukaryotic gene, the regulation of key genes by a restricted set of tissue-specific enhancers during development must be very precisely controlled in space and time because they encode proteins that specify cellular identities in the embryo (Caplan and Ordahl, 1978; Lewis, 1978). These critical developmental genes cannot therefore be expressed ubiquitously.

In addition to activators, another class of regulatory $TF$s, repressors (see Figure 2), are capable of binding directly to enhancers, in this case to prevent target gene transcription (Dearolf *et al.*, 1989; Stanojevic *et al.*, 1989). While the molecular roles of activators and repressors in promoting or preventing recruitment of RNA polymerase II to gene promoters are not completely understood, some mechanisms for the functional activity of enhancers have been characterized. The predominant theory is that activators

**Enhancer/cis-regulatory grammar:** the way in which the specific number, arrangement, and strength of binding sites contributes to the functional output of the enhancer. This is distinct from the grammar of protein assembly; it is a complex grammar of a transcriptional code.

**Transcription factor binding site (TFBS):** a sequence of DNA known to be bound by a specific transcription factor protein that influences transcription of nearby target genes.

**Activator:** a transcription factor that, when bound within a particular enhancer, is able to recruit the transcriptional machinery to upregulate transcription of a target gene under control of the enhancer.

**Repressor:** a transcription factor that, when bound within a particular enhancer, blocks transcription of the target gene.

**Eve stripe 2 enhancer (S2E):** an extensively studied embryonic enhancer of the even-skipped gene.

**Position-weight matrix (PWM):** generated from a compilation of experimentally-verified binding site sequences for a specific TF, it is a mathematical matrix that indicates the probability of finding a specific nucleotide at each position in the binding site.

**Cluster:** a group of closely spaced TFBSs thought to be the hub of enhancer activity. Clusters usually include binding sites for both activators and repressors.

**Orthologous gene:** a gene derived from the gene of a common ancestor.

**2-dimensional similarity plots:** a graphical method that identifies regions of similarity between two sequences.

**PATSER:** a pattern search program that identifies potential transcription factor binding sites in a given DNA sequence using a position-weighted matrix.

**Enhancer State:** a particular arrangement of transcription factors bound to their corresponding binding sites in an enhancer.

**Graph based probabilistic models:** a graph is used to denote conditional independence between random variables, encoding a complete joint-probability distribution in a compact representation. A common biological application contains nodes representing genes and edges representing regulatory interactions among these genes.

**Thermodynamic equilibrium:** when a system is in thermal, mechanical, and chemical equilibrium, resulting in no change in the population average or time average of all relevant product and reactant concentrations.

**Occupancy profile/distribution:** the probability distribution of all possible states of the enhancer. Often referred to as the Boltzmann Distribution in Chemistry and Physics.

**Binding affinity:** the equilibrium binding constant associated with the binding of a transcription factor to a binding site. This is calculated for the corresponding chemical reaction, as shown in Example 1, as the equilibrium concentration of the product divided by the product of the equilibrium concentrations of all reactants.

**Cooperativity:** an interaction taking place between two transcription factors (possibly at a preferred distance) which leads all states in which those two transcription factors are bound to have a modified binding energy compared to that expected under the assumption of independent binding.

**Quenching:** the repressive activity that takes place when a bound repressor blocks the ability of a nearby bound activator to communicate with the basal machinery.

**Figure 2:** Glossary of specialized terms.

directly interact with components of the basal transcription machinery via specific protein domains such as glutamine-rich, proline-rich and acidic domains or hydrophobic β sheets (McEwan *et al.*, 1993), for a detailed review, see (Kadonaga, 2004). There is also extensive evidence that sequence-specific binding of activator *TF*s to individual enhancer CRMs leads to recruitment, via protein interactions with co-activator enzymes, of an extensive number of components of the RNA polymerase II transcriptional machinery, including the Mediator complex. The Mediator complex is highly conserved in eukaryotes from yeast to humans, although its components can vary when assembled at individual enhancers (Kadonaga, 2004). The Mediator complex facilitates interactions between the enhancer and chromatin-modifying enzymes, such as histone acetyltransferases and nucleosome remodeling factors to establish a chromatin environment that facilitates transcription of the target gene (see Figure 1). In contrast, repressors may disrupt enhancer functional activity in one of two ways; (1) competition, where the binding sites for repressors and activators within an enhancer sequence overlap and as a result, repressor binding excludes activators, and (2) quenching, where repressors are able to inhibit the regulatory activity of activators bound to nearby sites within the enhancer (Levine and Manley, 1989; Small *et al.*, 1991b; Gray *et al.*, 1994; Kirchhamer *et al.*, 1996).

## 3.1    Gene Regulation in Early *Drosophila* Development (Borok, *et al.* (2010))

In metazoans, enhancers are major players in the developmental cascade that transforms the early embryo from a mass of uniform, undifferentiated cells into a segmented and highly organized structure of differentiated cells. In *Drosophila*, the dynamic developmental specification of the embryonic body plan and of differentiated cell fates is accomplished by a combination of early spatio-temporal expression gradients of activator and repressor *TF*s that act upon downstream embryonic enhancers. Based on the timing of their expression during embryonic development, the genes in this cascade represent four basic developmental *TF* families: maternal, gap, pair-rule and homeotic genes (described in detail in Figure 3), for a review, see (Sauer *et al.*, 1996). At the top of the cascade, maternal mRNAs are deposited in the unfertilized egg cell during oogenesis (Berleth *et al.*, 1988; Steward *et al.*, 1988). Spatially restricted translation of localized maternal mRNAs in the fertilized egg establishes *TF* gradients in the embryo. In turn, maternal *TF*s bind at target embryonic enhancers for gap genes, directing gap *TF* expression patterns in the developing embryo (Driever and Nüsslein-Volhard, 1988; Struhl *et al.*, 1989) (Figure 4a). Gap *TF*s further regulate downstream target genes, such as those for pair-rule and homeotic *TF*s (Stanojevic *et al.*, 1989; Qian *et al.*, 1991). At each step in the cascade, gene expression patterns are controlled by the binding of *TF*s to specific clusters of activator and repressor binding sites within embryonic enhancers. Fine-tuning of transcription is mediated by the specific molecular properties of individual enhancer CRMs. Whether a given *TF* acts as an activator or repressor when it binds to an embryonic enhancer can be context-dependent (Ip *et al.*, 1991; Small *et al.*, 1996). In addition, DNA sequences within embryonic enhancers may bind *TF*s with varying affinities (Struhl *et al.*, 1989; Jiang *et al.*, 1991). The functional consequence is that enhancers may require different specific threshold concentrations of interacting activators and repressors in order to regulate transcription of their target genes. The central role of enhancers in the regulatory cascade responsible for development of the *Drosophila* embryo makes an in-depth analysis of their function critical to the field of developmental biology.

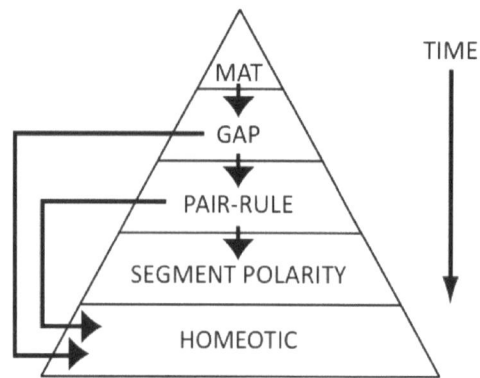

**Figure 3:** Key players in anterio-posterior patterning in early *Drosophila* development: Early in *Drosophila* embryonic development, the initial anterior to posterior morphogen gradient consists of maternally deposited (MAT) mRNAs in the unfertilized egg, including *bicoid* and *hunchback*. Translation produces the MAT transcription factors (*TF*s) which can activate or repress spatio-temporally restricted patterns of expression of GAP genes such as *kruppel*, *knirps* and *giant*. In turn, these GAP *TF*s regulate downstream expression of PAIR-RULE genes such as eve in stripes in the developing *Drosophila* embryo. PAIR-RULE *TF*s regulate SEGMENT POLAR-ITY genes further downstream in cascade. In addition, GAP and PAIR-RULE *TF*s both regulate the expression of the HOMEOTIC genes, which ultimately define segmental identity. (Figure obtained from: Borok, *et al.* (2010): http://dev.biologists.org/content/137/1/5)

### 3.2    A CRM Paradigm: *even-skipped* Stripe 2 Enhancer

Probably the best characterized embryonic CRM is the *even-skipped* (*eve*) stripe 2 enhancer (S2E) in *Drosophila melanogaster*. *eve* is a pair-rule gene expressed under the control of various neighboring CRMs in seven distinct stripes in the developing embryo (Macdonald *et al.*, 1986) (Figure 4b-d). The pattern of eve expression that S2E directs is entirely derived from the combination of transcription factor binding sites (TFBSs, see Figure 2) embedded within its DNA sequence (Small *et al.*, 1991b) (Figure 4). Pioneering studies in the laboratory of Michael Levine twenty years ago discovered that twelve different binding sites for KRUPPEL (KR), GIANT (GT), BICOID (BCD) and HUNCHBACK (HB) *TF*s are located in the minimal S2E, a 480 bp region of the CRM that is sufficient to drive stripe 2 expression (Figure 4c) (Goto *et al.*, 1989; Stanojevic *et al.*, 1989; Small *et al.*, 1991b). Notably, eight of the twelve TFBSs form two tight clusters at each end of the minimal S2E. Each cluster has closely spaced activator-binding sites, each of which strongly overlaps with a repressor-binding site (Figure 4c). These observations suggested two important ideas regarding the molecular architecture of an enhancer; (1) clustering of TFBSs is critical to enhancer function, and (2) the overlap between activator and repressor TFBSs enables the characteristically sharp boundaries between stripes of gene expression driven by many early embryonic enhancers (Figure 4d).

Analysis of the *TF* gradients present in the developing *Drosophila* embryo reveals how S2E directs eve expression with such sharp boundaries. Activation of S2E-driven expression of eve occurs through the binding of the HB and BCD activators (see Figure 2), which are present at high concentrations in the anterior of the embryo (Figure 4a). Binding of the KR and GT repressors (see Figure 2), which are present in

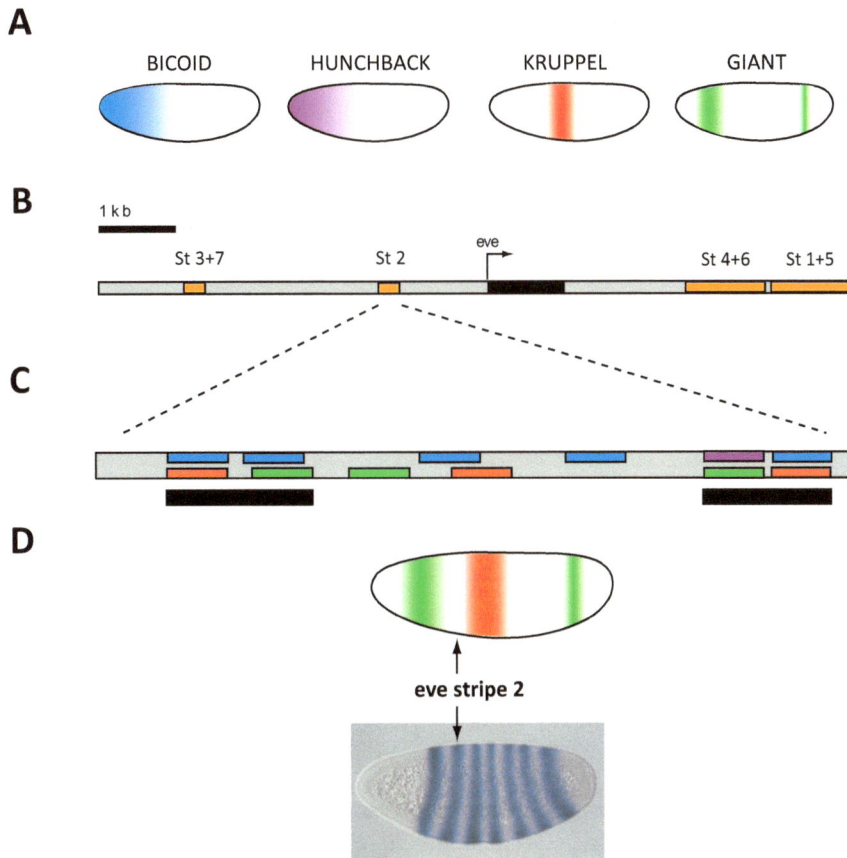

**Figure 4:** Transcription factor gradients activate *even-skipped expression*: (A) The localization patterns of four major transcription factors (*TF*s) in the early *Drosophila* embryo are shown. Embryos are oriented with anterior to the left and dorsal is up. The BICOID (blue) and HUNCH-BACK (purple) *TF*s are activators of the *even-skipped* (*eve*) stripe 2 enhancer, while the KRUP-PEL (red) and GIANT (green) *TF*s are repressors. The activators are both broadly expressed in the anterior half of the embryo, but repressor expression is more restricted. (B) Map of the *eve* genomic locus, including the embryonic enhancers (orange) responsible for eve *gene* (black) expression. Each enhancer drives *eve* expression in one or two developing parasegments of the embryo. Together, the enhancers drive expression in seven stripes (St 1-7) in odd numbered parasegments. (C) The minimal *eve* stripe 2 enhancer (St 2) of D. *melanogaster* contains twelve transcription factor binding sites. The locations of color coded binding sites for the activators and repressors shown in panel A are indicated. Two clusters of binding sites (black bars) at each end of the minimal St 2 module are thought to be particularly important for functional activity. (D) Sharp borders of eve stripe 2 directed-expression are established by high concentrations of GIANT (green) at the anterior boundary and KRUPPEL (red) at the posterior boundary. (Figure obtained from: Borok, *et al.* (2010): http://dev.biologists.org/content/137/1/5

distinct non-overlapping patterns in the anterior half of the embryo, prevents activation of S2E (Small *et al.*, 1991b) and thus delineates the boundaries of the second stripe of eve expression (Figure 4d). As a result, in the presumptive 2nd abdominal segment (the spatial interval in the embryo where HB and BCD activators are present and KR and GT repressors are absent) HB and BCD are able to occupy activator binding sites in S2E (Figure 4c) (Small *et al.*, 1991a). With strong activation and no repression, S2E only drives *eve* expression in a narrow 2-3 cell-wide region of the developing embryo (Figure 4d) (Macdonald *et al.*, 1986). By integrating the study of the spatial distribution of *TF*s in the embryo, the binding of these *TF*s at specific enhancers and the resulting patterns of target gene expression, we begin to see how an embryonic enhancer is analogous to a central processing unit. The enhancer must be capable of receiving input signals from *TF*s and of outputting a response in the form of directing a very specific spatio-temporal pattern of target gene expression.

### 3.3    Evolution of the eve Stripe 2 Embryonic Enhancer (Borok, *et al.* (2010))

Recent evolutionary analyses of TFBSs within enhancer sequences and their relative rate of evolutionary turnover are beginning to provide a useful perspective on the critical molecular mechanisms of enhancer function. Early comparative studies in the Kreitman laboratory concentrated on an evolutionary analysis of the sequence of S2E across several *Drosophila* species, including *D. melanogaster, D. yakuba, D. erecta and D. pseudoobscura* (see Figure 5a for phylogenetic relationship). Their studies revealed that all of the *Drosophila* species investigated possess an orthologous early embryonic enhancer (see Figure 2) capable of driving eve expression in a similar spatio-temporal stripe 2 pattern when tested in transgenic D. melanogaster (Ludwig *et al.*, 1998). This functional conservation partially extends to chimeric enhancers created by juxtaposing two halves of the S2E, each half taken from a different *Drosophila* species, which are capable of directing a similar pattern of gene expression in transgenic *D. melanogaster* (Ludwig *et al.*, 2000). However, the expression directed by the chimeric enhancers is not identical to the activity of the endogenous *eve* stripe 2 enhancer. In some embryos carrying the chimeric enhancers, reporter gene expression undergoes a posterior shift or expansion (Ludwig *et al.*, 2000), suggesting that nuanced enhancer architecture may be encoding important functional information.

Bioinformatic analysis revealed that the TFBSs contained within S2E are not well-conserved between orthologs (Ludwig and Kreitman, 1995; Ludwig *et al.*, 1998). There is, in fact, significant turnover of TFBSs between the *Drosophila* S2E orthologs studied: of the seventeen known binding sites analyzed in the 798bp full-length S2E from *D. melanogaster*, only three are completely conserved at the sequence level in the other three *Drosophila* species studied (Ludwig *et al.*, 1998) (Figure 5b). In addition, none of the sixteen surveyed binding sites from the full-length D. melanogaster S2E are conserved in all thirteen sequenced *Drosophila* species (Ludwig *et al.*, 2000). Detailed sequence alignment revealed that binding sites for BCD, HB, KR and GT identified in *D. melanogaster* are subject to extensive nucleotide substitutions in other *Drosophila* species (Ludwig *et al.*, 1998; Ludwig *et al.*, 2000). The key question therefore becomes: how is the functional activity of the enhancer preserved at all, despite the extensive evolutionary turnover of TFBSs within the CRM?

Some resolution to this intriguing issue is being provided by exciting new studies that have expanded the evolutionary scope of S2E analysis. These studies analyze evolutionarily divergent species outside of the *Drosophila* genus (Figure 5). *Drosophila* species generally have small, compact genomes with relatively uniformly conserved non-coding DNA. In comparison, species of the true fruit flies (Tephritidae family,

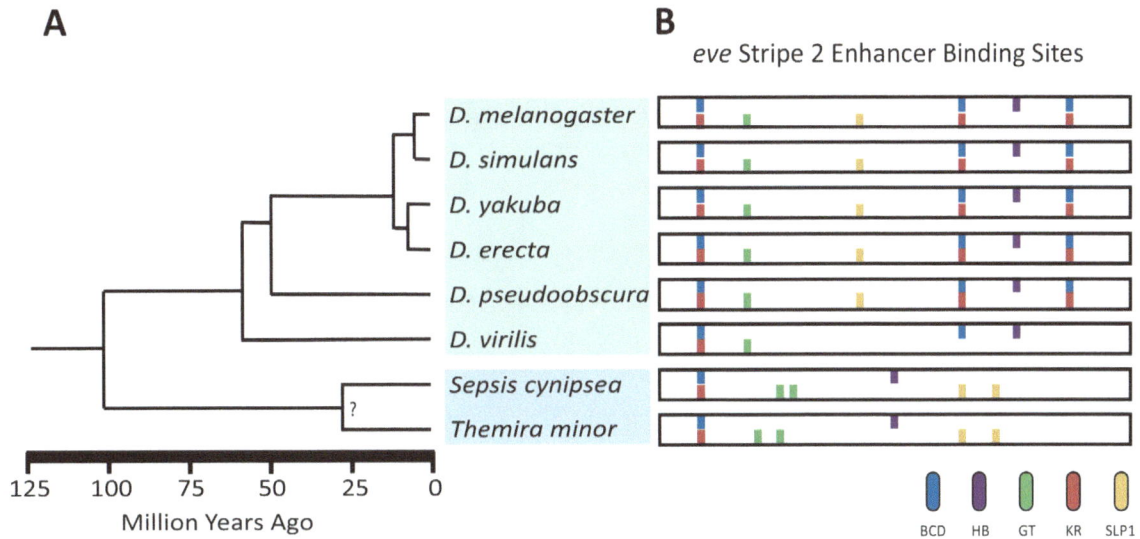

**Figure 5:** Phylogenetic relationship and eve stripe 2 enhancer architecture of *Drosophila* and *Sepsid* species: (A) The *Drosophila* (green box) diverged from the Sepsid family (blue box) approximately 100 million years ago (Mya). The distantly related *Drosophila* species, D. *melanogaster* and *D. virilis* diverged 60 Mya (Tamura *et al.*, 2004). (B) The organization of a subset of bioinformatically predicted binding sites for the transcription factors BICOID (BCD, blue), HUNCHBACK (HB, purple), GIANT (GT, green), KRUPPEL (KR, red) and SLOPPY-PAIRED 1 (SLP1, yellow) within the minimal *eve* stripe 2 enhancer (summarized from (Hare *et al.*, 2008a)) are shown for eight species; *D. melanogaster*, *D. simulans*, *D. yakuba*, *D. erecta*, *D pseudoobscura*, *D.virilis*, *Sepsis cynipsea* and *Themira minor*. (Figure obtained from: Borok, *et al.* (2010): `http://dev.biologists.org/content/137/1/5`

Sepsid species) have genomes that are between 4-6 times larger than that of *D. melanogaster* and which contain blocks of conserved non-coding sequence flanked by regions that are poorly conserved (Peterson *et al.*, 2009). The increased evolutionary divergence between these species, combined with these differences in overall genome structure, enable a more accurate measure of TFBS turnover and the functional significance of sequence conservation.

Recent studies compare the eve regulatory locus in *Drosophila* to that of Sepsid species, which diverged approximately 100 million years ago (Hare *et al.*, 2008a) (Figure 5a). Nevertheless, *eve* is expressed in the same seven transverse stripes in Sepsid embryos as in *Drosophila* embryos (Hare *et al.*, 2008a). In addition, many of the *TF*s upstream in the developmental cascade, including HB, GT and KR, are also expressed in conserved embryonic patterns in the Sepsid species *Themira minor*. Despite the fact that eve regulatory regions are found to be only minimally conserved between these groups, Sepsid *eve* enhancers identified through clusters of HB, CAUDAL (CAD), KNI, KR, and BCD binding sites are able to drive conserved gene expression patterns in transgenic *D. melanogaster*.

Functional conservation of the Sepsid and *Drosophila* S2E orthologs, despite relatively low sequence conservation, indicates that some other shared molecular property is responsible for their activity. The identity of this common molecular mechanism is currently the focus of active research and debate. Bioinformatic analysis in the Eisen laboratory demonstrates that there has been large-scale reorganization of the TFBSs in the eve enhancers from different *Drosophila* and Sepsid species (Figure 5b), indicating that the spatial organization of the binding sites within enhancer regions may not be critical (Hare *et al.*, 2008a). However, detailed analysis of the architecture of S2E orthologs reveals the existence of 20-30 bp blocks of highly conserved sequence enriched in pairs of neighboring or overlapping TFBSs. This discovery suggests that the relative position of binding sites to one another may be more important than their overall spatial arrangement within an enhancer (Figure 5b) (Hare *et al.*, 2008a).

Several critical issues were raised following the conclusions drawn from the initial studies of the orthologous insect S2Es (Hare *et al.*, 2008a). A primary concern is that the S2E sequences in *Drosophila* and *Themira* are not as diverged as originally indicated and therefore the lack of sequence homology does not indicate a lack of conserved transcription factor organization. Using 2D similarity plots (see Figure 2), Crocker and Erives aligned the S2Es from *Drosophila melanogaster* and *Themira putris* and found extensive homology between a series of specific 14-41 bp stretches of sequence. The order of these sequence blocks is conserved across the entire length of the enhancer, suggesting that their position relative to each other is critical. As a result, the authors argue that these sequences harbor binding sites for KR, BCD and GT and thus that the TFBS architecture is largely unchanged between these insect families (Crocker and Erives, 2008a). In response, Hare *et al.* note that the plots only align half of the minimal S2E region. In contrast, the other half of S2E exhibits little or no conservation despite its necessity for proper functional activity of the S2E module (Hare *et al.*, 2008b). Furthermore, computational studies utilizing PATSER (a bioinformatics tool that can be used to scan a given DNA sequence with a position-weighted matrix (PWM, see Figure 2) representing a binding motif for a specific transcription factor) to predict TFBSs within S2E orthologs reveal that an extensive genomic reorganization of binding sites has occurred between *Drosophila* and Sepsid families. Indeed, 24 of the TFBSs analyzed in this study are not conserved between *Drosophila* and Sepsids, despite the fact that many of these sites bind conserved proteins known to regulate eve expression through S2E, such as HB, BCD, GT, KR and an additional pair-rule repressor TF, SLOPPY PAIRED 1 (SLP1) (Andrioli *et al.*, 2002; Hare *et al.*, 2008b). The studies by Hare *et al.* suggest that TFBSs are the essential molecular components within enhancer regions that, even when extensively reorganized, can still function to produce the same patterns of expression.

Overall, there exist caveats to the use of sequence alignments, including similarity plots, which can overemphasize weak homology across short stretches of sequence that are sometimes near the threshold for statistical significance. Though sequence analysis and alignment approaches can be useful in the identification of potential regions of conservation, the biological relevance of such alignments is not easily deciphered. To date, no functional synthetic S2E has been built, which could support the idea that this CRM is a loose cluster of TFBSs with as yet undefined organizational requirements. Further functional analyses of S2E will continue to elucidate the molecular mechanisms of enhancer regulation. In the meantime, mathematical modeling of S2E as well as additional *Drosophila* CRMs is also beginning to shed light on this issue.

# 4    Mathematical Modeling to Understand Enhancer Function

In formulating an approach to understand how a biological process works, scientists develop models, a term which carries different connotations to researchers in different fields. Biologists may use a model to provide a non-quantitative, simplified interpretation of the processes taking place. Mathematicians, statisticians, and quantitative biologists use the term to refer to an equation or system of equations that precisely describes the physical aspects of the system. For experimentalists, developing hypotheses and executing experiments, such as those described in the previous sections, is often very time consuming. To streamline the process mathematical modeling is used to effectively target experimental biological studies. For example, mathematical modeling has been crucial in enhancer discovery: without having to perform genome-wide ChIP experiments, bioinformaticians have utilized statistical models based on DNA-protein binding site sequences to efficiently search the entire genome for clusters of binding sites (Bailey and Gribskov, 1998; Kazemian et al., 2011). These clusters then serve as 'predicted enhancer regions' that can be tested in transgenic assays.

The issues of guiding experimental design are critically important in the area of transcriptional regulation. System-wide insights are key to understanding enhancer function. Unfortunately, little is known about many of the proteins involved in regulation and their interactions, making the design of experiments very challenging. Mathematical models, however, are capable of using available enhancer information and quantitative expression data to fit parameter values, such as activator efficiency or $TF$ cooperativity, and predicting expression from additional enhancers, giving researchers a better idea of what proteins and enhancers should be further investigated experimentally.

In the field of gene regulation, two of the key mathematical models that have been applied are Boolean and thermodynamic-based (also termed "Fractional Occupancy") models. Both models have inherent strengths and weaknesses involving the amount of input data and the level of complexity. Boolean models are graph based probabilistic models used to find regulatory interactions and gene networks when looking at genome-wide data. They have the benefit of using large amounts of available gene array data to identify specific gene interaction networks, but a major drawback is their inability to explain complex interactions between the individual components of the transcriptional machinery (ie: $TF$ and polymerase interactions) (Sanchez and Thieffry, 2001; Yuh et al., 2001; Albert and Othmer, 2003). Thermodynamic-based models, on the other hand, can explain a great deal of the intricate machinery at the DNA-protein binding level. They utilize information on DNA sequence, protein binding specificity, and $TF$ concentrations using the laws of biophysical thermodynamics, and often include terms for specific $TF$ interactions and distance-dependent DNA binding events. Although many researchers believe that these fractional occupancy models will someday have the ability to decipher the *cis*-regulatory grammar behind enhancer architecture, the amount of data necessary to test current hypotheses is still lacking (Ackers et al., 1982; Bintu et al., 2005; Janssens et al., 2006; Zinzen et al., 2006; Segal et al., 2008; Gertz et al., 2009; Fakhouri et al., 2010; He et al., 2010; Ay and Arnosti, 2011). One limitation to using these approaches is that thermodynamic-based models are static in nature and Boolean models only represent time, state, or space with a discrete set of values. Whether they are adding insight into which gene products affect other genes or whether they are predicting expression patterns, these conclusions can only be made for specific time points or over some arbitrary time scale.

In this chapter we focus on the contributions of the most popular static model of transcriptional regulation for incorporating DNA level information, thermodynamic-based (or fractional occupancy) modeling. We first derive a simple thermodynamic-based model and discuss how it can be analyzed to produce biological insights on the limitations of DNA-sequence and $TF$ contributions to gene expression. We then show examples of how more complicated biochemical mechanisms, such as protein-protein cooperativity, can be incorporated into the model to allow for a more realistic picture of the regulatory system and generate hypotheses regarding the cis-regulatory grammar. The general equation for calculating gene expression from the protein occupancy profile of the enhancer is given by:

$$[mRNA] \propto \sum_{i \in G} \frac{S_i}{S}, \tag{1}$$

where $G = \{$all successful states of the enhancer$\}$, $S_i$ represents the contribution from state $i$, and $S$ represents the sum of the contributions from all possible states of the enhancer.

## 4.1   Thermodynamic-Based Modeling

Thermodynamic fractional occupancy models aim to predict gene expression output from the DNA sequence of the enhancer CRM and the concentration of $TF$s involved in regulation. The term "thermodynamic" itself is often misinterpreted; it only refers to the fact that the model has been derived with thermodynamic equilibrium assumptions. Historically, these calculations have been done using techniques derived from statistical physics which involve computing all possible states of $TF$s binding to a CRM and relating these states to gene expression (Shea and Ackers, 1985; Reinitz et al., 2003; Bintu et al., 2005; Janssens et al., 2006; Zinzen et al., 2006; Segal et al., 2008; Gertz et al., 2009; Fakhouri et al., 2010; He et al., 2010; Sherman and Cohen, 2012). During implementation, the model is derived in two separate parts. The first part is the true "thermodynamic" component of the model, which is derived using chemical stoichiometric and equilibrium equations. It is assumed that RNA polymerase II (RNAP), the driving force in gene transcription, is recruited by bound $TF$s. This requires the occupancy distribution of $TF$s on the DNA sequence to be computed using equilibrium constants (binding affinities) and concentration levels. The second part to thermodynamic-based modeling requires some scientific guesswork. There are two common ways to convert binding states into gene expression output. The first approach models transcriptional output as proportional to the probability of RNAP binding, which is related to the active, or successful, states of the enhancer (Zinzen et al., 2006; Fakhouri et al., 2010; Sherman and Cohen, 2012). The second approach represents it with a nonlinear sigmoidal function in which activators have a positive influence and repressors have a negative influence (Segal et al., 2008). For a thermodynamic-based modeling study in a eukaryote, the choice of sigmoidal function is arbitrary, and reflects the lower and upper bounds observed in the transcription process. Again, a shortfall of this approach is that this function is not chemically or physically derived. Here we will describe thermodynamic-based modeling using the first approach. Due to the lack of data relating RNAP binding to the state of an enhancer, we also assume that transcriptional output of an enhancer (measured as the concentration of mRNA) is directly proportional to the fraction of successful states. This leads one to formulate the equation used in simple thermodynamic-based models in the following way:

$$[mRNA] \propto \sum_{i \in G} \frac{S_i}{S}, \tag{2}$$

where $G = \{$all successful states of the enhancer$\}$, N is the number of all possible states of the enhancer, and $S = \sum_{i=1}^{N} S_i$. Here, and throughout the remainder of this chapter, $[.]$ denotes the concentration of the given product or reactant.

To calculate each state's contribution, $S_i$, one must rely on the assumption that the system is in thermodynamic equilibrium, using simple chemical stoichiometric and equilibrium equations. The following example serves as a guide to calculating the contribution of a state.

Example 1: Consider the case of a fragment of DNA (also referred to as a binding site or motif), $M$, which a protein (transcription factor), $TF$, can bind. The chemical equation for $TF$ binding to $M$ is:

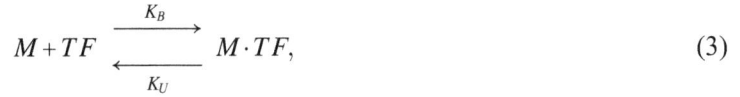

$$M + TF \xrightleftharpoons[K_U]{K_B} M \cdot TF, \tag{3}$$

where $K_B$ is the constant associated with the rate of binding and $K_U$ is the constant associated with the rate of dissociation. The rate equations associated with this chemical equation are:

$$\frac{d[M]}{dt} = K_U[M \cdot TF] - K_B[M][TF], \tag{4}$$

$$\frac{d[TF]}{dt} = K_U[M \cdot TF] - K_B[M][TF], \tag{5}$$

$$\frac{d[M \cdot TF]}{dt} = K_B[M][TF] - K_U[M \cdot TF], \tag{6}$$

Under the assumption that the system is in thermodynamic equilibrium,

$$\frac{d[M]}{dt} = K_U[M \cdot TF] - K_B[M][TF] = 0., \tag{7}$$

Thus, it follows that

$$K_U[M \cdot TF] = K_B[M][TF]. \tag{8}$$

Let

$$K_{TF} = \frac{K_B}{K_U} = \frac{[M \cdot TF]}{[M][TF]}. \tag{9}$$

Due to matter conservation (stoichiometry),

$$[M]_{total} = [M] + [M \cdot TF]. \tag{10}$$

Therefore, it follows that

$$P = \frac{[M \cdot TF]}{[M] + [M \cdot TF]} = \frac{\dfrac{[M \cdot TF][TF]}{[M][TF]}}{\dfrac{[M][TF]}{[M][TF]} + \dfrac{[M \cdot TF][TF]}{[M][TF]}} = \frac{K_{TF}[TF]}{1 + K_{TF}[TF]}, \tag{11}$$

where $K_{TF}$ is referred to as the binding affinity (equilibrium constant) of $TF$ and $P$ is the fractional occupancy, or the time-averaged occupancy of the $TF$ on the enhancer.

Relating Example 1 back to the earlier formulation, note that if the TF considered in the example is an activator protein:

$$[mRNA] \propto P = \sum_{i \in G} \frac{S_i}{S}, \tag{12}$$

with $S_i = 1$ when i corresponds to the state of the enhancer with nothing bound and $S_i = K_{TF}[TF]$ when $i$ corresponds to the state of the enhancer with the protein, $TF$, bound. In general, when considering an enhancer with multiple binding sites, and hence multiple possible states, the state of the enhancer with nothing bound (referred to as the empty state) is defined to have contribution 1, and each nonempty state consists of a product of protein concentrations and binding affinities, (ie: a product of terms of the form $K_{TF}[TF]$ ), derived from this same assumption that the system is in thermodynamic equilibrium. Note here that although the empty state has contribution 1, this state is not a successful state adding to the transcription of mRNA (i.e. the empty state is not included in the set $G$). Thus, the empty state's value of 1 only appears in the denominator as a possible state of the enhancer. The next example should further illustrate this point, as well as demonstrate the treatment of repressor proteins.

Example 2: Consider the case of an enhancer which contains two binding sites, one for a transcriptional activator, $A$, and one for a transcriptional repressor, $R$. Assume that the expression level of the gene (measured as the concentration of mRNA) is proportional to the fraction of successful states, where 'successful' is defined as having only the activator bound and not the repressor. The expression level is then calculated as:

$$[mRNA] \propto P_A(1-P_R) = \left(\frac{K_A[A]}{1+K_A[A]}\right)\left(\frac{1}{1+K_R[R]}\right) = \frac{K_A[A]}{1+K_A[A]+K_R[R]+K_A K_R[A][R]}. \tag{13}$$

With Example 2, one can start to see the high level of computation that must go into such a model as enhancers become more complicated, containing multiple $TF$ binding sites, due to the combinatorial nature of multiple $TF$s binding to a CRM. In addition, there are many important biological questions that have been posed in the case of more complicated thermodynamic-based models and their parameters (i.e., the effects of protein-protein cooperativity). However, we will begin by analyzing some mathematical properties of a simple thermodynamic-based model similar to the one depicted in Example 2.

## 4.2    Integrating Complexity in Thermodynamic-Based Models

When using a thermodynamic-based model in practice, each state is not solely based on the binding affinities and concentrations of the proteins bound to the enhancer, but also carries with it a statistical weight which can hold biological meaning within the system. In addition, successful states can include those with repressors bound, simply causing a reduction in the weight of the state. A state's weight can represent biological phenomena such as the activation efficiency of a particular protein, the cooperativity of multiple bound proteins, the quenching (or repressive) efficiency of a bound repressor on a bound activator, etc. In the following examples, cooperativity and quenching terms have been added to the weight of such states under the assumption that they have a multiplicative effect on the binding energy of the state or the 'success' of the state, respectively, due to interactions between adjacently bound $TF$s (Fakhouri et al., 2010; He et al., 2010; Sherman and Cohen, 2012).

Example 3: Consider the case of an enhancer which contains two binding sites, each for a transcriptional activator, A1 and A2. Assume that the expression level of the gene (measured as the concentration of mRNA) is proportional to the fraction of successful states, where 'successful' is defined as having at least one activator bound and that these two $TF$s are cooperating. The expression level is then calculated as:

$$[mRNA] \propto \frac{K_{A1}[A1]+K_{A2}[A2]+CK_{A1}K_{A2}[A1][A2]}{1+K_{A1}[A1]+K_{A2}[A2]+CK_{A1}K_{A2}[A1][A2]}, \tag{14}$$

where C represents the cooperative interaction between the $TF$s when they bind simultaneously.

The cooperativity of two proteins adjacently bound is assumed to affect the state's weight by modifying the binding energy of that state. Thus, a parameter $C \geq 1$, representing the cooperative interaction between the $TF$s when they bind simultaneously, is multiplied by the binding affinities of the adjacently bound proteins. Thus, as shown in Example 3, the state $i$ with $A1$ and $A2$ bound cooperatively is given by $S_i = CK_{A1}K_{A2}[A1][A2]$ . Again, in general, when considering an enhancer with multiple binding sites, and hence multiple possible interactions:

$$S_i = \prod_{j=1}^{n_i} K_j C_{j,j+1}[TF_j], \tag{15}$$

where $n_i$ is the number of binding sites bound by a $TF$ in state i, $K_j$ is the binding affinity of binding site $[TF_j]$ is the protein concentration corresponding to the $TF$ bound at binding site $j$, and $C_{j,j+1}$ is the cooperativity parameter representing the cooperative interaction between the $TF$s bound at the adjacent positions $j$ and $j+1$ in state $i$. We assume that $C_{n_i,n_i+1} = 1$ since there are only proteins bound in state $i$.

Example 4: Consider the case of an enhancer which contains two binding sites, one for a transcriptional activator, $A$, and one for a transcriptional repressor, $R$. Assume that the expression level of the gene (measured as the total mRNA) is proportional to the fraction of successful states, where 'successful' is defined as having the activator bound with the ability to communicate with the transcriptional machinery and that when the repressor is bound, it has some ability to quench the activator, or decrease its ability to communicate with the transcriptional machinery. The expression level is then calculated as:

$$[mRNA] \propto \frac{K_A[A] + QK_AK_R[A][R]}{1 + K_A[A] + K_R[R] + K_AK_R[A][R]}, \tag{16}$$

where $1 - Q$ represents the quenching ability of the bound repressor, $R$, on $A$ when both proteins are bound ( $Q = 0$ when $R$ is quenching at 100% efficiency).

The quenching efficiency of a bound repressor on an adjacently bound activator is assumed to affect a state only in whether it is 'successful' or not. Note that one can depict a state with activators and repressors bound adjacently as being divided into two sub-states, one successful state when the activators have the ability to activate the gene and one unsuccessful state when the repressors are blocking that ability. Since this is simply the division of a single state, the $Q$ parameter is always in the interval $[0,1]$ , representing the proportion of time the state is successful. This was illustrated in Example 4, and can be written in general as:

$$[mRNA] \propto \sum_{i \in G} \frac{S_i}{S} Q_i, \tag{17}$$

where $Q_i = \prod_{j=1}^{n_i} Q_{j,j+1}$ and $Q_{j,j+1}$ is the quenching parameter representing the repressive activity between the $TF$s bound at the adjacent positions $j$ and in state $i$, causing the proportion of time the state is successful to be reduced. We assume that since there are only proteins bound in state i and anytime the $TF$s bound at the adjacent positions $j$ and $j+1$ do not represent one repressor and one activator (or vice versa).

It is easy to imagine biological examples when such weights would be important. If a certain activator communicates strongly with the basal machinery of transcription, giving it a high activation efficiency, the gene expression should increase when this particular protein is bound. Thus a larger weight is given to this state. On the other hand, if a repressor is bound, a smaller weight is given to the state since the activator may be "quenched" by the repressor and with some probability lose the ability to communicate with the basal machinery. These weights, which hold such high biological relevance and have the ability to provide hypotheses on the mechanisms involved in transcriptional regulation, should therefore be incorporated in future work with thermodynamic-based models of transcriptional regulation in the early *Drosophila* embryo.

### 4.3   Modeling Cooperativity and Quenching at Enhancers

The two biological phenomena that have recently drawn the most attention in this field are cooperativity between pairs of $TF$s and quenching or repressive activity of repressors on activators. Some investigation of these weights has been carried out previously, but only very simple functions have been considered to date (Reinitz *et al.*, 2003; Janssens *et al.*, 2006; Zinzen *et al.*, 2006; Fakhouri *et al.*, 2010). Levine and colleagues tested a model on endogenous gene expression data in the early *Drosophila* embryo which incorporated terms for protein cooperativity, although one constant cooperativity value was given to each pair of proteins (Zinzen *et al.*, 2006). Later, a similar model, which incorporated terms for protein cooperativity, was tested by Arnosti and colleagues on synthetic gene expression data in the early *Drosophila* embryo (Fakhouri *et al.*, 2010). A discrete (very small) number of different cooperativity values were used to incorporate distance (in base pairs between binding sites)-dependent cooperativity (Fakhouri *et al.*, 2010). It is still unknown what the distance-dependent cooperativity function is for any given pair of proteins *in vivo*, although hypotheses can be made based upon what is known about the actual size of proteins, the helical shape of DNA, and the nucleosome positioning on DNA.

With regard to the quenching of short-range repressors on bound activator proteins, in 2003 a model which incorporated a distance-dependent quenching term into thermodynamic-based models was proposed, but not implemented (Reinitz et al., 2003). In this study, the quenching function proposed was a piecewise-defined monotonically decreasing function of distance. The function was constructed by taking two constant functions (1 and 0) and connecting them with a linear function. This was based on the notion that repressors have a given range over which they can repress bound activators. They quench with full (1) efficiency when activator sites are very close and do not quench at all (0) when they are out of range. In between these two distances, a linear interpolation was done, assuming that repressors can vary in their efficiency at intermediate distances (Reinitz *et al.*, 2003). Using this same idea, in 2006 two different studies were published using models with either a simple monotonic step-function or a linear function for distance-dependent quenching (Janssens et al., 2006; Zinzen *et al.*, 2006). In 2010, a study by Fakhouri *et al.* also incorporated quenching into their model. Since their study was conducted on synthetic enhancers in which the activity of short-range repressors was thoroughly investigated by creating enhancers with varying distances between repressor binding sites and activator binding sites, they were able to handle distance-dependent quenching with a bit more sophistication (Fakhouri *et al.*, 2010). In the Fakhouri *et al.* study, a step-function representing distance-dependent quenching was fit. Different step-functions were investigated by altering the binning strategy used (the intervals on which each step was defined) and fitting each function to the experimental data. One of the most surprising findings is that the best fit quenching function was non-monotonic, supporting the hypothesis that repressors have a preferred distance due to spatial constraints (Fakhouri *et al.*, 2010).

During implementation of thermodynamic-based models, another important consideration is how to calculate the occupancy distribution of $TF$s on an enhancer that contains overlapping binding sites with the ability to bind two different proteins. This is a common enhancer characteristic due to similarities in protein binding preferences. For example, $TF$s involved in early *Drosophila* development, such as BICOID and KRUPPEL (e.g. at the S2E) as well as TWIST and SNAIL, have been shown to bind the same region of DNA (Stanojevic *et al.*, 1991; Ip *et al.*, 1992). Thermodynamic-based models handle such binding sites by making the assumption that, due to spatial constraints, TFBSs may be occupied by only one protein at a time (competitive binding). This affects the total number of possible states since any overlapping binding sites have three possible states compared to binding sites for a single protein which have only two possible states. An example of the occupancy distribution of $TF$s on an enhancer that contains an overlapping binding site follows.

Example 5: Consider the case of an enhancer which contains two binding sites, one for a transcriptional activator, $A1$, and one overlapping binding site which can bind a transcriptional activator, $A2$, or a repressor, R. Assume that the expression level of the gene (measured as the concentration of mRNA) is proportional to the fraction of successful states. We will assume that the activators, $A1$ and $A2$, can cooperate, with C representing the cooperative interaction between the $TF$s when they bind simultaneously, and that $R$ can repress $A1$, with representing the quenching ability of $R$ on $A1$ when both proteins are bound. The expression level is then calculated as:

$$[mRNA] \propto \frac{K_{A1}[A1]+K_{A2}[A2]+CK_{A1}K_{A2}[A1][A2]+QK_{A1}K_R[A1][R]}{1+K_{A1}[A1]+K_{A2}[A2]+K_R[R]+CK_{A1}K_{A2}[A1][A2]+K_{A1}K_R[A1][R]}. \quad (18)$$

Note that with this formulation there are only six possible states of the enhancer (six terms in the denominator) since A2 and R cannot bind simultaneously.

## 5  Is Transcription Factor Binding Site Organization Critical for Enhancer Function? (Borok, *et al.* (2010))

The current debate over the functional significance of TFBS organization and interaction in CRMs reveals a key mystery in developmental biology: how exactly does an enhancer function at the molecular level? Without a doubt, the TFBSs within an enhancer are critically important. However, studies of S2E suggest that binding site turnover occurs frequently in evolution, resulting in changes to the overall number and architecture of TFBSs within orthologous enhancers. Surprisingly, these pronounced differences appear to have no significant effect on the regulation of target gene transcription, suggesting that enhancers are under selective pressure to be functionally robust to evolutionary changes at the sequence level. In general, enhancers from different species maintain their conserved functional activity despite significant modulation of their sequence architecture during evolution.

Can we use these observations of enhancer activity to develop a clearer idea of the molecular function of CRMs? Recent studies do in fact lend support to the information display/billboard model of enhancer function (Figure 6a). The information display/billboard model suggests that an enhancer functions not as a single large processor, but as a series of autonomous signals, each of which can have an effect on target gene transcription (Arnosti *et al.*, 1996b; Kulkarni and Arnosti, 2003). In this model, as long as there is never a net decrease in activator and repressor TFBSs, the enhancer can continue to function normally. The only requirement is for the presence of the 'correct' combination of TFBSs somewhere in the enhancer sequence (Figure 6a). Could this loose requirement be all that is needed to establish a precise response to the complex binding of multiple $TF$s at a CRM? Hare and colleagues concede that certain binding site clusters may not be so flexible (Hare *et al.*, 2008a). Functionally linked sites, such as the tight clusters at either end of the minimal S2E, may not be subject to an equivalent rate of evolutionary turnover as are more independent sites within the CRM. The most parsimonious explanation for these conflicting discoveries is that individual CRMs may in fact be very idiosyncratic. Enhancers may function differently depending upon the $TF$s by which they are bound and the genes they regulate. This may reflect the unique properties of specific $TF$s.

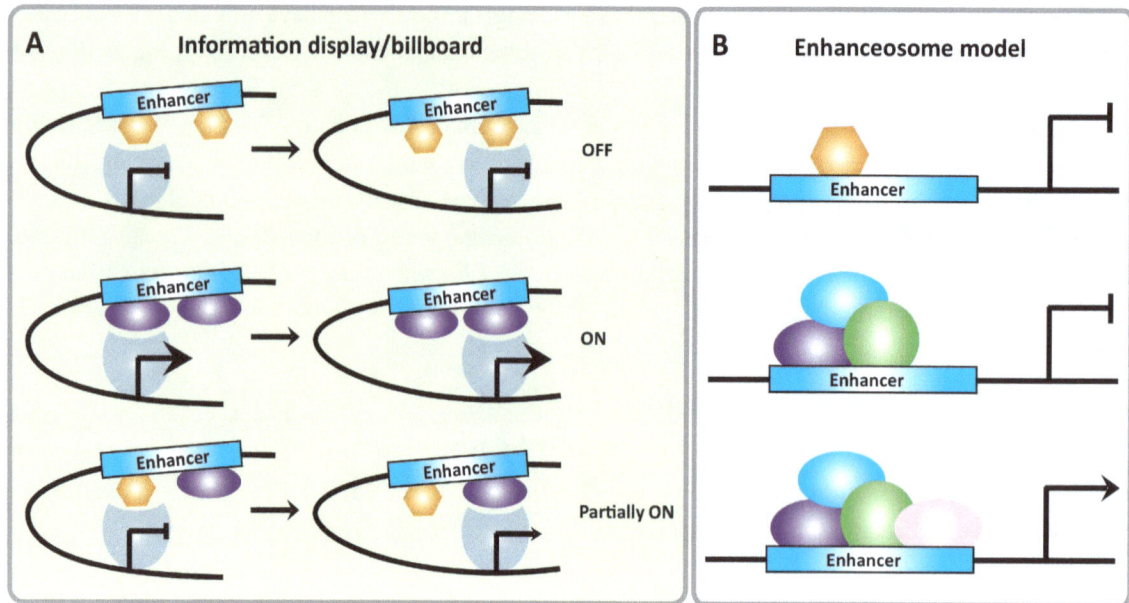

**Figure 6:** Information display/billboard and enhanceosome models of cis-regulatory module function: (A) In the information display/billboard model, the transcriptional machinery (gray polygon) samples the regulatory landscape found at an enhancer module (blue box) (Kulkarni and Arnosti, 2003). If the basal transcriptional machinery encounters only repressors (orange hexagons), the target gene will not be upregulated. The binding of only activators (purple ellipses) at the regulatory module will result in strong target gene expression. A combination of signals from specific DNA sites being bound by repressors and activators will lead to an intermediate (or more likely spatio-temporally restricted) level of target gene activity. An information display enhancer is tolerant of evolutionary binding site turnover because the transcriptional machinery samples only discrete regions of the enhancer and the output signal will not differ if transcription factor binding sites are located in different regions within the enhancer sequence. (B) In an enhanceosome, the enhancer can only function when a large regulatory protein complex has assembled (purple, blue, green and pink ellipses). If a repressor (orange hexagon) occludes binding sites, or if one of the components of the complex is absent, the enhancer will not drive target gene expression. An enhanceosome will not tolerate binding site turnover, as the protein complex is extremely stereospecific. (Figure obtained from: Borok, *et al.* (2010): http://dev.biologists.org/content/137/1/5

Different $TF$s will utilize distinct molecular interactions to bind to DNA and the mechanisms by which they promote transcription will also vary. Innovative work from the Carroll laboratory on CRMs regulating *yellow* gene expression in wing pigmentation in different *Drosophila* species has demonstrated that enhancers with novel regulatory activity can in fact be generated by modifications to $TF$ binding (Gompel *et al.*, 2005) (for a review see (Prud'homme *et al.*, 2007)).

The central idea of the information display/billboard model (that enhancers display regulatory information to the basal transcriptional machinery and that this information is interpreted and gene expression regulated accordingly) is also the central assumption in thermodynamic-based modeling. Thermodynamic-based models are created with the flexibility to incorporate a complex enhancer grammar. By including terms for binding affinity, cooperativity, and quenching this modeling approach allows for different numbers, strengths, positions, and combinations of TFBSs to drive similar or identical expression patterns. In other words, two divergent enhancer sequences can lead to the same transcriptional output. The recent application of thermodynamic-based modeling approaches in two independent studies demonstrated that incorporating cooperative $TF$ interactions gave their models the ability to correctly predict gene expression patterns, especially in areas of low TF concentrations and at genes with slight differences in expression pattern (Zinzen $et\ al.$, 2006; Segal $et\ al.$, 2008). Reinitz and colleagues (Janssens $et\ al.$, 2006) not only speculated on important $TF$ interactions using a thermodynamic-based model, but after successfully modeling eve stripe 2 expression, their results allowed them to correctly predict expression patterns induced by mutations in specific TFBSs. More recently, Arnosti and colleagues (Fakhouri $et\ al.$, 2010) modeled a data set comprised of synthetic enhancers designed to test important features of enhancer grammar, such as distance-dependent effects of short-range repressors and homotypic repressor cooperativity. They found that a distance-dependent quenching function was key to their model's ability to fit the expression data, which contained different expression patterns driven by enhancers that differed only in their arrangement of binding sites, not the overall number or strength of binding sites. Based on this model they were then able to successfully predict the expression regulated by the endogenous enhancer, $rho$ (Fakhouri $et\ al.$, 2010). In combination these studies have shown that thermodynamic-based models have the ability to correctly predict similar expression patterns from CRMs with variation in the position, strength, and number of binding sites. This strongly supports a billboard-type model, allowing architectural flexibility in an enhancer with respect to TFBS position and strength, opposed to a model with a low tolerance for TFBS turnover.

Despite these successes in modeling CRM function, there are examples of enhancers that do not appear to fit well with the information display/billboard model. In vertebrates, the number of well characterized enhancers is low, but few examples support the information display model perfectly. For example, mammalian sequences with multiple binding sites for the GATA-1 $TF$ continue to function as an enhancer if only a single binding site is intact. However, a very particular site must remain intact: eliminating two of the three GATA-1 sites in an enhancer may not have any effect on its function, but the single loss of the third critical site can completely abolish enhancer activity in mice (Cheng $et\ al.$, 2008). A genome-wide analysis of the occupancy of two $TF$s (CCAAT/enhancer binding protein and hepatocyte nuclear factor 4 alpha) in five different vertebrate species reveals that while each $TF$ has conserved binding preferences, most binding $in\ vivo$ is in fact species-specfic and can be explained by sequence changes to the bound sequence motifs (Schmidt $et\ al.$, 2010). These examples stress the functional importance of a subset of possible binding sites, while the issue of overall TFBS architecture at mammalian enhancers remains largely unexplored.

Perhaps the best studied counterexample to the information display/billboard model in vertebrates is the $interferon$-$\beta$($IFN$-$\beta$) enhanceosome. The $IFN$-$\beta$ gene is upregulated in mammals in response to viral infection and the enhancer that directs this expression requires a very specific set of $TF$s to carry out this regulatory activity (Thanos and Maniatis, 1995). Every $TF$ component is required for the enhanceosome to successfully form and mediate the upregulation of the $IFN$-$\beta$ gene (Panne $et\ al.$, 2007) (see Figure 6b). As a result of this highly structured enhancer-TF complex, there has been virtually no evolutionary binding site turnover at this CRM throughout 100 million years of mammalian evolution. These recent studies demonstrate that evolution can impact enhancers via a number of distinct mechanisms, including, but not limited to, reorganization of the total number, binding affinity and spatial arrangement of TFBSs.

# 6    Conclusions

Future studies now need to ask precisely what it is within the enhancer sequence, the genomic context, or the $TF$s themselves, that contributes to the differences in functional activity between enhancers. These questions will be answered largely through a combination of detailed bioinformatic analyses of genomic sequences, mathematical modeling of enhancer activity and functional tests across related eukaryotic species. As our knowledge of $TF$ binding activity during embryogenesis increases, computational tools, including position-weight matrices, can be used to find binding sites that are conserved between species and to compare their distribution in genomic DNA sequences. Thermodynamic-based models incorporating increased complexity, including cooperative and quenching interactions between $TF$s and regulatory sequences, will provide a rich foundation of hypotheses on enhancer functional activities. *In vivo* functional studies should follow such investigations, guided by rapid cell-based assays to screen potential sequences. While these types of experiments have been performed on a few enhancers, the next step is to apply the same techniques to the ever-growing array of other known enhancers. In addition, expanding our current catalog of known enhancer CRM orthologs in other insects and mammals/vertebrates would greatly contribute to our understanding of the evolution of CRM function. Only by exploring the evolution of a wide range of different enhancers can we hope to understand both their sequence architecture and exactly how these CRMs function in directing the precise patterns of gene expression that give rise to the elegant complexity of embryonic development.

# 7    Acknowledgments

Research in our laboratory is supported by funding to R.A.D. from the National Science Foundation and National Institutes of Health and Howard Hughes Medical Institute Undergraduate Science Education Program grants to the Biology department at Harvey Mudd College. J.M.D. is a Teaching and Research Postdoctoral Fellow at Harvey Mudd College and is supported in part by NSF Grant DMS-0839966.

Portions of this chapter (especially Section 3.1, 3.3, 5 and 6) were previously published in: Borok, M. J. *et al. Development* 137: 5-13 (2010) and Dresch, J.M. (2012) Multi-Scale, Multi-Dimension, DNA-Based Mathematical Modeling of Gene Expression. PhD dissertation, Michigan State University. (Publication No. 3506079)

# References

Ackers, G., Johnson, A. and Shea, M. (1982). Quantitative model for gene regulation by lambda phage repressor, PNAS 79: 1129-1133.

Albert, R. and Othmer, H. (2003). The topology of the regulatory interactions predicts the expression pattern of the segment polarity genes in Drosophila melanogaster, Journal of Theoretical Biology 223: 1-18.

Andrioli, L. P., Vasisht, V., Theodosopoulou, E., Oberstein, A. and Small, S. (2002). Anterior repression of a Drosophila stripe enhancer requires three position-specific mechanisms., Development 129: 4931-40.

Arnosti, D., Gray, S., Barolo, S., Zhou, J. and Levine, M. (1996a). The gap protein knirps mediates both quenching and direct repression in the Drosophila embryo, EMBO Journal 15(14): 3659-3666.

Arnosti, D. N., Barolo, S., Levine, M. and Small, S. (1996b). The eve stripe 2 enhancer employs multiple modes of transcriptional synergy., Development 122: 205-14.

Ay, A. and Arnosti, D. (2011). Mathematical modeling of gene expression: a guide for the perplexed biologist, Critical Reviews in Biochemistry and Molecular Biology 46(2): 137-151.

Bailey, T. and Gribskov, M. (1998). Combining evidence using p-values: application to sequence homology searches, Bioinformatics 14(1): 48-54.

Banerji, J., Olson, L. and Schaffner, W. (1983). A lymphocyte-specific cellular enhancer is located downstream of the joining region in immunoglobulin heavy chain genes, Cell 33: 729-740.

Banerji, J., Rusconi, S. and Schaffner, W. (1981). Expression of a beta-globin gene is enhanced by remote SV40 DNA sequences, Cell 27: 299-308.

Barkess, G. and West, A. (2012). Chromatin insulator elements: establishing barriers to set heterochromatin boundaries, Epigenomics 4(1): 67-80.

Bellen, H. J. (1999). Ten years of enhancer detection: lessons from the fly., Plant Cell 11: 2271-81.

Benoist, C. and Chambon, P. (1981). In vivo sequence requirements of the SV40 early promoter region, Nature 290: 304-310.

Bergman, C., Carlson, J. and Celniker, S. (2005). Drosophila DNase I footprint database: a systematic genome annotation of transcription factor binding sites in the fruitfly, Drosophila melanogaster, Bioinformatics 21(8): 1747-1749.

Berleth, T., Burri, M., Thoma, G., Bopp, D., Richstein, S., Frigerio, G., Noll, M. and Nüsslein-Volhard, C. (1988). The role of localization of bicoid RNA in organizing the anterior pattern of the Drosophila embryo, EMBO J. 7: 1749-1756.

Bintu, L., Buchler, N., Garcia, H., Gerland, U., Hwa, T., Kondev, J., Kuhlman, T. and Phillips, R. (2005). Transcriptional regulation by the numbers: applications, Current Opinion in Genetics and Development 15: 125-135.

Bonn, S., Zinzen, R., Girardot, C., Gustafson, E., Perez-Gonzalez, A., Delhomme, N., Ghavi-Helm, Y., Wilczynski, B., Riddell, A. and Furlong, E. (2012). Tissue-specific analysis of chromatin state identifies temporal signatures of enhancer activity during embryonic develoment, Nature Genetics 44(2): 148-156.

Borok, M. J., Tran, D. A., Ho, M. C. W. and Drewell, R. A. (2010). Dissecting the regulatory switches of development: lessons from enhancer evolution in Drosophila. Development 137: 5-13.

Buecker, C. and Wysocka, J. (2012). Enhancers as information integration hubs in development: lessons from genomics., Trends Genet. 28(6): 276-284.

Caplan, A. I. and Ordahl, C. P. (1978). Irreversible gene repression model for control of development, Science 201: 120-130.

Celniker, S. E., Sharma, S., Keelan, D. J. and Lewis, E. B. (1990). The molecular genetics of the bithorax complex of Drosophila: cis-regulation in the Abdominal-B domain., EMBO J. 9: 4277-86.

Cheng, Y., King, D. C., Dore, L. C., Zhang, X., Zhou, Y., Zhang, Y., Dorman, C., Abebe, D., Kumar, S. A., Chiaromonte, F. *et al*. (2008). Transcriptional enhancement by GATA1-occupied DNA segments is strongly associated with evolutionary constraint on the binding site motif, Genome Research 18: 1896-1905.

Choi, O. R. and Engel, J. D. (1986). A 3 enhancer is required for temporal and tissue-specific transcriptional activation of the chicken adult beta-globin gene, Nature 323: 731-734.

Crocker, J. and Erives, A. (2008a). A closer look at the eve stripe 2 enhancers of Drosophila and Themira, PLoS Genetics 4: e1000276.

Dearolf, C. R., Topol, J. and Parker, C. S. (1989). Transcriptional control of Drosophila fushi tarazu zebra stripe expression, Genes Dev. 3: 384-398.

Driever, W. and Nüsslein-Volhard, C. (1988). A gradient of bicoid protein in Drosophila embryos, Cell 54: 83-93.

Fakhouri, W., Ay, A., Sayal, R., Dresch, J., Dayringer, E. and Arnosti, D. (2010). Deciphering a transcriptional regulatory code: modeling short-range repression in the Drosophila embryo, Molecular Systems Biology 6: 341.

Gertz, J., Siggia, E. and Cohen, B. (2009). Analysis of combinatorial cis-regulation in synthetic and genomic promoters, Nature 457: 215-218.

Gompel, N., Prudhomme, B., Wittkopp, P. J., Kassner, V. A. and Carroll, S. B. (2005). Chance caught on the wing: cis-regulatory evolution and the origin of pigment patterns in Drosophila, Nature 433: 481-487.

Gorkin, D., Lee, D., Reed, X., Fletez-Brant, C., Bessling, S., Loftus, S., Beer, M., Pavan, W. and McCallion, A. (2012). Integration of ChIP-seq and machine learning reveals enhancers and a predictive regulatory sequence vocabulary in melanocytes, Genome Research.

Goto, T., Macdonald, P. and Maniatis, T. (1989). Early and late periodic patterns of even skipped expression are controlled by distinct regulatory elements that respond to different spatial cues, Cell 57: 413-422.

Gray, S., Szymanski, P. and Levine, M. (1994). Short-range repression permits multiple enhancers to function autonomously within a complex promoter., Genes Dev. 8: 1829-38.

Harding, K., Hoey, T., Warrior, R. and Levine, M. (1989). Autoregulatory and gap gene response elements of the even-skipped promoter of Drosophila., EMBO J. 8: 1205-12.

Hare, E. E., Peterson, B. K. and Eisen, M. B. (2008b). A careful look at binding site reorganization in the even-skipped enhancers of Drosophila and sepsids, PLoS Genetics 4: e1000268.

Hare, E. E., Peterson, B. K., Iyer, V. N., Meier, R. and Eisen, M. B. (2008a). Sepsid even-skipped enhancers are functionally conserved in Drosophila despite lack of sequence conservation, PLoS Genetics 4: e1000106.

He, Q., Bardet, A., Patton, B., Purvis, J., Johnston, J., Paulson, A., Gogol, M., Stark, A. and Zeitlinger, J. (2011). High conservation of transcription factor binding and evidence for combinatorial regulation across six Drosophila species, Nature Genetics 21: 414-421.

He, X., Samee, M., Blatti, C. and Sinha, S. (2010). Thermodynamics-based models of transcriptional regulation by enhancers: the roles of synergistic activation, cooperative binding and short-range repression, PLoS Computational Biology 6(9): e1000935.

Heintzman, N., Stuart, R., Hon, G., Fu, Y., Ching, C., Hawkins, R., Barrera, L., Van Calcar, S., Qu, C., Ching, K. et al. (2007). Distinct and predictive chromatin signatures of transcriptional promoters and enhancers in the human genome., Nature Genetics 39(3): 311-318.

Hiromi, Y., Kuroiwa, A. and Gehring, W. J. (1985). Control elements of the Drosophila segmentation gene fushi tarazu, Cell 43: 603-613.

Ip, Y., Park, R., Kosman, D., Yazdanbakhsh, K. and Levine, M. (1992). dorsal-twist interactions establish snail expression in the presumptive mesoderm of the Drosophila embryo, Genes and Development 6: 1518-1530.

Ip, Y. T., Kraut, R., Levine, M. and Rushlow, C. A. (1991). The dorsal morphogen is a sequence-specific DNA-binding protein that interacts with a long-range repression element in Drosophila, Cell 64: 439-446.

Jaeger, J., Surkova, S., Blagov, M., Janssens, H., Kosman, D., Kozlov, K., Manu, Myasnikova, E., Vanario-Alonso, C., Samsonova, M. et al. (2004). Dynamic control of positional information in the early Drosophila embryo, Nature 430: 368-371.

Janssens, H., Hou, S., Jaeger, J., Kim, A., Myasnikova, E., Sharp, D. and Reinitz, J. (2006). Quantitative and predictive model of transcriptional control of the Drosophila melanogaster even skipped gene, Nature Genetics 38: 1159-1165.

Jiang, J., Kosman, D., Ip, Y. T. and Levine, M. (1991). The dorsal morphogen gradient regulates the mesoderm determinant twist in early Drosophila embryos, Genes Dev. 5: 1881-1891.

Jiang, J. and Levine, M. (1993). Binding affinities and cooperative interactions with bHLH activators delimit threshold responses to the dorsal gradient morphogen, Cell 72: 741-752.

Kadonaga, J. T. (2004). Regulation of RNA polymerase II transcription by sequence-specific DNA binding factors, Cell 116: 247-257.

Karch, F., Weiffenbach, B., Peifer, M., Bender, W., Duncan, I., Celniker, S., Crosby, M. and Lewis, E. B. (1985). The abdominal region of the bithorax complex., Cell 43: 81-96.

Kazemian, M., Zhu, Q., Halfon, M. and Sinha, S. (2011). Improved accuracy of supervised CRM discovery with interpolated Markov models and cross-species comparison, Nucleic Acids Research 39(22): 9463-9472.

Kirchhamer, C. V., Yuh, C. H. and Davidson, E. H. (1996). Modular cis-regulatory organization of developmentally expressed genes: two genes transcribed territorially in the sea urchin embryo, and additional examples, Proceedings of the National Academy of Sciences of the United States of America 93: 9322-8.

Kulkarni, M. and Arnosti, D. (2005). cis-Regulatory Logic of Short-Range Transcriptional Repression in Drosophila melanogaster, Molecular Cell Biology 25(9): 3411-3420.

Kulkarni, M. M. and Arnosti, D. N. (2003). Information display by transcriptional enhancers, Development 130: 6569-6575.

Levine, M. and Manley, J. L. (1989). Transcriptional repression of eukaryotic promoters., Cell 59: 405-8.

Lewis, E. B. (1978). A gene complex controlling segmentation in Drosophila, Nature 276: 565-570.

Ludwig, M. Z., Bergman, C., Patel, N. H. and Kreitman, M. (2000). Evidence for stabilizing selection in a eukaryotic enhancer element, Nature 403: 564-567.

Ludwig, M. Z. and Kreitman, M. (1995). Evolutionary dynamics of the enhancer region of even-skipped in Drosophila, Mol. Biol. Evol. 12: 1002-1011.

Ludwig, M. Z., Patel, N. H. and Kreitman, M. (1998). Functional analysis of eve stripe 2 enhancer evolution in Drosophila: rules governing conservation and change, Development 125: 949-58.

MacArthur, S. L., XY; Li, J; Brown, JB; Chu, HC; Zeng, L; Grondona, BP; Hechmer, A; Simirenko, L; Kernen, SVE; Knowles, DW; Stapleton, M; Bickel, P; Biggin, MD; Eisen, MB (2009). Developmental roles of 21 Drosophila transcription factors are determined by quantitative differences in binding to an overlapping set of thousands of genomic regions, Genome Biology 10: R80.

Macdonald, P. M., Ingham, P. and Struhl, G. (1986). Isolation, structure, and expression of even-skipped: a second pair-rule gene of Drosophila containing a homeo box, Cell 47: 721-734.

McEwan, I. J., Wright, A. P., Dahlman-Wright, K., Carlstedt-Duke, J. and Gustafsson, J. A. (1993). Direct interaction of the tau 1 transactivation domain of the human glucocorticoid receptor with the basal transcriptional machinery, Mol. Cell. Biol. 13: 399-407.

Nobrega, M. A., Ovcharenko, I., Afzal, V. and Rubin, E. M. (2003). Scanning human gene deserts for long-range enhancers., Science 302(413).

Noyes, M., Meng, X., Wakabayashi, A., Sinha, S., Brodsky, M. and Wolfe, S. (2008). A systematic characterization of factors that regulate Drosophila segmentation via a bacterial one-hybrid system, Nucleic Acids Research 36(8): 2547-2560.

Ong, C. and Corces, V. (2012). Enhancers: emerging roles in cell fate specification., EMBO 13(5): 423-430.

Ozdemir, A., Fisher-Aylor, K., Pepke, S., Samanta, M., Dunipace, L., McCue, K., Zeng, L., Ogawa, N., Wold, B. and Stathopoulos, A. (2011). High resolution mapping of Twist to DNA in Drosophila embryos: Efficient functional analysis and evolutionary conservation., Genome Research 21(4): 566-577.

Pan, D., Huang, J. and Courey, A. (1991). Functional analysis of the Drosophila twist promoter reveals a dorsal-binding ventral activator region, Genes and Development 5: 1892-1901.

Panne, D., Maniatis, T. and Harrison, S. C. (2007). An atomic model of the interferon-beta enhanceosome, Cell 129: 1111-1123.

Peterson, B. K., Hare, E. E., Iyer, V. N., Storage, S., Conner, L., Papaj, D. R., Kurashima, R., Jang, E. and Eisen, M. B. (2009). Big genomes facilitate the comparative identification of regulatory elements, PLoS ONE 4: e4688.

Prudhomme, B., Gompel, N. and Carroll, S. B. (2007). Emerging principles of regulatory evolution, Proceedings of the National Academy of Sciences of the United States of America 104: 8605-8612.

Qian, S., Capovilla, M. and Pirrotta, V. (1991). The bx region enhancer, a distant cis-control element of the Drosophila Ubx gene and its regulation by hunchback and other segmentation genes, EMBO J. 10: 1415-1425.

Reinitz, J., Hou, S. and Sharp, D. (2003). Transcriptional Control in Drosophila, ComPlexUs 1: 54-64.

Sanchez, L. and Thieffry, D. (2001). A logical analysis of the Drosophila gap-gene system, Journal of Theoretical Biology 211: 115-141.

Sandmann, T., Girardot, C., Brehme, M., Tongprasit, W., Stolc, V. and Furlong, E. (2007). A core transcriptional network for early mesoderm development in Drosophila melanogaster, Genes and Development 21: 436-449.

Sauer, F., Rivera-Pomar, R., Hoch, M. and Jäckle, H. (1996). Gene regulation in the Drosophila embryo, Philos. Trans. R. Soc. Lond. B. Biol. Sci. 351: 579-587.

Schmidt, D., Wilson, M., Ballester, B., Schwalie, P., Brown, G., Marshall, A., Kutter, C., Watt, S., Martinez-Jimenez, C., Mackay, S. *et al.* (2010). Five-Vertebrate ChIP-seq Reveals the Evolutionary Dynamics of Transcription Factor Binding, Science 328(5981): 1036-1040.

Segal, E., Raveh-Sadka, T., Schroeder, M., Unnerstall, U. and Gaul, U. (2008). Predicting expression patterns from regulatory sequence in Drosophila segmentation, Nature 451: 535-540.

Shea, M. and Ackers, G. (1985). The OR control system of bacteriophage lambda. A physical-chemical model for gene regulation, Journal of Molecular Biology 181: 211-230.

Shepherd, B., Garabedian, M. J., Hung, M. C. and Wensink, P. C. (1985). Developmental control of Drosophila yolk protein 1 gene by cis-acting DNA elements, Cold Spring Harb. Symp. Ouant. Biol. 50: 521-526.

Sherman, M. and Cohen, B. (2012). Thermodynamic State Ensemble Models of cis-Regulation, PLoS Computational Biology 8(3): e1002407.

Sinkkonen, L., Hugenschmidt, T., Berninger, P., Gaidatzis, D., Mohn, F., Artus-Revel, C., Zavolan, M., Svoboda, P. and Filipowicz, W. (2008). MicroRNAs control de novo DNA methylation through regulation of transcriptional repressors in mouse embryonic stem cells., Nat Struct Mol Biol. 15(3): 259-267.

Small, S., Blair, A. and Levine, M. (1991a). Regulation of even-skipped stripe 2 in the Drosophila embryo, EMBO J. 11: 4047-4057.

Small, S., Blair, A. and Levine, M. (1996). Regulation of two pair-rule stripes by a single enhancer in the Drosophila embryo, Dev. Biol. 175: 314-324.

Small, S., Kraut, R., Hoey, T., Warrior, R. and Levine, M. (1991b). Transcriptional regulation of a pair-rule stripe in Drosophila, Genes Dev. 5: 827-839.

Spitz, F. and Furlong, E. (2012). Transcription factors: from enhancer binding to developmental control., Nat Rev Genet. 13(9): 613-626.

Stanojevic, D., Hoey, T. and Levine, M. (1989). Sequence-specific DNA-binding activities of the gap proteins encoded by hunchback and Krüppel in Drosophila, Nature 341: 331-335.

Stanojevic, D., Small, S. and Levine, M. (1991). Regulation of a segmentation stripe by overlapping activators and repressors in the Drosophila embryo, Science 254(5036): 1385-1387.

Steward, R., Zusman, S. B., Huang, L. H. and Schedl, P. (1988). The dorsal protein is distributed in a gradient in early Drosophila embryos, Cell 55: 487-495.

Struhl, G., Struhl, K. and Macdonald, P. M. (1989). The gradient morphogen bicoid is a concentration-dependent transcriptional activator, Cell 57: 1259-1273.

Struhl, K. (1984). Genetic properties and chromatin structure of the yeast gal regulatory element: an enhancer-like sequence, Proceedings of the National Academy of Sciences of the United States of America 81: 7865-7869.

Szymanski, P. and Levine, M. (1995). Multiple modes of dorsal-bHLB transcriptional synergy in the Drosophila embryo, EMBO Journal 14: 2229-2238.

Tamura, K., Subramanian, S. and Kumar, S. (2004). Temporal patterns of fruit fly (Drosophila) evolution revealed by mutation clocks., Molecular Biology and Evolution 21: 36-44.

Thanos, D. and Maniatis, T. (1995). Virus induction of human IFN beta gene expression requires the assembly of an enhanceosome, Cell 83: 1091-1100.

Thisse, C., Perrin-Schmitt, F., Stoetzel, C. and Thisse, B. (1991). Sequence-Specific Transactivation of the Drosophila twist Gene by the dorsal Gene Product, Cell 65: 1191-1201.

Visel, A., Blow, M. J., Li, Z., Zhang, T., Akiyama, J. A., Holt, A., Plajzer-Frick, I., Shoukry, M., Wright, C., Chen, F. *et al.* (2009a). ChIP-seq accurately predicts tissue-specific activity of enhancers., Nature 457: 854-8.

Visel, A., Rubin, E. and Pennacchio, L. (2009b). Genomic Views of Distant-Acting Enhancers, Nature 10(461): 199-205.

Wildeman, A. G., Sassone-Corsi, P., Grundstr□m, T., Zenke, M. and Chambon, P. (1984). Stimulation of in vitro transcription from the SV40 early promoter by the enhancer involves a specific trans-acting factor, EMBO J. 3: 3129-3133.

Yuh, C., Bolouri, H. and Davidson, E. (2001). Cis-regulatory logic in the endo16 gene: switching from a specification to a differentiation mode of control, Development 128: 617-629.

Zeitlinger, J., Zinzen, R. P., Stark, A., Kellis, M., Zhang, H., Young, R. A. and Levine, M. (2007). Whole-genome ChIP-chip analysis of Dorsal, Twist, and Snail suggests integration of diverse patterning processes in the Drosophila embryo., Genes Dev. 21: 385-90.

Zinzen, R., Girardot, C., Gagneur, J., Braun, M. and Furlong, E. (2009). Combinatorial binding predicts spatio-temporal cis-regulatory activity, Nature 462: 65-70.

Zinzen, R., Senger, K., Levine, M. and Papatsenko, D. (2006). Computational models for neurogenic gene expression in the Drosophila embryo, Current Biology 16: 1358-1365.

# Strategies for Genetic Screening of Multiple Samples Using PCR-Based Targeted Sequence Enrichment

Paola Benaglio
*Department of Medical Genetics*
*University of Lausanne, Switzerland*

Carlo Rivolta
*Department of Medical Genetics*
*University of Lausanne, Switzerland*

# 1    Introduction

## 1.1    Next Generation Sequencing Technologies: An Overview

Biological research has been revolutionized by the introduction of dideoxy DNA sequencing, developed by Frederick Sanger et al. in the late '70s (Sanger *et al.*, 1977). This technique, that essentially dominated the field of DNA analysis for the following 3 decades, was instrumental for the sequencing of the human genome in 2004 (International Human Genome Consortium, 2004) and still is very heavily used. The succeeding advent and rapid development of the so-called "next generation" or "ultra high throughput" sequencing (NGS or UHTS) technologies ushered in an era in which reading an organism's genome has almost become a routine practice. In addition to the sequencing of whole genomes, the development of different NGS methods and protocols has enabled a wide range of applications. The most used and best established ones are the sequencing of entire transcriptomes (RNA-seq), the sequencing of DNA from chromatin immunoprecipitation assays (ChIP-seq), DNA methylation profiling, and the analysis of genetic variations, especially in the field of medical genetics.

The distinctive feature of next generation sequencing is the possibility of producing very high number of sequences (or *reads*) in a fast and cost-effective manner. The most used platforms are currently commercialized by Roche 454 (GS FLX and GS Junior), Illumina (HiSeq, Genome Analyzer and MiSeq), and Life Technologies (SOLiD System and Ion Torrent sequencers). Each platform is characterized by a combination of different strategies for template preparation, amplification and sequencing, which lead in all cases to the parallelization underlying the drastic drop of the per-base cost of sequencing.

Template preparation is mostly based on a "shotgun cloning" approach (used to sequence long fragments of DNA) and includes the random shearing of the input DNA, usually through nebulization or sonication, followed by the clonal amplification of the fragments obtained. "Emulsion PCR", for example, is the method of library amplification used by Roche 454, SOLiD, and Ion Torrent technologies. Fragments of DNA, ligated to universal adaptors, are captured and amplified on individual beads in a water-in-oil mixture (Metzker, 2010). The enriched beads are then fixed on a glass surface (SOLiD) or deposited into PicoTiterPlate (PTP) wells (Roche 454). In the Illumina platforms, the enrichment step occurs on a glass slide, where high-density primers are attached, and clonally amplified clusters are produced from the templates.

The sequencing reactions rely on different principles, based on either DNA polymerase or DNA ligase. Roche 454 uses pyrosequencing, in which the incorporation of complementary dNTPs results in the emission of photons (Margulies *et al.*, 2005). The Illumina technology relies on a sequencing-by-synthesis approach, based on the cyclic incorporation of fluorescent nucleotides with reversible termination. Ion Torrent employs a similar approach, but uses non-modified dNTPs and a silicon chip that detects hydrogen ions released during each cycle of polymerization (Rothberg *et al.*, 2011). In contrast to the previous methods, depending on the activity of DNA polymerase, SOLiD uses a ligase-based chemistry consisting of cycles of hybridization and ligation (McKernan *et al.*, 2009).

The sequences produced by NGS are first collected as raw images and then processed to generate a readable output that has to be either aligned to a reference genomic sequence or assembled to form a "de novo" DNA sequence. In all cases, assembly, mapping, and analysis of sequences require the use of dedicated software.

Typically, NGS platforms produce reads of shorter length than those produced by Sanger sequencing, in the range of 50 to 400 nucleotides, depending on the platform. The throughput of these machines varies from several Megabases to hundreds of Gigabases per run and the time needed to produce such reads from a few hours to a few days. All of these features have to be taken into account and selected according to the desired output, in particular with respect to the desired *coverage*. The coverage is defined as the number of reads that interrogate a given DNA base and indicates how "deeply" a sample is sequenced. A rough way to estimate the average coverage of a sequencing experiment is to divide the total throughput (in base pairs) by the size of the DNA fragment that has to be sequenced. Sequencing redundancy, or high coverage, is necessary to reconstruct a correct sequence since NGS reads contain a higher proportion of errors than sequences obtained by the Sanger method and therefore every base has to be interrogated multiple times. In principle, the more accurate an instrument is, the less coverage is needed. Typical NGS errors are represented by an incorrect base call or small insertion and deletions. They can occur randomly or systematically in certain DNA regions that are more difficult to sequence, such as GC rich regions and homopolymeric stretches (i.e. TTTT..., AAAA..., etc) (Harismendy *et al.*, 2009; Huse *et al.*, 2007).

NGS companies are putting constant effort into improving the accuracy, the throughputs, and the flexibility of their systems. It is therefore rather difficult to give a contemporary picture of their technical features, due to the continuing evolution of the technology and specialization of these instruments.

## 1.2   Enrichment Strategies

The analysis and interpretation of genome-wide sequencing results is currently a step behind the technology that produces them. For certain applications it is more interesting -and economically more convenient- to concentrate the study only to a limited part of the genome. In medical genetics, for example, it is still a common practice to screen for genetic variants only a limited number of genes (for example a genomic interval associated to an inheritable disease) or all the coding sequences of a genome (the so-called exome) (Gilissen *et al.*, 2011).

For this purpose, various strategies for enrichment of target DNA have been developed in recent years (Mamanova *et al.*, 2010; Mertes *et al.*, 2011). They can be divided mainly into PCR-, hybridization-, or circularization-based approaches. The choice of the enrichment strategy to be used depends on specific requirements of the project, and in particular on the target DNA size and the number of samples to be sequenced.

### 1.2.1   PCR-Based Enrichment Techniques

Polymerase chain reaction (PCR) is certainly the most reliable method for target enrichment, due to its high specificity, sensitivity and reproducibility. However, while this technique is very well suited to capillary electrophoresis (Sanger) sequencing, in which each amplicon is directly and separately analyzed, it is not completely adapted to NGS approaches. In fact, to exploit the full throughput of NGS and to perform an analysis that is economically viable, many samples and amplicons must be run at the same time. As it will be detailed in the next paragraph (1.3), the sequencing of multiple samples is limited by the long time and the relatively high costs required for library preparation. Multiple amplicons may be obtained via multiplex PCRs or pooling of single-plex PCRs. In both cases, the danger is an uneven representation of the amplicons forming the pool. This can occur from unequal PCR efficiency across the various amplicons or from unbalanced pooling of the fragments. Both of these events, if present, are in general difficult to correct. The manual production of PCRs is feasible for less than a hundred thousand bases of target DNA by using standard PCRs of few hundred bases, or by using long range PCR (LR-PCR) of approximately 10 Kbases. For larger target regions, the workflow involving primers design, optimization of robust PCRs, and generation and pooling of the products becomes less time- and cost- effective.

An automated solution for preparation of multiple PCRs (in this case standard PCRs) is provided by the RainStorm platform, produced by RainDance Technologies. In this system, emulsion-like PCR reactions occur as single-plexes in microdroplets, which are mechanically generated and assembled in a microfluidic system (Tewhey *et al.*, 2009). Up to 20,000 primer pairs and corresponding number of reactions can be supported at the same time by this machine, which allows a relatively uniform enrichment of up to 10 Mb regions.

Some PCR-based approaches allow the simultaneous generation of short PCRs and library preparations by means of the incorporation of sequencing adaptors to the PCR primers, which must amplify fragments shorter than the sequencing reads. The advantage of this strategy is to avoid the cleaning, pooling, and shotgun library preparation required for longer DNA fragments (Mertes *et al.*, 2011). The Fluidigm "Access Array System" employs this approach and allows, for example, the automatic preparation of 48 sample libraries using a microfluidic device that assembles and hosts 2,304 parallel separated PCR reactions.

Finally, certain platforms, such as Illumina Miseq and Life Technologies IonTorrent PGM, provide panels of ready-to-use highly multiplexed short PCR reactions to amplify target regions ranging from 1 Kb to 1 Mb, for up to 96 samples.

### 1.2.2   Hybrid Capture Enrichment Techniques

To select larger DNA regions (from 1 to 50 Mb of cumulative sequence), the hybrid capture method is preferred to the PCR method for its simplicity and rapidity, rather than for its specificity. The principle of sequence capture is based on the hybridization of a shotgun library to complementary probes of 60-150 nucleotides, designed to cover the target region. The hybridization reaction can occur in solution, or on a solid phase, where the probes are fixed on a microarray. The in-solution capture has the advantage of not requiring special equipment but a thermocycler, and of being more easily scalable. The main vendors of hybrid capture kits are NimbleGene (Roche) and Agilent; the first uses DNA probes, while the second longer RNA probes. The most used application of this technique is the enrichment of all the transcribed regions of the human genome, the so-called *whole exome capture*. One of the drawbacks of the hybrid capture method is the relatively high proportion of off-target and pseudogenes sequences, which have a negative effect on the coverage and the variant calling of the target region.

### 1.2.2   Circularization-based Enrichment Techniques

Another type of enrichment strategy is based on the use of custom molecular inversion probes (MIPs) or "gap-fill padlock", adapted from a SNP genotyping protocol (Akhras *et al.*, 2007). MIPs are synthetic DNA oligonucleotides that contain a common linker sequence flanked by two single-stranded sequences designed to anneal to two nonconsecutive parts of a genomic target region. Such a region can be of up to 191 bp in length (Turner *et al.*, 2009) or 500 bp when using longer padlock probes (LPPs) (Shen *et al.*, 2011). Once hybridized, the gap between the two specific sequences is filled by the DNA polymerase and closed by a ligase reaction. These circular products are then amplified by PCR with primers annealing to the common linker. Since this latter sequence contains NGS adaptors as well, ready-to sequence templates that do not require further steps for library preparation are produced. A slightly different approach involves the use of "selector probes" which differ from the previous one because the genomic DNA is first digested by restriction enzymes and the resulting fragments circularize after the hybridization to the probes (Dahl *et al.*, 2007). The advantages of these capture methods include high specificity and reproducibility, the characteristic of being library-free, and low input DNA (Turner *et al.*, 2009). Disadvantages are represented by a poorer uniformity of the captured targets and high initial costs of the probes (Mamanova *et al.*, 2010).

## 1.3    Multiplexing Strategies

The number of samples that can be simultaneously sequenced and resolved represents an important issue in NGS. While capillary electrophoresis sequencing offers the highest degree of scalability, with hundreds of samples and Kilobases sequenced per run, NGS platforms easily produce Gigabases of sequences, but typically distributed among few samples or only one. The reason for this is mainly physical: a capillary electrophoresis sequencer contains a few dozen capillaries that can be used simultaneously; NGS reactions occur on array-like surfaces with almost no separation to host different samples. The ideal application for NGS is therefore the sequencing of large amounts of DNA from an individual sample (e.g. a genome or an exome). In case of targeted resequencing, a smaller sequencing throughput is required and this is obtained either by using lower scale sequencers (the very new "benchtop sequencers" like Ion Torrent PGM, Illumina MiSeq and Roche 454 GS Junior) or by distributing the sequencing capacity of a big platform across many samples, to be sequenced at the same time. If such samples correspond to non-overlapping DNA sequences (e.g. each sample is constituted by an individual PCR product, representative of a unique genomic region), sample/sequence identification is performed a posteriori, when reads are assembled or mapped. Conversely, if each sample is constituted by a PCR product that originates from the DNA of a given individual and pairs of primers targeting the same DNA region for all samples, "multiplexing" procedures aimed at identifying individual samples become necessary. Such multiplexing is achieved during library preparation, via a step in which a sequence of DNA of 4-8 nt (the so-called *barcode*), unique to each sample, is ligated to all DNA fragments composing the library (Craig *et al.*, 2008; Smith *et al.*, 2010). Multiple libraries are then pooled in equal amounts and sequenced at once, along with their barcodes. The identification of samples occurs after the sequencing, thanks to the information contained in the genetic barcode tags.

Rather than technical, the real limitations of multiplexing are the high costs and the labor associated to sample preparation, which must be carried out separately for each sample in order to add individual nucleotide barcodes. As mentioned before, recent developments of PCR-based enrichment kits allow a greater automation in library preparation and a high level of multiplexing (up to 96 samples). However, this workflow is integrated for the moment only to low throughput sequencers (MiSeq, IonTorrent) or requires special equipment dedicated only to this process (Flugidim Access Array). Alternatively, other methods that do not require library preparation like MIPs can be appealing for processing many samples. Specifically, with MIPs barcodes can be directly inserted in the primers that will amplify the captured sequences and the NGS adaptors (Akhras *et al.*, 2007).

In case of recurrent genetic screenings performed on a same cohort of samples, a different strategy would be to initially tag the genomic DNA from different individuals with specific barcodes and NGS adaptor oligonucleotides, and then pool the barcoded fragments. Any downstream manipulation would be then performed on a single tube, which contains separable information of many individuals after the sequencing. This approach is available since the beginning of 2012 and is commercialized by PopulationGenetics, which also patented this workflow under the name of GenomePooling. In this approach, the regions of interest are extracted from the pool through specific primers and inverse simplex PCRs. Since they contain already both the individual barcode and sequences for NGS processing, they could be directly sequenced as a pool of samples (Casbon *et al.*, 2011). If this technique demonstrates to have sensitivity and specificity comparable to other enrichment methods, it will represent a very powerful tool for genetic screenings via NGS.

Many scientists have tried to bypass the step of individual barcoding by using as a strategy the "anonymous" pooling (i.e. with no tagging nucleotides) of target DNA from different samples and the creation of a unique library for sequencing (Calvo *et al.,* 2010; Lee *et al.*, 2011; Otto *et al.*, 2011; Out *et al.*, 2009). Obviously, by this approach it is not possible to assign any direct relationship between reads and samples to which they belong, and further validations are required to track back the carrier of the variations via capillary sequencing or other methods. For some purposes, sample identification may not represent a primary necessity, for example if the aim of the project is to estimate the allele frequency of certain alleles in a population (Ingman & Gyllensten, 2009).

The mixed information contained in the results of such sequencing projects, in fact, must be interpreted based on the expected frequency of a single allele in a pool of chromosomes. For example, if 100 human samples have been pooled together, each autosomal allele will represent the 0.5% of the total sequence reads. In projects aiming at the identification of novel or rare variations (like disease causing mutations), the detection threshold of DNA changes must be therefore set at a frequency as low as 0.5%, depending on the number of individuals pooled together. For such experiments, it is important that the error rate of the sequencing platform does not exceed the expected frequency of one variation present in one individual. The risk is to produce many false positives, if the variant detection threshold is set too low, or false negatives, if this is set too high. This point will be elucidated in the following paragraphs through the description of a real example.

Two main different ways of obtaining pooled libraries are to group samples before or after target enrichment. For example, in case of PCR-based enrichment, template DNA can be quantified, pooled and amplified in a unique reaction. Alternatively, PCR fragments must be generated for each samples and pooled in a second time. The first approach is by far quicker and cheaper, but on the other hand the second one allows assessing the product of each reaction and produce a more balanced pool across all different samples (Otto *et al.*, 2011; Out *et al.*, 2009).

## 1.4   Genetic Screenings of Multiple Samples in Medical Genetics

In medical genetics, the discovery of genes causing Mendelian diseases has been classically achieved through linkage analysis of families or through the screening of candidate genes in large cohorts of patients. Linkage analysis and sequencing of the genomic region harboring the mutation are very powerful techniques if large families are available. In absence of large families to study, the candidate gene approach can be chosen. The hypothesis that a gene may cause the disease, based on its biological relevance and other known data, is tested through the screening of many patients with the same disease. Nowadays, with high throughput sequencing being progressively more affordable, the use of the new technologies simplifies and accelerates the discovery process.

Before NGS technologies emerged, candidate gene sequencing for detection of disease causing mutations was carried out through the Sanger dideoxy method, which is still the gold-standard method for molecular diagnosis in many hereditary diseases. However, the high costs and time required for sequencing entire genes in many patients by this method forced many laboratories to apply cheaper screening techniques such as single-strand conformation polymorphism (SSCP) and denaturing high-pressure liquid chromatography (DHPLC) prior to Sanger sequencing. NGS has the potential of substituting these procedures and offers a cost effective and accurate alternative to the Sanger method.

The workflow of a NGS application is mostly defined by the enrichment and multiplexing strategies that are used, as described before. Successful examples include the use of commercial solutions such as the Raindance droplet-based multiplex PCR, or the Fluidigm microfluidic chip to test 86 known genes responsible for X-linked intellectual disability in 24 samples (Hu *et al.*, 2009), or 3 known familial hypercholesterolemia genes in 144 samples (Hollants *et al.*, 2012). Others have developed in-house methods to implement NGS in clinical diagnosis. For example, a pipeline based on a multiplex PCR enrichment step followed by a second PCR round to add sequencing adaptors was successfully applied to identify novel and known mutations in 3 genes responsible for the Marfan and Loeys-Dietz syndromes, in 87 patients (Baetens *et al.*, 2011). The anonymous pooling strategy described before was also proven to be efficient in mutation discovery (Benaglio *et al.*, 2011; Calvo *et al.*, 2010; Otto *et al.*, 2011; Out *et al.*, 2009). In general, based on published data, it appears that the majority of NGS efforts aimed at analyzing multiple patients at once have been devoted to molecular diagnosis of known disease-genes, rather than to the discovery of new genes. Furthermore, it seems that a uniformed protocol for sequencing a small target region in many patients is not yet present.

Conversely, whole exome and genome sequencing are the most used and best-established strategies to discover new disease genes. Thanks to these approaches, discovery occurs through an unbiased analysis of the variants that are present in the entire genome or exome, in many cases helped by genotyping or sequencing information from family members. Whole exome or genome sequencing are more successful for discovering new genes associated with recessive conditions, since homozygous (or compound heterozygous) rare variations are less frequent in the genome with respect to heterozygous changes, and therefore are easier to identify and verify in terms of possible pathogenicity.

In the cases presented below we applied the candidate gene approach to identify new mutations in a cohort of patients affected with autosomal dominant retinitis pigmentosa (adRP), a diseases leading to progressive retinal blindness. RP may be caused by mutations in more than 100 genes, each of them responsible for a small fraction of the cases (Hartong *et al.*, 2006). Diagnostic screening of known mutations are performed by using an arrayed primer extension chip by Asper Biotech or, more recently, by NGS of known genes after solid-phase capture arrays enrichment (Neveling *et al.*, 2011; Simpson *et al.*, 2010). Because of the high genetic heterogeneity displayed by RP, a very effective strategy for the identification of new disease genes, which are calculated to account for almost the half of RP patients, consists in the screening of candidate genes in large cohorts of patients (Dryja, 1997). Also, due to this genetic heterogeneity, the screening of single genes in a cohort of patients is expected to identify only a few individuals who are positive for a particular mutation.

We present two examples of single-gene screening in multiple patients (~100) using two different NGS strategies: the anonymous pooling approach and the tagged libraries pool approach. We chose long range PCR based methods, because of its high specificity, a crucial element to consider when many samples are processed together.

## 2  Anonymous Pooling Approach

The method presented here was applied to screen for heterozygous mutations an RP-associated gene (*SNRNP200*) and allowed us identifying new likely pathogenic DNA variants (Benaglio *et al.*, 2011). Because of the elevated number of exons to be analyzed (45), we adopted a protocol consisting in the parallel sequencing of pooled and untagged DNA samples and evaluated it as a potential method for studying rare diseases with elevated genetic heterogeneity, such as RP. We sequenced this gene with the Roche 454 GS FLX Titanium instrument, by using as template a pool of individually-obtained LR-PCRs from 96 unrelated patients with adRP, accounting for a total of 4,320 exons, 4,224 introns, or ~3.5 Mb.

## 2.1    Experimental Methodology

### 2.1.1    Enrichment and Sequencing Method

The candidate gene of interest was amplified in a cohort of 96 patients by 4 overlapping LR-PCRs of 5 to 12 kbases in length, spanning in total approximately 35 contiguous kbases of the human genome. We quantified the resulting 384 PCR products by using pre-casted agarose gels and densitometry, before pooling them in equimolar amounts. Library preparation and sequencing was performed in agreement with the specific protocols for Roche 454 GS FLX Titanium. Two runs of such platform were performed.

### 2.1.2    Sequence Analysis

The analysis of the sequencing results was performed with the CLC Genomics Workbench software package (CLC bio, Denmark). We first polished the raw sequences by trimming the low-quality extremities of the reads and by eliminating the reads shorter than 25 nucleotides. Mapping was restricted to reads that could align to the reference sequence with at least 98% identity for more than 98% of their size. For reliable detection of single-nucleotide substitutions, we considered only high quality reads of the assembly, in highly-covered regions. Specifically, we set a minimum of 99% average base call accuracy (or 20 PHRED score) and allowed a maximum of 3 mismatches or insertions/deletions, calculated on a region of eleven nucleotides spanning the called variant. The variation detection frequency threshold was set to 0.5% over a minimum of 1,000 reads, which corresponded roughly to the identification of one heterozygous change in a pool of 96 samples (192 chromosomes), each allele being theoretically represented by at least 5 reads of relatively good quality. Finally, we used the information of the two independent sequencing runs as technical replicates and selected only DNA variants that were detected in both processes. Changes detected by UHTS were validated by sequencing individual PCR products from each patient's DNA by capillary electrophoresis, only for selected exons. Moreover, if a likely pathogenic change could be confirmed, we screened for that particular change an additional cohort of 95 unrelated individuals presenting with the same disease. Potential effects of amino acid substitutions were evaluated by the web-based software PolyPhen (Ramensky *et al.*, 2002), while the involvement of isocoding DNA changes on gene splicing was tested by using NNSPLICE (Reese *et al.*, 1997).

## 2.2    Results and Discussion

Each run of Roche 454 FLX produced roughly 1.2 million raw sequences of 314 nt in size on average. After quality trimming and filtering, 87% of the raw reads aligned to the 35-kb reference sequence, producing an average base coverage of about 3,750 fold, with a minimum coverage of 500 reads for the 96% of the targeted region. If we assume that each sample is equally represented in the pool, we obtain a ~20x average coverage per single allele per patient, which is in the range of coverage recommended for confident DNA analysis (Bentley *et al.*, 2008; McKernan *et al.*, 2009).

The joint analysis of variant detection resulting from the two sequencing runs identified 79 DNA changes. We prioritized the analysis of candidate mutations according to the functional effect of such variations on the protein product of the gene. We therefore discarded all known polymorphisms (33), intronic and synonymous changes (24), and variations located within homopolymeric stretches (18), where pyrosequencing-based platforms are particularly prone to introduce errors (Huse *et al.*, 2007) (Table 1). Validation of DNA changes by Sanger sequencing of individual DNA samples and the subsequent identification of the patient(s) carrying putative mutations was restricted to four non-synonymous substitutions, located in 4 different exons.

| # Variants | Associated with homopolymers | Annotated SNPs | Intronic or non-coding | Synonymous | Nonsynonymous | Total |
|---|---|---|---|---|---|---|
| Merged | 110 | 37 | 63 | 5 | 7 | 222 |
| Intersection | 18 | 33 | 20 | 4 | 4 | 79 |

**Table 1:** Number of single nucleotide variations identified in the pooled sequences with a frequency higher than 0.5%. Results obtained by either the assembly generated by merging the sequences of the two runs (Merged) or by retaining only those identified in both runs (Intersection - used in our experiment) are presented.

Of the four putative missense mutations detected in both sequencing runs, only two were confirmed by Sanger sequencing. They had an allele frequency detected via NGS of 0.7% and 1.4%, corresponding to one and two actual carriers, respectively. The other two missense variations identified by NGS with a frequency of 0.5% were false positives. Additionally, we identified two new missense variations through Sanger sequencing but not by NGS (false negatives). These variants, affecting the same codon, were initially not detected by NGS because they were present in the pool with frequency values that were below the 0.5% threshold (0.1% and 0.4%) and therefore were not included in the list of candidate variants.

These novel missense changes, were likely pathogenic mutations. Specifically, they involved highly conserved residues, were not detected in 350 control chromosomes, and were found in few additional unrelated patients after the screening of a second cohort. Moreover, for two of them the co-segregation of the DNA variant in the affected family members could be performed and was consistent with that of a pathogenic allele.

In addition to the clinical relevance of these findings, this study gave us the possibility of exploring the anonymous pooling method and to point out its advantages and limitations. One marked limitation of our screening was the high rate of false positive and false negative variation calls with respect to the true signals. The reason for this was mainly attributable to the low frequency that we set for calling variants, which inevitably brought to detection of mismatches due to sequencing or mapping errors.

To test the behavior of this method with respect to false positive discovery, we made a comparison between the number of variations detected by Sanger and NGS for 6 exons, covering in total ~3% of the entire gene. We were interested in ascertaining the number of false positives (i.e. variants detected by NGS but not by Sanger sequencing) at different thresholds of detection, ranging from a frequency of 0.1% to 2.0%. As predictable, false positives were detected in large amounts at low frequency thresholds. However, they were drastically reduced starting from a frequency threshold of 0.3% and virtually eliminated when such frequency was 1% or higher, according to an exponential curve (Figure 1).

Interestingly, we observed that the number of false positives was significantly lower when we counted only signals detected independently in both sequencing runs (i.e. the strategy that we adopted), with respect to merging the sequences obtained by the two runs. Similarly, we could also reduce by more than five folds the number of DNA changes that were present in homopolymeric stretches (Table 1), corresponding almost certainly to sequencing errors.

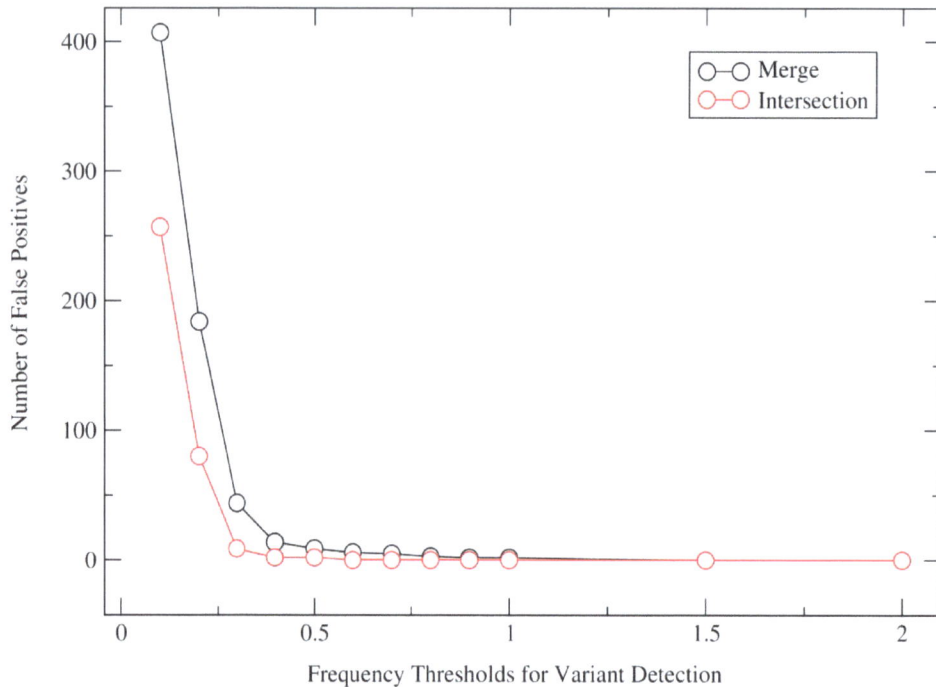

**Figure 1:** False positive variants as a function of different detection thresholds. Variations that were identified in the pooled sequencing experiments (merged dataset or intersection of the two sequencing runs) but not in the Sanger sequencing of the corresponding exons were considered as false positives. The comparison was performed over 6 exons of the gene.

Using higher thresholds of detection to correct the problem of false positives would also lead to the misidentification of potentially real variants, as we showed with our example. We could not in fact identify two true variations with an actual frequency of 0.4% and 0.1%, which were under the 0.5% limit that we chose for our analysis. While we can consider the first as a false negative (0.4%) because of stochastic deviation from the expected value, the second change (0.1%) was likely missed due to its underrepresentation with respect to the other alleles of the pool, rather than because of a sequencing error. This can happen for example when PCR products are pooled in an unbalanced quantity or when the two alleles from the same sample are differentially amplified due to the presence of a SNP near or inside the binding site of the PCR primers (Benaglio & Rivolta 2010; Ikegawa *et al.*, 2002).

It seems therefore that the correct balance between low noise from false positive and sensitive detection of true variants is a fine process that cannot be predicted a priori. A feasible strategy to overcome this issue, also adopted in similar works (Calvo *et al.*, 2010; Otto *et al.*, 2011), is to pool a lower number of samples and increase the detection frequency threshold consequently. For example, as it was showed by our simulation with different frequencies of detection, a marked improvement in specificity could be already observed at a frequency as low as 1%. This threshold could be used for variant detection of pools of 48 samples instead of 96 and theoretically allow the identification of 1 allele out of 96 with a lower noise due to sequencing errors.

To summarize, the DNA screening strategy presented here showed to be very efficient in finding new mutations, if compared to classical methods involving the individual sequencing and analysis of all the exons of a gene in hundreds of patients and controls. However, as a disadvantage with respect to classical exon-PCR analyses by Sanger sequencing or to UHTS of single samples, the results obtained with the pooled approach depend on stochastic variables that are difficult to control. The use of smaller pools of samples and more accurate sequencing platforms should almost certainly help increasing the efficiency of this method.

# 3   Tagged Libraries Pool Approach

Given the risk of missing potential mutations experienced in the anonymous pooling approach, we decided to test a safer, although more expensive technique involving the pool of tagged libraries. Tagged libraries should reduce the number of false positive and negative changes because the analysis is performed individually for each sample. A higher detection threshold for variant detection can therefore be used, and areas of potential errors can be more easily identified in those presenting low coverage. The target DNA in this screening consisted in two candidate adRP genes of 51 and 20 kb in size, amplified by 5 and 2 LR-PCRs, respectively. In order to achieve the parallelization required for library preparation of 95 samples, we chose a transposase-based method of fragmentation, described below. Moreover, we run a pilot test to evaluate the fragmentation protocol, the conditions for normalization of LR-PCRs, and the feasibility of merging untagged samples in single library preparations.

## 3.1   Experimental Methodology

### 3.1.1   Enrichment and Sequencing Method

Similar to the previous screening, long range PCR products of ~10 kb in length were individually obtained to target and amplify two candidate genes in a cohort of patients. The total number of exons and introns analyzed was 43 and 41, respectively. Prior to the screening of 95 samples, we conducted a pilot experiment on 18 libraries to test two methods of PCR product normalization. The first method, used for 8 samples, consisted in an approximate visual quantification of the 7 (5+2) long range PCRs on agarose gel and in an equimolar pooling that took into account their different PCR sizes. The PCR pools were subsequently purified and quantified. For 6 samples the purification and normalization of PCR products were performed with a commercial 96-well normalization plate (Invitrogen), which allows obtaining the same quantity of DNA for each product. Moreover, in the pilot test we wanted to assess the efficiency of variant detection when using the same barcode for multiple samples, in comparison with the results of individual sequencing. For this purpose, we included four libraries obtained by merging the pools of LR-PCRs from 2 or 4 samples, purified by the two methods just described (Figure 2).

For each sample (pool of LR-PCRs), a library was obtained by using a commercial transposase-based kit (Nextera), starting from 50 ng of input DNA. The protocol consisted in two thermocycler reactions. In the first reaction, an enzyme fragments and tags the DNA by means of appended transposon ends ("tagmentation"). After on-column purification of such product, a limited-cycle PCR is performed to add the barcoded adaptors, compatible with the sequencing platform. Eighteen different adaptors were used for the pilot study. After their purification and quantification, the libraries were pooled together and run on one lane of Illumina GAII platform sequencer.

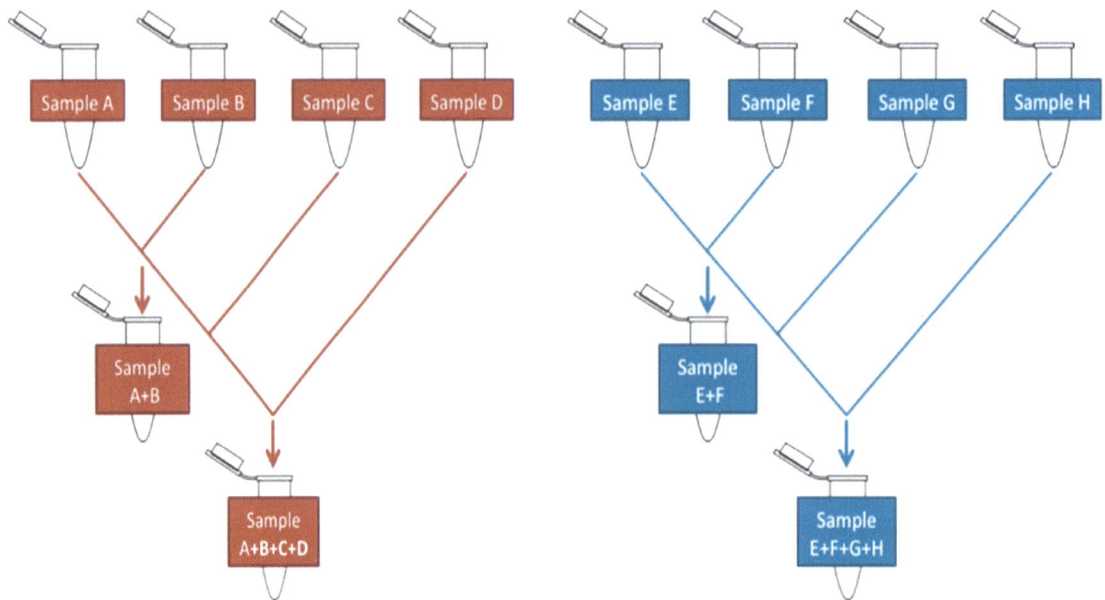

**Figure 2:** Design of the pilot study. LR-PCRs from samples in red were pooled by the "manual method" while the ones in blue by the "normalization method". We also merged two or four samples in order to test variant detection performance in non-tagged pools.

For the actual screening, we chose the first method of normalization ("manual method"), for reasons that will be detailed below. Libraries were again prepared for each sample via the commercial tagmentation protocol (Nextera), using 48 different barcoded adaptors optimized to allow the highest difference in sequence also in case of miscalled bases (Meyer & Kircher 2010). The 48 libraries were individualy purified and quantified, and then pooled together and sequenced. The same procedure was repeated for another set of 47 samples, to complete the sequencing of 95 different samples.

### 3.1.2   Sequence Analysis

The resulting sequences for each sample, separated according to the barcode that identified them (but which is not considered in the mapping), were aligned to the human genomic reference sequence of the two target genes (71 kb). We considered only reads having at least 95% identity for the 95% of their length. For confident variation calling (single nucleotide substitutions and small insertions and deletions), we set the threshold of detection to at least 20% of reads having a different base with respect to the reference sequence, and having a minimum coverage of 15 reads. In the experiments of pooled samples, the detection thresholds were set to 15% and 8% in the 2-sample and 4-sample pools, respectively.

## 3.2   Results and Discussion

The global metrics resulting from the pilot run, as well as the two discovery runs, are summarized in Table 2.

|  | Run #0 (Pilot) | Run #1 | Run #2 |
|---|---|---|---|
| **Instrument** | Illumina GAII | Illumina Hiseq | Illumina Hiseq |
| **Number of multiplexed samples** | 18* | 48 | 47 |
| **Number of Reads** | 22.7 M | 143 M | 149 M |
| **Read length** | 77 nt | 51 nt | 101 nt |
| **Average number of reads per sample** | 1.26 M | 2.9 M | 3.1 M |
| **Target DNA size** | 71 kb | 71 kb | 71 kb |
| **Total mapped reads** | 19 M (84%) | 120 M (84%) | 125 M (84%) |
| **Average number of mapped reads per sample** | 1 M | 2.5 M | 2.6 M |
| **Average base coverage per sample** | 1,140x | 1,800x | 3,900x |
| **Percentage of target DNA covered at least 1000x** | 52% | 80% | 98% |
| **Percentage of target DNA covered at least 500x** | 87% | 95% | 100% |

**Table 2:** Summary of the results of the sequencing runs described in this section. (*) Eight samples were obtained by manual normalization of PCRs, 6 samples by commercial normalization, and 4 samples corresponded to the pools of untagged samples.

### 3.2.1   Pilot Run

The pilot run (one lane of Illumina GA II flow cell) produced a total of 22.7 million reads of 77 nt (1.7 Gbases) that could be assigned to a specific sample according to the index sequence. For each sample this resulted in 1.3 million raw on average, with a standard deviation of 380,000; i.e. there was on average 25% variation between the number of reads assigned to each sample. This indicated that the libraries were pooled in a relatively balanced proportion and there was no major over-representation of a sample with respect to another.

Due to the shorter length of the sequences produced by the Illumina with respect to the Roche 454 sequencer, we decided neither to trim nor to filter the reads before the alignment process. Indeed, we observed that using trimmed or raw reads gave similar results in terms of percentage of mapped reads, even by using stringent parameters. We also confirmed that reads that did not align to the reference sequence were automatically discarded from the mapping, thus avoiding creating noise in subsequent variation detection. Nineteen millions reads (84%) aligned to the reference sequence of the two genes analyzed, with one million reads per sample on average. The percentage of reads that are used in a mapping procedure gives an indication of the accuracy of the platform (depending on the stringency of the used parameters), but it also reflects the specificity of the enrichment procedure. PCR enrichment results in general in high sequence specificity, if primers are well designed and no off-target amplification occurs. Nevertheless, for long range PCR it is often difficult to optimize robust conditions to specifically amplify DNA of different qualities and therefore failure rate of amplification is relatively high. For all experiments performed, we checked each PCR product on agarose gels and selected for sequencing only those displaying good quality of bands. Even though this procedure ensures in principle to have a high level of specificity in the final sequencing results, for very few samples we still had mapping percentages that were significantly below the average. For example, one sample of the pilot run produced only 39% of the reads mapping on the target genes, while 54% of them mapped to other chromosomes. Such aspecific enrichment was likely due to the lower yield of PCR amplification for certain DNA samples of inferior quality, rather than to environmental genomic contamination, which nonetheless cannot be excluded.

The average coverage per base per sample was about 1,000x, a very high figure for analysis of single samples. We were therefore confident that pooling a higher number of samples for the real screening would guarantee a sufficient coverage for these analyses.

As mentioned, we also tested the efficiency of two different techniques for the normalization of PCR products before pooling (visual inspection vs. commercial normalization kit). The efficiency of these procedures was scored by using the coefficient of variation of the average coverages calculated for each long range PCR of one sample (i.e the standard deviation of the coverage of LR-PCRs divided by the mean of the average coverage of LR-PCRs). This value was on average 0.4 with no significant differences across the groups of samples normalized manually or by the commercial plates. In this latter system, the DNA is normalized according to the total amount of DNA, not to the number of molecules. Consequently, an equimolar normalization occurs only for DNA molecules of the same size, but not for long range PCR products of different sizes. When we then measured the coefficient of variation of the average coverage of a given long range PCR across different samples, we obtained indeed a slightly better level of normalization of products with the commercial respect to the manual method (mean coefficients of variation = 0.30 vs. 0.42). These concepts are more clearly represented in Figure 3, showing specifically that in the manual normalization method (panel A) the coverage of long range PCR products are almost randomly variable, despite the effort of visual quantification, while in the commercial normalization method (panel B) the coverage is more consistent across the same LR-PCRs but varies with an inverse proportion with respect to their size. Specifically, shorter fragments (such as fragment #3) tend to have a higher coverage than longer ones (e.g. fragments #2 and #4). From the same plots we can also observe peaks of higher coverage where contiguous LR-PCR fragments overlap and therefore artificially create DNA intervals having a higher number of copies.

Taken together, these observations indicate that there is no real advantage in using commercial normalization kits such as the one that we tested, especially if we consider that the coverage obtained with high throughput platforms is very high and allows a confident detection of variations also at depths that are inferior to the average. This said, for other applications such as detection of structural variants or copy number variations, in which the analysis of the local changes in coverage is important, it will be necessary to operate a reliable normalization step.

Another element that we wanted to test was variant calling sensitivity in pooled samples. The rationale was the same as the one used in the previous experiment, i.e. to save on library preparation reagents by merging different samples into a unique library. Unlike in the previous project, we tried to pool only two or four samples together, instead of 96 (we had previously concluded that the main limitations of the test was lack of accuracy due to the high number of pooled samples). We also used a different sequencing platform (Illumina instead of Roche 454). To perform this new test we sequenced four samples separately and as a pool of 2 or 4 samples, and then compared whether there were any differences in the variants detected by the two sequencing strategies. Four samples were purified by using the normalization kit and four others by manual pooling (Figure 2).

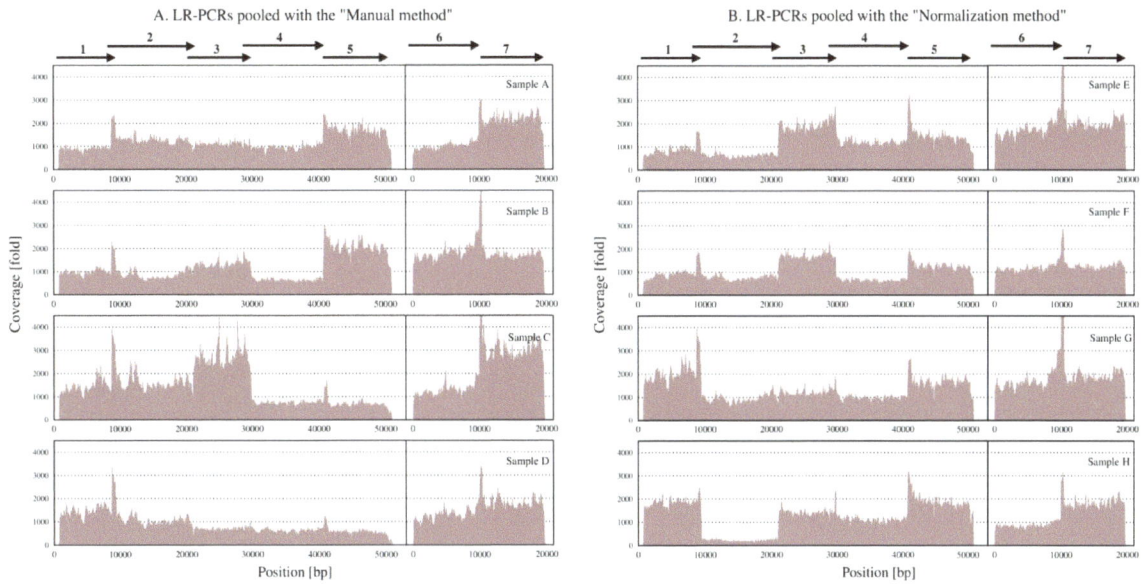

**Figure 3:** Coverage Plots. Base coverage values are represented for each point of the target regions that were amplified by the 7 LR-PCRs drawn at the top of the plots. The exact lengths of LR-PCRs are: 8.6, 12.2, 8.8, 11.6, 10.2, 10.3, and 9.7 kb. Panels on the left are examples form LR-PCRs that were pooled with the manual method, while those on the right show LR-PCRs normalized by the commercial kit.

The results of such test are reported in Table 3, and examples of the output in Table 4. The minimum frequency of reads expected for one allelic change in a two-sample pool is 25% and in a four-sample pool is 12.5%. Therefore, we set compatible thresholds of detection (15% and 8%) to take into account normal experimental fluctuations as well. When we compared the results obtained from single nucleotide substitution analyses, we observed that globally the values at which polymorphic alleles were detected in the pools were very close to the expected frequency (Table 4, examples 1 and 2). Some exceptions were however present and resulted to be due to an uneven pooling or to an unbalanced amplification of specific long range PCRs. When such events are particularly intense, false negative results tend to occur, and the effect is larger when the number of samples increases (Table 4, examples 3). For example, in the manual pool experiment with four samples, we observed that false negatives were almost exclusive of one particular sample, which was likely under-represented in the pool with respect to the other three. Conversely, unbalanced allelic amplification, which occurs when the two alleles are differentially amplified, is recognizable while analyzing the frequency of detection in individual samples. For instance, a clear indicator for this event is a substantial deviation from the 50/50 proportion for heterozygous SNP alleles. False positive variations (Table 4, example 4) were also present with a frequency of detection immediately above the threshold, likely because of an effect of sub-optimal sequencing or mapping events.

We performed the same analysis for the detection of small insertions and deletions, using the same parameters. The rate of false positives for detection of these variant resulted to be significantly higher. These errors, which consisted in the wrong incorporation of a base during sequencing, were especially localized in long DNA stretches of the same nucleotide, similar to the phenomenon observed

| | Samples | Frequency of detection | Single Nucleotide Substitutions | | | | Small Insertions/Deletions | | | |
|---|---|---|---|---|---|---|---|---|---|---|
| | | | # Detected Variants | # Expected Variants* | # False + | # False - | # Detected Variants | # Expected Variants* | # False + | # False - |
| **Manual pooling** | A | 20% | 91 | | | | 12 | | | |
| | B | 20% | 100 | | | | 10 | | | |
| | C | 20% | 70 | | | | 12 | | | |
| | D | 20% | 70 | | | | 11 | | | |
| | A+B | 15% | 112 | 115 | 1 | 4 | 28 | 16 | 12 | 0 |
| | A+B+C+D | 8% | 151 | 148 | 12 | 9 | 44 | 22 | 22 | 0 |
| **Normalization pooling** | E | 20% | 82 | | | | 9 | | | |
| | F | 20% | 96 | | | | 9 | | | |
| | G | 20% | 59 | | | | 10 | | | |
| | H | 20% | 112 | | | | 18 | | | |
| | E+F | 15% | 106 | 107 | 1 | 2 | 23 | 12 | 11 | 0 |
| | E+F+G+H | 8% | 158 | 171 | 4 | 17 | 42 | 24 | 24 | 6 |

**Table 3:** Number of variants identified in individual samples and in pools of two or four of them, using appropriate detection frequency thresholds for single alleles. (*)Expected variants were calculated as the sum of unique variants found in the individual samples used for the pools.

with the Roche 454 sequencer. It seems therefore that Illumina platforms are as well sensitive to this problem, at least when insertions or deletions are considered.

Based on all these observation, we concluded that the strategy of pooling samples might be an efficient technique; however, it does not guarantee perfect mutation detection, even when a few samples are pooled. Consequently, we chose to sequence individual samples as separate libraries for the screening of new candidate disease genes.

### 3.2.2  Screening Runs

The screening was performed with two lanes of Illumina Hiseq flowcells, each one processing 48 different samples that were multiplexed with barcoded adaptors. As reported in Table 2, each run yielded in total about 150 million reads, almost 6 times higher than the ones obtained with previous version of the platform (GAII) for the pilot experiment. After mapping procedures, 84% of the reads aligned to the reference sequence of the two genes and produced an average coverage of about 2,000 and 4,000x for each sample of the first and the second run, respectively. This was largely due to the fact that in the first run reads were 51 nt long while in the second they were 101 nt long (Table 2). The coefficients of variation calculated over the average coverages of every LR-PCR were 0.46 and 0.38, respectively, indicating that PCRs were pooled with less than half a fold difference on average. If we consider the coefficient of variation of the average coverage for each sample, we obtain 0.23 and 0.16 for the first and second round, respectively, suggesting a good balance among samples.

| Samples | Alleles | Alleles Frequencies | Read Count per Allele | Coverage | Alleles | Alleles Frequencies | Read Count Per Allele | Coverage |
|---|---|---|---|---|---|---|---|---|
| | | Example 1 | | | | Example 2 | | |
| A | T/C | 54.1/45.9 | 396/336 | 732 | C/A | 50.3/49.5 | 518/509 | 1029 |
| B | T/C | 51.1/48.9 | 393/376 | 769 | C | 99.9 | 1442 | 1444 |
| C | T/C | 50.9/49.1 | 556/536 | 1092 | C | 99.4 | 1108 | 1115 |
| D | T/C | 54.7/45.3 | 594/491 | 1085 | C | 99.9 | 999 | 1000 |
| A+B | T/C | 52.8/47.2 | 293/262 | 555 | C/A | 77.4/22.6 | 727/212 | 939 |
| A+B+C+D | C/T | 50.5/49.3 | 464/453 | 918 | C/A | 89.9/10.1 | 1118/126 | 1244 |
| | | Example 3 (False Negative) | | | | Example 4 (False Positive) | | |
| A | A | 100 | 692 | 692 | T | 100 | 677 | 677 |
| B | A | 100 | 575 | 575 | T/C | 98.5/1.5 | 535/8 | 543 |
| C | A | 99.8 | 633 | 634 | T/C | 99.3/0.7 | 550/4 | 554 |
| D | A/G | 54.3/45.7 | 238/200 | 438 | T/C | 99.1/0.9 | 422/4 | 426 |
| A+B | A | 99.7 | 664 | 666 | T/C | 88.5/11.0 | 554/69 | 626 |
| A+B+C+D | A/G | 93.1/6.9 | 471/35 | 506 | T/C | 87.5/12.4 | 474/67 | 542 |

**Table 4:** Examples of SNP alleles detected in individual and pooled samples. The thresholds for variant detection are the same as in Table 3. In Example 1 all samples have the same heterozygous change, which was correctly detected with ~50% frequency in both pooled samples. In Example 2 one sample out of four carries a SNP that was detected at the corresponding frequency in the two-sample (~25%) and in the four-sample (~12.5%) pools. Example 3 shows a false negative: allele G of sample D was detected in the pooled sample at a lower frequency (6.9%, highlighted) than the detection threshold, set at 8%. Example 4 shows a false positive detection in the four-sample pool (highlighted), in which reads carrying likely a sequencing error were counted as carrying a variant, due to the lower frequency threshold set in the pooled sample.

We then performed variant detection on every sample to look for candidate mutations. When we excluded all variants reported in dbSNP, a database of human polymorphisms, we obtained a list of 139 unique variants. We also excluded 48 changes that were judged to be in stretches of bad alignment or low coverage by visual inspection of the mapping. Among the remainder 91 novel variants, we did not find any good candidate mutations, for the main reason that they were almost all intronic changes with no obvious effects on splicing of the gene transcripts, as predicted by the program NNSPLICE. The only novel nonsynonymous substitution was also predicted by PolyPhen to be non-pathogenic.

Although we could not identify any variants with possible implication in the disease that we were studying, we could get some insights on the sequencing methods that we selected for the screening of candidate disease genes. In particular, preparing many libraries in parallel through the "tagmentation" method was proven to be extremely fast (only a few hours needed to process 96 samples) and reliable. While at the time of this experiment reagents were still rather expensive (the cost was comparable to the one for normal library preparation via nebulization and size selection), their price is now starting to drop considerably, making screenings of few genes for many samples more affordable. This latter feature, together with the time effectiveness of such kits, renders the multiplexed barcode method a better choice with respect to the anonymous pooling screening. In fact, with a relatively limited amount of additional effort and, likely, of costs, the results produced by this new approach contain ready-to-use information for a complete panel of individuals, with minimal necessities of validation by additional methods. Moreover, if sufficient coverage and sequencing quality are ensured, false discovery rates should be in principle very low.

The biggest limitations that we could observe about this approach, but which are nonetheless present in the anonymous pooling approach as well, are mainly related to long range PCR robustness and scalability. For our purpose, which was based on the sequencing of a small region for many samples, LR-PCR was the best choice for several reasons. It (i) allowed very specific amplification of the target region, (ii) required relatively few reactions to cover up to 100 kbases, (iii) included non-coding region, and (iv) could be achieved by using standard laboratory procedures and equipment. On the other hand, long range PCRs are not as robust as short range PCRs and are very sensitive to the quality of the template. Optimization of robust PCRs may require a certain effort, and even when the right conditions are found it is still possible to observe failure in amplification of certain DNAs, which must be re-amplified or discarded from the screening. The time and effort necessary to obtain a complete panel of LR-PCRs for many samples to be processed at once can be indeed relatively long with respect for example to enrichment by hybridization. Additionally, PCRs must be individually checked, pooled in equimolar amounts, cleaned and quantified before starting the library preparation. Automated or semi-automated PCR-based enrichment methods, such as the ones outlined in the Introduction, could offer an interesting alternative to overcome these issues.

# 4 Conclusions

The two methods described in this chapter represent two different ways of addressing the scientific question of whether several patients affected by a specific disease carry pathogenic mutations in a given gene. Both approaches, the anonymous pooling and the tagged multiplexing, can lead to an answer. The first method is faster and cheaper, but provides positive answers only when mutations in a candidate gene have a relatively high frequency in the cohort that is analyzed. Furthermore, in case of negative results, it is not possible to rule out that the screening was poisoned by false negative events. Since the differences in costs and time required to perform the first vs. the second method are progressively diminishing, it may be worthier using tagged multiplexed libraries. Moreover, the rapid evolution of high throughput sequencing technologies and associated equipment is predicted to further facilitate the sequencing of many samples together.

# Acknowledgements

We would like to thank Dr. Keith Harshman for precious technical support with NGS library preparation and sequencing, and Dr. Andrea Prunotto for helping in revising the manuscript. This research was supported in part by the Swiss National Science Foundation (Grants #320030-121929 and 310030_138346) and the Gebert Rüf Foundation (Rare Diseases - New Technologies grant).

# References

Akhras, M. S., Unemo, M., Thiyagarajan, S., Nyren, P., Davis, R. W., Fire, A. Z. & Pourmand, N. (2007). Connector inversion probe technology: a powerful one-primer multiplex DNA amplification system for numerous scientific applications. PLoS One, 2(9), e915.

Baetens, M., Van Laer, L., De Leeneer, K., Hellemans, J., De Schrijver, J., Van De Voorde, H., Renard, M., Dietz, H., Lacro, R. V., Menten, B. and others (2011). Applying massive parallel sequencing to molecular diagnosis of Marfan and Loeys-Dietz syndromes. Hum Mutat

Benaglio, P., McGee, T. L., Capelli, L. P., Harper, S., Berson, E. L. & Rivolta, C. (2011). Next generation sequencing of pooled samples reveals new SNRNP200 mutations associated with retinitis pigmentosa. Hum Mutat, 32(6), E2246-58.

Benaglio, P. & Rivolta, C. (2010). Ultra high throughput sequencing in human DNA variation detection: a comparative study on the NDUFA3-PRPF31 region. PLoS One, 5(9),

Bentley, D. R., Balasubramanian, S., Swerdlow, H. P., Smith, G. P., Milton, J., Brown, C. G., Hall, K. P., Evers, D. J., Barnes, C. L., Bignell, H. R. and others (2008). Accurate whole human genome sequencing using reversible terminator chemistry. Nature, 456(7218), 53-9.

Calvo, S. E., Tucker, E. J., Compton, A. G., Kirby, D. M., Crawford, G., Burtt, N. P., Rivas, M., Guiducci, C., Bruno, D. L., Goldberger, O. A. and others (2010). High-throughput, pooled sequencing identifies mutations in NUBPL and FOXRED1 in human complex I deficiency. Nat Genet, 42(10), 851-8.

Casbon, J. A., Osborne, R. J., Brenner, S. & Lichtenstein, C. P. (2011). A method for counting PCR template molecules with application to next-generation sequencing. Nucleic Acids Res, 39(12), e81.

Craig, D. W., Pearson, J. V., Szelinger, S., Sekar, A., Redman, M., Corneveaux, J. J., Pawlowski, T. L., Laub, T., Nunn, G., Stephan, D. A. and others (2008). Identification of genetic variants using bar-coded multiplexed sequencing. Nat Methods, 5(10), 887-93.

Dahl, F., Stenberg, J., Fredriksson, S., Welch, K., Zhang, M., Nilsson, M., Bicknell, D., Bodmer, W. F., Davis, R. W. & Ji, H. (2007). Multigene amplification and massively parallel sequencing for cancer mutation discovery. Proc Natl Acad Sci U S A, 104(22), 9387-92.

Dryja, T. P. (1997). Gene-based approach to human gene-phenotype correlations. Proc Natl Acad Sci U S A, 94(22), 12117-21.

Gilissen, C., Hoischen, A., Brunner, H. G. & Veltman, J. A. (2011). Unlocking Mendelian disease using exome sequencing. Genome Biol, 12(9), 228.

Harismendy, O., Ng, P. C., Strausberg, R. L., Wang, X., Stockwell, T. B., Beeson, K. Y., Schork, N. J., Murray, S. S., Topol, E. J., Levy, S. and others (2009). Evaluation of next generation sequencing platforms for population targeted sequencing studies. Genome Biol, 10(3), R32.

Hartong, D. T., Berson, E. L. & Dryja, T. P. (2006). Retinitis pigmentosa. Lancet, 368(9549), 1795-809.

Hollants, S., Redeker, E. J. & Matthijs, G. (2012). Microfluidic amplification as a tool for massive parallel sequencing of the familial hypercholesterolemia genes. Clin Chem, 58(4), 717-24.

Hu, H., Wrogemann, K., Kalscheuer, V., Tzschach, A., Richard, H., Haas, S. A., Menzel, C., Bienek, M., Froyen, G., Raynaud, M. and others (2009). Mutation screening in 86 known X-linked mental retardation genes by droplet-based multiplex PCR and massive parallel sequencing. Hugo J, 3(1-4), 41-9.

Huse, S. M., Huber, J. A., Morrison, H. G., Sogin, M. L. & Welch, D. M. (2007). Accuracy and quality of massively parallel DNA pyrosequencing. Genome Biol, 8(7), R143.

Ikegawa, S., Mabuchi, A., Ogawa, M. & Ikeda, T. (2002). Allele-specific PCR amplification due to sequence identity between a PCR primer and an amplicon: is direct sequencing so reliable? Hum Genet, 110(6), 606-8.

Ingman, M. & Gyllensten, U. (2009). SNP frequency estimation using massively parallel sequencing of pooled DNA. European Journal of Human Genetics, 17(3), 383-386.

International Human Genaome Consortium (2004). Finishing the euchromatic sequence of the human genome. Nature, 431(7011), 931-45.

Lee, J. S., Choi, M., Yan, X., Lifton, R. P. & Zhao, H. (2011). On optimal pooling designs to identify rare variants through massive resequencing. Genet Epidemiol, 35(3), 139-47.

Mamanova, L., Coffey, A. J., Scott, C. E., Kozarewa, I., Turner, E. H., Kumar, A., Howard, E., Shendure, J. & Turner, D. J. (2010). Target-enrichment strategies for next-generation sequencing. Nat Methods, 7(2), 111-8.

Margulies, M., Egholm, M., Altman, W. E., Attiya, S., Bader, J. S., Bemben, L. A., Berka, J., Braverman, M. S., Chen, Y. J., Chen, Z. and others (2005). Genome sequencing in microfabricated high-density picolitre reactors. Nature, 437(7057), 376-80.

McKernan, K. J., Peckham, H. E., Costa, G. L., McLaughlin, S. F., Fu, Y., Tsung, E. F., Clouser, C. R., Duncan, C., Ichikawa, J. K., Lee, C. C. and others (2009). Sequence and structural variation in a human genome uncovered by short-read, massively parallel ligation sequencing using two-base encoding. Genome Res, 19(9), 1527-41.

Mertes, F., Elsharawy, A., Sauer, S., van Helvoort, J. M., van der Zaag, P. J., Franke, A., Nilsson, M., Lehrach, H. & Brookes, A. J. (2011). Targeted enrichment of genomic DNA regions for next-generation sequencing. Brief Funct Genomics, 10(6), 374-86.

Metzker, M. L. (2010). Sequencing technologies - the next generation. Nat Rev Genet, 11(1), 31-46.

Meyer, M. & Kircher, M. (2010). Illumina sequencing library preparation for highly multiplexed target capture and sequencing. Cold Spring Harb Protoc, 2010(6), pdb prot5448.

Neveling, K., Collin, R. W., Gilissen, C., van Huet, R. A., Visser, L., Kwint, M. P., Gijsen, S. J., Zonneveld, M. N., Wieskamp, N., de Ligt, J. and others (2011). Next-generation genetic testing for retinitis pigmentosa. Hum Mutat, 33(6), 963-72.

Otto, E. A., Ramaswami, G., Janssen, S., Chaki, M., Allen, S. J., Zhou, W., Airik, R., Hurd, T. W., Ghosh, A. K., Wolf, M. T. and others (2011). Mutation analysis of 18 nephronophthisis associated ciliopathy disease genes using a DNA pooling and next generation sequencing strategy. J Med Genet, 48(2), 105-16.

Out, A. A., van Minderhout, I. J., Goeman, J. J., Ariyurek, Y., Ossowski, S., Schneeberger, K., Weigel, D., van Galen, M., Taschner, P. E., Tops, C. M. and others (2009). Deep sequencing to reveal new variants in pooled DNA samples. Hum Mutat, 30(12), 1703-12.

Ramensky, V., Bork, P. & Sunyaev, S. (2002). Human non-synonymous SNPs: server and survey. Nucleic Acids Res, 30(17), 3894-900.

Reese, M. G., Eeckman, F. H., Kulp, D. & Haussler, D. (1997). Improved splice site detection in Genie. J Comput Biol, 4(3), 311-23.

Rothberg, J. M., Hinz, W., Rearick, T. M., Schultz, J., Mileski, W., Davey, M., Leamon, J. H., Johnson, K., Milgrew, M. J., Edwards, M. and others (2011). An integrated semiconductor device enabling non-optical genome sequencing. Nature, 475(7356), 348-52.

Sanger, F., Nicklen, S. & Coulson, A. R. (1977). DNA sequencing with chain-terminating inhibitors. Proc Natl Acad Sci U S A, 74(12), 5463-7.

Shen, P., Wang, W., Krishnakumar, S., Palm, C., Chi, A. K., Enns, G. M., Davis, R. W., Speed, T. P., Mindrinos, M. N. & Scharfe, C. (2011). High-quality DNA sequence capture of 524 disease candidate genes. Proc Natl Acad Sci U S A, 108(16), 6549-54.

Simpson, D. A., Clark, G. R., Alexander, S., Silvestri, G. & Willoughby, C. E. (2010). Molecular diagnosis for heterogeneous genetic diseases with targeted high-throughput DNA sequencing applied to retinitis pigmentosa. J Med Genet, 48(3), 145-51.

Smith, A. M., Heisler, L. E., St Onge, R. P., Farias-Hesson, E., Wallace, I. M., Bodeau, J., Harris, A. N., Perry, K. M., Giaever, G., Pourmand, N. and others (2010). Highly-multiplexed barcode sequencing: an efficient method for parallel analysis of pooled samples. Nucleic Acids Res, 38(13), e142.

Tewhey, R., Warner, J. B., Nakano, M., Libby, B., Medkova, M., David, P. H., Kotsopoulos, S. K., Samuels, M. L., Hutchison, J. B., Larson, J. W. and others (2009). Microdroplet-based PCR enrichment for large-scale targeted sequencing. Nat Biotechnol, 27(11), 1025-31.

Turner, E. H., Lee, C., Ng, S. B., Nickerson, D. A. & Shendure, J. (2009). Massively parallel exon capture and library-free resequencing across 16 genomes. Nat Methods, 6(5), 315-6.

# Finding and Characterizing Small Group I Introns in rRNA Genes

Lorena B. Harris
*Department of Biological Sciences*
*Bowling Green State University, USA*

Scott O. Rogers
*Department of Biological Sciences*
*Bowling Green State University, USA*

# 1 Introduction

Introns are common features in eukaryotic genomes. They have been found in eukaryotic mRNA, tRNA and rRNA genes, as well as in the genes of chloroplasts, mitochondria, archaea, bacteria and viruses. Group I introns have the widest distribution at the kingdom level, being absent only from the genomes of Archaea (Cavalier-Smith, 1991; Jackson *et al.*, 2002; Johansen *et al.*, 2007; Moreira *et al.*, 2012). They are among the most ancient introns. They are ribozymes (i.e., self-splicing) and exhibit great variation and diversity ranging in length from 63 nucleotides (nt) to several kilobases (Doudna *et al.*, 1989; Shinohara *et al.*, 1996; Simon *et al.*, 2005), some of which are stabilized by chaperone proteins (Coetzee *et al.*, 1994). Some genes contain multiple group I introns (Gargas *et al.*, 1995; Simon *et al.*, 2005). These characteristics indicate a long and plastic evolutionary history for these ribozymes.

Many group I introns in eukaryotic nuclear genomes have been described in the rRNA gene loci of fungi (Gargas *et al.*, 1995; Haugen *et al.*, 2004, 2005; Nikoh & Fukatsu 2001; Shinohara *et al.*, 1996). They contain most or all of the pairing regions, P1 - P10, as well as joining regions, some of which are thought to be essential for splicing. P2 appears to be optional, as it is absent from many group I introns. P6 and P8 also are variable in length, including some that are extremely short. All group I introns have an internal guide sequence (IGS) and functional sites that accomplish folding and two trans-esterification reactions. Detailed models of group I ribozymes have been proposed on the basis of nucleotide hydrogen bonding to form regions of stable secondary structure (Cech, 1990; Davila-Aponte *et al.*, 1991; DeWachter *et al.*, 1992; Simon *et al.*, 2005; Gast *et al.*, 1994; Johansen & Voigt 1994; Rangan *et al.*, 2003; Shinohara *et al.*, 1996), by analysis of deletion mutants (Doudna & Cech 2002; Doudna & Szostak 1989), and by X-ray crystallographic analysis (Adams *et al.*, 2004; Golden *et al.*, 2004). Some of the longer introns contain open reading frames (ORFs), containing gene sequences for insertion site-specific endonucleases, although most lack ORFs, and fall within the range of 200 to 600 nt.

A small functional group I ribozyme of 164 nt in length was constructed as a deletion mutant of the T4 *sunY* intron (Doudna & Szostak 1989). However, natural introns one-third that size were subsequently described from ascomycetous fungi within the small subunit genes of the ribosomal RNA gene (rRNA SSU) locus (Bhattacharya *et al.*, 2000; Cubero *et al.*, 2000; Gargas *et al.*, 1995; Harris & Rogers, 2008, 2011; Rogers *et al.*, 1993). The short group I intron-like elements in fungal rRNA genes are unusual, in that they are devoid of most of the core sequences conserved in all other larger group I introns. They range in size from 63-78 nt (from the rRNA SSU genes of *Arthonia lapidicola*, *Phialophora americana*, *P. richardsiae*, *P. verrucosa*, *P. parasitica*, and *Porpidia crustulata*) and appear to contain only P1, P10 and P7. They have been described as degenerate introns, but research indicates that they are capable of accurate splicing *in vivo* and *in vitro* via a group I intron mechanism (Rogers *et al.*, 1993; Harris & Rogers, 2008).

Here, we describe the detailed methodology used to locate, characterize and test these small introns (reported previously in Harris, 2007; Harris & Rogers, 2008, 2011). They are challenging to find because they are short and rare. Therefore, it is often difficult to define their precise 5' and 3' splice borders. Also, because of their short lengths, automated determination of secondary structure and other base interactions is problematic. The small introns appear to contain only P1, P7, and P10. The P7 region has been derived from a fragment of the P9 region of a larger group I intron (Harris & Rogers, 2008). Nonetheless, splicing occurs *in vitro* via a group I intron ribozyme reaction pathway, except that the final nucleotide in the intron is a U rather than the canonical G. However, more than just the 63-74 nt of the intron appears to be necessary for splicing, because *in vitro* splicing reactions failed to occur when only the intron and

20 nt on either side of the intron were present. However, when 300 nucleotides of the 3' exon were included (which consisted of ITS1 and the 5' half of the 5.8S gene), *in vitro* splicing proceeded. Inclusion of longer pieces of the 5' end had no effect on splicing. This was the first indication that these small introns might be discontinuous, and that functions provided by the 3' transcript were necessary for splicing.

## 2 Materials and Methods (Summarized in Figure 1)

### 2.1 Source of Nucleic Acids

Cultures of *Phialophora americana* (isolates 1046, 3504, 8730, 10507, 10508, CDC-5, CDC-10 and NYS323-90), *P. europa* (isolate NIH B1214), *P. parasitica* (isolate 2509), *P. richardsiae* (isolate 1207) and *P. verrucosa* (isolates NIH 8701 and NIH 8702) were obtained from Prof. CJK Wang (State University of New York, College of Environmental Science and Forestry, Syracuse, NY). All are human pathogens, except *P. americana*, which is a plant pathogen. The fungi were grown on malt extract agar (MEA; 2% malt extract, 1.5% agar, pH 7.5) for 14 days at 22°C in 9 cm Petri plates. Morphological confirmations were performed using light microscopy (Leica DME, Bannockburn, IL), electron scanning microscopy (HITACHI, S-2700, SEM), and confocal microscopy (Olympus FluoView Confocal microscope). Hyphae, conidia and conidiophores were examined to confirm taxonomic characters specific for each species.

### 2.2 DNA Extraction and PCR Amplification

Mycelia were excised from the culture plates and ground to a powder in a mortar and pestle with dry ice. DNA was extracted using a CTAB (cetyltrimethylammonium bromide) preparation method (Rogers, *et al.* 1989). The DNA was quantified on 1% agarose gels in TBE (89 mM Tris base, 89 mM borate, 2 mM EDTA, pH 8.0), containing 5 μg /ml ethidium bromide at 5 V/cm for 1 hr, and photographed using UV illumination. Polymerase Chain Reaction (PCR) was performed to amplify targets from the 3' end of the SSU gene through the 5' one-third of the 5.8S rRNA gene (Figure 2). PCR was performed using primers ITS2 (GCTGCGTTCTTCATCGATGC) and ITS5 (GGAAGTAAA-GTCGTAACAAGG) (White, *et al.* 1990). Each reaction consisted of 5-10 ng of genomic DNA, 25 pmol of each primer, 5 pmol of each dNTP, 1 U Ampli*Taq* DNA polymerase, 10 mM Tris-HCl (pH 8.2), 50 mM KCl, 1.5 mM MgCl$_2$, and 0.0001% (w/v) gelatin. The total volume of each reaction was 25 μl. The thermal cycling program (GeneAmp PCR System 9700, Applied Biosystems, Foster City, CA) was: 94°C for 2 min; then 35 cycles of 1 min at 94°C, 2 min at 54°C, and 2 min at 72°C. This was followed by a final extension of 10 min at 72°C. Amplification was confirmed by subjecting aliquots to electrophoresis on 2% agarose gels (with TBE and ethidium bromide, as described above). The PCR products were purified using a QIAquick PCR purification kit (QIAGEN, Valencia, CA). Sequencing was performed by Gene Gateway, LLC (Hayward, CA).

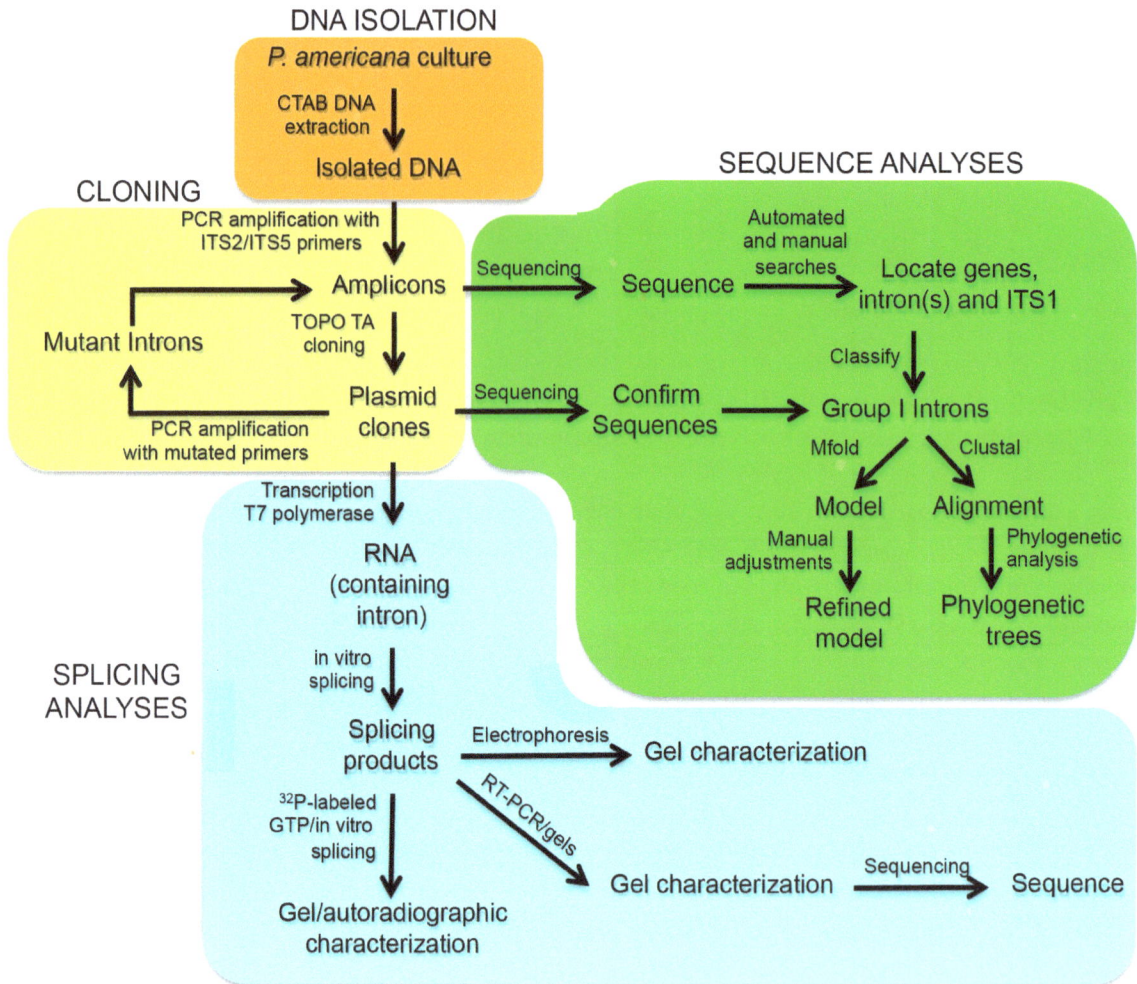

**Figure 1:** Summary of methods used. Cultivation and DNA extraction are highlighted in orange. PCR amplification and cloning, including construction of mutant clones, are highlighted in yellow. Sequencing analysis, including sequence determination, alignment, locating introns, model building and phylogenetic analyses is highlighted in green. *In vitro* transcription, splicing, and assay of their results are indicated in blue. Details are provided in text, as well as in Harris, 2007, and Harris & Rogers, 2008, 2011.

## 2.3    Cloning of the PCR Products

Only amplicons of *P. americana* (isolate 1046) were cloned and transcribed for *in vitro* splicing assays. The PCR product (above) was cloned (Figure 2) into expression vector pCR2.1-TOPO using a TOPO TA cloning kit (Invitrogen Corporation, Carlsbad, CA). Additional constructs were produced. One (Figure 2b) contained a larger portion of the 5' exon (amplified using primers NS5 (White *et al.* 1990) and ITS2, and cloned into pCR2.1). Another (Figure 2c) consisted of the intron and only 20 nt of each of the two exons[1]. A third (Fig. 2d) contained a long 5' exon and a short 3' exon (amplified with NS5 and NSITSr). These were sequenced to confirm cloning and the direction of the insert, using the M13 forward primer in the pCR2.1 vector. Clones with inserts in the forward (sense direction with respect to the T7 promoter) were used for *in vitro* transcription and splicing reactions. A clone with the reverse insert that included 20 nt of the 5' exon, the intron, and the 300 nt 3' exon was used as an antisense control (Figure 2a).

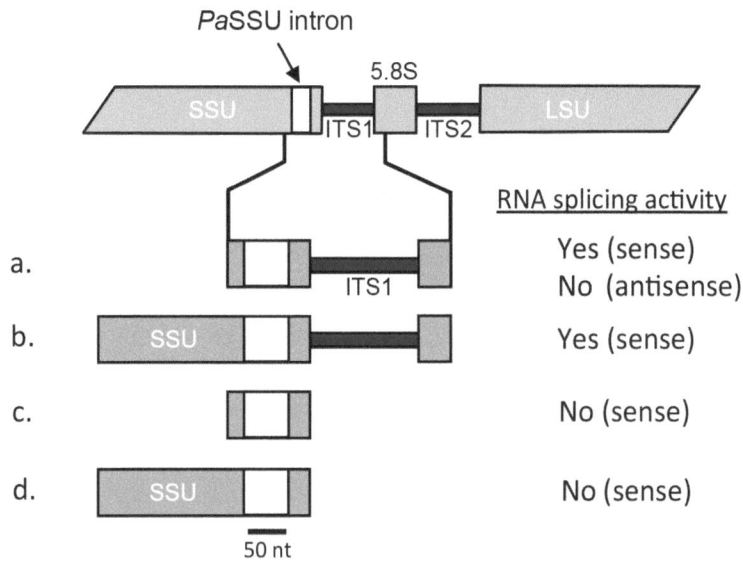

**Figure 2:** Portion of the rRNA gene locus, including parts of the SSU and LSU genes, ITS1, the PaSSU intron, the 5.8S gene and ITS2. **a.** Primary clone used for study. It includes 20 nt of the 5' exon (part of the rRNA SSU gene), the 67 nt intron, the remainder of the 3' end of the rRNA SSU gene, ITS1, and the 5' one-third of the 5.8S rRNA gene. The sense strand RNA exhibited splicing activity, while the antisense strand failed to exhibit splicing activity. **b.** A clone that contained a longer portion (200 nt) of the 5' exon. The sense strand RNA exhibited splicing activity. **c.** A clone that contained only 20 nt of each of the exons. No splicing activity was detected. **d.** A clone containing the longer 5' exon, but a short (20 nt) 3' exon. It failed to exhibit splicing activity.

## 2.4    *In vitro* Transcription

Linearization of the recombinant plasmids was performed by digestion with *Spe*I (to produce RNA with the intron), then treated with proteinase K (1200 $\mu$g/ml) and 0.5% SDS for 1 h at 37°C, followed by phenol/chloroform extraction, and ethanol purification. The *Spe*I site is 36 nt upstream from the site of insertion of the intron-containing amplicons. The DNA was subjected to electrophoresis on 1% agarose gels to determine concentration. RNA was synthesized from the recombinant plasmid DNA templates, using T7 RNA polymerase (MEGAscript T7 Kit, Applied Biosystems, Foster City). Initiation of *in vitro* transcription experiments proceeded as follows: 0.5 – 1.0 $\mu$g of DNA, 7.5 mM of ATP, GTP, UTP, and CTP, 2 $\mu$l

---

[1] Amplified using primers ITS5 and NSITSr: GCAGGTTCACCTATATATACCGTTAGTATAACTGTCAAAC, and cloned into pCR2.1

of 10X reaction buffer (according to the manufacturer), and 2 $\mu$l 10X T7 RNA polymerase were gently mixed in a 20 $\mu$l volume. Then, the reaction was incubated at 37°C for 5 h. After the transcription was completed, an aliquot was immediately either loaded in an agarose gel to confirm transcription, or was frozen at -80°C for later agarose gel assay. Once the transcription experiments began, it was important to store the RNA at -80°C, in order to avoid degradation. Additionally, the splicing reaction often initiated while transcription was in progress. Therefore, limiting time and increases in temperature were important in controlling both the degree of degradation as well as the amount of splicing that occurred prior to the *in vitro* splicing assay.

## 2.5   Splicing Assays

*In vitro* splicing reactions were performed in 30 $\mu$l reaction volumes containing 1.0 – 2.0 $\mu$g of single stranded RNA (denatured at 85°C for 10 min), 100 mM Tris-HCl, 500 mM KCl, 15 mM MgCl$_2$, 0.01% w/v gelatin, incubated at 55°C for 10 min. Then, the MgCl$_2$ concentration was adjusted to 25 mM, followed by incubation at 37°C for 5 min, addition of 10 mM GTP, and incubation at 32°C for 60 min. The splicing reactions were stopped by adding 2X RNA loading dye solution (98% formamide, 10 mM EDTA, 0.1% xylene cyanol FF, 0.1% bromophenol blue, pH 7.3), followed by denaturation of the nucleic acids by heating at 85°C for 10 min. Splicing was confirmed by subjecting 18 $\mu$l of the splicing product to electrophoresis on 8% polyacrylamide gels (19:1 acrylamide:bisacrylamide; Amresco, Solon, OH) with 8 M urea, or on 2.5% agarose gels (BioRad, Hercules, CA) with TBE (89 mM Tris-base, 89 mM borate, 2 mM EDTA, pH 8.0), and stained with 0.1 $\mu$l/ml SYBR Gold (Molecular Probes, Eugene, OR). Reverse transcription (RT) PCR was performed on each of the resulting bands using a single RT step to synthesize DNA, followed by subsequent PCR amplification with primers ITS2, ITS5, NS5 and/or NSITSr (depending on the specific clone used) using GeneAmp reagents from an EZ rTth RNA PCR Kit (Applied Biosytems, Branchburg, NJ). At least 100 ng/$\mu$l of template was required in a 30 $\mu$l RT-PCR reaction to obtain a robust product. The following reagents were used: 30 pmol of each primer, 6 pmol of each dNTP, 2.5 U/$\mu$l rTh DNA polymerase, 50 mM bicine (pH 8.2), 115 mM potassium acetate, 8% w/v glycerol, and 25 mM Mn(OAc)$_2$. The thermal cycling program (GeneAmp PCR System 9700, Applied Biosystems, Foster City, CA) was: 60°C for 30 min; then 45 cycles of 94°C for 30 s, 54°C for 45 s, and 72°C for 2 min; followed by 10 min of incubation at 72°C. The amplicons were separated on 2% agarose gels in TBE with 0.5 $\mu$g/ml ethidium bromide, at 5 – 12 V/cm for 1 – 2 h. The bands retrieved after RT-PCR were cloned pCR2.1-TOPO. After transformation, growth, and purification, each plasmid was linearized by digestion with *Spe*I prior to sequencing using the T7 primer, which is 69 nt upstream from the amplicon insertion site.

## 2.6   Mutant Construction and Testing

Several mutant introns were constructed by PCR using synthesized primers with differences from the wild type intron. The single mutations were (numbers correspond to the nucleotide relative to 5' position 1 of the intron): -2 G $\Rightarrow$ C, -1 U $\Rightarrow$ A, -1 U $\Rightarrow$ C, 1 G $\Rightarrow$ C, 4 U $\Rightarrow$ G, 7 A $\Rightarrow$ del; 15 G $\Rightarrow$ A, 15 G $\Rightarrow$ C, 41 G $\Rightarrow$ A, 43 C $\Rightarrow$ U, 45 G $\Rightarrow$ A, 45 G $\Rightarrow$ C, 45 G $\Rightarrow$ U, 45/46 GU $\Rightarrow$ AC, 57 G $\Rightarrow$ U. Each was sequenced (as above) to confirm the mutation and orientation. The mutant introns were cloned using pCR2.1 vectors (as above). RNA was transcribed from these mutant plasmids (as above), and subjected to *in vitro* splicing (as above).

### 2.7  $^{32}$P-GTP Labeling Splicing Experiment

*In vitro* splicing conditions were prepared, as above, except [α-$^{32}$P] GTP (40 $\mu$Ci, 6000 Ci/mmole) was used to replace unlabeled GTP, in a total reaction volume of 10 $\mu$l. In group I introns, the free guanosine becomes covalently bound to the 5' end of the intron in the first step of splicing. The reaction was incubated for 1 h at 32 °C. RNA denaturation was at 75 °C for 10 min. Then, the samples were chilled on ice for 2 min, prior to loading the samples into the gel. Electrophoresis was performed at 5 V/cm for 1 hour using a 2.5% agarose gel, with SYBR gold (Molecular Probes, Eugene, OR), and then sealed in a plastic bag. The RNA bands were visualized in the gel using a UV transilluminator. Detection of the radioactivity was performed by placing the gel for a few seconds up to one minute in a Phosphor imager (Storm 860, Molecular Dynamics, Piscataway, NJ).

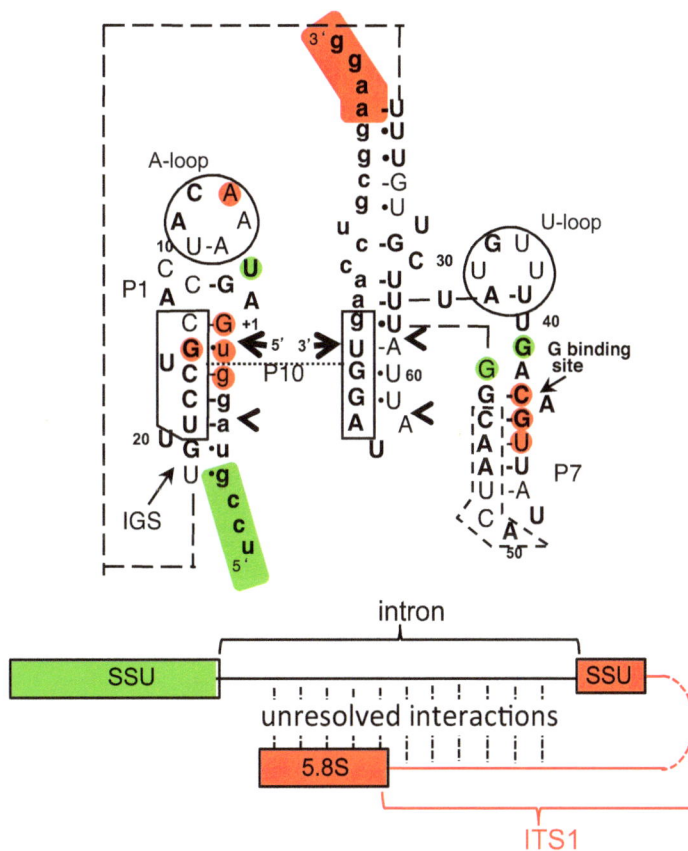

**Figure 3:** Structure of the PaSSU intron as determined using Mfold (Zucker 2003) and adjusted based on standard group I introns. The intron has a P1, P10 and P7. The P1 contains the G•U pair at the 5' exon-intron border; P10 contains the 3' exon-intron border, and P7 contains the guanosine binding site. Results of mutational and splicing assays are provided. Nucleotide changes that resulted in loss of splicing activity are indicated in red. Changes that had little or no effect on splicing are indicated in green. Part of ITS1/5.8S rRNA region appears to aid splicing, but the specific region has not yet been identified (lower portion of figure).

### 2.8  Structural Analysis

The intron sequence was subjected to secondary structure analysis using Mfold (Zuker, 2003). Because of the short length of the intron, after the initial determinations of secondary structure, parts of the sequence were removed and reanalyzed separately. Manual adjustments were made based on maximization of base pairing, while considering the P1 possibilities and long range interactions based on previous models, to produce the final structures (Adams *et al.*, 2004, 2005; Cech, 1990; Michel & Westof, 1990; Shinohara *et al.*, 1996). The *Cg*SSU group I intron from *Cenococcum geophilum* was used as the primary model, although comparisons to other introns also were made.

### 2.9    Sequence Analysis and Phylogenetic Analysis

Sequences of introns from subgroups IC1, IC2, IC3, ID, as well as two other small introns that were previously uncategorized from fungi were selected for comparison to the *Pa*SSU intron. Only the P1, P9.2, and P10 regions that were considered to be orthologous regions were used in the analysis. The P7-like region of *Pa*SSU (as well as the analogous regions of the *Arthonia lapidicola* and *Porpidia crustulata*) was aligned with all of the P9.2 sections, because we concluded previously that it originated as a part of that region (Harris & Rogers, 2008). Following alignment using ClustalW2 (http://www.ebi.ac.uk/Tools/clustalw2/index.html), the sequences were examined, and manual adjustments were made as needed. Phylogenetic analyses were performed with PAUP (Phylogenetic Analysis Using Parsimony; Swofford, 2001) using Maximum Parsimony (with bootstrapping).

# 3    Results

Splicing using RNA from the clone with only 20 nt of each exon (Figure 2c) failed to splice *in vitro* in any of the numerous attempts. However, when clones included the 3' exon (that consisted of ITS1 and the 5' one-third of the 5.SS rRNA; Figure 2a & 2b) splicing occurred, whether or not the longer 5' exon was present. When the 3' exon (including ITS1 and the 5' one-third of the 5.8S rRNA) was deleted, no splicing was observed (Figure 2d; details in Harris, 2007; Harris & Rogers, 2008). Splicing occurred via a group I intron splicing pathway (Harris & Rogers, 2008). The first nucleophilic attack at the 5' exon-intron border was indistinguishable from that of standard group I introns. In the experiments with $^{32}$P-GTP, the labeled guanosine comigrated with the intron in gels (Harris & Rogers, 2008), indicating covalent attachment to the intron. The attack was at the G•U wobble pair, the exon was separated from the intron, and it was concluded that the free guanosine became covalently bonded to the 5' end of the intron (Figure 3). The second step also appeared to be a nucleophilic attack, but the 3' exon-intron border differed from usual group I introns, in that the final nucleotide of the intron was a U rather than the canonical G. Part of ITS1 and or the 5.8S rRNA appeared to stabilize the conformation of the intron so that splicing can proceed, because splicing only occurred if these regions were included in the RNA.

### 3.1    Mutant Introns

Several mutant introns were subjected to *in vitro* splicing testing. Splicing occurred whether or not the 200 nt of the 5' exon was present (Figure 3). When nucleotides in or near the 5' splice site were changed, splicing was negatively affected (Figure 3). Changing a single A residue in the A-loop of P1 caused a cessation of splicing, while changing an unpaired U residue within P1 had no affect on splicing. Changes in the proposed P7 region also had mainly detrimental effects on splicing, although changes in nucleotides that appeared to have no interactions with other nucleotides (41G and 57G) had no effect on splicing. This region may interact with ITS1 and/or the 5.8S rRNA, but the interaction is unresolved at this time. A general model for sequence and structure conservation is presented in Figure 4.

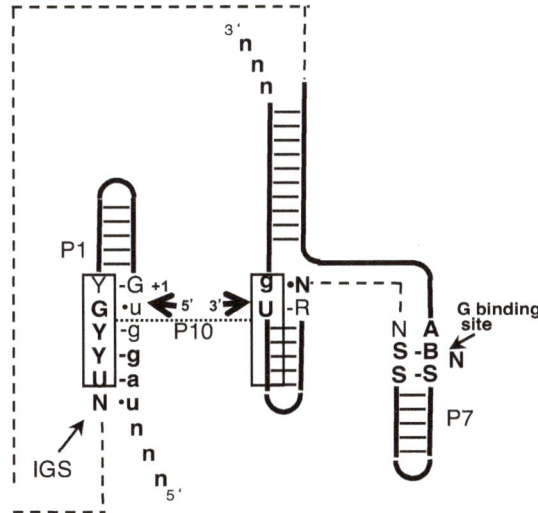

**Figure 4**: Model of the small intron based on sequence conservation (Harris 2007; Harris and Rogers 2008, 2011). The primary regions of sequence conservation are at the two splice sites and P7. Other regions are more variable in sequence, but the overall intron structures are preserved. Y = C or U; R = A or G; S = G or C; B = C, G or U; N = A, G, C, or U.

## 3.2  Sequence Analysis

Alignment of sequences allowed an analysis of nucleotide changes (Table 1). The rates of change compared to isolate 1046 ranged from 30% to 73%. The transversion to transition ratio ranged from 1:1 to approximately 3:1.

| Isolates | Similarity | Mutations | Tv/Ts |
|----------|-----------|-----------|-------|
| *Pa*SSU 1046 | 100% | N/A | N/A |
| *Pa*SSU CDC5 | 73% | 18 | 3:1 |
| *Pa*SSU 10507 | 55% | 30 | 1:1 |
| *Pa*SSU CDC10 | 35% | 43 | 1:1 |
| *Pv*SSU 8701 | 35% | 43 | 1.5:1 |
| *Pv*SSU 8702 | 35% | 43 | 2:1 |
| *Pp*SSU 2509 | 30% | 47 | 1:1 |

**Table 1:** Percent of similarity among isolates, number of mutations and the ratios of transversions to transitions.

## 3.3  Phylogenetic analysis

The small introns lie within a single clade within the IC1 subgroup (Figure 5).

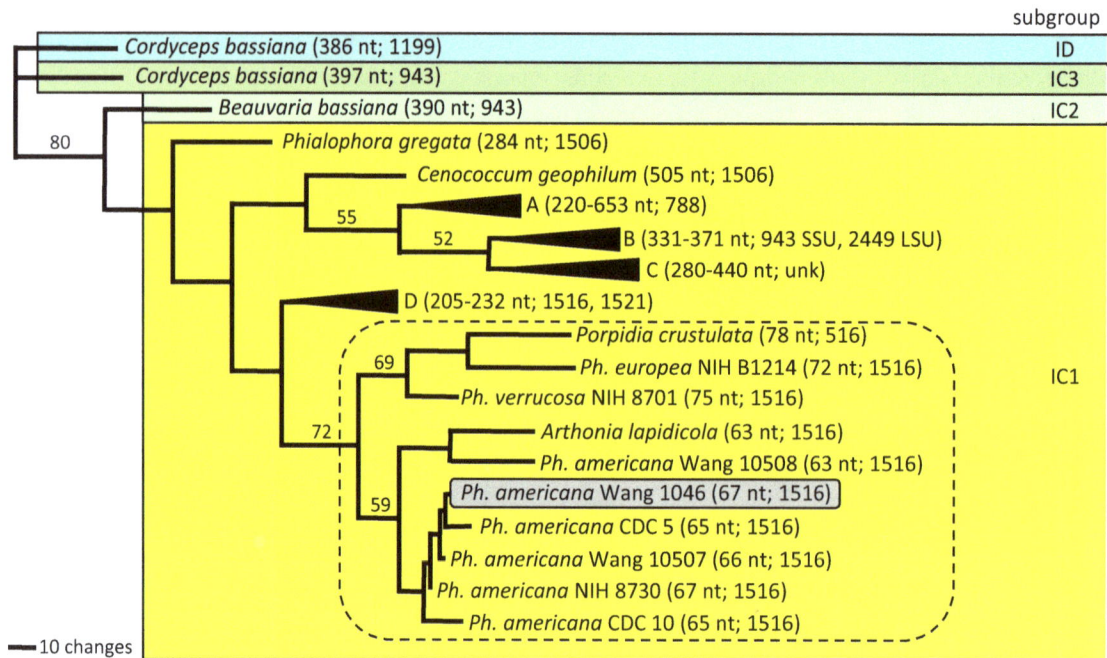

**Figure 5:** Unrooted phylogenetic tree of group IC and ID introns, including the small introns (inside dashed lines). Triangles labeled A, B, C and D indicate summaries of groups of related group IC1 introns. Lengths of the introns are indicated in nucleotides (nt). Positions are listed in relation to the *E. coli* rRNA genes. All are within the SSU rRNA gene, except where noted (LSU or unk = unknown).

# 4   Discussion

Small group I introns exhibit many of the key features of larger group I introns, but have unique features and evolutionary histories. Group I introns, in general, are taxonomically widespread, have a long evolutionary history and have influenced the evolution of many types of organisms and organelles. However, our knowledge of their structures, functions and evolution remain rudimentary. They appear to have originated as mobile genetic elements. Many have been described that contain open reading frames that have been identified as site-specific endonucleases that recognize sequences on double-stranded DNAs and form a double-stranded break a dozen or more nucleotides from the recognition site. A DNA version of the intron is then inserted into the site. This explains part of their ability to insert into intron-less sites and convert genetic loci. Most group I introns have lost their ability to produce these endonucleases, but some still are capable of inserting into intron-less sites as long as the endonuclease activity is supplied by a version that expresses the endonuclease activity in trans. Many of the group I introns insert into gene regions, where there are selective pressures that assure continued accurate splicing activity. Retention of the small introns in the rRNA gene locus of fungi is the result of this necessity to maintain splicing activity, and therefore produce functional rRNAs and ribosomes.

The core region has been very well studied in *Tetrahymena thermophila* by Cech and coworkers since 1980 (see e.g., Cech, 1988) and it was synthesized and studied to show by chemical mapping that it folds into a stable tertiary structure (Murphy & Cech, 1993). Subsequent studies concluded that the P4-P5-P6 region is an independently folding domain, and that mutations in the P4-P5-P6 core regions disrupt the stability and conformation of the molecule (Murphy & Cech, 1994). Similarly, it has been concluded that P1, P3, P7, P9, and P10 are essential for splicing. P1 and P10 hold the two exons, as well as the 5' and 3' splice sites (respectively), while the P3/P7/P8/P9 domain adds stability to P1 and P10. It is assumed that some of the tertiary binding interactions have important influences on intron function and autocatalytic activity. P2 is absent from many group I introns, and therefore appears to be non-essential. Magnesium ions and guanosine held by P7 and joining region J7/8, are required for intron activity, both of which influence the final structure of the active ribozyme. These interactions have roles in positioning the substrate for the reactions, probably by lowering the entropic barrier of the reaction (Cech & Herschlag, 1996), or perhaps interacting with magnesium, which optimally positions the guanosine to allow the initial nucleophilic attack on the RNA chain at a specific U residue (at the end of the 5' exon) of a G•U pair within P1 (Cech & Herschlag, 1996; Johnson *et al.*, 2003). The second reaction usually is initiated by the guanosine in the last position of the intron (the omega guanosine, $\omega$G) in standard group I introns (although the last nucleotide for all of the *Phialophora* small introns is a U).

Detailed analyses of a set of small (63-75 nt) group I introns within these small rRNA subunit gene of species of *Phialophora* (*P. americana*, *P. richardsiae*, *P. verrucosa* and *P. parasitica*), a genus of fungi that infect both plants and animals (including humans) indicated that only P1, P10 and a modified P7 were present in these introns (Figure 2 & 3; Harris, 2007; Harris & Rogers, 2008, 2010; Shinohara *et al.*, 1993; Rogers *et al.*, 1993). The P7 element had originated from part of the P9.2 element of a larger ancestral group I intron. While no other core regions were present, portions of ITS1 and/or the 5.8S rRNA (included within the 3' exon) stabilized the splicing reaction (Figure 2a & 2b). Constructs that were missing this 3' region failed to splice *in vitro* (Figure 2c & 2d). RNA without longer portions of the 5' exon spliced normally *in vitro* (Figure 2a). Because the intron probably is spliced out of the rRNA prior to ribosome assembly, the ITS1/5.8S region may have two functions in the maturation process for loci that contain these small introns.

Mutation analyses of the regions of the *P. americana* small intron confirmed the importance of some of the regions (Figure 3; Harris, 2007; Harris & Rogers, 2008). First, deletion of most of the 5' exon had no effects on splicing, while deletion of the 3' exon completely halted splicing activity. It is unclear at this time, which parts of the 3' exon (which includes the entire ITS1 region, as well as the 5' one-third of the 5.8S rRNA) are important to the splicing reaction. Other point mutations indicated the importance of other structures in the intron. In particular, the clones that contained mutations in and around the proposed 5' splice site (position -2 G⇒C; -1 U⇒A or C; 1 G⇒C) all led to cessation of splicing at that site. Change of the U to a G at position 4 had no effect on splicing, but might have further stabilized P1, because of the possible pairing with a C at position 11. The deletion of a single A at position 7 caused this mutant to fail to splice *in vitro*. It is proposed that this A-rich loop (nucleotides 5-10) might pair with the U-rich loop (nucleotides 34-39) to stabilize parts of the intron. However, the three adjacent residues (5-7) might be important for other reasons. Changes in the putative P7 region also led to the loss of splicing activity in the mutant RNAs. Specifically, changes in the proposed guanosine binding site (positions 43 C⇒U, 45⇒A, C, or U, and 45/46 GU⇒AC) all produced RNAs that failed to splice *in vitro*. However, changes at positions 41 (G⇒A) and 57 (G⇒U) appeared to splice normally. The mutational analyses are consistent with the model presented in Figs. 3 & 4, which includes a P1, P10 and P7 regions. However, as stated previously, the P7 appears to have been formed from a P9.2 region of a larger ancestral group I intron (Harris, 2007; Harris & Rogers, 2008).

While structure and function among these small introns are maintained, a great deal of sequence divergence is permissible (Figure 4; Harris 2007; Harris & Rogers, 2008, 2011). Some isolates contained introns with more than 50% sequence conservation (Table 1) to *Pa*SSU1046 (*Pa*SSU CDC5 - 73%; *Pa*SSU 10507 - 55% and *Pa*SSU 8730 - 91%). Others exhibit much less sequence conservation, such as *Pa*SSU CDC10 (45%), *Pv*SSU NIH8701 (35%), *Pv*SSU NIH8702 (35%) and *Pp*SSU2509 (30%). However, these introns have retained the P1, P10 and P7 structures, as well as the 3' and 5' splice sites (Harris & Rogers, 2011). Mutations or variability in the intron may be directly affecting the variability of their phenotype by altering expression of the SSU rRNA, and consequently cell growth, although this awaits further examination.

Variations observed in the SSU rRNA base composition are almost entirely due to fixation of point mutations. Curiously, a higher rate of transversions than transitions was found among these introns. For example, *Pa*SSU CDC5 has 73% of sequence conservation with *Pa*SSU 1046, and a transversion:transition rate of 3:1. The isolates such as *Pa*SSU CDC10, *Pa*SSU 8701, *Pa*SSU 8702 and *Pa*SSU 2509 sequence conservation is from 30-35 % to *Pa*SSU 1046, with ratios of 1:1. This is in contrast to general rates of transitions and transversions, where transitions usually occur approximately 1.5 to 3 times more often than do transversions, partly due to C-to-T transitions that are elevated in regions with high concentrations of 5-methylcytosines (Lindahl 1993). These changes often lead to mutations where a T-A pair is substituted for a C-G pair. The high rates of transversions may reflect selective pressures to maintain sufficient hydrogen bonding within the introns. Selection would favor replacements of A-U and G•U pairs with G-C pairs in order to compensate for the loss of structure stabilizing hydrogen bonds. Many of these changes would require transversions.

Recombination probably was the mechanism that led to the shortening these introns (Figure 6). Almost all of the small introns are located at the 1516 position of the rRNA SSU gene (relative to the *E. coli* rRNA SSU gene), which likely occurred as a single event. However, in *Porpidia crustulata*, a similar small related intron occurs at the 516 position of the same gene (Figure 5). Because of the sequence and length similarities, it may represent a translocation event in this species. However, a transposition event requiring a site-specific endonuclease would have had to occur. Another scenario is that an independent recombination event led to the formation of this small intron. Recombination and gene conversion are common within the rRNA gene locus (Rogers & Bendich, 1987a, 1987b), which would favor the second scenario. No other group I introns of this size have been described. All of the other standard group I introns in the rRNA genes of fungi are 200 nt and larger, and none have ORFs. Introns of intermediate size may be incapable of forming a structure that is conducive to splicing. Although recombination may have produced such intermediate-sized introns, splicing may be interrupted, which would produce a faulty SSU rRNA, leading to a lethal condition for that cell and for the organism, thus leading to extinction of any intermediate-sized intron. The small introns were favored by selection because splicing was maintained through interactions with ITS1 and/or 5.8S rRNA (for the intron at 516, analogous interactions with the SSU rRNA or with ITS1/5.8S region must occur). Therefore, there appears to be a window of nucleotides within the P7 region of the intron that interacts with another window of nucleotides within the ITS1/5.8S rRNA region that retains splicing of the intron. The fact that the size of the small introns is restrained indicates that formation of these functional discontinuous introns is rare events. Another outcome of recombination to form these small introns would be the formation of a longer putative intron (Figure 6) that would contain a nearly complete version of the intron (lacking P9, P10 and the 3' intron-exon border) fused to another nearly complete intron (lacking the 5' intron-exon border and P1). This has not been observed, and therefore may have led to lethality for these rRNA regions. Duplicate copies of most of the pairing regions may have led to severely altered intron structures.

The similarities in intron sequences among the isolates and their similarities to the other group I introns in the same region of the SSU rRNA gene (the 1506-1521 nt region, with respect to the *E. coli* rRNA SSU gene) indicates that these introns were inserted into this location at a time that predated the separation of these taxa. Also, phylogenetic analyses resulted in a single clade for all of the small introns, including one from *Porpidia crustulata*, which is inserted at the 516 nt position, indicating a common origin (Figure 5; Harris & Rogers, 2008). The sequence conservation among most isolates of *P. americana*, and the high sequence variation among the other small introns indicates a long history for these small introns. Point mutations, gene conversion and recombination have resulted in an incredible high variation and diversity among group I introns in the 1506-1521 region of the rRNA SSU genes in fungi, including the small putative group I intron here presented.

The evolutionary pathways that led to the formation of the small group I-like ribozymes have proceeded in several steps. Initially, ancestral elements (i.e., introns or related ancestral elements) invaded the rRNA gene locus early in fungal evolution (or within a fungus ancestor). At that time, the ORF containing the site-specific endonuclease gene would have been necessary. After the initial transformation of the genes, the introns then spread to other locations of the rRNA locus (Gargas *et al.*, 1995). During this time, the ORFs were gradually lost, but the splicing functions were retained, partly due to the selective pressures that required the retention of the ability to construct rRNAs and ribosomes. Later, a small intron was formed by non-homologous recombination between two full-length introns. This occurred between introns located at or near the 1516 position (details discussed in Harris & Rogers, 2011), and may have occurred many times during the past 500 million years. However, few of the recombinants were viable. The evolutionary success of the small introns was due to a characteristic of the ITS1/5.8S region that was able to complement for some of the intron functions. This region would have to substitute for some of the functions of the P4/P5/P6 and P3/P7/P8/P9 domains, which function as stabilizing scaffolds in the intron. This event caused the formation of these discontinuous group I-like introns. Another recombination event likely created one of the small introns in an ancestor of *Porpidium crustulata*. This might have occurred from a single crossover event, similar to the one that led to the formation of the other small introns at the 1516 position. However, because the *P. crustulata* small intron groups with the other small introns in the phylogenetic analysis, it might have been formed by a double crossover event between a large intron at the 516 position and a small intron at the 1516 position. It is unknown whether these introns have led to the evolution and physiology of these species, but their continued presence indicates that their maintenance as functional introns has been important to the survival of these species. Some ribosomal repeats have lost the intron completely, some of which occur in the same isolates (Rogers *et al.*, 1993; Yan *et al.*, 1995; Shinohara *et al.*, 1996). This might be the final step in the evolution of the intron-containing rRNA genes within these fungi, that of losing the introns completely.

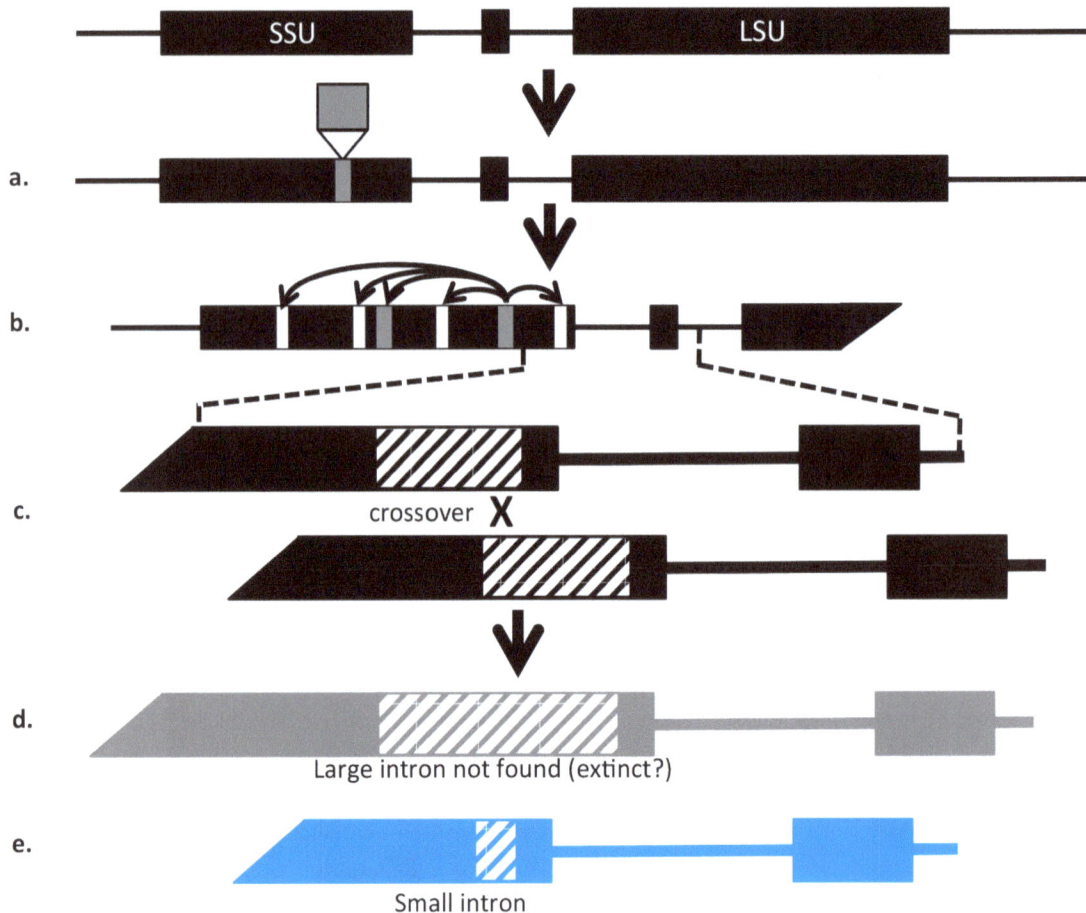

**Figure 6:** Proposed evolution of the small group I introns. **a.** Insertion of the introns began with a group I intron (gray box) that contained a site-specific endonuclease gene that recognized sequences in the rRNA genes of the ancestral genes. **b.** After establishment of the first intron, insertion of additional copies into the same genes occurred. Gene conversion would rapidly convert all of the copies (an average of 100-200 in fungi) to a single (or small number) of gene repeat versions. Eventually, all of the introns lost their endonuclease genes (white boxes), likely through genetic drift and selection. **c.** Next, in an ancestor of *Phialophora* (and related genera), a non-homologous recombination event occurred that formed a longer (**d**) and a shortened version (**e**) of the intron at the 1516 location of the SSU rRNA gene. The longer version may have disabled the SSU gene, and thus went extinct, because the longer versions have not been found. The small version survived and became established as the organisms speciated, which led to the current situation. It is unknown whether movement to the 516 position occurred prior to insertion into the 1516 position, although they appear to be monophyletic in phylogenetic analyses (Figure 5).

# References

Adams, P. L., Stahley, M. R., Gill, M. L., Kosek, A. B., Wang, J., & Strobel, S. A. (2004) Crystal structure of a group I intron splicing intermediate. RNA, 10, 1867-1887.

Bhattacharya, D., Lutzoni, F., Reeb, V., Simon, D., Nason, J., & Fernandez, F. (2000) Widespread occurrence of spliceosomal introns in the rDNA genes of ascomycetes. Molecular Biology & Evolution, 17, 1971-1984.

Cavalier-Smith, T. (1991) Intron evolution: a new hypothesis. Trends in Genetics, 7, 145-148.

Cech, T. R. (1988) Conserved sequences and structures of group I introns: Binding an active site for RNA catalysis – a review. Gene, 73, 259-271.

Cech, T. R. (1990) Self-splicing group I introns. Annual Review of Biochemistry, 59, 543-568.

Cech, T. R., & Herschlag, D. (1996) Group I ribozymes: Substrate recognition, catalytic strategies, and comparative mechanistic analysis. In Nucleic Acids and Molecular Biology, eds. Eckstein, F., & Lilley, D.M.J. (Springer-Verlag, Berlin, Germany), 10, 1–17.

Coetzee, T., Herschlag, D., & Belfort, M. (1994) Escherichia coli proteins, including ribosomal protein S12, facilitate in vitro splicing of phage T4 introns by acting as RNA chaperones. Genes & Development, 8, 1575-1588.

Cubero, O. F., Bridge, P. D., & Crespo, A. (2000) Terminal-sequence conservation identifies spliceosomal introns in ascomycete 18S RNA genes. Molecular Biology & Evolution, 17, 751-756.

Dávila-Aponte, J. A., Huss, V. A. R., Sogin, M. L., & Cech, T. R. (1991) A self-splicing group I intron in the nuclear pre-rRNA of the green alga, Ankistrodesmus stipitatus. Nucleic Acids Research, 19, 4429-4436.

De Wachter, R., Neefs, J-M., Goris, A., & de Peer, Y. V. (1992) The gene coding for small ribosomal subunit RNA in the basidiomycete Ustilago maydis contains a group I intron. Nucleic Acids Research, 20, 1251-1257.

Doudna, J. A., & Cech, T. R. (2002) The chemical repertoire of natural ribozymes. Nature, 418, 222-228.

Doudna, J. A., Cormack, B., & Szostak, J. W. (1989) RNA structure, not sequence, determines the 5' splice-site specificity of a group I intron. Proceedings of the National Academy of Sciences USA, 86, 7402-7406.

Doudna, F., & Szostak, J. W. (1989) Miniribozymes, small derivatives of the sunY intron, are catalytically active. Molecular and Cellular Biology, 9, 5480-5483.

Gargas, A., DePriest, P., & Taylor, J. (1995) Positions of multiple insertions in SSU rDNA of lichen-forming fungi. Molecular Biology and Evolution, 12, 208-218.

Golden, B. L., Kim, H., & Chase, E. (2005) Crystal structure of an active group I ribozyme-product complex. Nature Structural Molecular Biology, 12, 82-89.

Harris, L. B. (2007) Characterization of a small ribozyme with self-splicing activity. PhD Dissertation, Department of Biological Sciences, Bowling Green State University, Bowling Green, OH.

Harris, L. B., & Rogers, S. O. (2008) Splicing and evolution of an unusually small group I intron. Current Genetics, 54, 213-222.

Harris, L. B., Rogers, S. O, (2011) Evolution of small putative group I introns in the SSU rRNA gene locus of Phialophora species. BioMed Central Research Notes, 4, 258.

Haugen, P., Runge, H. J., & Bhattacharya, D. (2004) Long-term evolution of the S788 fungal nuclear small subunit rRNA group I introns. RNA, 10, 1084-1096.

Haugen, P., Simon, D. M., & Bhattacharya, D. (2005) The natural history of group I introns. Trends in Genetics, 21, 111-119.

Jackson, S. A., Cannone, J. J., Lee, J. C., Gutell, R. R., & Woodson, S. A. (2002) Distribution of rRNA introns in the three-dimensional structure of the ribosome. Journal of Molecular Biology, 323, 35–52.

Johansen, S. D., Haugen, P., & Nielsen, H. (2007) Expression of protein-coding genes embedded in ribosomal DNA. Biological Chemistry, 388, 679–686.

Johnson, A. K., Baum, D. A., Tye, J., Bell, M. A., & Testa, S. M. (2003) Molecular recognition properties of IGS-mediated reactions catalyzed by a Pneumocystis carinii group I intron. Nucleic Acids Research, 31, 1921-1934.

Lindahl, T. (1993) Instability and decay of the primary structure of DNA. Nature, 362, 709-715.

Michel, F., & Westhof, E. (1990) Modeling of the three-dimensional architecture of group I catalytic introns based on comparative sequence analysis. Journal of Molecular Biology, 216, 585-610.

Moreira, S., Breton, S., & Burger, G. (2012) Unscrambling genetic information at the RNA level. WIREs RNA, 3, 213-228.

Murphy, F. L., & Cech, T. R. (1993) An independently folding domain of RNA tertiary structure within the Tetrahymena ribozyme. Biochemistry, 3, 5291-5300.

Murphy, F. L., & Cech, T. R. (1994) GAAA tetraloop and conserved bulge stabilize tertiary structure of a group I intron domain. Journal of Molecular Biology, 236, 49-63.

Nikoh, N., & Fukatsu, T. (2001) Evolutionary dynamics of multiple group I introns in nuclear ribosomal RNA genes of endoparasitic fungi of the genus Cordyceps. Molecular Biology and Evolution, 18, 1631-1642.

Rogers, S. O., & Bendich, A. J. (1987a) Heritability and variability in ribosomal RNA genes of Vicia faba. Genetics, 117, 285-295.

Rogers, S. O., & Bendich, A. J. (1987b) Ribosomal RNA genes in plants: variability in copy number and in the intergenic spacer. Plant Molecular Biology, 9, 509-520.

Rogers, S. O., Rehner, S., Bledsoe, C., Mueller, G. J., & Ammirati, J. F. (1989) Extraction of DNA from Basidiomycetes for ribosomal DNA hybridizations. Canadian Journal of Botany, 67, 1235-1243.

Rogers, S. O., Yan, Z., Shinohara, M., LoBuglio, K., & Wang C. J. K. (1993) Messenger RNA intron in the nuclear 18S ribosomal RNA gene of deuteromycetes. Current Genetics, 23, 338-342.

Shinohara, M., LoBuglio, K., & Rogers, S. O. (1996) Group I intron family in the nuclear ribosomal RNA small subunit genes of Cenococcum geophilum isolates. Current Genetics, 29, 377-387.

Simon, D., Moline, J., Helms, G., Friedl, T., & Bhattacharya, D. (2005) Divergent histories of rDNA group I introns in the lichen family Physciaceae. Journal of Molecular Evolution, 60, 434-446.

Swofford, D. (2001) PAUP: phylogenetic analysis using parsimony, Version 4, Sinaur Academic Publishers.

White, T. J., Bruns, T., Lee, S., & Taylor, J. (1990) Amplification and direct sequencing of fungal ribosomal RNA genes for phylogenteics. In: Innis M. A., Gelfand D. H., Sninsky J. J., & White T. J., editors, PCR Protocols, a Guide to Methods and Applications. Academic Press, Inc., Harcourt Brace Janovich Publishers, New York. pp 315-322.

Yan, Z. H., Rogers, S. O. & Wang, C. J. K. (1995) Assessment of Phialophora species based on ribosomal DNA internal transcribed spacers and morphology. Mycologia, 87, 72-83.

Zuker, M. (2003) Mfold Web server for nucleic acid folding and hybridization prediction. Nucleic Acids Research, 31, 1-10.

# Variant Antigen Expression Control in *Plasmodium* Parasites

Fernanda Janku Cabral, Wesley Luzetti Fotoran and Gerhard Wunderlich
*Department of Parasitology, Institute for Biomedical Sciences*
*University of São Paulo, Brazil*

# 1   General Introduction to Malaria

Malaria is still an important cause of morbidity and mortality in tropical areas of the world. From the epidemiologic perspective, the most important causative agents of malaria are *Plasmodium falciparum* and *Plasmodium vivax*, while *Plasmodium malariae* and *Plasmodium ovale* are less frequent in many regions, and *Plasmodium knowlesi* is present only Southeast Asian rain forests. It is estimated that approximately 2,4 billion people are at risk of *P. falciparum* transmission with 300 to 500 million clinical episodes and 1 million deaths per year (Guerra *et al.*, 2008). At the same time, 2,9 billion people live in areas where vivax malaria is transmitted (Guerra *et al.*, 2010) and actually an estimated 80 to 300 million cases occur annually (Mueller *et al.*, 2009).

The life cycle of *P. falciparum* initiates when sporozoites are injected in the host dermis by anopheline mosquitoes. After migrational events, some of these sporozoites enter the blood stream and reach the liver where they invade (Vaughan *et al.*, 2008). Inside parenchymal hepatocytes, sporozoites differentiate to a replicative form termed liver schizonts and after 6-13 days depending on the infecting species, merozoites are released into the bloodstream as membrane-surrounded merosomes (Sturm *et al.*, 2006) and start invading the erythrocytes. After an active invasion of erythrocytes which involves several receptor-ligand interactions (reviewed in (Cowman & Crabb, 2006) and (Farrow *et al.*, 2011)), merozoites differentiate in young trophozoites (rings), trophozoites and schizonts. After 48 hours (*P. malariae* 72 h), the infected red blood cell (IRBC) is lysed and 8 to 32 new merozoites are released and each lysis causes the typical fever attacks felt by malaria patients (for a review on malaria pathogenesis, see (Miller *et al.*, 2002)). Eventually, gametocytes develop from invaded merozoites and these can be ingested by anophelines during the next blood meal. Inside the mosquito host, gametes develop and after zygote formation and migration to the outside of the intestinal epithelium, meiosis occurs and finally thousands of sporozoites are released in the hemolymph of the mosquito host which then actively invade the salivary gland (Ghosh & Jacobs-Lorena, 2009) and become transmittable to the next mammalian host.

One of the major complications of human infections with *P. falciparum* is the expression of ligand proteins at the erythrocyte surface which cause the IRBC to interact with endothelial cell receptors such as CD36, ICAM-1, Chondroitin sulphate A (CSA) and others (reviewed in (Rowe *et al.*, 2009) and (Pasternak & Dzikowski, 2009)) and potentially mediate severe disease outcomes by accumulation of IRBC in deep capillaries (reviewed in (van der Heyde *et al.*, 2006)). While the cytoadhesive properties of *P. falciparum* IRBC could be associated to large and highly variant proteins termed PfEMP1 (*Plasmodium falciparum* erythrocyte membrane protein 1 (Leech *et al.*, 1984)), the ligands and receptors in other adhesive species of *Plasmodium* such as strains of *P. berghei* (Kaul *et al.*, 1994) and *P. vivax* (Carvalho *et al.*, 2010) remain elusive although the variant *P. vivax* VIR proteins were recently suspected to be involved (Bernabeu *et al.*, 2011; Carvalho *et al.*, 2010). In *P. falciparum,* other variant protein families in addition to PfEMP1 were identified at the IRBC surface and these include variant protein family members such as RIFIN (Cheng *et al.*, 1998), STEVOR (Cheng *et al.*, 1998; Weber, 1988), and perhaps SURFIN (Winter *et al.*, 2005). With the exception of PfEMP1, all these proteins have in common that we do not know what their function might be in *P. falciparum*. The same is true for the PIR (*Plasmodium* interspersed repeats) family of proteins (Janssen *et al.*, 2004), such as the VIR (*vivax* interspersed repeats) proteins in *P. vivax*, and the CIR, BIR and YIR (*chabaudi, berghei, yoelii* interspersed repeats, respectively) found in the rodent *Plasmodium* species *P. chabaudi, P. berghei* and *P. yoelii*, respectively.

The number of genes discussed here varies from a few (11 *surf* genes) to hundreds (*pir* genes of non-falciparum *Plasmodium*) per haploid genome and takes us to the central issue: If these genes code for antigens which are targets for the immune response, then the simultaneous expression and exposition of all possible antigen variants would lead to a rapid recognition of the circulating parasites. On the other hand, the failure to express any variant antigen would be detrimental since its function – in the case of PfEMP1 the cytoadherence to endothelial cells avoiding spleen passage – would not be exerted. Many pathogenic organisms, including *Giardia*, *Trypanosoma brucei*, *Plasmodium* and others have developed complex and differing mechanisms to control the expression of sometimes very large gene variant antigen encoding gene families (reviewed in (Donelson, 1995; Prucca *et al.*, 2008)). The result is in almost all cases the sequential expression of one or a few alleles out of a large repertoire of antigenically different molecules. This mode of expression is termed antigenic variation and ensures that the pathogen is always "one step ahead" of the immune response. In the following, we discuss the mechanisms by which different *Plasmodium* species seem to control the expression of their different variant gene families, most of which involved in antigenic variation.

## 2  *Plasmodium Falciparum Var* Gene Transcription

The phenomenon that mature forms of *Plasmodium falciparum* are rarely detected in the peripheral blood of infected individuals was observed many years ago. In end of the 1960s it was discovered that these forms adhere to the endothelium of organs (Miller, 1969). In the following years, the adhesive properties of infected IRBC were characterized and in 1984 Leech and colleagues identified a large parasite encoded antigen at the IRBC surface as a main ligand and termed it *P. falciparum* membrane protein 1 (PfEMP1, (Leech *et al.*, 1984)). It was also observed that the adhesive properties and antigenic properties of IRBC change over time even in cloned parasite lines in continuous culture, turning evident that the expression of the adhesion-causing ligands changed during reinvasion cycles (Roberts *et al.*, 1992). However, it was not known at that time if these phenotypic switches occurred as a consequence of genetic rearrangements, transcriptional or translational changes. Also, it was unclear if these phenotypic changes occurred with the same dynamics in natural infections. The identification of the PfEMP1-encoding *var* genes only occurred in 1995 (Baruch *et al.*, 1995; Smith *et al.*, 1995; Su *et al.*, 1995). Three years later, two groups showed that during the trophozoite stage of phenotypically homogenous parasites expressing one PfEMP1 version, only one dominant *var* transcript out of the 50 to 60 existing *var* genes per haploid genome was present. This process was termed allelic exclusion. Also, the authors showed that in contrast to *Trypanosoma brucei* (Barry *et al.*, 1998; Rudenko *et al.*, 1994) no genetic rearrangement of *var* genes[1] was associated when switching occurred (Chen *et al.*, 1998; Scherf *et al.*, 1998; Scherf *et al.*, 2008). Later, two independent groups showed that *var* transcription switching took place as a consequence of changing promoter activity, meaning that silenced *var* genes showed no significant full length transcription (Kyes *et al.*, 2007; Schieck *et al.*, 2007). These transcriptional switches were also observed in parasites from natural or experimental infections (Kaestli *et al.*, 2004; Peters *et al.*, 2002; Wunderlich *et al.*, 2005). Many attempts were conducted to measure the velocity of transcriptional switching between reinvasions and early results showed that there are slowly switching *var* genes and fast-switching *var* genes (Horrocks *et al.*, 2004). There is evidence that transcriptional switching occurs

---

[1] Notably, and independently from transcriptional events, the genetic recombination of *var* genes does occur at a high rate most probably during meiosis in the mosquito host (Freitas-Junior *et al.* 2000) explaining why *var* gene repertoires are vastly different between strains (eg. (Bull *et al.*, 2005; Fowler *et al.*, 2002)).

following an organized pattern (Enderes *et al.*, 2011; Recker *et al.*, 2011) and that chromosomal position (telomeric versus centromeric position, see Figure 1) also plays a role in the switching dynamic (Frank *et al.*, 2007).

## 2.1   Sequence Elements in the *Var* 5' Untranslated Region and the *Var* Intron Play a Crucial Role for Allelic Exclusion

In general, the 5' untranslated regions of *var* genes can be classified in three general groups depending on which type of *var* gene is controlled by this region (Lavstsen *et al.*, 2003; Rask *et al.*, 2010). These groups were termed upsA, B and C and mixtures thereof (see figure 1). Due to the very high AT content, it is very difficult to identify canonic regulatory sequences in these promoters. Two observations were very important to shed a light on the mechanism of allelic exclusion in *var* transcription in *P. falciparum*: First, it was shown that the *var* intron present in all *var* genes which participate in allelic exclusion (this is, they can assume different states of activation) is a very strong silencing element (Deitsch *et al.*, 2001) and this property is at least partly due to its intrinsic bi-directional promoter activity (Calderwood *et al.*, 2003). The second finding was that a given *var* promoter itself present as a transgenic construct can participate in the allelic exclusion process and its activation can lead to the silencing of all other *var* loci (Voss *et al.*, 2006) - uncoupled from the existence of a PfEMP1 product (Dzikowski *et al.*, 2006). In studies using gel shift assays, some canonic sequence elements (SPE1 and SPE2) could be identified in *var* promoters which bind to only partially characterized nuclear proteins (Voss *et al.*, 2003). The sequence motif which is crucial for the crosstalk of promoter activation and silencing was recently discovered by the group of Till Voss (Brancucci *et al.*, 2012). However, the definition of this element still does not *per se* explain why some promoters are silenced and why only one or two promoters are active per parasite. An additional layer of regulation seems to exist at least for specific *var* genes: When working with parasites expressing the CSA-binding PfEMP1 VAR2CSA by transcribing the relatively conserved *var2csa*  gene (PlasmoDB: PF3D7_1200600)*,* Amulic and colleagues detected that an additional 5'-untranslated ORF was present in the transcript which after several reinvasions led to the translational repression of VAR2CSA production, while maintaining *var2csa* transcription at previous levels (Amulic *et al.*, 2009), meaning that at least this *var* can be controlled at the transcriptional and translational level.

## 2.2   Histone modifications and nuclear factors involved in *var* transcription

In *P. falciparum*, several lines of evidence have shown that epigenetic events – understood as the dynamic modification of histone tails - play a major role in the control of not only *var* genes but also other gene families involved in antigenic variation (Salcedo-Amaya *et al.*, 2009). It is estimated that at least 60 different histone posttranslational modifications may occur in eukaryotic cells (Berger, 2007). Actually, the role of all these modifications is not totally understood, but it is well-known that acetylation, methylation, ubiquitination, SUMOylation, glycosylation and phosphorylation play a role in gene expression control in eukaryotic cells in general (Berger, 2007) as well as in protozoan parasites (Croken *et al.*, 2012). Post-translational modification (PTMs) of histones is a reversible process which depends on enzymes called histone acetyl transferases (HAT), histone deacetylases (HDACs), histone methyltransferases (HMTs) and histone demethylases. In *P. falciparum,* MYST (<u>M</u>OZ, <u>Y</u>bf1/<u>S</u>as3, Sas2 and <u>T</u>ip60) and GCN5 are two important HATs proteins that have been characterized. In the erythrocytic stages, MYST mRNA is expressed in higher levels in rings and schizonts and lower levels in trophozoites (Miao *et al.*, 2010). It was also established that recombinant purified MYST is able to acetylate histone H4 in vitro at lysine K4, K8, K12 and K16 and is located in the nucleus. MYST is enriched at the transcriptional start site (TSS) of *var* genes, probably playing a role in regulation of antigenic variation. In addition, the overexpression of MYST seems to severely interfere in the cell cycle (Miao *et al.*, 2010). The other known plasmodial HATs belongs to the GCN5 (general control non-repressed protein 5) family and PfGCN5 mRNA is expressed constitutively in all stages of the cycle, suggesting a role in the parasite's differentiation process. It was also established that PfGCN5 preferentially acetylates core histones *in vitro* at K8 and K14 (H3). Further results have shown that PfGCN5 has the ability to interact with other nuclear transcriptional coactivators in *P. falciparum* (Fan *et al.*, 2004).

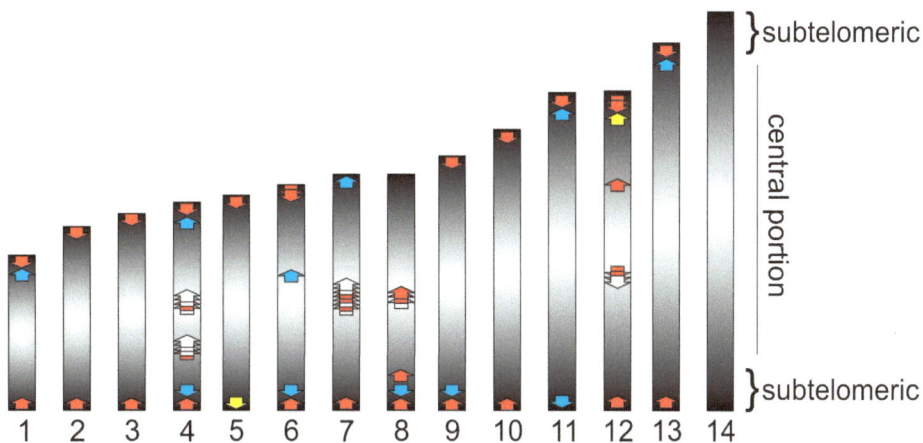

**Figure 1:** A: The var gene distribution along the 14 chromosomes from the *P. falciparum* strain 3D7 (modified from (Deitsch & Hviid, 2004)). The color of the arrows indicates the var/promoter type following the classification of Lavstsen et al. (Lavstsen *et al.*, 2003). Note that type A var genes (with an upsA type promoter) are depicted in blue while upsB type loci are in red and type C appear white. The two yellow arrows indicate former type D and E promoters, which were reclassified to the upsA type (Rask *et al.*, 2010).

Whereas HAT activity is to reversibly acetylate histones, HDACs catalyze the deacetylation of histones. HDACs form a family of histone modifying enzymes and are divided in four classes according with yeast counterparts: classes I, II and IV are related to the zinc-dependent yeast proteins (Yang & Seto, 2008). The Class III HDAC consists of the NAD-dependent sirtuin family related to the yeast silencing information regulator 2 (SIR2) which mediates gene silencing at telomeres (Gasser & Cockell, 2001). The first HDAC that has been characterized for *P. falciparum* was PfHDAC1 and it can be classified as a class I enzyme. Immunomicroscopy experiments have shown that PfHDAC1 is located in the nucleus (Joshi *et al.*, 1999). Although few studies exist that clearly describe HDAC activity, several reports have shown the importance of HDACs to control gene expression in *P. falciparum*. Recently, a study using the potent HDAC inhibitor apicidin has shown that parasites treated with this compound suffer a severe developmental arrest, which is the result of transcriptional deregulation of one half of the parasite genome (Chaal *et al.*, 2010). Hyperacetylation and consequently demethylation of the nucleosomes at different *P. falciparum* gene loci was observed (Chaal *et al.*, 2010). Also, the treatment with apicidin caused the up-regulation of Apicomplexa Apetala 2 (ApiAP2) genes - which encode probable plant-like transcription factors - in the specific developmental stages in which they are commonly repressed (Chaal *et al.*, 2010). Notably, histone modifying enzymes including HDACs are of major importance as drug targets (reviewed by (Andrews *et al.*, 2012)). Recently, the specific inhibition of a plasmodial Histone methyltransferase led to the rapid death of *P. falciparum* and *P. berghei* erythrocytic forms (Malmquist *et al.*, 2012).

The Class III SIR2 proteins have been widely studied in *P. falciparum* due their role in regulation of antigenic variation. Biochemical studies have shown that PfSIR2 is able to modify acetylated H3 and H4 histones, with the concomitant oxydation of NADH+H$^+$ (French *et al.*, 2008). Maybe the most important role for PfSir proteins is in the regulation of mutually exclusive expression of *var* genes. Freitas-Junior and colleagues and Duraisingh and colleagues have shown the role of PfSIR2, annotated as the PlasmoDB gene PF3D7_1328800, in the control of mutual expression of *var* genes (Duraisingh *et al.*, 2005; Freitas-Junior *et al.*, 2005). In this work, it was shown that PfSIR2 is located in the telomeric foci and in the nucleolus, similar to what was observed in yeast (Gotta *et al.*, 1997). In *P. falciparum* parasites selected for *var2csa* transcription, it was found that chromatin in the region of the upsA/E *var2csa* promoter was immunoprecipitated by anti-acetylated H4 antibody when the *var2csa* gene was active, but not when *vas2csa* was inactive. In the latter situation, it became immunoprecipitable with anti-PfSIR2, suggesting that PfSIR2 is intrinsically related to the silencing of *var* genes (Freitas-Junior *et al.*, 2005). Knockout of PfSIR2 led to a general derepression of several *var* genes (Duraisingh *et al.*, 2005). Later, Chookajorn and colleagues (Chookajorn *et al.*, 2007) associated silent *var* sites to H3K9me3 (trimethylated lysine 9 at Histone 3). In a detailed ChIP analysis using a panel of different anti-Histone antibodies, Lopez-Rubio and colleagues confirmed H3K9ac with activation and H3K9me3 with silencing of *var* loci. In the same study, a timeline for modifications at active and silent loci was suggested ((Lopez-Rubio *et al.*, 2007) and Figure 2). During the intraerythrocytic development, even active *var* genes become silenced in maturing parasites at around 20 h after reinvasion, however, the same *var* genes begin to be transcribed again after reinvasion by default (epigenetic memory). In their work, Lopez-Rubio and colleagues found a correlation of H3K4me2 modification and locus activation in the next cycle. This means that *var* loci of parasites in schizont stage are modified with H3K4me2 and are prone to be activated after the next reinvasion (poised status)(Lopez-Rubio *et al.*, 2007). The H3K9 and H3K4 modifications are not limited to *var* loci but seem to associate to other variant gene families and may even identify novel variant genes in a genome wide scan (Lopez-Rubio *et al.*, 2009; Salcedo-Amaya *et al.*, 2009). The spectrum of histone modifications in *Plasmodium* were thoroughly reviewed in the excellent report of Cui and Miao (Cui & Miao, 2010).

In another work the function of the two paralogs PfSIR2A and PfSIR2B was reported and these have distinct roles in the control of *var* genes (Tonkin *et al.*, 2009). Applying targeted disruption of either PfSIR2A and/or PfSIR2B, Tonkin and colleagues showed that different *var* gene promoters are controlled by these proteins. In the ΔPfSIR2A lineages the activation of the telomeric/subtelomeric upsB *var* genes was observed (see Figure 1 and 2), while in PfSIR2B knockouts the telomeric upsA and centromeric C *var* promoters were highly active. Importantly, in these deleted ΔPfSIR2A/B parasites, multiple *var* genes were expressed, suggesting that mutually exclusive expression was interrupted in these lineages. This corroborates with the idea that both proteins somehow cooperate in the silencing of *var* promoters (Tonkin *et al.,* 2009). A recent study examined the correlation of *var* transcription, disease and the expression levels of PfSIR2A and B (Merrick *et al.*, 2012) and the authors showed that external factors such as fever or starvation lead to an upregulation of PfSIR2A expression. In turn, higher PfSIR2A expression resulted in the selective upregulation of *var* genes of the upsB type, which were also higher expressed in the group consisting of severe malaria infections (Merrick *et al.*, 2012). Their data indicate that higher quantities of the histone deacetylase PfSIR2A does not result in stronger silencing but selective upregulation of a group of *var* genes.

In addition to the roles of acetylation and deacetylation in gene activation and repression through modification of H3 or H4 histones, methylation is also important in the silencing or maintenance of poised states of *P. falciparum* gene loci. Methylases are enzymes that add methyl groups in lysine or arginine residues of histones. *P. falciparum* contains members of the methylase domain SET (*Drosophila* suppressor of variegation – Su(var), the Polycomb-group protein Enhancer of zeste – E(z) and Trithorax (TRX) group proteins) family, some of which have been characterized (Cui *et al.*, 2008; Volz *et al.*, 2012). Cui and colleagues have shown that in the *P. falciparum* genome, there are 9 annotated genes which encode proteins with the SET domain and these probably play a role in the regulation of gene expression. In the same study, the expression of the putative SET domains was found throughout the erythrocytic cycle. Further, phylogenetic analyses have inferred that PfSET domains may potentially methylate H3K4, H3K27, K3K36, H3K9 and H3K36 (Cui *et al.*, 2008). This *in silico* approach was also able to identify JmJC (Jumonji demethylase domain), which are demethylases in *Saccharomyces cerevisiae* (Fang *et al.*, 2007) and HeLa cells (Tsukada *et al.*, 2006). During an approach to map putative epigenetic factors in the *P. falciparum* nucleus which associate to active *var* loci, a protein containing a plant-like SET domain was identified in *P. falciparum* (Volz *et al.*, 2012). The factor termed PfSET10, annotated as PF3D7_1221000, is a H3K4 methyltransferase and in transgenic parasites overexpressing PfSET10, the transcription and allelic exclusion of *var* genes is maintained. Using ChIP-qPCR, it was found out that the H3K4me2 mark is enriched in higher levels, leading also to a stronger transcription of "switched-on" *var* genes in these parasite lineage. Intriguingly, the PfSET10 methyltransferase did not colocalize with H2A.Z (see below and (Volz *et al.*, 2012)).

Recent studies have underscored the importance of histone variants in *P. falciparum* gene regulation. Bartfai and colleagues determined the content of histone H2A.Z in intergenic regions of the *P. falciparum* genome. It was estimated that the average width of H2A.Z marked regions is 1248bp spanning 6 or 8 nucleosomes, suggesting a demarcation of intergenic regions (Bartfai *et al.*, 2010). Further ChIP and PCR analysis of the H2A.Z enrichment have shown that H2A.Z is concentrated at the transcription start site (TSS) of active *var2csa* genes. In contrast, in parasites where *var2csa* is inactive, H2A.Z is clearly not enriched. This indicates that H2A.Z occupancy in the promoter region results in the activation of transcription of *var* genes (Petter *et al.*, 2011). H2A.Z recruiting to promoters directly seems to correlate with transcriptional activity since the initial enrichment of H2A.Z at the TSS of active *var* promoters in ring stage decreases while the parasite develops to schizonts (Figure 2). This clearly reinforces the idea of promoter architecture remodeling at TSS regions related to *var* transcription (Petter *et al.*, 2011).

Besides histone modifications, other factors contribute to the silencing of *var* loci: Perez-Toledo and colleagues identified that heterochromatin protein 1 (HP1) associated to silenced chromatin attracted by H3K9me3 (see Figure 2, (Perez-Toledo *et al.*, 2009)). Great interest was caused by the detection of novel putative plant-like transcription factors ApiAP2 ((Balaji *et al.*, 2005), reviewed in (Painter *et al.*, 2011)). In a genome wide scan for binding sites of many members of the 27-member ApiAP2 family, three members consistently showed binding to sequences present in *var* promoters. While one (PfSIP2, PF3D7_0604100) seems to redirect certain *var* promoters via SPE2 motif binding to the nuclear periphery and has no influence on the activity of recognized *var* loci (Flueck *et al.*, 2010), the function of two other factors (PF3D7_1466400, PF3D7_1141100) which also bind elements in *var* promoters (Campbell *et al.*, 2010) were not reported so far. Obviously, the latter are strong candidates for being key regulators of *var* transcription and perhaps even mediators of allelic exclusion and should be tested by the available methods such as epitope tagging and conditional knockdown (de Azevedo *et al.*, 2012).

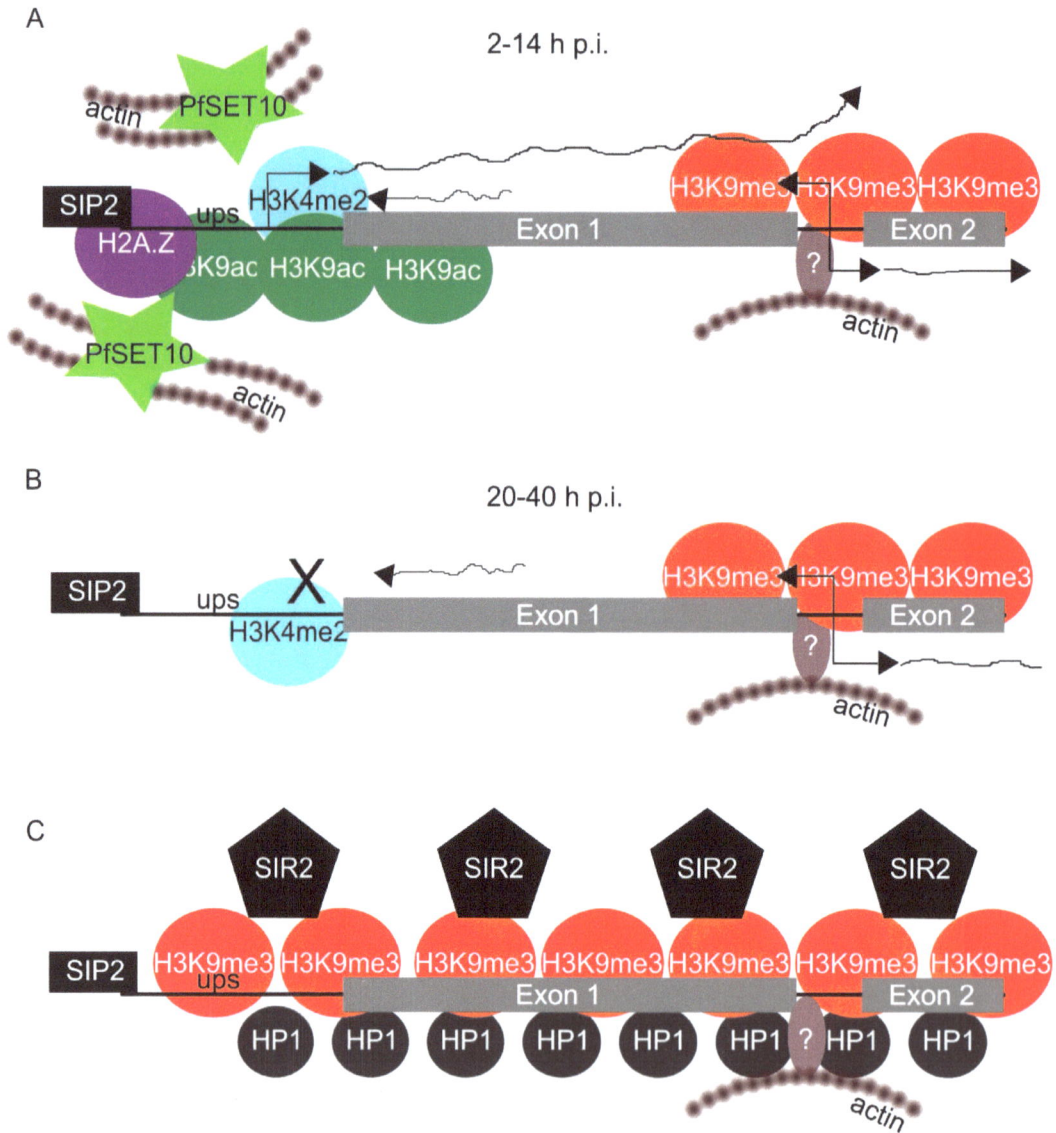

**Figure 2:** Hypothetical model of events at *var* loci, based on the data of different groups cited throughout the text. A: An active *var* locus (in ring stage parasites) with the presence of H3K9ac, H3k4me2, H2.AZ and PfSET10. Note that PfSIP2 associates to only upsB promoters. PfSET10 is associated to the active site and probably interacts with plasmodial actin as does a short sequence in the *var* intron, possibly via an unknown factor (marked as such). B: The same locus is shown now in late trophozoite/schizont stage parasites (20-40 h post reinvasion) with decreased H3K9ac (but also few H3K9me3) and the continued presence of H3K4me2 ("poised mark"). H2.AZ falls off the temporarily silenced but "poised" locus. C: A silenced *var* locus with the tight packing of H3K9me3 throughout the promoter and coding region with the co-association of PfSIR2 and HP1. Note that the *var* intron transcribes bi-directionally and possibly leads to dsRNA at some point in the active locus. There is experimental evidence for the indicated antisense *var* transcript in the 5' region of exon 1 (Raabe *et al.*, 2010). Transcripts are shown as irregular lines, while active promoters are indicated as straight lines with arrows. The model does not discern which unknown factor(s) lead to the transformation of an active to a silenced locus and vice-versa (switching) and does also not show spatial movements of *var* loci.

## 2.3  Nuclear Architecture, *Var* Loci Movement and Their Role in Allelic Exclusion

The human sleeping sickness parasite *Trypanosoma brucei* also employs variant surface glycoproteins (VSA) to escape the immune system (reviewed in (Rudenko, 2011)). This parasite developed a sophisticated system of genetic rearrangements by translocation of *vsg* genes into one of the 20 telomeric transcriptional activation sites, of which one is in fact active (mechanism reviewed in (Horn & McCulloch, 2010)). This exclusive transcription is apparently guaranteed by the fact that *vsg* genes are transcribed by RNA-polymerase 1 in the nucleolus. Thus, it is believed that there are spatial constraints which limit the access to transcription to one single transcription site (Navarro & Gull, 2001) and chromatin modifications at the active transcriptions site lead to the recruiting to the nucleolus (Rudenko, 2010). In *P. falciparum,* more than half of the *var* loci are in subtelomeric or telomeric position ((Fischer *et al.*, 1997; Gardner *et al.*, 2002), see Figure 1), and telomeres appear organized in "bouquets" in the nucleus (Freitas-Junior *et al.*, 2000). These also localize to heterochromatic regions and are linked via proteic factors (Marty *et al.*, 2006). Activation of loci involves movement out of a bouquet to a site in the nucleus where transcription may occur (Duraisingh *et al.*, 2005; Ralph *et al.*, 2005b). Recently, Zhang and colleagues showed that the *var* intron has a crucial role in the repositioning process, since they contain a short 18 bp segment which is able to recruit an actin-containing complex (Zhang *et al.*, 2011). Additionally, the Histone methyltransferase PfSET10, apparently a marker of the active transcription site of *var* genes, also associated to actin (Volz *et al.*, 2012). Telomeric regions were thoroughly studied in *P. falciparum* due to the massive presence of *var* genes and because they contain important repetitive regions that are not transcriptionally silent (Broadbent *et al.*, 2011; Sierra-Miranda *et al.*, 2012). Several novel factors, such as Alba proteins, are being detected that may play a role in variant gene regulation (Chene *et al.*, 2012; Goyal *et al.*, 2012). Despite of great advances in the visualization of nuclear structures (Weiner *et al.*, 2011) the visual mapping of transcription factories where *var* genes are transcribed is only becoming available now and will permit progress regarding this issue (Mancio-Silva & Scherf, 2013). It is also possible that there is a spatial link of the nuclear pores and *var* transcription sites, although no specific data are available yet. The simultaneous visualization of active *var* loci by Bromouracil staining and their co-localization with possibly involved nuclear factors such as Alba, ApiAP2 and other yet to be defined factors would be helpful to dissect events leading to the observed allelic exclusion.

## 2.4  Gene Silencing When There Is No RNAi: Are Non-Coding RNAs Involved in Plasmodial Variant Gene Regulation?

Another mostly unexplored mechanism for the regulation of gene expression in *Plasmodium sp.* is perhaps noncoding RNA. ncRNAs can be divided into structural ncRNAs and regulatory ncRNAs. Structural ncRNAs include ribosomal, transfer, small nuclear, and small nucleolar RNAs. Regulatory ncRNAs can be classified into microRNAs (miRNAs), Piwi-interacting RNAs (piRNAs), small interfering RNAs (siRNAs), and long non-coding RNAs (lncRNAs)(Ponting *et al.*, 2009). At least in *P. falciparum*, until now no hard evidence has been provided for miRNAs, piRNAs and siRNAs as well as for the related biochemical machinery (Baum *et al.*, 2009; Xue *et al.*, 2008) despite of earlier studies showing a putative RNAi-like effect in dsRNA-treated parasites (Gissot *et al.*, 2005; Malhotra *et al.*, 2002; McRobert & McConkey, 2002). On the other hand, there is significant antisense RNA production in the parasite (Patankar *et al.*, 2001; Raabe *et al.*, 2010) and the deep analysis of non-coding RNAs revealed that most of the *var* gene and *rif* gene loci showed antisense transcripts complementary to sequences near the 5' end of *var* and *rif* open reading frames ((Raabe *et al.*, 2010), see figure 2). Recent studies have shown that noncoding RNAs may play a role as transcriptional regulators in *P. falciparum*, regulating virulence genes (Broadbent *et al.*, 2011). Further, the association of noncoding RNAs with chromatin was accessed through ChIP-qPCR experiments, and this has revealed that anti-H3 antibodies efficiently co-immunoprecipitate RNA. This suggests that noncoding RNAs do play a role as regulators of *var* transcription (Epp *et al.*, 2009) by perhaps creating a link between DNA sequence, and chromatin-binding proteins as found in *Schizosaccharomyces pombe* (Harrison *et al.*, 2009). Two groups described the existence of long noncoding RNAs in *P. falciparum* and suggested a role in variant gene regulation at least in telomeric *var* genes (Broadbent *et al.*, 2011; Sierra-Miranda *et al.*, 2012). The picture however is far from clear and one can only speculate about mechanisms given the fact that antisense RNAs are detected from the majority of *var* loci including loci with active transcription (Ralph *et al.*, 2005a). Perhaps the formation of short double-strand products recruits the corresponding loci indirectly to PfSET10 proteins, while solely short antisense transcripts maintain *var* loci silent. The determination of localization and function of RNA and DNA-binding proteins, present in the plasmodial genome, may provide more insights into the complex regulation of the *var* gene family. Based on the information given before, we suggest in Figure 2 a hypothetical and still incomplete model for factors which contribute to activation or silencing of *var* promoters.

## 3    The Regulation of *P. Falciparum* Non-*Var* Gene Families: *Rif*, *Stevor*, Pfmc-TM2 and *Surf*

The largest variant gene family in *P. falciparum* is the *rif* (repetitive interspersed family) gene family, discovered in 1988 by Weber (Weber, 1988). The *rif* genes were recently classified based on sequence similarities and presence or absence of specific sequence motifs into two major groups (Joannin *et al.*, 2008). Initially described as exposed at the IRBC surface, this concept has been revised and it appears that one of the two subgroups of RIFIN is localized to the parasite built secretory machinery in the IRBC termed Maurer's clefts instead of the IRBC surface. Additionally, there is expression of several RIFINs at a time showing that strict allelic exclusion does not occur (Petter *et al.*, 2007). Several groups have addressed the transcription mode of *rif* genes which is much more difficult due to their similarity and their number: more than 200 *rif* genes are annotated in the *P. falciparum* 3D7 genome (plasmodb.org) and there is no phenotypic selection method as exists for the phenotypic selection of parasites which then transcribe determined *var* genes (Golnitz *et al.*, 2008; Salanti *et al.*, 2003). An initial report which detected simultaneously transcripts from *rif, stevor* and *var* genes postulated that *rif* genes are transcribed in a tightly period 16-24h in the erythrocytic cycle (Kyes *et al.*, 2000; Kyes *et al.*, 1999). This concept was revised when genome wide analysis methods became available. In fact, several *rif* genes were simultaneously transcribed in parasites and the majority of *rif* genes is potentially transcribed in young trophozoite stage or schizont stage parasites (Wang *et al.*, 2009). In an attempt to understand control aspects of *rif* regulation, Tham and colleagues mapped sequence elements in a *rif* promoter. In the region −870 to −860 upstream of the *rif* TSS, the *CGCACAACAC* element appears to function as a repressor element since its absence led to an increase of transcription. Using EMSA, it was shown that yet unknown binding factor(s) may exert repressive effects. In addition, another repressive element, *TATGCAatgATT* was characterized in the region −356 to −562 upstream of the TSS, and this is also a target of proteic transcriptional regulators (Tham *et al.*, 2007). This work also provided evidence that *rif* transcription is not related to *var* transcription although it is also regulated by PfSIR2 (Duraisingh *et al.*, 2005) suggesting that even in the neighborhood of a transcriptionally active *var* gene, *rif* genes may not be transcribed maintaining their chromatin in a closed state (Tham *et al.*, 2007). Intriguingly, the study by Campbell *et al.* regarding ApiAP2 factors did not depict specifically any ApiAP2-binding sites in *rif* promoters/5' upstream regions (Campbell *et al.*, 2010).

Clonally variant families in *P. falciparum* are frequently subjected to transcriptional switching and *rif* genes are no exception. When monitoring *rif* transcription in a RT-qPCR approach using *rif* specific primers in differently adhesive 3D7 *P. falciparum* parasite lines, we could show that a number of different or identical *rif* genes are simultaneously transcribed in each adhesive phenotype and a high rate of switching was observed after several reinvasions, much higher than described for any experiment looking at *var* gene transcription, although persistence of some *rif* transcripts was also observed (Cabral & Wunderlich, 2009). Importantly, we and others observed the persistence of PFD0070c - a type rif2A - in different adhesive phenotypes (Cabral & Wunderlich, 2009; Wang *et al.*, 2009). Given the fact that i) *rif* transcription occurs at different times throughout the asexual erythrocytic cycle, ii) a number of *rif* transcripts are found at any given timepoint, and iii) transcription may even extend to other stages such as the sporozoite stage where RIFINs were detected (Lasonder *et al.*, 2002) it is suggestive that *var* and *rif* controlling factors may differ. In two other gene families, namely *stevor* and *Pfmc-2TM* switching rates were also measured. Although both gene families belong to the same superfamily (Sam-Yellowe *et al.*, 2004), switching rates were quite lower than those that we observed for *rif* genes (Lavazec *et al.*, 2007). In genome wide ChIP-on-Chip assays, *rif* (as also *stevor* and *Pfmc-2TM*, but not *surf*) genes showed similar histone marks as *var* genes (Lopez-Rubio *et al.*, 2009; Salcedo-Amaya *et al.*, 2009), indicating that *rif* promoter associated factors recruit the same histone modifying factors as *var*-locus associated factors, while *surf* genes are regulated in another manner. It was recently investigated that *rif* neighboring chromatin regions are also under control of the PfSIR2B histone deacetilase, indicating the reversible character of histone modification in *rif* promoters (Tonkin *et al.*, 2009). In another study, it was shown that reversible histone modification also controls *rif* expression, and the modification remains stable after several reinvasions (Cabral *et al.*, 2012). In our hands, *rif* genes which showed high transcript quantities were associated dominantly with acetylated H3K9. In contrast, silent *rif* loci seemed preferentially methylated (H3K9me3), coinciding with the previous epigenome results (Lopez-Rubio *et al.*, 2009; Salcedo-Amaya *et al.*, 2009). We also tested the possibility for poised states controlling *rif* transcription. After ChIP using H3K4me2, the mark for poised *var* genes in schizont stage parasites, we observed that dimethylation at H3K4 in trophozoites was correlated to active transcription in the later schizont stages, reminiscent of the modifications observed for *var* genes.

Two important studies addressed the question if *var* and *rif* transcription could be cross-influenced in parasites transfected with constructs containing either *var, rif, stevor* or *Pfmc-2TM* promoters driving transcription of drug resistance genes, similar to the approach used by Voss and colleagues in their 2006 paper (Voss *et al.*, 2006). A cross-influence would favor the hypothesis of a common variant gene transcription site in the nucleus, keeping in mind that *var* loci move to specific regions during their activation and that this site may pose a spatial limit to the transcription of several variant genes perhaps carrying the same "marked for transcription" recruiting factors. While one study showed that dominant transcription from a *var* promoter also suppressed endogenous *rif* and *stevor* transcripts and vice versa, but not *Pfmc-2TM* (Howitt *et al.*, 2009), another study did not find such a relation (Witmer *et al.*, 2012). The study by Witmer et al. also clearly showed that there is really no strict allelic exclusion neither in *rif* nor in *stevor* transcription (Lopez-Rubio *et al.*, 2009; Salcedo-Amaya *et al.*, 2009). However, both studies used transfected parasite lines with episomal bi-cistronic plasmid constructs which are known to concatemerize into multiple-copy molecules (Frank *et al.*, 2006), which then leads to the artificial increase of active promoter loci per cell. Different studies have found up to 20 plasmid copies per transfected cell (for example (Epp *et al.*, 2008)). Also, none of the studies took into account that different *rif* genes are transcribed at different time points, turning it possible that *rif* genes are regulated in clusters. For example, it is possible the *rif* genes which encode erythrocyte surface localized RIFINs are regulated independently from *rif* genes that encode Maurer's clefts-resident RIFINs. Another possibility is that ring stage/schizont stage-transcribed *rif* genes are transcribed in a coordinated way and independently from trophozoite-transcribed *rif* genes, which are accordingly transcribed in a coordinated way. An accurate way to unambiguously show the interplay between any given promoter would be the use of different *rif* promoters in the context of the recently described artificial chromosome (Iwanaga *et al.,* 2010; Iwanaga *et al.*, 2012) which occur mostly as a single copy per cell. Any variant gene promoter driving an antibiotic resistance gene would then be present and transcribed in genuine quantities upon addition of the specific antibiotic. This would permit realistic comparisons between *rif* transcript quantities from all loci and the artificial locus at different time points in the erythrocytic cycle. The artificial chromosome approach would also permit FISH-colocalization experiments showing if proteins involved in *var* transcription (HP1, PfSET10, Alba and others) do associate or not to active *rif* promoters.

The small family of *surf* genes was described for the first time in 2005 (Winter *et al.*, 2005) has not yet been the object of more detailed studies regarding their transcription. It is unclear if SURFIN form typical variant antigen families since different SURFINs are much more conserved between different strains than *var, rif* and *stevor* genes. The role of the SURFIN antigens is far from clear and to date the localization of only 2 alleles, SURFIN 4.1 e 4.2, has been thoroughly studied (Mphande *et al.*, 2008; Winter *et al.*, 2005). The knockout of SURFIN 4.2 (PF3D7_0424400) slightly reduced the rigidity of IRBC (Maier *et al.*, 2008). Preliminary and unpublished results from our lab point to the possibility of constitutive expression of SURFIN 4.1 and transcriptional switching of at least two other *surf* genes when parasites were grown *in vitro* for 20-40 reinvasions. Taking into account that *surf* genes are not marked by the variant gene family-typical histone modifications H3K9me3/H3K9ac, additional mechanisms would be at work if there is a phenomenon such as transcriptional switching and/or allelic exclusion.

### 3.1   PIR Family Expression in *P. Vivax* and Murine Species

In comparison to *var* genes the expression of *pir* genes in species other than *P. falciparum* has been studied in much less detail. The most widely distributed parasite species *P. vivax* possesses variant proteins of the PIR superfamily, and these were termed VIR antigens (del Portillo *et al.*, 2001). The sequencing of the *P. vivax* genome (Salvador 1 strain) revealed that there are 346 *vir* genes which can be clustered in 5 different subfamilies (Carlton *et al.,* 2008), some of which contain genes with and others without the canonic IRBC export signal VTS/PEXEL (**V**acuolar **t**ransport **s**ignal/*Plasmodium* **ex**port **el**ement, (Hiller *et al.*, 2004; Marti *et al.*, 2004) indicating that similar to RIFINs VIR proteins may localize partially inside the cytosol of the IRBC and at its surface, which was indeed found (Bernabeu *et al.*, 2011). Due to the difficulty of culturing *P. vivax*, to date there is only one study that approached the transcription of *vir* genes using PCR with degenerated primers for different *vir* subfamilies followed by clone sequencing (Fernandez-Becerra *et al.*, 2005). Using single cell PCR and subfamily specific antibodies to VIR subfamilies, this study showed an expression pattern similar to RIFINs and different VIRs were identified in single IRBC. Again, due to the difficulty of *in vitro* culture, no study exists regarding transcriptional switching, epigenetic aspects or factors involved in the control of *vir* genes although ApiAP2 proteins are also conserved in this species (Painter *et al.*, 2011).

Relatively few data exist on the regulation of murine *Plasmodium* species *pir* control, which are present in all currently used murine models. Given the cytoadhesive properties of species such as *P. berghei* (Kaul *et al.*, 1994) or *P. chabaudi* (Mota *et al.*, 2000), it is still unclear if BIR or CIR proteins mediate this effect. However, it was shown that *pir* transcription is modulated and may change depending on the site (e.g. parasites in different organs transcribe different *pir* genes (Ebbinghaus & Krucken, 2011)) and over time (Cunningham *et al.*, 2009). Also, there is transcriptional switching apparently driven by the murine immune response (Cunningham *et al.*, 2005). In a recent attempt using a proteomic approach and transgenic parasites, the receptor for cytoadherence in *P. berghei* was not identified, but proteins which are responsible for the transport of proteins, including possible ligands, to the IRBC surface *(Fonager et al.*, 2012). The transcription mode of *pir* genes is somehow similar to *rif* genes with a group of genes being expressed schizont stage parasites (*cir, bir* (Janssen *et al.*, 2002)) or in ring stage and schizonts (*vir, cir, bir* (Carlton *et al.*, 2008; Cunningham *et al.*, 2009)) and others in trophozoites (*yir*, (Fonager *et al.*, 2007)), while the remaining loci remain silenced. Fonager and colleagues detected alternative splicing in the *yir* family and suggest epigenetic mechanisms of expression control (Fonager *et al.*, 2007), however, to our knowledge no ChIP experiments were performed with any murine *Plasmodium* species. It is tempting to speculate that *pir* genes from different species are controlled by similar factors and the elucidation of these factors may ultimately lead to a novel point of intervention against *P. vivax*.

# 4    Conclusion and Future Directions

The expression of variant proteins by *Plasmodium* has evolved as a strategy for survival or persistence in at least the mammalian host. Although only for one variant protein family the function seems clear (PfEMP1 encoded by *var* genes), several reports showed that there is immune recognition of RIFINs (Abdel-Latif *et al.*, 2002) and PIR and that absence of the latter proteins leads to a decrease in parasite survival in the host (Fonager *et al.*, 2012). The absence of PfEMP1 in natural infections was never tested for ethical reasons but it can be estimated that PfEMP1 is absolutely necessary for the survival in an immune competent human host with an intact spleen. As shown above, many data were accumulated regarding the *var* gene transcription, permitting to formulate a hypothesis explaining how *var* transcription is orchestrated. However, the picture for the other variant gene families with apparent relevance in antigenic variation is still largely undefined. We expect that the factors involved in *rif* or *pir* transcription will be identified and validated, probably by the use of novel techniques such as artificial chromosomes or more efficient knockdown/conditional knockouts. Finally, the detection of factors that control expression, especially the novel plant-like transcription factors of the ApiAP2 family, are expected to produce tools for intervention against the parasite. The perturbation specifically of the antigenic variation either by i) breaking the transcriptional repression of all variant antigens leading to a fast antigenic exhaustion of circulating parasites or ii) the complete repression of any variant gene expression leading probably to accelerated spleen clearance, would in turn help the infected host to rapidly eliminate circulating parasites.

## Acknowledgements

Research in GWs lab is/was supported by grants from FAPESP, PRONEX-CNPq and CAPES and FJC and WLF are supported by fellowships from CAPES and FAPESP, respectively.

## References

Abdel-Latif, M. S., Khattab, A., Lindenthal, C., Kremsner, P. G., Klinkert, M. Q. (2002). Recognition of variant Rifin antigens by human antibodies induced during natural Plasmodium falciparum infections. Infection and Immunity, 70, 7013-7021.

Amulic, B., Salanti, A., Lavstsen, T., Nielsen, M. A., Deitsch, K. W. (2009). An upstream open reading frame controls translation of var2csa, a gene implicated in placental malaria. PLoS Pathogens, 5, e1000256.

Andrews, K. T., Tran, T. N., Fairlie, D. P. (2012). Towards histone deacetylase inhibitors as new antimalarial drugs. Current Pharmaceutical Design, 18, 3467-3479.

Balaji, S., Babu, M. M., Iyer, L. M., Aravind, L. (2005). Discovery of the principal specific transcription factors of Apicomplexa and their implication for the evolution of the AP2-integrase DNA binding domains. Nucleic Acids Research, 33, 3994-4006.

Barry, J. D., Graham, S. V., Fotheringham, M., Graham, V. S., Kobryn, K., Wymer, B. (1998). VSG gene control and infectivity strategy of metacyclic stage Trypanosoma brucei. Molecular and Biochemical Parasitology, 91, 93-105.

Bartfai, R., Hoeijmakers, W. A., Salcedo-Amaya, A. M., Smits, A. H., Janssen-Megens, E., Kaan, A., Treeck, M., Gilberger, T. W., Francoijs, K. J., Stunnenberg, H. G. (2010). H2A.Z demarcates intergenic regions of the plasmodium falciparum epigenome that are dynamically marked by H3K9ac and H3K4me3. PLoS Pathogens, 6, e1001223.

Baruch, D. I., Pasloske, B. L., Singh, H. B., Bi, X., Ma, X. C., Feldman, M., Taraschi, T. F., Howard, R. J. (1995). Cloning the P. falciparum gene encoding PfEMP1, a malarial variant antigen and adherence receptor on the surface of parasitized human erythrocytes. Cell, 82, 77-87.

Baum, J., Papenfuss, A. T., Mair, G. R., Janse, C. J., Vlachou, D., Waters, A. P., Cowman, A. F., Crabb, B. S., de Koning-Ward, T. F. (2009). Molecular genetics and comparative genomics reveal RNAi is not functional in malaria parasites. Nucleic Acids Research, 37, 3788-3798.

Berger, S. L. (2007). The complex language of chromatin regulation during transcription. Nature, 447, 407-412.

Bernabeu, M., Lopez, F. J., Ferrer, M., Martin-Jaular, L., Razaname, A., Corradin, G., Maier, A. G., Del Portillo, H. A., Fernandez-Becerra, C. (2011). Functional analysis of Plasmodium vivax VIR proteins reveals different subcellular localizations and cytoadherence to the ICAM-1 endothelial receptor. Cellular Microbiology, 14, 386-400.

Brancucci, N. M., Witmer, K., Schmid, C. D., Flueck, C., Voss, T. S. (2012). Identification of a cis-acting DNA-protein interaction implicated in singular var gene choice in Plasmodium falciparum. Cellular Microbiology. doi: 10.1111/cmi.12004. [Epub ahead of print].

Broadbent, K. M., Park, D., Wolf, A. R., Van Tyne, D., Sims, J. S., Ribacke, U., Volkman, S., Duraisingh, M., Wirth, D., Sabeti, P. C., Rinn, J. L. (2011). A global transcriptional analysis of Plasmodium falciparum malaria reveals a novel family of telomere-associated lncRNAs. Genome Biology, 12, R56.

Bull, P. C., Berriman, M., Kyes, S., Quail, M. A., Hall, N., Kortok, M. M., Marsh, K., Newbold, C. I. (2005). Plasmodium falciparum variant surface antigen expression patterns during malaria. PLoS Pathogens, 1, e26.

Cabral, F. J., Wunderlich, G. (2009). Transcriptional memory and switching in the Plasmodium falciparumrif gene family. Molecular and Biochemical Parasitology, 168, 186-190.

Cabral, F. J., Fotoran, W. L., Wunderlich, G. (2012). Dynamic activation and repression of the plasmodium falciparum rif gene family and their relation to chromatin modification. PLoS ONE, 7, e29881.

Calderwood, M. S., Gannoun-Zaki, L., Wellems, T. E., Deitsch, K. W. (2003). Plasmodium falciparum var genes are regulated by two regions with separate promoters, one upstream of the coding region and a second within the intron. Journal of Biochemical Chemistry, 278, 34125-34132.

Campbell, T. L., De Silva, E. K., Olszewski, K. L., Elemento, O., Llinas, M. (2010). Identification and genome-wide prediction of DNA binding specificities for the ApiAP2 family of regulators from the malaria parasite. PLoS Pathogens, 6, e1001165.

Carlton, J. M., Adams, J. H., Silva, J. C., Bidwell, S. L., Lorenzi, H., Caler, E., Crabtree, J., Angiuoli, S. V., Merino, E. F., Amedeo, P., Cheng, Q., Coulson, R. M., Crabb, B. S., Del Portillo, H. A., Essien, K., Feldblyum, T. V., Fernandez-Becerra, C., Gilson, P. R., Gueye, A. H., Guo, X., Kang'a, S., Kooij, T. W., Korsinczky, M., Meyer, E. V., Nene, V., Paulsen, I., White, O., Ralph, S. A., Ren, Q., Sargeant, T. J., Salzberg, S. L., Stoeckert, C. J., Sullivan, S. A., Yamamoto, M. M., Hoffman, S. L., Wortman, J. R., Gardner, M. J., Galinski, M. R., Barnwell, J. W., Fraser-Liggett, C. M. (2008). Comparative genomics of the neglected human malaria parasite Plasmodium vivax. Nature, 455, 757-763.

Carvalho, B. O., Lopes, S. C., Nogueira, P. A., Orlandi, P. P., Bargieri, D. Y., Blanco, Y. C., Mamoni, R., Leite, J. A., Rodrigues, M. M., Soares, I. S., Oliveira, T. R., Wunderlich, G., Lacerda, M. V., del Portillo, H. A., Araujo, M. O., Russell, B., Suwanarusk, R., Snounou, G., Renia, L., Costa, F. T. (2010). On the cytoadhesion of Plasmodium vivax-infected erythrocytes. Journal of Infectious Diseases, 202, 638-647.

Chaal, B. K., Gupta, A. P., Wastuwidyaningtyas, B. D., Luah, Y. H., Bozdech, Z. (2010). Histone deacetylases play a major role in the transcriptional regulation of the Plasmodium falciparum life cycle. PLoS Pathogens, 6, e1000737.

Chen, Q., Fernandez, V., Sundstrom, A., Schlichtherle, M., Datta, S., Hagblom, P., Wahlgren, M. (1998). Developmental selection of var gene expression in Plasmodium falciparum. Nature, 394, 392-395.

Chene, A., Vembar, S. S., Riviere, L., Lopez-Rubio, J. J., Claes, A., Siegel, T. N., Sakamoto, H., Scheidig-Benatar, C., Hernandez-Rivas, R., Scherf, A. (2012). PfAlbas constitute a new eukaryotic DNA/RNA-binding protein family in malaria parasites. Nucleic Acids Research, 40, 3066-3077.

Cheng, Q., Cloonan, N., Fischer, K., Thompson, J., Waine, G., Lanzer, M., Saul, A. (1998). stevor and rif are Plasmodium falciparum multicopy gene families which potentially encode variant antigens. Molecular and Biochemical Parasitology, 97, 161-176.

Chookajorn, T., Dzikowski, R., Frank, M., Li, F., Jiwani, A. Z., Hartl, D. L., Deitsch, K. W. (2007). Epigenetic memory at malaria virulence genes. Proceedings of the National Academy of Sciences U S A, 104, 899-902.

Cowman, A. F., Crabb, B. S. (2006). Invasion of red blood cells by malaria parasites. Cell, 124, 755-766.

Croken, M. M., Nardelli, S. C., Kim, K. (2012). Chromatin modifications, epigenetics, and how protozoan parasites regulate their lives. Trends in Parasitology, 28, 202-213.

Cui, L., Fan, Q., Cui, L., Miao, J. (2008). Histone lysine methyltransferases and demethylases in Plasmodium falciparum. International Journal of Parasitology, 38, 1083-1097.

Cui, L., Miao, J. (2010). Chromatin-mediated epigenetic regulation in the malaria parasite Plasmodium falciparum. Eukaryot Cell, 9, 1138-1149.

Cunningham, D., Fonager, J., Jarra, W., Carret, C., Preiser, P., Langhorne, J. (2009). Rapid changes in transcription profiles of the Plasmodium yoelii yir multigene family in clonal populations: lack of epigenetic memory? PLoS One, 4, e4285.

Cunningham, D. A., Jarra, W., Koernig, S., Fonager, J., Fernandez-Reyes, D., Blythe, J. E., Waller, C., Preiser, P. R., Langhorne, J. (2005). Host immunity modulates transcriptional changes in a multigene family (yir) of rodent malaria. Molecular Microbiology, 58, 636-647.

de Azevedo, M. F., Gilson, P. R., Gabriel, H. B., Simoes, R. F., Angrisano, F., Baum, J., Crabb, B. S., Wunderlich, G. (2012). Systematic analysis of FKBP inducible degradation domain tagging strategies for the human malaria parasite Plasmodium falciparum. PLoS One, 7, e40981.

Deitsch, K. W., Calderwood, M. S., Wellems, T. E. (2001). Malaria. Cooperative silencing elements in var genes. Nature, 412, 875-876.

Deitsch, K. W., Hviid, L. (2004). Variant surface antigens, virulence genes and the pathogenesis of malaria. Trends Parasitol, 20, 562-566.

del Portillo, H. A., Fernandez-Becerra, C., Bowman, S., Oliver, K., Preuss, M., Sanchez, C. P., Schneider, N. K., Villalobos, J. M., Rajandream, M. A., Harris, D., Pereira da Silva, L. H., Barrell, B., Lanzer, M. (2001). A superfamily of variant genes encoded in the subtelomeric region of Plasmodium vivax. Nature, 410, 839-842.

Donelson, J. E. (1995). Mechanisms of antigenic variation in Borrelia hermsii and African trypanosomes. Journal of Biochemical Chemistry, 270, 7783-7786.

Duraisingh, M. T., Voss, T. S., Marty, A. J., Duffy, M. F., Good, R. T., Thompson, J. K., Freitas-Junior, L. H., Scherf, A., Crabb, B. S., Cowman, A. Г. (2005). Heterochromatin silencing and locus repositioning linked to regulation of virulence genes in Plasmodium falciparum. Cell, 121, 13-24.

Dzikowski, R., Frank, M., Deitsch, K. (2006). Mutually exclusive expression of virulence genes by malaria parasites is regulated independently of antigen production. PLoS Pathogens, 2, e22.

Ebbinghaus, P., Krucken, J. (2011). Characterization and tissue-specific expression patterns of the Plasmodium chabaudi cir multigene family. Malaria Journal, 10, 272.

Enderes, C., Kombila, D., Dal-Bianco, M., Dzikowski, R., Kremsner, P., Frank, M. (2011). Var Gene promoter activation in clonal Plasmodium falciparum isolates follows a hierarchy and suggests a conserved switching program that is independent of genetic background. Journal of Infectious Diseases, 204, 1620-1631.

Epp, C., Raskolnikov, D., Deitsch, K. W. (2008). A regulatable transgene expression system for cultured Plasmodium falciparum parasites. Malaria Journal, 7, 86.

Epp, C., Li, F., Howitt, C. A., Chookajorn, T., Deitsch, K. W. (2009). Chromatin associated sense and antisense noncoding RNAs are transcribed from the var gene family of virulence genes of the malaria parasite Plasmodium falciparum. RNA, 15, 116-127.

Fan, Q., An, L., Cui, L. (2004). Plasmodium falciparum histone acetyltransferase, a yeast GCN5 homologue involved in chromatin remodeling. Eukaryotic Cell, 3, 264-276.

Fang, J., Hogan, G. J., Liang, G., Lieb, J. D., Zhang, Y. (2007). The Saccharomyces cerevisiae histone demethylase Jhd1 fine-tunes the distribution of H3K36me2. Molecular and Cellular Biology, 27, 5055-5065.

Farrow, R. E., Green, J., Katsimitsoulia, Z., Taylor, W. R., Holder, A. A., Molloy, J. E. (2011). The mechanism of erythrocyte invasion by the malarial parasite, Plasmodium falciparum. Seminars in Cellular and Developmental Biology, 22, 953-960.

Fernandez-Becerra, C., Pein, O., de Oliveira, T. R., Yamamoto, M. M., Cassola, A. C., Rocha, C., Soares, I. S., de Braganca Pereira, C. A., del Portillo, H. A. (2005). Variant proteins of Plasmodium vivax are not clonally expressed in natural infections. Molecular Microbiology, 58, 648-658.

Fischer, K., Horrocks, P., Preuss, M., Wiesner, J., Wunsch, S., Camargo, A. A., Lanzer, M. (1997). Expression of var genes located within polymorphic subtelomeric domains of Plasmodium falciparum chromosomes. Molecular and Cellular Biology, 17, 3679-3686.

Flueck, C., Bartfai, R., Niederwieser, I., Witmer, K., Alako, B. T., Moes, S., Bozdech, Z., Jenoe, P., Stunnenberg, H. G., Voss, T. S. (2010). A major role for the Plasmodium falciparum ApiAP2 protein PfSIP2 in chromosome end biology. PLoS Pathogens, 6, e1000784.

Fonager, J., Cunningham, D., Jarra, W., Koernig, S., Henneman, A. A., Langhorne, J., Preiser, P. (2007). Transcription and alternative splicing in the yir multigene family of the malaria parasite Plasmodium y. yoelii: identification of motifs suggesting epigenetic and post-transcriptional control of RNA expression. Molecular and Biochemical Parasitology, 156, 1-11.

Fonager, J., Pasini, E. M., Braks, J. A., Klop, O., Ramesar, J., Remarque, E. J., Vroegrijk, I. O., van Duinen, S. G., Thomas, A. W., Khan, S. M., Mann, M., Kocken, C. H., Janse, C. J., Franke-Fayard, B. M. (2012). Reduced CD36-dependent tissue sequestration of Plasmodium-infected erythrocytes is detrimental to malaria parasite growth in vivo. Journal of Experimental Medicine, 209, 93-107.

Fowler, E. V., Peters, J. M., Gatton, M. L., Chen, N., Cheng, Q. (2002). Genetic diversity of the DBLalpha region in Plasmodium falciparum var genes among Asia-Pacific isolates. Molecular and Biochemical Parasitology, 120, 117-126.

Frank, M., Dzikowski, R., Costantini, D., Amulic, B., Berdougo, E., Deitsch, K. (2006). Strict pairing of var promoters and introns is required for var gene silencing in the malaria parasite Plasmodium falciparum. Journal of Biochemical Chemistry, 281, 9942-9952.

Frank, M., Dzikowski, R., Amulic, B., Deitsch, K. (2007). Variable switching rates of malaria virulence genes are associated with chromosomal position. Molecular Microbiology, 64, 1486-1498.

Freitas-Junior, L. H., Bottius, E., Pirrit, L. A., Deitsch, K. W., Scheidig, C., Guinet, F., Nehrbass, U., Wellems, T. E., Scherf, A. (2000). Frequent ectopic recombination of virulence factor genes in telomeric chromosome clusters of P. falciparum. Nature, 407, 1018-1022.

Freitas-Junior, L. H., Hernandez-Rivas, R., Ralph, S. A., Montiel-Condado, D., Ruvalcaba-Salazar, O. K., Rojas-Meza, A. P., Mancio-Silva, L., Leal-Silvestre, R. J., Gontijo, A. M., Shorte, S., Scherf, A. (2005). Telomeric heterochromatin propagation and histone acetylation control mutually exclusive expression of antigenic variation genes in malaria parasites. Cell, 121, 25-36.

French, J. B., Cen, Y., Sauve, A. A. (2008). Plasmodium falciparum Sir2 is an NAD+-dependent deacetylase and an acetyllysine-dependent and acetyllysine-independent NAD+ glycohydrolase. Biochemistry, 47, 10227-10239.

Gardner, M. J., Hall, N., Fung, E., White, O., Berriman, M., Hyman, R. W., Carlton, J. M., Pain, A., Nelson, K. E., Bowman, S., Paulsen, I. T., James, K., Eisen, J. A., Rutherford, K., Salzberg, S. L., Craig, A., Kyes, S., Chan, M. S., Nene, V., Shallom, S. J., Suh, B., Peterson, J., Angiuoli, S., Pertea, M., Allen, J., Selengut, J., Haft, D., Mather, M. W., Vaidya, A. B., Martin, D. M., Fairlamb, A. H., Fraunholz, M. J., Roos, D. S., Ralph, S. A., McFadden, G. I., Cummings, L. M., Subramanian, G. M., Mungall, C., Venter, J. C., Carucci, D. J., Hoffman, S. L., Newbold, C., Davis, R. W., Fraser, C. M., Barrell, B. (2002). Genome sequence of the human malaria parasite Plasmodium falciparum. Nature, 419, 498-511.

Gasser, S. M., Cockell, M. M. (2001). The molecular biology of the SIR proteins. Gene, 279, 1-16.

Ghosh, A. K., Jacobs-Lorena, M. (2009). Plasmodium sporozoite invasion of the mosquito salivary gland. Current Opinion in Microbiology, 12, 394-400.

Gissot, M., Briquet, S., Refour, P., Boschet, C., Vaquero, C. (2005). PfMyb1, a Plasmodium falciparum transcription factor, is required for intra-erythrocytic growth and controls key genes for cell cycle regulation. Journal of Molecular Biology, 346, 29-42.

Golnitz, U., Albrecht, L., Wunderlich, G. (2008). Var transcription profiling of Plasmodium falciparum 3D7: assignment of cytoadherent phenotypes to dominant transcripts. Malaria Journal, 7, 14.

Gotta, M., Strahl-Bolsinger, S., Renauld, H., Laroche, T., Kennedy, B. K., Grunstein, M., Gasser, S. M. (1997). Localization of Sir2p: the nucleolus as a compartment for silent information regulators. EMBO J, 16, 3243-3255.

Goyal, M., Alam, A., Iqbal, M. S., Dey, S., Bindu, S., Pal, C., Banerjee, A., Chakrabarti, S., Bandyopadhyay, U. (2012). Identification and molecular characterization of an Alba-family protein from human malaria parasite Plasmodium falciparum. Nucleic Acids Research, 40, 1174-1190.

Guerra, C. A., Gikandi, P. W., Tatem, A. J., Noor, A. M., Smith, D. L., Hay, S. I., Snow, R. W. (2008). The limits and intensity of Plasmodium falciparum transmission: implications for malaria control and elimination worldwide. PLoS Medicine, 5, e38.

Guerra, C. A., Howes, R. E., Patil, A. P., Gething, P. W., Van Boeckel, T. P., Temperley, W. H., Kabaria, C. W., Tatem, A. J., Manh, B. H., Elyazar, I. R., Baird, J. K., Snow, R. W., Hay, S. I. (2010). The international limits and population at risk of Plasmodium vivax transmission in 2009. PLoS Neglected Tropical Diseases, 4, e774.

Harrison, B. R., Yazgan, O., Krebs, J. E. (2009). Life without RNAi: noncoding RNAs and their functions in Saccharomyces cerevisiae. Biochemical Cell Biology, 87, 767-779.

Hiller, N. L., Bhattacharjee, S., van Ooij, C., Liolios, K., Harrison, T., Lopez-Estrano, C., Haldar, K. (2004). A host-targeting signal in virulence proteins reveals a secretome in malarial infection. Science, 306, 1934-1937.

Horn, D., McCulloch, R. (2010). Molecular mechanisms underlying the control of antigenic variation in African trypanosomes. Current Opinion in Microbiology, 13, 700-705.

Horrocks, P., Pinches, R., Christodoulou, Z., Kyes, S. A., Newbold, C. I. (2004). Variable var transition rates underlie antigenic variation in malaria. Proceedings of the National Academy of Sciences U S A, 101, 11129-11134.

Howitt, C. A., Wilinski, D., Llinas, M., Templeton, T. J., Dzikowski, R., Deitsch, K. W. (2009). Clonally variant gene families in Plasmodium falciparum share a common activation factor. Molecular Microbiology, 73, 1171-1185.

Iwanaga, S., Khan, S. M., Kaneko, I., Christodoulou, Z., Newbold, C., Yuda, M., Janse, C. J., Waters, A. P. (2010). Functional identification of the Plasmodium centromere and generation of a Plasmodium artificial chromosome. Cell Host & Microbe, 7, 245-255.

Iwanaga, S., Kato, T., Kaneko, I., Yuda, M. (2012). Centromere plasmid: a new genetic tool for the study of Plasmodium falciparum. PLoS ONE, 7, e33326.

Janssen, C. S., Barrett, M. P., Turner, C. M., Phillips, R. S. (2002). A large gene family for putative variant antigens shared by human and rodent malaria parasites. Proceedings in Biological Sciences, 269, 431-436.

Janssen, C. S., Phillips, R. S., Turner, C. M., Barrett, M. P. (2004). Plasmodium interspersed repeats: the major multigene superfamily of malaria parasites. Nucleic Acids Research, 32, 5712-5720.

Joannin, N., Abhiman, S., Sonnhammer, E. L., Wahlgren, M. (2008). Sub-grouping and sub-functionalization of the RIFIN multi-copy protein family. BMC Genomics, 9, 19.

Joshi, M. B., Lin, D. T., Chiang, P. H., Goldman, N. D., Fujioka, H., Aikawa, M., Syin, C. (1999). Molecular cloning and nuclear localization of a histone deacetylase homologue in Plasmodium falciparum. Molecular and Biochemical Parasitology, 99, 11-19.

Kaestli, M., Cortes, A., Lagog, M., Ott, M., Beck, H. P. (2004). Longitudinal assessment of Plasmodium falciparum var gene transcription in naturally infected asymptomatic children in Papua New Guinea. Journal of Infectious Diseases, 189, 1942-1951.

Kaul, D. K., Nagel, R. L., Llena, J. F., Shear, H. L. (1994). Cerebral malaria in mice: demonstration of cytoadherence of infected red blood cells and microrheologic correlates. American Journal for Tropical Medicine and Hygiene, 50, 512-521.

Kyes, S., Pinches, R., Newbold, C. (2000). A simple RNA analysis method shows var and rif multigene family expression patterns in Plasmodium falciparum. Molecular and Biochemical Parasitology, 105, 311-315.

Kyes, S., Christodoulou, Z., Pinches, R., Kriek, N., Horrocks, P., Newbold, C. (2007). Plasmodium falciparum var gene expression is developmentally controlled at the level of RNA polymerase II-mediated transcription initiation. Molecular Microbiology, 63, 1237-1247.

Kyes, S. A., Rowe, J. A., Kriek, N., Newbold, C. I. (1999). Rifins: a second family of clonally variant proteins expressed on the surface of red cells infected with Plasmodium falciparum. Proceedings of the National Academy of Sciences U S A, 96, 9333-9338.

Lasonder, E., Ishihama, Y., Andersen, J. S., Vermunt, A. M., Pain, A., Sauerwein, R. W., Eling, W. M., Hall, N., Waters, A. P., Stunnenberg, H. G., Mann, M. (2002). Analysis of the Plasmodium falciparum proteome by high-accuracy mass spectrometry. Nature, 419, 537-542.

Lavazec, C., Sanyal, S., Templeton, T. J. (2007). Expression switching in the stevor and Pfmc-2TM superfamilies in Plasmodium falciparum. Molecular Microbiology, 64, 1621-1634.

Lavstsen, T., Salanti, A., Jensen, A. T., Arnot, D. E., Theander, T. G. (2003). Sub-grouping of Plasmodium falciparum 3D7 var genes based on sequence analysis of coding and non-coding regions. Malaria Journal, 2, 27.

Leech, J. H., Barnwell, J. W., Miller, L. H., Howard, R. J. (1984). Identification of a strain-specific malarial antigen exposed on the surface of Plasmodium falciparum-infected erythrocytes. Journal of Experimental Medicine, 159, 1567-1575.

Lopez-Rubio, J. J., Gontijo, A. M., Nunes, M. C., Issar, N., Hernandez Rivas, R., Scherf, A. (2007). 5' flanking region of var genes nucleate histone modification patterns linked to phenotypic inheritance of virulence traits in malaria parasites. Molecular Microbiology, 66, 1296-1305.

Lopez-Rubio, J. J., Mancio-Silva, L., Scherf, A. (2009). Genome-wide analysis of heterochromatin associates clonally variant gene regulation with perinuclear repressive centers in malaria parasites. Cell Host & Microbe, 5, 179-190.

Maier, A. G., Rug, M., O'Neill, M. T., Brown, M., Chakravorty, S., Szestak, T., Chesson, J., Wu, Y., Hughes, K., Coppel, R. L., Newbold, C., Beeson, J. G., Craig, A., Crabb, B. S., Cowman, A. F. (2008). Exported proteins required for virulence and rigidity of Plasmodium falciparum-infected human erythrocytes. Cell, 134, 48-61.

Malhotra, P., Dasaradhi, P. V., Kumar, A., Mohmmed, A., Agrawal, N., Bhatnagar, R. K., Chauhan, V. S. (2002). Double-stranded RNA-mediated gene silencing of cysteine proteases (falcipain-1 and -2) of Plasmodium falciparum. Molecular Microbiology, 45, 1245-1254.

Malmquist, N. A., Moss, T. A., Mecheri, S., Scherf, A., Fuchter, M. J. (2012). Small-molecule histone methyltransferase inhibitors display rapid antimalarial activity against all blood stage forms in Plasmodium falciparum. Proceedings of the National Academy of Sciences U S A, 109, 16708-16713.

Mancio-Silva, L., Scherf, A. (2013). In Situ Fluorescence Visualization of Transcription Sites and Genomic Loci in Blood Stages of Plasmodium falciparum. Methods Molecular Biology, 923, 335-351.

Marti, M., Good, R. T., Rug, M., Knuepfer, E., Cowman, A. F. (2004). Targeting malaria virulence and remodeling proteins to the host erythrocyte. Science, 306, 1930-1933.

Marty, A. J., Thompson, J. K., Duffy, M. F., Voss, T. S., Cowman, A. F., Crabb, B. S. (2006). Evidence that Plasmodium falciparum chromosome end clusters are cross-linked by protein and are the sites of both virulence gene silencing and activation. Molecular Microbiology, 62, 72-83.

McRobert, L., McConkey, G. A. (2002). RNA interference (RNAi) inhibits growth of Plasmodium falciparum. Molecular and Biochemical Parasitology, 119, 273-278.

Merrick, C. J., Huttenhower, C., Buckee, C., Amambua-Ngwa, A., Gomez-Escobar, N., Walther, M., Conway, D. J., Duraisingh, M. T. (2012). Epigenetic dysregulation of virulence gene expression in severe Plasmodium falciparum malaria. Journal of Infectious Diseases, 205, 1593-1600.

Miao, J., Fan, Q., Cui, L., Li, X., Wang, H., Ning, G., Reese, J. C., Cui, L. (2010). The MYST family histone acetyltransferase regulates gene expression and cell cycle in malaria parasite Plasmodium falciparum. Molecular Microbiology, 78, 883-902.

Miller, L. H. (1969). Distribution of mature trophozoites and schizonts of Plasmodium falciparum in the organs of Aotus trivirgatus, the night monkey. American Journal for Tropical Medicine and Hygiene, 18, 860-865.

Miller, L. H., Baruch, D. I., Marsh, K., Doumbo, O. K. (2002). The pathogenic basis of malaria. Nature, 415, 673-679.

Mota, M. M., Jarra, W., Hirst, E., Patnaik, P. K., Holder, A. A. (2000). Plasmodium chabaudi-infected erythrocytes adhere to CD36 and bind to microvascular endothelial cells in an organ-specific way. Infection and Immunity, 68, 4135-4144.

Mphande, F. A., Ribacke, U., Kaneko, O., Kironde, F., Winter, G., Wahlgren, M. (2008). SURFIN4.1, a schizont-merozoite associated protein in the SURFIN family of Plasmodium falciparum. Malaria Journal, 7, 116.

Mueller, I., Galinski, M. R., Baird, J. K., Carlton, J. M., Kochar, D. K., Alonso, P. L., del Portillo, H. A. (2009). Key gaps in the knowledge of Plasmodium vivax, a neglected human malaria parasite. Lancet Infect Diseases, 9, 555-566.

Navarro, M., Gull, K. (2001). A pol I transcriptional body associated with VSG mono-allelic expression in Trypanosoma brucei. Nature, 414, 759-763.

Painter, H. J., Campbell, T. L., Llinas, M. (2011). The Apicomplexan AP2 family: integral factors regulating Plasmodium development. Molecular and Biochemical Parasitology, 176, 1-7.

Pasternak, N. D., Dzikowski, R. (2009). PfEMP1: an antigen that plays a key role in the pathogenicity and immune evasion of the malaria parasite Plasmodium falciparum. International Journal for Biochemistry and Cell Biology, 41, 1463-1466.

Patankar, S., Munasinghe, A., Shoaibi, A., Cummings, L. M., Wirth, D. F. (2001). Serial analysis of gene expression in Plasmodium falciparum reveals the global expression profile of erythrocytic stages and the presence of anti-sense transcripts in the malarial parasite. Molecular Biology of the Cell, 12, 3114-3125.

Perez-Toledo, K., Rojas-Meza, A. P., Mancio-Silva, L., Hernandez-Cuevas, N. A., Delgadillo, D. M., Vargas, M., Marti-nez-Calvillo, S., Scherf, A., Hernandez-Rivas, R. (2009). Plasmodium falciparum heterochromatin protein 1 binds to tri-methylated histone 3 lysine 9 and is linked to mutually exclusive expression of var genes. Nucleic Acids Research, 37, 2596-2606.

Peters, J., Fowler, E., Gatton, M., Chen, N., Saul, A., Cheng, Q. (2002). High diversity and rapid changeover of expressed var genes during the acute phase of Plasmodium falciparum infections in human volunteers. Proceedings of the National Academy of Sciences U S A, 99, 10689-10694.

Petter, M., Haeggstrom, M., Khattab, A., Fernandez, V., Klinkert, M. Q., Wahlgren, M. (2007). Variant proteins of the Plasmodium falciparum RIFIN family show distinct subcellular localization and developmental expression pat-terns. Molecular and Biochemical Parasitology, 156, 51-61.

Petter, M., Lee, C. C., Byrne, T. J., Boysen, K. E., Volz, J., Ralph, S. A., Cowman, A. F., Brown, G. V., Duffy, M. F. (2011). Expression of P. falciparum var genes involves exchange of the histone variant H2A.Z at the promoter. PLoS Pathogens, 7, e1001292.

Ponting, C. P., Oliver, P. L., Reik, W. (2009). Evolution and functions of long noncoding RNAs. Cell, 136, 629-641.

Prucca, C. G., Slavin, I., Quiroga, R., Elias, E. V., Rivero, F. D., Saura, A., Carranza, P. G., Lujan, H. D. (2008). Antigenic variation in Giardia lamblia is regulated by RNA interference. Nature, 456, 750-754.

Raabe, C. A., Sanchez, C. P., Randau, G., Robeck, T., Skryabin, B. V., Chinni, S. V., Kube, M., Reinhardt, R., Ng, G. H., Manickam, R., Kuryshev, V. Y., Lanzer, M., Brosius, J., Tang, T. H., Rozhdestvensky, T. S. (2010). A global view of the nonprotein-coding transcriptome in Plasmodium falciparum. Nucleic Acids Research, 38, 608-617.

Ralph, S. A., Bischoff, E., Mattei, D., Sismeiro, O., Dillies, M. A., Guigon, G., Coppee, J. Y., David, P. H., Scherf, A. (2005a). Transcriptome analysis of antigenic variation in Plasmodium falciparum--var silencing is not dependent on antisense RNA. Genome Biology, 6, R93.

Ralph, S. A., Scheidig-Benatar, C., Scherf, A. (2005b). Antigenic variation in Plasmodium falciparum is associated with movement of var loci between subnuclear locations. Proceedings of the National Academy of Sciences U S A, 102, 5414-5419.

Rask, T. S., Hansen, D. A., Theander, T. G., Gorm Pedersen, A., Lavstsen, T. (2010). Plasmodium falciparum erythrocyte membrane protein 1 diversity in seven genomes--divide and conquer. PLoS Computational Biology, 6.

Recker, M., Buckee, C. O., Serazin, A., Kyes, S., Pinches, R., Christodoulou, Z., Springer, A. L., Gupta, S., Newbold, C. I. (2011). Antigenic variation in Plasmodium falciparum malaria involves a highly structured switching pattern. PLoS Pathogens, 7, e1001306.

Roberts, D. J., Craig, A. G., Berendt, A. R., Pinches, R., Nash, G., Marsh, K., Newbold, C. I. (1992). Rapid switching to multiple antigenic and adhesive phenotypes in malaria. Nature, 357, 689-692.

Rowe, J. A., Claessens, A., Corrigan, R. A., Arman, M. (2009). Adhesion of Plasmodium falciparum-infected erythrocytes to human cells: molecular mechanisms and therapeutic implications. Expert Reviews in Molecular Medicine, 11, e16.

Rudenko, G., Blundell, P. A., Taylor, M. C., Kieft, R., Borst, P. (1994). VSG gene expression site control in insect form Trypanosoma brucei. EMBO J, 13, 5470-5482.

Rudenko, G. (2010). Epigenetics and transcriptional control in African trypanosomes. Essays in Biochemistry, 48, 201-219.

Rudenko, G. (2011). African trypanosomes: the genome and adaptations for immune evasion. Essays in Biochemistry, 51, 47-62.

Salanti, A., Staalsoe, T., Lavstsen, T., Jensen, A. T., Sowa, M. P., Arnot, D. E., Hviid, L., Theander, T. G. (2003). Selective upregulation of a single distinctly structured var gene in chondroitin sulphate A-adhering Plasmodium falciparum involved in pregnancy-associated malaria. Molecular Microbiology, 49, 179-191.

Salcedo-Amaya, A. M., van Driel, M. A., Alako, B. T., Trelle, M. B., van den Elzen, A. M., Cohen, A. M., Janssen-Megens, E. M., van de Vegte-Bolmer, M., Selzer, R. R., Iniguez, A. L., Green, R. D., Sauerwein, R. W., Jensen, O. N., Stunnenberg, H. G. (2009). Dynamic histone H3 epigenome marking during the intraerythrocytic cycle of Plasmodium falciparum. Proceedings of the National Academy of Sciences U S A, 106, 9655-9660.

Sam-Yellowe, T. Y., Florens, L., Johnson, J. R., Wang, T., Drazba, J. A., Le Roch, K. G., Zhou, Y., Batalov, S., Carucci, D. J., Winzeler, E. A., Yates, J. R., 3rd (2004). A Plasmodium gene family encoding Maurer's cleft membrane proteins: structural properties and expression profiling. Genome Research, 14, 1052-1059.

Scherf, A., Hernandez-Rivas, R., Buffet, P., Bottius, E., Benatar, C., Pouvelle, B., Gysin, J., Lanzer, M. (1998). Antigenic variation in malaria: in situ switching, relaxed and mutually exclusive transcription of var genes during intraerythrocytic development in Plasmodium falciparum. EMBO J, 17, 5418-5426.

Scherf, A., Lopez-Rubio, J. J., Riviere, L. (2008). Antigenic variation in Plasmodium falciparum. Annual Reviews in Microbiology, 62, 445-470.

Schieck, E., Pfahler, J. M., Sanchez, C. P., Lanzer, M. (2007). Nuclear run-on analysis of var gene expression in Plasmodium falciparum. Molecular and Biochemical Parasitology, 153, 207-212.

Sierra-Miranda, M., Delgadillo, D. M., Mancio-Silva, L., Vargas, M., Villegas-Sepulveda, N., Martinez-Calvillo, S., Scherf, A., Hernandez-Rivas, R. (2012). Two long non-coding RNAs generated from subtelomeric regions accumulate in a novel perinuclear compartment in Plasmodium falciparum. Molecular and Biochemical Parasitology, 185, 36-47.

Smith, J. D., Chitnis, C. E., Craig, A. G., Roberts, D. J., Hudson-Taylor, D. E., Peterson, D. S., Pinches, R., Newbold, C. I., Miller, L. H. (1995). Switches in expression of Plasmodium falciparum var genes correlate with changes in antigenic and cytoadherent phenotypes of infected erythrocytes. Cell, 82, 101-110.

Sturm, A., Amino, R., van de Sand, C., Regen, T., Retzlaff, S., Rennenberg, A., Krueger, A., Pollok, J. M., Menard, R., Heussler, V. T. (2006). Manipulation of host hepatocytes by the malaria parasite for delivery into liver sinusoids. Science, 313, 1287-1290.

Su, X. Z., Heatwole, V. M., Wertheimer, S. P., Guinet, F., Herrfeldt, J. A., Peterson, D. S., Ravetch, J. A., Wellems, T. E. (1995). The large diverse gene family var encodes proteins involved in cytoadherence and antigenic variation of Plasmodium falciparum-infected erythrocytes. Cell, 82, 89-100.

Tham, W. H., Payne, P. D., Brown, G. V., Rogerson, S. J. (2007). Identification of basic transcriptional elements required for rif gene transcription. International Journal of Parasitology, 37, 605-615.

Tonkin, C. J., Carret, C. K., Duraisingh, M. T., Voss, T. S., Ralph, S. A., Hommel, M., Duffy, M. F., Silva, L. M., Scherf, A., Ivens, A., Speed, T. P., Beeson, J. G., Cowman, A. F. (2009). Sir2 paralogues cooperate to regulate virulence genes and antigenic variation in Plasmodium falciparum. PLoS Biology, 7, e84.

Tsukada, Y., Fang, J., Erdjument-Bromage, H., Warren, M. E., Borchers, C. H., Tempst, P., Zhang, Y. (2006). Histone demethylation by a family of JmjC domain-containing proteins. Nature, 439, 811-816.

van der Heyde, H. C., Nolan, J., Combes, V., Gramaglia, I., Grau, G. E. (2006). A unified hypothesis for the genesis of cerebral malaria: sequestration, inflammation and hemostasis leading to microcirculatory dysfunction. Trends in Parasitology, 22, 503-508.

Vaughan, A. M., Aly, A. S., Kappe, S. H. (2008). Malaria parasite pre-erythrocytic stage infection: gliding and hiding. Cell Host & Microbe, 4, 209-218.

Volz, J. C., Bartfai, R., Petter, M., Langer, C., Josling, G. A., Tsuboi, T., Schwach, F., Baum, J., Rayner, J. C., Stunnenberg, H. G., Duffy, M. F., Cowman, A. F. (2012). PfSET10, a Plasmodium falciparum methyltransferase, maintains the active var gene in a poised state during parasite division. Cell Host & Microbe, 11, 7-18.

Voss, T. S., Kaestli, M., Vogel, D., Bopp, S., Beck, H. P. (2003). Identification of nuclear proteins that interact differentially with Plasmodium falciparum var gene promoters. Molecular Microbiology, 48, 1593-1607.

Voss, T. S., Healer, J., Marty, A. J., Duffy, M. F., Thompson, J. K., Beeson, J. G., Reeder, J. C., Crabb, B. S., Cowman, A. F. (2006). A var gene promoter controls allelic exclusion of virulence genes in Plasmodium falciparum malaria. Nature, 439, 1004-1008.

Wang, C. W., Magistrado, P. A., Nielsen, M. A., Theander, T. G., Lavstsen, T. (2009). Preferential transcription of conserved rif genes in two phenotypically distinct Plasmodium falciparum parasite lines. International Journal of Parasitology, 39, 655-664.

Weber, J. L. (1988). Interspersed repetitive DNA from Plasmodium falciparum. Molecular and Biochemical Parasitology, 29, 117-124.

Weiner, A., Dahan-Pasternak, N., Shimoni, E., Shinder, V., von Huth, P., Elbaum, M., Dzikowski, R. (2011). 3D nuclear architecture reveals coupled cell cycle dynamics of chromatin and nuclear pores in the malaria parasite Plasmodium falciparum. Cellular Microbiology, 13, 967-977.

Winter, G., Kawai, S., Haeggstrom, M., Kaneko, O., von Euler, A., Kawazu, S., Palm, D., Fernandez, V., Wahlgren, M. (2005). SURFIN is a polymorphic antigen expressed on Plasmodium falciparum merozoites and infected erythrocytes. Journal of Experimental Medicine, 201, 1853-1863.

Witmer, K., Schmid, C. D., Brancucci, N. M., Luah, Y. H., Preiser, P. R., Bozdech, Z., Voss, T. S. (2012). Analysis of subtelomeric virulence gene families in Plasmodium falciparum by comparative transcriptional profiling. Molecular Microbiology, 84, 243-259.

Wunderlich, G., Alves, F. P., Golnitz, U., Tada, M. S., Camargo, E. F., Pereira-da-Silva, L. H. (2005). Rapid turnover of Plasmodium falciparum var gene transcripts and genotypes during natural non-symptomatic infections. Revista do Instituto de Medicina Tropical de São Paulo, 47, 195-201.

Xue, X., Zhang, Q., Huang, Y., Feng, L., Pan, W. (2008). No miRNA were found in Plasmodium and the ones identified in erythrocytes could not be correlated with infection. Malaria Journal, 7, 47.

Yang, X. J., Seto, E. (2008). The Rpd3/Hda1 family of lysine deacetylases: from bacteria and yeast to men and men. Nat Rev Molecular and Cellular Biology, 9, 206-218.

Zhang, Q., Huang, Y., Zhang, Y., Fang, X., Claes, A., Duchateau, M., Namane, A., Lopez-Rubio, J. J., Pan, W., Scherf, A. (2011). A critical role of perinuclear filamentous actin in spatial repositioning and mutually exclusive expression of virulence genes in malaria parasites. Cell Host & Microbe, 10, 451-463.

www.ingramcontent.com/pod-product-compliance
Lightning Source LLC
Chambersburg PA
CBHW050803220326
41598CB00006B/104